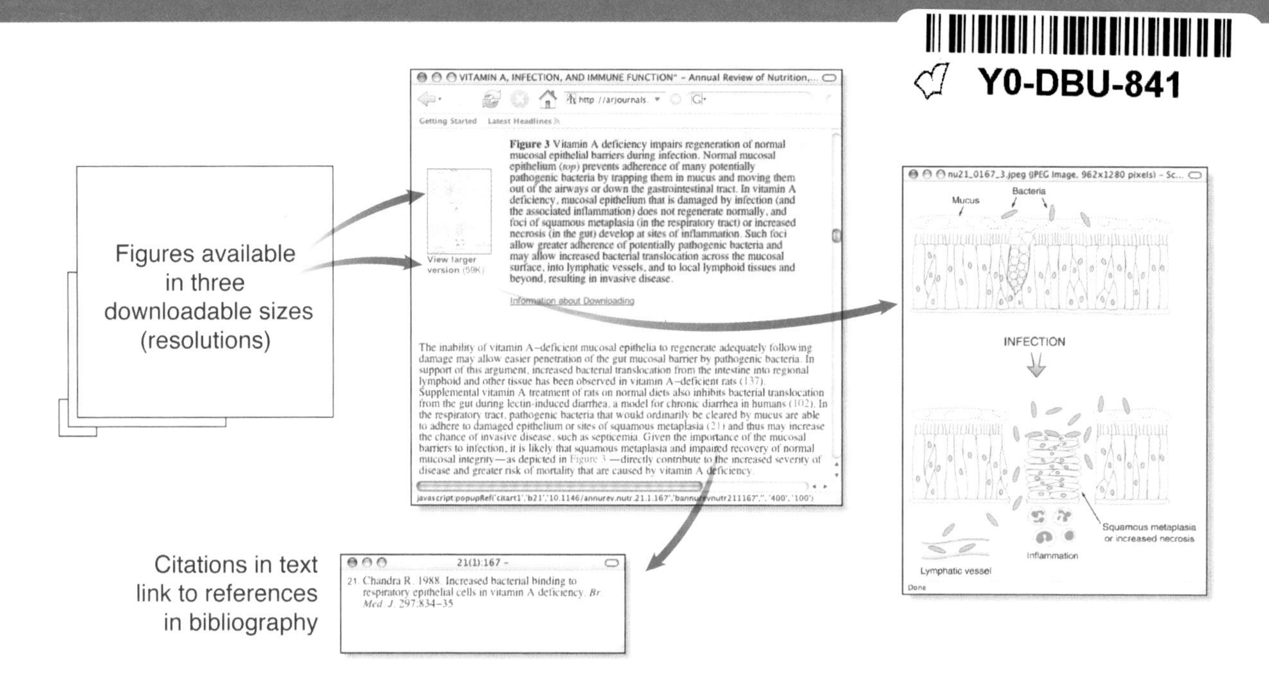

Y0-DBU-841
Figures available in three downloadable sizes (resolutions)
VITAMIN A, INFECTION, AND IMMUNE FUNCTION* - Annual Review of Nutrition,...
Figure 3 Vitamin A deficiency impairs regeneration of normal mucosal epithelial barriers during infection. Normal mucosal epithelium (top) prevents adherence of many potentially pathogenic bacteria by trapping them in mucus and moving them out of the airways or down the gastrointestinal tract. In vitamin A deficiency, mucosal epithelium that is damaged by infection (and the associated inflammation) does not regenerate normally, and foci of squamous metaplasia (in the respiratory tract) or increased necrosis (in the gut) develop at sites of inflammation. Such foci allow greater adherence of potentially pathogenic bacteria and may allow increased bacterial translocation across the mucosal surface, into lymphatic vessels, and to local lymphoid tissues and beyond, resulting in invasive disease.
View larger version (59K)
Information about Downloading
Mucus
Bacteria
INFECTION
Squamous metaplasia or increased necrosis
Inflammation
Lymphatic vessel
Citations in text link to references in bibliography
21. Chandra R. 1988. Increased bacterial binding to respiratory epithelial cells in vitamin A deficiency. Br Med J. 297:834–35

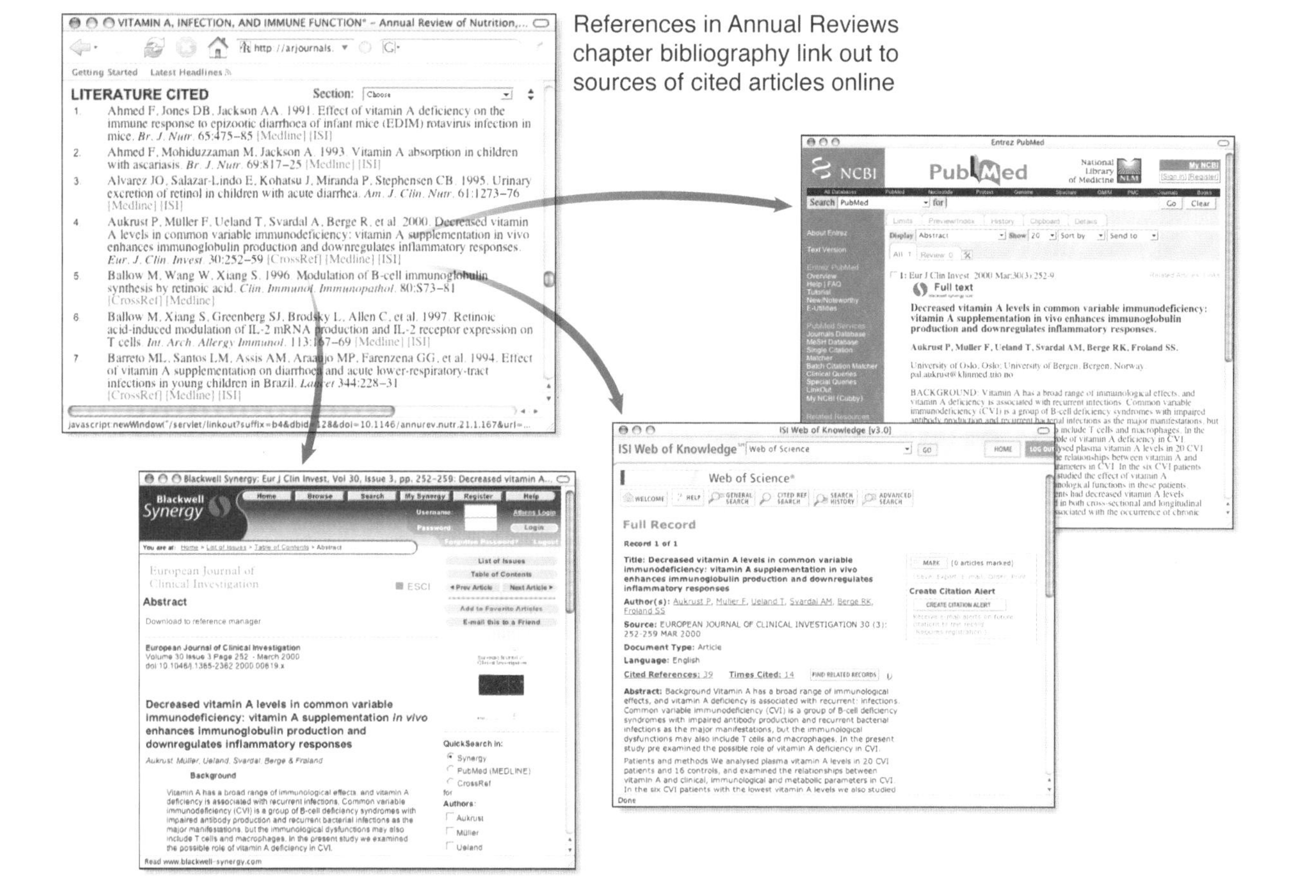

References in Annual Reviews chapter bibliography link out to sources of cited articles online
LITERATURE CITED
Entrez PubMed
ISI Web of Knowledge
Web of Science
Full Record
Blackwell Synergy
Decreased vitamin A levels in common variable immunodeficiency: vitamin A supplementation in vivo enhances immunoglobulin production and downregulates inflammatory responses

Annual Review of
Nutrition

Production Editor: Lisa Dean
Managing Editor: Veronica Dakota Padilla
Bibliographic Quality Control: Mary A. Glass
Electronic Content Coordinator: Suzanne K. Moses

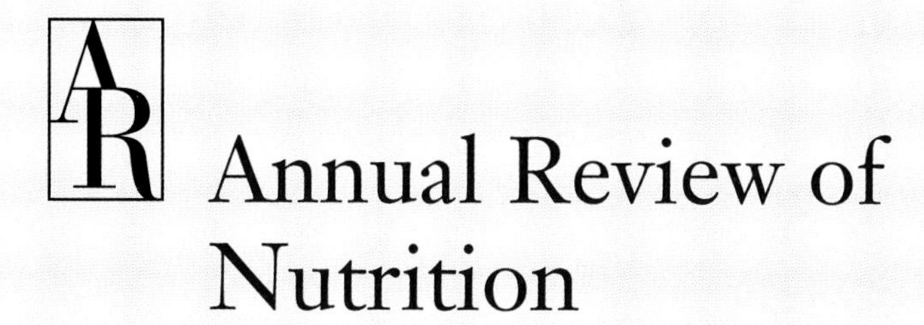

Annual Review of Nutrition

Volume 27, 2007

Robert J. Cousins, *Editor*
University of Florida

Dennis M. Bier, *Associate Editor*
Baylor College of Medicine

Barbara A. Bowman, *Associate Editor*
Centers for Disease Control and Prevention

www.annualreviews.org • science@annualreviews.org • 650-493-4400

Annual Reviews
4139 El Camino Way • P.O. Box 10139 • Palo Alto, California 94303-0139

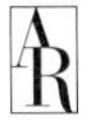

Annual Reviews
Palo Alto, California, USA

International Standard Serial Number: 0199-9885
International Standard Book Number: 978-0-8243-2827-6

∞ The paper used in this publication meets the minimum requirements of American National Standards for Information Sciences—Permanence of Paper for Printed Library Materials, ANSI Z39.48-1992.

TYPESET BY APTARA, INC.
PRINTED AND BOUND BY EDWARDS BROTHERS, ANN ARBOR, MICHIGAN

Preface

Volume 27 of the *Annual Review of Nutrition* continues the tradition of providing critical authoritative reviews of topics covering all aspects of the nutrition field. Barbara Bowman and Dennis Bier shared editorial duties for Volume 27 with me. The other editorial committee members who generated the topics for this volume were Kathleen Rasmussen, Dale Romsos, Rima Rozen, John Suttie, and Steven Ziesel. We are pleased that the *Annual Review of Nutrition* continues to have an extremely high ranking among citation-monitoring services.

The prefatory chapter offers readers of this volume the special opportunity to share Nevin Scrimshaw's reflection on his half-century-plus involvement in the worldwide nutrition community. He highlights his role in establishing INCAP and the Nutrition and Food Science Department at MIT as well as his work with the United Nations University and other groups that address nutrition issues in developing countries. Also in this volume, Forsum & Löf discuss energy requirements during pregnancy and the need to base these requirements on accurate energy intake data. Rasmussen reviews the negative relationship between obesity in women of reproductive age and successful breastfeeding outcomes. Sellen presents a hypothesis that humans evolved a flexible neonatal feeding strategy as an adaptation, but under contemporary conditions, this strategy may produce imbalances that prevent optimal feeding practices for infants and children. In their chapter on brain evolution among primates, Leonard and coauthors suggest that humans have an energetically expensive brain that dictates their low-muscle/high-fat body composition.

Votruba & Jensen review the hypothesis regarding regional differences in body fat deposition and discuss evidence suggesting that these differences do not appear to be gender specific. Wahren & Ekberg review the latest understanding of the liver's dynamic roles in glucose processing/production and how these events are differentially altered in Type 1 and Type 2 diabetes. The chapter by Tremblay et al. outlines the evidence that the high quality of dietary protein from fish, operating through the mTOR transcription factor, modulates insulin action. Yudkoff and coauthors describe the evidence suggesting that ketogenic diets promote glutamine syntheses yielding an antiseizure effect in epileptics. Brosnan & Brosnan review the evidence that creatine plays a role beyond that of an ATP buffer by also serving as an energy shuttle that requires a dietary source to supplement endogenous synthesis. The molecular genetics of anorexia nervosa is reviewed by Bulik and coauthors within the context of the familial component as supported with twin studies.

Waterland & Michels review evidence supporting epigenetic mechanisms in health and disease origins and the role of nutrition as one of the environmental stimuli involved. The coordination of energy homeostasis with circadian gene networks and sleep/wakefulness cycles is discussed in the chapter by Ramsey et al. Taste receptor genes, T1R and T2R, and their adaptation to feeding-behavior differences of vertebrate species is the subject of the chapter by Bachmanov & Beauchamp. The neurophysiology surrounding the rejection (by animals) of diets that lead to deficiency of indispensable amino acids is presented by Gietzen and coauthors. Mizushima & Klionsky review recent information on how autophagy responds to nutrient limitations to maintain intracellular protein metabolism. The critical role of the selenium-requiring enzyme glutathione peroxidase 1 in oxidant defense as demonstrated with transgenic mice is placed in perspective by Lei et al.

In a review of copper, iron, and zinc transporter genes that are expressed in the mammary gland, Lönnerdal provides evidence on how the abundance of these micronutrients in milk is regulated during lactation. Traber describes how the liver, through synthesis of tocopherol transfer protein, regulates the distribution of body vitamin E levels. The influence of the carbohydrate-responsive element-binding protein, ChREBP, on hepatic lipid synthesis is presented in the review by Postic and coauthors. Control of adipocyte lipolysis for energy substrate generation via novel lipases including desnutrim/ATGL and nonenzymatic proteins is described by Duncan et al. Spindler & Dhahbi present evidence that the genomics of dietary calorie restriction to increase lifespan point to genes involved in apoptosis and autophagy.

The *Annual Review of Nutrition* editors are confident that the reviews in volume 27—written by recognized authorities—will provide extremely valuable aids for teaching and research purposes. As always, these volumes are only possible through the efforts and support of our Production Editor, Lisa Dean, and the President of Annual Reviews, Samuel Gubins.

Robert J. Cousins
Editor

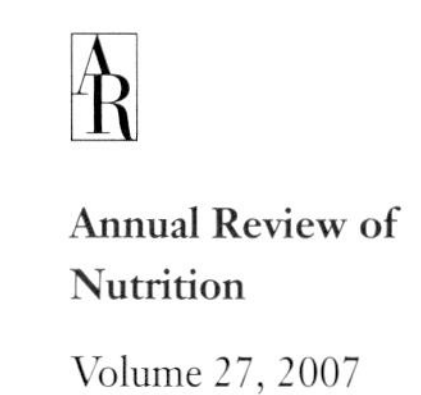

Annual Review of Nutrition

Volume 27, 2007

Contents

Indexes

Errata

An online log of corrections to *Annual Review of Nutrition* chapters (if any, 1997 to the present) may be found at http://nutr.annualreviews.org/errata.shtml

Notice

Cow's Milk and Linear Growth in Industrialized and Developing Countries
Camilla Hoppe, Christian Mølgaard, Kim F. Michaelsen
Annual Review of Nutrition 26:131–73

In the course of preparing this review for last year's volume, the authors consulted Andrea S. Wiley's article "Does Milk Make Children Grow? Relationships Between Milk Consumption and Height in NHANES 1999–2002" [*American Journal of Human Biology*, 17:425–41 (2005)]. While we then cited Dr. Wiley's article in our review, we also unintentionally merged into our text a considerable number of phrases and sentences from Dr. Wiley's paper, without proper attribution. We deeply regret this serious error and apologize to Dr. Wiley.

Camila Hoppe, Christian Mølgaard, and Kim F. Michaelsen

Related Articles

From the ***Annual Review of Biochemistry***, Volume 76, 2007

The Eyes Absent Family of Phosphotyrosine Phosphatases: Properties and Roles in Developmental Regulation of Transcription
Jennifer Jemc and Ilaria Rebay

Translocation of Proteins into Mitochondria
Walter Neupert and Johannes M. Herrmann

From the ***Annual Review of Cell and Developmental Biology***, Volume 23, 2007

Cerebellar Development
Alexandra Joyner and Roy Sillitoe

Muscle Cell Progenitors and Tissue Regeneration
Margaret Buckingham

Transcriptional Control of Wound Repair
Matthias Schafer and Sabine Werner

From the ***Annual Review of Medicine***, Volume 58, 2007

Kidney Disease and Cardiovascular Risk
Marcello Tonelli and Marc A. Pfeffer

Cardiovascular Risks of Antiretroviral Therapies
Kristin Mondy and Pablo Tebas

From the ***Annual Review of Physiology***, Volume 69, 2007

Iron Homeostasis
Nancy C. Andrews and Paul J. Schmidt

Transporters as Channels
Louis J. DeFelice and Tapasree Goswami

Regulation of Intestinal Cholesterol Absorption
David Q.-H. Wang

Annual Reviews is a nonprofit scientific publisher established to promote the advancement of the sciences. Beginning in 1932 with the *Annual Review of Biochemistry*, the Company has pursued as its principal function the publication of high-quality, reasonably priced *Annual Review* volumes. The volumes are organized by Editors and Editorial Committees who invite qualified authors to contribute critical articles reviewing significant developments within each major discipline. The Editor-in-Chief invites those interested in serving as future Editorial Committee members to communicate directly with him. Annual Reviews is administered by a Board of Directors, whose members serve without compensation.

Annual Reviews of

Anthropology
Astronomy and Astrophysics
Biochemistry
Biomedical Engineering
Biophysics and Biomolecular Structure
Cell and Developmental Biology
Clinical Psychology
Earth and Planetary Sciences
Ecology, Evolution, and Systematics
Entomology
Environment and Resources
Fluid Mechanics
Genetics
Genomics and Human Genetics
Immunology
Law and Social Science
Materials Research
Medicine
Microbiology
Neuroscience
Nuclear and Particle Science
Nutrition
Pathology: Mechanisms of Disease
Pharmacology and Toxicology
Physical Chemistry
Physiology
Phytopathology
Plant Biology
Political Science
Psychology
Public Health
Sociology

SPECIAL PUBLICATIONS
Excitement and Fascination of Science, Vols. 1, 2, 3, and 4

Fifty-Five-Year Personal Experience with Human Nutrition Worldwide

Nevin S. Scrimshaw

Massachusetts Institute of Technology, Cambridge, Massachusetts 02139; International Nutrition Foundation, Boston, Massachusetts 02111; Friedman School of Nutrition, Tufts University, Boston, Massachusetts 02111; and United Nations University, Tokyo, Japan; email: nscrimshaw@inffoundation.org

Annu. Rev. Nutr. 2007. 27:1–18

The *Annual Review of Nutrition* is online at http://nutr.annualreviews.org

This article's doi:
10.1146/annurev.nutr.27.061406.093746

0199-9885/07/0821-0001$20.00

Key Words

protein, amino acids, kwashiorkor, infection, atherosclerosis, single-cell protein, cholesterol, Incaparina, iron deficiency

Abstract

By 1950 the vitamins had been identified, but little was known of their functions. Beriberi, pellagra, and ariboflavinosis were disappearing, but kwashiorkor and/or marasmus were common in most developing countries. Requirements for protein were still uncertain, and those for essential amino acids or essential fatty acids were unknown. The author's contributions in the field of vitamins began in the 1950s and have been reported in more than 650 publications and in 20 books or monographs. These contributions include establishing the Institute of Nutrition of Central America and Panama, the Department of Nutrition and Food Science at the Massachusetts Institute of Technology, the World Hunger Program of the United Nations University, and the International Nutrition Foundation. His scientific contributions include identification of synergistic interactions of nutrition and infection, use of potassium iodate for fortifying crude moist salt, research in the epidemiology of kwashiorkor and marasmus, development of a successful low-cost protein-rich food for infants and young children, establishment of human protein requirements, and investigation of single-cell protein for food use.

Contents

PROLOGUE

The attack on Pearl Harbor on December 7, 1941, found me an instructor for advanced biology courses at Ohio Wesleyan University after obtaining a PhD in Biology at Harvard University the preceding June. I was already admitted to the University of Rochester Medical School with a research assistantship and laboratory in the Department of Vital Economics (Nutrition and Endocrinology).

In June 1942, I arrived in Rochester, New York, to find most departments pioneering in nutrition. Dean G. Whipple (Pathology) was demonstrating the role of amino acids in protein synthesis through plasmaphoresis studies in dogs, K. Mason (Anatomy) was studying vitamin E, W.R. Bloor (Biochemistry) was describing the metabolism of fatty acids, and S. Clausen (Pediatrics) was researching vitamin A in children. In Vital Economics, E. Nasset was exploring the metabolic role of intestinal flora, and R. Sealock was developing microbiological methods for amino acid analysis. The department head, J.R. Murlin, had obtained an army contract to study nitrogen balance and exercise capacity with various diets. My role was to analyze B vitamins in the diets using recently developed microbiological methods.

After I graduated from medical school in 1945, a rotating internship in Gorgas Hospital, Panama Canal Zone, enabled me to review dietary differences among socioeconomic and racial groups in relation to complications of pregnancy in the records of 10,000 patients seen by a single physician. Contrary to expectations, nutrition did not account for the sharp differences in hypertension and pre-eclampsia among groups (47).

Upon my return to the University of Rochester in 1946 as a postdoctoral fellow, I obtained support for studying the effect of nutrition on complications of pregnancy among women in the City of Rochester. Again, no nutritional effect on pre-eclampsia was found. During this period, I interacted closely with I.M. Hoobler, director of the Children's Fund of Michigan, and W.J. Darby, who were conducting studies that yielded similar results.

Stimulating acquaintances in those early years were H. Sebrell, who had worked with J. Goldberger in demonstrating the role of diet in pellagra; C.A. Elvehjem, who described niacin as the cause of "black-tongue" in dogs, triggering recognition of its role in pellagra; P. Gyorgy, who identified pyridoxine and biotin; W.R. Rose, who determined human requirements for individual essential amino acids;

and C.G. King, who identified the structure of ascorbic acid. Other acquaintances included R.R. Williams, who synthesized thiamine; H. VonDam, the discoverer of vitamin K; E.V. McCollum, the discoverer of vitamin A; W. Aykroid, the first director of the Nutrition Division of the Food and Agriculture Organization (FAO); Cicely Williams, who first described kwashiorkor, HAPC Oomens, who crusaded against avitaminosis A and keratomalacia in Indonesia, R.A. McCance and Elsie Widdowson, who investigated starvation in prisoners of the Germans at the end of World II; G. Goldsmith, who did classical clinical studies of pellagra; and A. Keys, who studied human starvation. Later, Keys and my lifelong friend, M. Hegsted, would quantify the influence of lipids on cholesterol levels. The aforementioned as well as many other pioneers in the field strengthened my commitment to nutrition.

INCAP YEARS: 1949–1961

Beginnings

After three years of fellowship and residency at the University of Rochester, I agreed to organize and direct an Institute of Nutrition of Central America and Panama (INCAP), based in Guatemala. My medical school professors felt that I was throwing away a promising academic career. How wrong they were! Although we started in September 1949 in an adobe building with only three laboratories, three offices, and a conference room/library, an operating budget of $37,500, and no PhDs, the discoveries and publications followed rapidly. By 1955, we had a large, new, permanent building, which was provided by Guatemala. In 12 years—with increased country quotas and National Institutes of Health (NIH), foundation, and industry research grants—the annual budget was about $900,000, and the heads of seven divisions had doctorates. By its 25th anniversary, INCAP had published 695 scientific papers in English and as many in Spanish.

Kwashiorkor and Marasmus

Cicely Williams first described kwashiorkor (K) in what is now Ghana in 1933 (73). Her excellent publication was overlooked until J. Brock (World Health Organization; WHO) and M. Autret (FAO) toured Africa and reported to the second FAO/WHO Expert Committee in 1951 that the disease described by Williams was widespread throughout Africa. At the meeting, I recognized it as a condition common in Central America.

We began to study intensively both K and marasmus (M) using one cot and one crib for six children on an overcrowded pediatric ward in the general hospital. With a nutritionist to supervise their food intake, the K children rapidly lost edema, skin lesions, anorexia, and apathy. However, they failed to gain weight for many more weeks (41). After we acquired a research unit of six individual cubicles in a private pediatric hospital, we never again saw a stationary period in the treatment of K. We then realized that it was the adverse nutritional impact of multiple cross-infections in an open ward that prevented these children from gaining weight (42).

We found that the signs and symptoms of K (edema, pigmented skin lesions, pale pluckable hair, profound apathy, and serum biochemical changes) disappeared with skim milk alone administered by gastric tube. Of course, it then became necessary to add vitamins and minerals for further recovery (44). Concurrently, J. Brock and J. Hanson in South Africa achieved initial recovery with an amino acid mixture and energy source. We developed guidelines for treatment of K and M that nearly eliminated deaths in the hospital, which previously had a high rate (4, 5). Since nearly all patients had concurrent diarrhea and pneumonia, we routinely administered penicillin.

As we explored the epidemiology of K, we concluded that in Central America it was always acutely superimposed, mainly as the result of preceding infection(s), on some degrees of chronic undernutrition (41). M usually developed slowly over months or years before death threatened, whereas K could develop in a few weeks and was often fatal soon after the classical symptoms appeared. We conceptualized severe malnutrition in Central America as a triangle; the hypotenuse represented increasing degrees of chronic undernutrition, with K superimposed as an acute episode on any degree of marasmus (38).

M alone was characterized by wasting but did not show the clinical signs and symptoms of K. Nor were the abnormal biochemical changes present characteristic of severe protein deficiency.[1] We concluded that the child with M was wasting from lack of food and living on his or her own tissues. The latter supplied a balance of energy and good-quality protein. At first both body fat and muscle are metabolized, but once all of the fat has been consumed, lean body mass must supply both energy and protein, and the end is near.

The Incaparina Story

The most frustrating aspect of field visits at this time was our inability to help women with severely malnourished children who approached us in the villages we visited. They could not afford the protein sources we could suggest. Milk was too expensive and their diets had almost no meat. An egg could be exchanged for corn to provide a meal for the entire family. We set about to develop a culturally acceptable plant-based complementary food for older infants and young children at the lowest possible cost.

Soy, a potential protein source, was not grown in the American tropics, and peanut meal, another protein source, was too costly. Cottonseed meal was being shipped to Europe in large quantities for feeding ruminants. It was cheap and its protein quality was an excellent complement to the amino acid pattern of maize protein. However, it contained unacceptable amounts of the toxic pigment gossypol. With guidance from A. Altshul, a specialist at the United States Department of Agriculture (USDA) Southern Regional Research Laboratory, we worked with a large mill in Nicaragua to press the seed at a lower temperature and pressure so that the gossypol was expressed with the oil. A mixture containing approximately one-third cottonseed meal and two-thirds maize meal with added vitamins and minerals had essentially the same protein value and more complete micronutrient content in comparison with milk, at one-third the cost. Guatemalan mothers cooked and flavored it as traditional maize gruel (atole) (34).

Although it was intended as a complementary food for infants and young children when breast milk was not sufficient, it is still extremely popular among Guatemalans of all ages and is recognized as nutritious. The concept of Incaparina was patented for free use with the indigenous protein resources of any developing country.

In 1967, India was experiencing famine and was dependent on wheat donated by United States. This provided for older children and adults, but not for infants and young children. I was invited by the government of India to develop an acceptable food for young children, patterned after Incaparina, using the donated wheat and local complementary protein sources.

My first day in India was spent in New Delhi with Venkatachalam, Deputy Director of the Indian Council of Medical Research, working out an agreement on the nutritional composition of the new food based on United Nations (UN) Protein Advisory Group (PAG) recommendations. The second day was spent in Hyderabad, looking at potential sources of oil seed meals. Suitable cottonseed flour was not available, but peanut meal was abundant. The problem was aflatoxin produced by a ubiquitous soil mold under conditions of

[1] So-called classical kwashiorkor without chronic weight loss was not seen in Central America and was exceedingly rare even in Jamaica, where it was first described. The "mehlnahrschaden" or "starch dystrophy" of 19th- and early 20th-century Europe was the development of severe protein deficiency with little or no loss of weight for length because of abundant calories.

high humidity. Although chemical processing to remove it was too costly, a solution was provided through using conveyor belts with workers on each side picking out moldy peanuts. With strict supervision and sampling of each batch before use, meal could be produced that met PAG standards for cottonseed flour in complementary food mixtures for child feeding.

I spent the third and fourth days at the Central Food Technology Laboratory in Mysore, developing various formulas that would meet specifications and testing the formulas with female staff. The name "balahar" was chosen for the new food source because it meant "child food" in most of the Indian languages. At the beginning of the next week, the Ministry of Health in New Delhi approved the proposal, and construction began promptly on factories to produce balahar for relief purposes. Balahar proved valuable in the emergency and continued to be available as a relief food for many decades. An instant form, balamul, is commercially available. Some years later I led a team to assist Thailand with complementary food development (38). The concept of Incaparina and balahar has been the basis for the development of similar low-cost nutritious complementary foods in many other developing countries.

Nutrition and Infection

In the 1950s, no textbook mentioned a relationship between nutrition and infection, except for tuberculosis. My colleagues and I began to document the greater severity of infections in malnourished subjects. We soon concluded that nearly all cases of kwashiorkor were precipitated by preceding infections (64). Measles, chicken pox, whooping cough, rubella, diarrheal disease, and even staphylococcal skin infections were capable of precipitating kwashiorkor in malnourished children (31). It is common for Central American villages to have a composite child growth curve at the third percentile of normal. Growth of a breastfed village child during the first six months of life is usually satisfactory, but when breast milk is no longer sufficient as the sole source of food, infants are more exposed to pathogens, and growth begins to falter in response to multiple infections. As an example of the impact of infections, the time required for poorly nourished children to regain their weight at the onset of whooping cough was 13–24 weeks in 25% of children and 25 weeks or more in another 25% (22).

Our metabolic studies demonstrated a decrease in nitrogen balance during the acute, catabolic phase of an infection, followed by rapid anabolic recovery if the diet has enough protein. Otherwise, children lose nitrogen during the acute phase of the illness and will fail to catch up after the acute illness has passed. We determined through metabolic balance studies that any infection—no matter how mild, or even subclinical—has an adverse effect on nutritional status (12).

A variety of mechanisms contribute to the adverse effect of infections on nutritional status. Decreased food intake due to anorexia plays a role, as do metabolic losses in the urine, internal diversion of protein for synthesis of immune proteins (e.g., antibodies, globulins, cytokines), decreased absorption (if infection affects the gastrointestinal tract), increased metabolic rate (related to altered cytokine profile), and direct nutrient losses in the stool, if diarrhea is present.

The notion that improved nutritional status could reduce the frequency and severity of infections was based, in part, on a previous investigation into the causes of death in children in four Guatemalan Highland villages (3). Kwashiorkor, respiratory infections, and diarrhea were each associated with approximately one-third of the postneonatal deaths. However, kwashiorkor deaths would not have occurred without precipitating infections, and few of the diarrheal and respiratory deaths would have occurred in well-nourished children. Our conclusion was that nearly all of the postneonatal young child deaths were due to the synergistic interaction of malnutrition and infection and not to either alone.

The results stimulated an investigation into hospital deaths in Latin American public hospitals, which found that nutrition was a factor in more than half of all deaths, although most of these were officially attributed to infection (29).

Research in three Guatemalan highland villages from 1959 to 1964 was designed to test whether improved nutrition alone or health care alone was more effective in improving nutritional status, lowering morbidity and mortality, and promoting growth and development in children younger than five years old (53). Children fed Incaparina made with dried skim milk daily to supply 16 g protein and micronutrients had significantly fewer diarrheal and respiratory illnesses than did those in health care and placebo villages. Our funds did not allow us to explore the effects of both interventions in the same village because the NIH study section members said "the results were obvious." This study demonstrated a close relationship between growth and infections. Later studies confirmed a relationship between early growth retardation and lasting cognitive impairment (10, 20).

As evidence from our Central American field studies of the synergistic interactions between nutrition and infection accumulated during the 1950s, it was met with skepticism or indifference. This reaction, along with the encouragement of epidemiologist John Gordon, motivated me to assemble evidence for the concept of synergism between nutrition and infection in the scientific literature (59). With added material, it became the 1968 WHO monograph with the same title (60). The role of infection in worsening nutritional status was documented (37). Important concepts such as "weanling diarrhea" and "second-year death rate" were introduced and became widely accepted. A great deal of information has accumulated since 1968 in support of these relationships, and the subsequent knowledge explosion of cell-mediated immune mechanisms has led to an understanding of how malnutrition lowers resistance. Today, recognition of the synergistic relationship between nutrition and infection is a driving force in public health interventions to reduce the burden of infections and malnutrition.

Early Protein and Amino Acid Requirement Studies

Working with Ricardo Bressani and others, I conducted a long series of metabolic studies in young children that explored the protein quality and limiting amino acids in plant protein sources in the region. With wheat, lysine supplementation alone restored its protein value to that of milk (45). This was replicated later by studies at the Massachusetts Institute of Technology (MIT) (61).

Lysine partially restored the protein utilization of maize, but only with added tryptophan did the nitrogen utilization per gram of protein from maize approach that of milk (6, 8). One variety analyzed had an essential amino acid pattern and protein value similar to that of egg or milk (7). This variety was later developed at CIMMYT in Mexico, and we found it had high protein quality for consumption by children (7) and adults (74).

Other essential amino acids were not significantly limiting in cereal protein. Methionine was observed to be the limiting amino acid in legumes, and the complementarity of the essential amino patterns of an appropriate mix of protein from cereal and legumes was confirmed. Retention was always higher after a period of deficiency of either total nitrogen or of one or more essential amino acids, confirming the importance of the anabolic recovery period after an infection.

Endemic Goiter and Potassium Iodate

As we began to work in the Guatemala villages, we observed that goiters were readily visible in many villagers. Consequently, endemic goiter surveys were conducted in all of the INCAP member countries. It was determined through palpation of the thyroid gland (27) that the prevalence of goiters in Guatemala was 38%, with comparable prevalence levels in the other INCAP member countries surveyed. The United States and Canada had addressed the problem of goiters by adding potassium iodide to salt. However, such a solution was not feasible in Central America because potassium iodide could be used only with refined, dry salt, with an added stabilizer and moisture-proof packaging. Such salt would be unrecognizable and prohibitively expensive in Central America, where crude salt was sold, often from moist open piles in the marketplace.

After consulting a chemical handbook, we identified a compound, potassium iodate, that was not hygroscopic, but there was no information on its bioavailability. We conducted trials in schoolchildren in two villages in Guatemala and El Salvador. Schoolchildren were given identical-looking tablets with no iodine, potassium iodide, or iodate in amounts simulating that provided by iodized salt (46). The fall in goiter prevalence was identical with iodide and iodate. Potassium iodate mixed into salt and stored in burlap bags in the humid, tropical Pacific coast of Guatemala remained well distributed after nine months (1).

With this information, the governments of Central America passed legislation requiring the iodation of salt for human consumption. INCAP helped the governments set up control laboratories and provided manufacturers with technical help. In Guatemala the prevalence of endemic goiter dropped to 7% three years after iodation began (49). Iodation was soon adopted by all of the Central American countries as well as a number of countries in South America. Today it is making possible the campaign of the UN and other agencies and foundations to eliminate goiter as a public health problem in developing countries.

Inter-American Atherosclerosis Study

The growing interest in serum cholesterol and lipoprotein levels in the United States prompted us to explore these levels in Central America. We found that the levels were much lower in local populations (19, 24–26, 62). Virtually no overlap existed among children from rural areas, urban areas, and the privileged children in private schools in Guatemala (37). Deaths from heart disease were rare in the public hospitals of Central America. These observations were sufficient for a large NIH grant to determine the frequency and severity of atherosclerosis in comparisons of autopsies from 13 Latin American (LA) hospitals with those from Charity Hospital in New Orleans. The lead investigators were two pathologists from Louisiana State University, one from the Universidad del Valle, Colombia, and one from INCAP. The statistician, M. Guzman, and I looked for nutritional correlations. The project lasted from 1960 to 1964; during that time, we obtained aortas and coronary and cerebral vessels stained for fat from more than 14,000 male and nearly 8000 female autopsies.

The degree of atherosclerosis was evaluated independently by each of the four pathologists, with samples mixed and blinded. In New Orleans, the severity of lesions increased rapidly after age 20, but in the LA hospitals, it increased only slowly and rarely became significant at any age. The only factor that we could identify as correlating significantly was the total fat in the diet (52). Unfortunately, we did not have sufficient dietary data to relate the findings to the type of fat.

Transition

In 1960, James Killian, the president of MIT and chairman of the trustees of the Nutrition Foundation, was persuaded by Glen King, president of the Nutrition Foundation, to invite me to establish a Department of Nutrition and Food Science at MIT, absorbing a small Department of Food Technology. I agreed, but it was another year before I reluctantly left INCAP. The competence and leadership capabilities of the senior INCAP staff indicated that it was time. This judgment was confirmed by INCAP's continued productivity and growth for the next 30 years. Unfortunately, a civil war, a terrorist kidnapping of the director and administrator, and Pan American Health Organization policies have since caused the loss of key staff and research capacity.

THE MIT YEARS: 1961–1986

Establishing a Department

In July 1961, I arrived at MIT to establish the new graduate Nutrition and Food Science department. The opportunity provided the resources to select and hire an outstanding faculty and the freedom to determine the research mission and graduate training programs of the department. As the first department to combine nutrition, food science and technology, and food toxicology, it became a successful model for other institutions. It soon provided in-depth multidisciplinary graduate degree training in nutritional biochemistry and metabolism, clinical nutrition, food toxicology, food science and technology, industrial and food microbiology, and biochemical engineering.

Within a year, we started an outpatient unit for metabolic balance studies. Within three years, an NIH grant established the only Clinical Research Center (CRC) outside a teaching hospital. An NIH clinical training grant and other support concurrently attracted a long series of exceptionally well-qualified and motivated MDs to obtain PhDs in nutritional biochemistry and metabolism. The CRC facilities provided 24-hour nursing and medical coverage for clinical research, and the MDs in the program had major medical responsibility for the center and the quality of its research.

With faculty of the Nutrition and Food Science Department, clinicians from Harvard and Boston universities, and physicians in the PhD program, the center became extremely productive. MDs in the program pioneered the concept of nutrition support services in hospitals. Everyone in the clinical nutrition training program spent time on nutrition support services established in area teaching hospitals. Graduates of the MD-PhD program are now leaders in nutrition investigation and research administration in the United States and many foreign countries.

In 1971, the International Nutrition Program was established with its own MA and PhD track. After my retirement as department head in 1988, I became its director and obtained support for fellowships from the United Nations University (UNU). The MA and PhD programs were unique for North American students, and most are now leaders in national and international agencies and nongovernmental organizations.

Single-Cell Protein Studies

Talented students and I carried out a long series of studies of protein requirements under various physiological and pathological conditions, including an examination of the value of a variety of protein sources. Using students and staff as subjects, we investigated torula yeast as a dietary protein source and soon learned that despite good biological value, its use for this purpose was limited by its high nucleic acid content, which induced elevated uric acid levels and increased the risk of gout (11).

An N balance study to evaluate the biological value of food yeast shocked at high temperature to reduce its nucleic acid to acceptable limits was favorable in the study's six subjects. However, a large-scale study to evaluate its acceptability and tolerance in a group of 50 students had to be suspended because of both intestinal and cutaneous allergic reactions. We learned that, to reduce the cost, the second batch had been heat shocked at a lower temperature for a longer time. French MD graduate student Jean Claude Dillon developed an in vitro immunological method using leucocytes of sensitized subjects to show that the culprit was a polypeptide of approximately 50,000 molecular weight produced only at the lower temperature (35, 48).

We soon became the world center for the evaluation of single-cell protein and work with yeast and bacteria produced by different companies on a variety of substrates. Processing to reduce the RNA content was necessary and often made the product allergenic. We used the in vitro method to guide processing. However, the development of bacterial and yeast protein was ultimately suspended on economic grounds. The production requirements are now known, and work can be resumed when financial prospects become favorable.

Fungi as a food protein source do not need processing to reduce RNA (57). No problems were encountered with filamentous microfungi produced on sulfite paper waste in Finland or starch in the United Kingdom (69). Unfortunately, the former was doomed when industry discontinued the sulfite process, but the latter is in British and U.S. markets, labeled as Quorn™.

Protein and Amino Acid Requirements

Vernon Young came to MIT in 1965 as a research associate and rapidly rose in the academic ranks to full professor, became a National Academy member, and won prestigious awards. We soon had joint laboratories and research conferences with our graduate students. Although we each had projects of our own, many were shared. I obtained a grant from US AID to explore the extent to which milk protein could be diluted by the less expensive nonessential N sources glycine and diamonium citrate. If the essential amino acid pattern proposed by Rose and accepted by FAO/WHO was valid, the proportion of N from essential amino acids required for optimum utilization was much less than that contained in milk, meat, and eggs. The results of my research were not consistent with the Rose pattern, but an explanation of the discrepancy had to wait until after my retirement, when Vernon Young determined amino acid requirements with a powerful new approach using stable isotopes. He demonstrated that essential amino acid requirements were about double the previous estimates (75).

Following my INCAP work on the effects of infection on nitrogen balance and confirmation at MIT of significant negative effects of even yellow fever vaccine despite the lack of febrile response (12), we explored effects of other causes of stress on N balance. We found that freshmen but not upper-class MIT students had increased nitrogen losses during the final exam period (54). Our N balance studies that had the greatest practical consequences concerned the protein requirements of normal adults.

Prior to 1971, diets of developing country populations were usually found to be limiting in protein relative to calories based on FAO/WHO estimates of protein and energy requirements. In an effort to put protein requirements on a more quantitative basis, MIT professor Hamish Munro proposed a factorial approach at the 1971 committee meeting (17). This assumed that human protein requirements must be the sum of obligatory urinary, fecal, and miscellaneous N losses (hair, nails, skin, etc.) $\times$ 6.25 in subjects reaching equilibrium on a free diet. This could not be applied for lack of data. Instead, by rather tortuous reasoning, the committee arrived at an allowance of 0.71 g of egg or milk protein per kg, but then suggested 0.8 to 1.1 for a good mixed diet, as consumed in the United States and Europe.

Soon afterward, we placed 100 MIT students on a nitrogen-free diet for 28 days. Within eight days, they reached a plateau that gave us stable figures for "obligatory" urinary and fecal losses and their variances (55). We later obtained similar data for women and elderly subjects. Our data for men were almost exactly confirmed by Callaway et al. (9), who also measured losses for hair, skin, nails, etc. (9). The 1971 Expert Consultation used these data to arrive at a factorial estimate of 0.57 g protein per kg as sufficient to meet the requirements of almost all normal adults.

Before the report was published, graduate student Cuthbert Garza began a three-month

N balance study with six MIT students at this level. At the end of one month, three were in negative N balance. At the end of the three months, all six had two or more of the following: loss of lean body mass, lower creatinine excretion, and cumulative negative N balance elevated serum transaminase (13). The study was replicated immediately with four subjects, three of whom had had a cumulatively negative N balance at 50 days, and one of whom had had abnormally elevated serum amylase (14). In one subject, N loss was the equivalent of 1.5 kg lean body mass. Losses were corrected by giving 250–500 calories more than the estimated energy requirement, although this resulted in weight gain. The results of these two studies suggested that the 1973 committee had made a serious mistake to which the obligatory N data had contributed. In a third study with six subjects, N balance was negative in five of six subjects until above-requirement N balance was achieved with progressive caloric additions (15).

Getting protein requirements right became a priority of the UNU. A working group was convened in Costa Rica in 1977 (71) to analyze the problem and determine how best to approach it. The recommendation, based on our work at MIT, was to select individuals in many different countries and determine their nitrogen balance at four different levels of protein when consuming their usual diets adjusted to their energy requirement. The zero nitrogen balance intercept of a line through the four points gave the individual protein requirement under these conditions, and the multiple intercepts gave their variance (36). The preliminary findings, which were reviewed during a workshop, indicated that the results from all of the countries were remarkably uniform, and the mean requirement was close to the value recommended by the 1971 committee as sufficient for nearly all normal adults (67).

Longer-term N balance studies were planned at the new mean plus two standard deviations of 0.8 g protein/kg, and additional countries were recruited for the shorter studies. A final workshop of the project was held in 1981 to summarize the data in advance of the next FAO/WHO/UNU Expert Group on Protein and Energy Requirements (30). The combined data for 10 countries indicated a mean requirement of 0.63 g protein/kg, with a standard deviation of 0.20. The next Expert consultation accepted these data as definitive and with some minor adjustment for additional data, proposed an adult protein allowance of 0.75 g/kg body weight (18). This correction returned the estimated protein requirement to previous levels, but economists and nutritionists had already accepted the erroneous low value, recalculated developing country diets, and announced that calories were limiting in developing country diets, not protein. Unfortunately, this error still lingers. The first N balance study in elderly subjects suggested there is a higher protein requirement for this group than for younger adults (68).

Other Activities

A long series of investigations of symptoms from milk consumption in lactose malabsorbers led to a definitive monograph on the subject (56). Among other significant studies was the demonstration that hemoglobin is linearly related to the take-home pay of rubber tappers in Indonesia who are paid by the amount they collect (2). The same was true for women tea pickers. In both cases, iron supplementation increased take-home pay.

In studies in both Indonesia and Egypt, young children who were iron deficient performed more poorly on cognitive tests, and scores improved with iron supplementation (28).

During the MIT period, the convening of major international conferences opened new fields. Two were particularly influential. In 1967, there were almost no interactions between professionals studying behavior in rats and in children, and nutrition and cognition was not a recognized field. After an international conference on malnutrition, learning, and behavior supported by the Nutrition Foundation and publication of the resulting book (51), nutrition and cognition became an increasingly recognized discipline.

A 1967 workshop focused on the possibility of producing edible protein from yeasts, bacteria, and microfungi (23). The term "single cell protein" was used for the first time in its title and was soon universally adopted. Academic and industrial research was stimulated, and a larger conference was held only six years later (66).

INTERNATIONAL UNION OF NUTRITION SCIENCES

In 1972, Glen King asked for my help in developing a system of commissions with specialized committees for the International Union of Nutrition Sciences (IUNS), of which he had become president. Soon three commissions with multiple committees were functioning. Although some did little, others produced valuable recommendations and publishable reports. IUNS was changed from an organization inactive between triennial International Congresses to a continuous international influence. As president of IUNS from 1978 to 1981, I expanded the committee structure. Later, the UNU World Hunger Program was able to support and make use of a number of IUNS committees for specific objectives. IUNS continues to have a network of active committees and task forces and to work closely with the International Nutrition Foundation.

UNITED NATIONS UNIVERSITY

In the mid 1970s, the government of Japan contributed an endowment of 100 million dollars for a United Nations University in Tokyo, plus building space and upkeep. Its mission was to apply instruments of scholarship (research, advanced training, and dissemination of knowledge) to the solution of pressing global problems of human survival and welfare. It was to have no faculty or students but instead to work through existing institutions, with special emphasis on developing countries. In its approval, the General Assembly of the United Nations stipulated that one of its three initial programs should be focused on world hunger.

Fourteen years after I established the Nutrition and Food Science Department at MIT, I was invited to come to Tokyo as one of three program vice rectors, each with an annual budget of one million dollars, plus an equal amount for an overall fellowship program. I felt that I could not leave MIT, but I agreed to help initially. I ended up as de facto vice rector for the program for the next six years, and when it became the UNU's Food and Nutrition Program, I continued to direct it for an additional 12 years.

Initially, an International Advisory Committee for the Hunger Program selected three priorities: "Human Protein Needs Under Conditions of Developing Countries," "Post Harvest Food Conservation," and "Food and Nutrition Policy." A network of 36 associated and cooperating institutions and a larger number of institutional research collaborations was established. In its first six years, more than 500 fellowships were awarded to developing country scientists for advanced training in areas related to food and nutrition wherever in the world seemed most appropriate. Fellowships were limited to two years, but those doing well in doctoral programs found ways to complete them.

THE INTERNATIONAL NUTRITION FOUNDATION

Another institution for which I am responsible is the International Nutrition Foundation (INF). It was organized in 1983 to carry on some of the programs of the UNU/WFP at a time when it was threatened by a change in rectors. Fortunately, the UNU Council valued the program and would not allow its termination. The primary role of INF became facilitating the nutrition programs of UNU. I have served as president since the founding of INF, which has a governing board of distinguished academics. With support from international agencies, bilateral and nongovernmental agencies, and industry, INF now has an extensive fellowship program, edits and publishes the UNU *Food and Nutrition Bulletin*, and supports research.

Over the past few years I have designed INF field studies in Pakistan (16), China (76), and Syria, in which the lysine fortification of wheat flour improved immune status as judged by T-cell increase and enhanced complement C3 response. In Syria, it also reduced indicators of anxiety and stress in family members (65). The impact of lysine supplementation on diarrhea incidence is currently being investigated in Bangladesh, and the stress effect is being researched in Ghana.

OTHER INTERNATIONAL ACTIVITIES

Some of the international activities that I was instrumental in founding deserve mention. In 1966, a report I prepared for the United Nations Economic and Social Council, "International Action to Avert the Impending Protein Crisis," became the basis for a meeting convened by the UN Secretary-General (70). In the same year, I became involved in establishing and guiding the UN PAG to advise on the development of complementary foods for young children in developing countries. It produced much-needed specifications for possible components of weaning foods and their preclinical and clinical evaluation and served its purpose well. When its task of developing guidelines and standards for the development of complementary foods was completed, it was replaced in 1977 by the UN Subcommittee on Nutrition and its Scientific Advisory Committee.

The International Dietary Energy Consultative Group reflected the growing recognition of the consequences of chronic energy deficiency. I served as chair, but Nestle Foundation (NF) Director Beat Schurch, as its technical secretary, was responsible for much of its success. Meetings supported largely by UNU and NF produced a series of valuable monographs widely distributed by NF without charge (21, 32, 33, 58, 63).

Three committees that I chaired from the start had gratifying impact. The first was the International Committee of the U.S. Food and Nutrition Board, which is still active. The second was the Committee on International Centers for Medical Research, which was supported by program grants from NIH. Centers were in Cali, Colombia; San Jose, Costa Rica; Kuala Lumpur, Malaysia; Lahore, Pakistan, and Calcutta, India. The entire committee visited each site annually for several days during the 10 years of the program. The third was the Malnutrition Panel of the U.S. Cooperative Medical Science program. Beginning in 1973, the panel met alternately in Japan and the United States to develop a network of nutrition research projects in Southeast Asia; it still continues.

I chaired two missions for the U.S. Senate Subcommittee on Refugees headed by Senator Ted Kennedy. One was a visit to five countries with food shortages—Egypt, Pakistan, India, Indonesia, and Philippines—to develop recommendations for U.S. policy (70). The other was a mission of five physicians to determine the needs of Vietnam for rebuilding its health and social infrastructure when the peace treaty under negotiation in Paris was concluded. The destruction caused by air raids on the industrial periphery of Hanoi, the largest hospital, and a residential area were recent and painfully evident. To our surprise, however, levels of sanitation were high and unlike all of the rest of Southeast and South Asia, diarrhea was not a health problem even in rural villages. Moreover, sufficient vaccines were being produced for the entire child population (50). We made constructive suggestions for helping Vietnam after the war, but the United States was too bitter to ever implement them.

My most memorable foreign trip was with Senator Ted Kennedy. By September 1971, the number of refugees in India from the war in what is now Bangladesh had escalated to ten million. We visited camps around the entire periphery of Bangladesh in torrential monsoon rains and found the Indian government doing an outstanding job of feeding the refugees from its own grain stores and with dried milk contributed by the United Nations Children's Fund (UNICEF). A team from the All-India Institute of Medical Sciences had observed that infant mortality rates in the camps were extremely high, in part because infants who were severely malnourished and dehydrated with diarrheal or respiratory disease needed a special formula to survive. This recommendation had been agreed upon by UNICEF and the Indian Council of Medical Research but was ignored by authorities in New Delhi, who were overwhelmed by other problems. Kennedy's prestige supported by my recommendation as an international nutrition authority was sufficient to overcome the bureaucratic barrier, and a few weeks later the special food provided by UNICEF began arriving in the camps.

LIFE-SPAN HEALTH OF U.S. CIVIL WAR VETERANS

In 1989, Robert Fogel, the economic historian at the University of Chicago who later received a Nobel Prize and whom I had met at a conference in Bellagio, revealed a grand design for collecting life-span health and social information on 40,000 U.S. Civil War veterans. Data were available from physicians' examinations at induction, when sick or wounded, when reporting for pension examinations, and at death. The problem posed was how to enable student coders in the National Archives to interpret the often illegible handwriting, arcane and inconsistent medical terminology, overly detailed description of wounds, and lack of quantitative measures.

With the help of I. Rosenberg, the coding task was accomplished over a period of years, and the resulting public use tapes have been the bases of dozens of seminal articles. In general, the data reveal a much earlier onset of chronic disease in nineteenth-century males compared with a similar contemporary sample and point to the economic implications. Recently data from 6000 African American Civil War veterans have been added and are available for analysis.

INTERNATIONAL INVOLVEMENT

The foregoing account does not capture the full extent of my international life. After spending nine months in Panama from 1945 to 1946 and two months in 1947, I lived for 12 years in Guatemala. However, during this period, I visited other Central American countries almost monthly, and I was sent by the Pan American Health Organization as a consultant to every Latin American country except Uruguay. I made frequent trips to Geneva and Rome to represent WHO as the Secretariat of Expert Committees and attended joint FAO/WHO nutrition meetings. I have continued to spend much of my time in travel for international nutrition activities.

During the first six years with UNU, I traveled to Tokyo every two months and lived in Tokyo for 12 months. In addition to travel to congresses, workshops, and meetings and work in Latin America, I designed and supervised field studies in Egypt, Indonesia, and Kazakhstan on the effects of iron supplementation in rural communities, of lysine fortification of wheat flour in Pakistan, China, and Syria, and currently of lysine supplementation in Bangladesh and Ghana. Outside of Latin America, countries I have visited for nutrition activities 10 to 30 or more times include China, India, Italy (FAO), Japan, Kazakhstan (ADB/UNICEF), Malaysia, Pakistan, Philippines, Switzerland (WHO), Thailand, and the United Kingdom. I have traveled nearly as many times to Bangladesh, Malaysia, Sri Lanka, and other countries. I have participated in some kind of nutrition-related activity in more than 90 countries and have worked extensively for UN agencies.

EPILOGUE

The most prestigious of the honors I have received was the 1991 World Food Prize Laureate for the development of Incaparina, the demonstration of the feasibility of adding potassium iodate to crude moist salt, and the identification of the synergism between nutrition and infection. My scientific career has been characterized by superb collaborators, outstanding and close friends in a large number of countries, constant participation in a wide range of nutrition-related international activities, and remarkable opportunities for developing human capacity and building institutions. With this, along with the strong personal and professional support of my anthropologist wife of 65 years, five successful children who have been tolerant of their father's travels and overcommitments, as well as eight grandchildren, no one could ask for more.

LITERATURE CITED

1. Arroyave G, Pineda O, Scrimshaw NS. 1956. The stability of potassium iodate in crude table salt. *Bull. World Health Organ.* 14:183–85
2. Basta SS, Soekirman S, Karyadi D. 1979. Iron deficiency anemia and the productivity of adult males in Indonesia. *Am. J. Clin. Nutr.* 32(4):916–25
3. Behar M, Ascoli W, Scrimshaw NS. 1958. An investigation into the causes of death in children in four rural communities in Guatemala. *Bull. World Health Organ.* 19:1093–102
4. Behar M, Bressani R, Scrimshaw NS. 1959. Treatment and prevention of kwashiorkor. *Am. J. Clin. Nutr.* 1:73–101
5. Behar M, Viteri F, Scrimshaw NS. 1957. Treatment of severe protein deficiency in children (kwashiorkor). *Am. J. Clin. Nutr.* 5:506–15
6. Bressani R, Behar M, Viteri F. 1958. Supplementation of cereal proteins with amino acids. I. Effect of amino acid supplementation of corn-masa at high levels of protein intake on the nitrogen retention of young children. *J. Nutr.* 66:485–99
7. Bressani R, Elias LG, Scrimshaw NS, Guzman MA. 1962. Nutritive value of Central American corns. VI. Varietal and environmental influence on the nitrogen, essential amino acid, and fat content of ten varieties. *Cereal Chem.* 39:59–67
8. Bressani R, Scrimshaw NS, Behar M, Viteri F. 1958. Supplementation of cereal proteins with amino acids II. Effect of amino acid supplementation of corn-masa at intermediate levels of protein intake on the nitrogen retention of young children. *J. Nutr.* 66:501–13
9. Calloway DH, Odell AC, Margen S. 1971. Sweat and miscellaneous nitrogen losses in human balance studies. *J. Nutr.* 101(6):775–86
10. Chavez A, Martinez C, Soberanes B. 1995. The effect of malnutrition on human development: a 24-year study of well-nourished and malnourished children living in a poor Mexican village. In *Community-Based Longitudinal Nutrition and Health Studies*, ed. NS Scrimshaw, pp. 1–28. Boston, MA: Int. Found. Dev. Countries
11. Clifford AJ, Riumallo JA, Young VR, Scrimshaw NS. 1976. Effect of oral purines on serum and urinary uric acid of normal, hyperuricemic and gouty humans. *J. Nutr.* 106:428–34
12. Gandra YR, Scrimshaw NS. 1961. Infection and nutritional status. II. Effect of mild virus infection induced by 17-D yellow fever vaccine on nitrogen metabolism in children. *Am. J. Clin. Nutr.* 9:159–63
13. Garza C, Scrimshaw NS. 1976. Human protein requirements: the effect of variations in energy intakes within the maintenance range. *Am. J. Clin. Nutr.* 29:280–87

14. Garza C, Scrimshaw NS, Young VR. 1977. Human protein requirements: evaluation of the 1973 FAO/WHO safe level of protein intake for young men at high energy intakes. *Br. J. Nutr.* 37:403–20
15. Garza C, Scrimshaw NS, Young VR. 1978. Human protein requirements: interrelationships between energy intake and nitrogen balance in young men consuming the 1973 FAO/WHO safe level of egg protein, with added non-essential amino acids. *J. Nutr.* 108:90–96
16. Hussain T, Abbas S, Khan MA, Scrimshaw NS. 2004. Lysine fortification of wheat flour improves selected indices of the nutritional status of predominantly cereal-eating families in Pakistan. *Food Nutr. Bull.* 25:114–23
17. Joint FAO/WHO Expert Committee. 1973. Energy and protein requirements. Report of a Joint FAO/WHO Expert Committee. *WHO Tech. Rep.* Ser. 522. Geneva: World Health Org.
18. Joint FAO/WHO/UNU Expert Consultation. 1985. Energy and protein requirements. Report of a Joint FAO/WHO/UNU Expert Consultation. *WHO Tech. Rep.* Ser. 724. Geneva: World Health Org.
19. Mann GV, Munoz JA, Scrimshaw NS. 1955. The serum lipoprotein and cholesterol concentrations of Central and North Americans with different dietary habits. *Am. J. Med.* 19:25–32
20. Martorell R. 1995. The INCAP Longitudinal Study (1969–77) and its follow up (1988–89): an overview of results. In *Community-Based Longitudinal Nutrition and Health Studies*, ed. NS Scrimshaw, pp. 125–42. Boston, MA: Int. Nutr. Found.
21. Martorell R, Scrimshaw NS, eds. 1990. The effects of improved nutrition in early childhood: the Institute of Nutrition of Central America and Panama (INCAP) follow-up study. *Proc. IDECG Workshop, Bellagio, Italy*. Lausanne, Switzerland: Int. Dietary Energy Consult. Group, Nestle Found.
22. Mata LJ. 1978. The children of Santa Maria Cauque: a prospective field study of health and growth. Cambridge, MA: MIT Press
23. Mateles R, Tannenbaum S. 1968. *Single Cell Protein*. Cambridge, MA: MIT Press
24. Mendez J, Savits BS, Flores M, Scrimshaw NS. 1959. Cholesterol levels of maternal and fetal blood at parturition in upper and lower income groups in Guatemala City. *Am. J. Clin. Nutr.* 7:595–98
25. Mendez J, Scrimshaw NS, Abrams MD, Forman EN. 1960. Serum lipids and protein-bound iodine levels of Guatemalan pregnant women from two different socioeconomic groups. *Am. J. Obstet. Gynecol.* 80:114–18
26. Munoz JA, Scrimshaw NS. 1955. The serum lipoprotein and cholesterol concentrations of Central and North Americans with different dietary habits. *Am. J. Med.* 19:25–32
27. Perez C, Scrimshaw NS. 1958. Classification of goitre and techniques of endemic goitre surveys. *Bull. World Health Organ.* 18:217–32
28. Pollitt E, Soemantri AG, Yunis F, Scrimshaw NS. 1985. Cognitive effects of iron-deficiency anaemia. *Lancet* 325(8421):158
29. Puffer RR, Serrano CV. 1976. The inter-American investigation of mortality in childhood. *World Health Stat. Rep.* 29:493–542
30. Rand WM, Uauy R, Scrimshaw NS, eds. 1984. Protein energy-requirement studies in developing countries: results of international research. Tokyo: United Nations Univ.
31. Salomon JB, Gordon JE, Scrimshaw NS. 1966. Studies of diarrheal disease in Central America: X. Associated chickenpox, diarrhea and kwashiorkor in a highland Guatemalan village. *Am. J. Trop. Med. Hyg.* 15:997–1002

32. Schurch B, Scrimshaw NS, eds. 1987. Chronic energy deficiency: consequences and related issues. *Proc. IDECG Workshop, Guatemala City, Guatemala City*. Lausanne, Switzerland: Int. Dietary Energy Consult. Group, Nestle Found.
33. Schurch B, Scrimshaw NS, eds. 1989. Activity, energy expenditure and energy requirements of infants and children. *Proc. IDECG Workshop, Cambridge, MA, USA*. Lausanne, Switzerland: Int. Dietary Energy Consult. Group, Nestle Found.
34. Scrimshaw NS. 1980. The background and history of Incaparina. *Food Nutr. Bull.* 2(2):1–2
35. Scrimshaw NS. 1986. Nutritional and tolerance considerations in the feeding of single cell protein. In *Journal of the Proceedings of the International Symposium*, ed. J de La Noue, G Goulet, J Amiot, pp. 197–214. Québec: Québec Centre de la Recherce en Nutrition, Université Laval
36. Scrimshaw NS. 1996. Appendix: criteria for valid nitrogen balance measurement of protein requirements. *Eur. J. Clin. Nutr.* 50(Suppl. 1):196–97
37. Scrimshaw NS. 2003. Historical concepts of interactions, synergism and antagonism between nutrition and infection. *J. Nutr.* 133(1):316–21S
38. Scrimshaw NS, Austin JE, Harris JR, Rha CK, Sinskey AJ. 1973. *High-Protein Product Development in Thailand*. Cambridge, MA: MIT Press
39. Scrimshaw NS, Balsam A, Arroyave G. 1957. Serum cholesterol levels in school children from three socio-economic groups. *Am. J. Clin. Nutr.* 5:629–33
40. Scrimshaw NS, Behar M. 1961. Protein malnutrition in young children. *Science* 133:2039–47
41. Scrimshaw NS, Behar M, Arroyave G, Viteri F. 1957. Kwashiorkor in children and its response to protein therapy. *J. Am. Med. Assoc.* 164:555–61
42. Scrimshaw NS, Behar M, Arroyave G, Viteri F, Tejada C. 1956. Characteristics of kwashiorkor (sindrome pluricarencial de la infancia). *Fed. Proc.* 15:977–85
43. Scrimshaw NS, Behar M, Viteri F, Arroyave G, Tejada C. 1957. Epidemiology and prevention of severe protein malnutrition (kwashiorkor) in Central America. *Am. J. Public Health* 47:53–67
44. Scrimshaw NS, Bressani R, Behar M, Viteri F. 1958. Supplementation of cereal proteins with amino acids. I. Effect of amino acid supplementation of corn-masa at high levels of protein intake on the nitrogen retention of young children. *J. Nutr.* 66:485–99
45. Scrimshaw NS, Bressani R, Wilson D, Behar M, Chung M. 1963. Supplementation of cereal proteins with amino acids. IV. Lysine supplementation of wheat flour fed to young children at different levels of protein intake in the presence and absence of other amino acids. *J. Nutr.* 79:333–39
46. Scrimshaw NS, Cabezas A, Castillo F, Mendez J. 1953. Effect of potassium iodate on endemic goitre and protein-bound iodine levels in school-children. *Lancet* 265(6778):166–68
47. Scrimshaw NS, Culver GA, Stevenson RA. 1947. Toxic complications of pregnancy in Gorgas hospital, Panama Canal Zone, 1931–1945. *Am. J. Obstet. Gynecol.* 54:428–44
48. Scrimshaw NS, Dillon JC. 1979. Allergic responses to some single-cell proteins in human subjects. In *Single-Cell Proteins: Safety for Animal and Human Feeding*, ed. S Garattini, S Paglialunga, NS Scrimshaw, pp. 171–78. Oxford/New York: Pergamon
49. Scrimshaw NS, Franco LV, Arellano R, Sagastume C, Mendez JI, de Leon R. 1966. Efecto de la yodacion de la sal de la prevalencia de bocio endemico en ninos escolares de Guatemala. *Bol. Oficina Sanit. Panam.* 60:222–28
50. Scrimshaw NS, French D, Halberstan M, Levinson J. 1973. *Report of the Indochina Study Mission on Humanitarian Needs for Rehabilitation and Reconstruction of North Vietnam. March 10–17, 1973*. Washington, DC: US Govt. Print. Off.

51. Scrimshaw NS, Gordon JE. 1968. *Malnutrition, Learning, and Behavior*. Cambridge, MA: MIT Press
52. Scrimshaw NS, Guzman MA. 1968. Diet and atherosclerosis. *Lab. Invest.* 18:623–28
53. Scrimshaw NS, Guzman MA. 1995. A comparison of supplementary feeding and medical care of preschool children in Guatemala. In *Community-based Longitudinal Nutrition and Health*, ed. NS Scrimshaw, pp 1–28. Boston, MA: Int. Nutr. Found.
54. Scrimshaw NS, Habicht JP, Piche ML, Cholakos B, Arroyave G. 1966. Protein metabolism in young men during university examinations. *Am. J. Clin. Nutr.* 18:321–24
55. Scrimshaw NS, Hussein MA, Murray E, Rand WM, Young VR. 1972. Protein requirements of man: variations in obligatory urinary and fecal nitrogen losses in young men. *J. Nutr.* 102:1595–604
56. Scrimshaw NS, Murray EB. 1988. The acceptability of milk and milk products in populations with a high prevalence of lactose intolerance. *Am. J. Clin. Nutr.* 48(4):1079–159
57. Scrimshaw NS, Murray EB. 1995. Nutritional value and safety of single cell protein. In *Biotechnology*, ed. G Reed, TW Nagodawithana, 9:221–37. New York: Weinheim
58. Scrimshaw NS, Schurch B, eds. 1991. Protein-energy interactions. *Proc. IDECG Workshop, Waterville Valley, NH, USA*. Lausanne, Switzerland: Int. Dietary Energy Consult. Group, Nestle Found.
59. Scrimshaw NS, Taylor CE, Gordon JE. 1959. Interactions of nutrition and infection. *Am. J. Med. Sci.* 237:367–403
60. Scrimshaw NS, Taylor CE, Gordon JE. 1968. Interactions of nutrition and infection. *World Health Org. Monog. Ser.* 57. Geneva: World Health Organ.
61. Scrimshaw NS, Taylor Y, Young VR. 1973. Lysine supplementation of wheat gluten at adequate and restricted energy intakes in young men. *Am. J. Clin. Nutr.* 26(9):965–72
62. Scrimshaw NS, Trulson M, Tejada C, Hegsted DM, Stare FJ. 1957. Serum lipoprotein and cholesterol concentrations. Comparison of rural Costa Rican, Guatemalan, United States populations. *Circulation* 15:805–13
63. Scrimshaw NS, Waterlow JC, Schurch B, eds. 1994. Energy and protein requirements. *Proc. IDECG Workshop, London, England, UK*. Lausanne, Switzerland: Int. Dietary Energy Consult. Group, Nestle Found.
64. Scrimshaw NS, Wilson D, Bressani R. 1960. Infection and kwashiorkor. *J. Trop. Pediatr.* 6:37–43
65. Smriga M, Ghosh S, Mouneimne Y, Pellett P. 2004. Lysine fortification reduces anxiety and lessens stress in family members in economically weak communities in northwest Syria. *Proc. Natl. Acad. Sci. USA* 101(22):8285–88
66. Tannenbaum SR, Wang DIC, eds. 1975. *Single-Cell Protein*. Cambridge, MA: MIT Press
67. Torun B, Young VR, Rand WM, eds. 1981. Protein-energy requirements of developing countries: evaluation of new data. Tokyo: United Nations Univ.
68. Uauy RN, Scrimshaw NS, Young VR. 1978. Human protein requirements: nitrogen balance response to graded levels of egg protein in elderly men and women. *Am. J. Clin. Nutr.* 31(5):779–85
69. Udall J, Lo CW, Young VR, Scrimshaw NS. 1984. The tolerance and nutritional value of two micro fungal foods in human subjects. *Am. J. Clin. Nutr.* 40(2):285–92
70. United Nations. 1971. Strategy statement on action to avert the protein crisis in the developing countries. New York: United Nations
71. United Nations Univ. 1979. Protein requirements under conditions prevailing in developing countries. Tokyo: United Nations Univ.
72. U.S. Senate Subcommittee. *Summary of Special Study Mission to Asia and the Middle East, January* 1975. Washington, DC: US Govt. Print. Off.

73. Williams CD. 1933. A nutritional disease of children associated with a maize diet. *Arch. Dis. Child.* 8:423
74. Young VR, Ozalp I, Cholakos BV, Scrimshaw NS. 1971. Protein value of Colombian opaque-2 corn for young adult men. *J. Nutr.* 101:1475–82
75. Young V, Pellet PL. 1990. Current concepts concerning indispensable amino acid needs in adults and their implications for international nutrition planning. *Food Nutr. Bull.* 12:289–300
76. Zhao W, Zhai F, Zhang D, An Y, Liu Y, et al. 2004. Lysine-fortified wheat flour improves the nutritional and immunological status of wheat-eating families in northern China. *Food Nutr. Bull.* 25(2):123–30

Protein Turnover Via Autophagy: Implications for Metabolism*

Noboru Mizushima[1,2] and Daniel J. Klionsky[3]

[1]Department of Physiology and Cell Biology, Tokyo Medical and Dental University, Tokyo 113-8519, Japan; email: nmizu.phy2@tmd.ac.jp

[2]SORST, Japan Science and Technology Corporation, Kawaguchi 332-0012, Japan

[3]Life Sciences Institute, and Departments of Molecular, Cellular and Developmental Biology and Biological Chemistry, University of Michigan, Ann Arbor, Michigan 48109; email: klionsky@umich.edu

Annu. Rev. Nutr. 2007. 27:19–40

First published online as a Review in Advance on February 20, 2007

The *Annual Review of Nutrition* is online at http://nutr.annualreviews.org

This article's doi: 10.1146/annurev.nutr.27.061406.093749

0199-9885/07/0821-0019$20.00

*Both authors contributed equally in the preparation of this review.

Key Words

amino acids, neurodegeneration, protein degradation, proteolysis, starvation

Abstract

Autophagy is a process of cellular "self-eating" in which portions of cytoplasm are sequestered within double-membrane cytosolic vesicles termed autophagosomes. The autophagosome cargo is delivered to the lysosome, broken down, and the resulting amino acids recycled after release back into the cytosol. Autophagy occurs in all eukaryotes and can be up-regulated in response to various nutrient limitations. Under these conditions, autophagy may become essential for viability. In addition, autophagy plays a role in certain diseases, acting to prevent some types of neurodegeneration and cancer, and in the elimination of invading pathogens. We review the current information on the mechanism of autophagy, with a focus on its role in protein metabolism and intracellular homeostasis.

Contents

INTRODUCTION

Autophagy/macroautophagy: the sequestration of cytoplasm within double-membrane vesicles for delivery to, and degradation within, the lysosome followed by recycling

When most people consider the topic of nutrition, the first thoughts that come to mind concern the types of food we eat. Of course, we also know that food is consumed as a fuel source and as such it must be broken down to provide energy and building blocks for anabolism. When nutrients become limiting, the biosynthetic needs may alter, but they must still be met to maintain viability. The carbohydrate stores of most organisms can supply nutrients only for a few hours; during the initial phase of fasting, it is generally thought that proteins are broken down to provide substrates for gluconeogenesis (9, 125). Accordingly, once these stores are exhausted during starvation conditions, the cell employs autophagy as a means of reutilizing existing macromolecules to preserve essential functions (49). Autophagy involves the dynamic rearrangement of cellular membranes to allow portions of the cytoplasm to be delivered to the degradative compartment, broken down, and recycled. Protein degradation via autophagy therefore plays a major role in the body's response to nutritional stress. Autophagy, however, is more than a starvation response. For example, this process is involved in cellular remodeling, including modifications that adapt the cell to changes in the types of available nutrients. This role of autophagy is seen when particular organelles such as peroxisomes are rapidly and specifically degraded in response to shifting carbon sources (15, 30).

Autophagy also has important roles beyond nutrition, and it has been linked to various pathophysiological conditions. For example, autophagy is involved in tumor suppression, in eliminating invading viruses and bacteria from host cells, in antigen presentation, neurodegeneration, and some myopathies. In addition, autophagy can function as a type of programmed cell death, distinct from apoptosis. Many of these aspects of autophagy have recently been the subject of reviews (11, 12, 59, 68, 79, 98, 106). In this review, we focus our discussion on the connections between autophagy and nutrition. We elaborate on the recent advances in mammalian cells that reveal the importance of autophagy in cellular metabolism.

OVERVIEW OF AUTOPHAGY

Morphology and Different Types of Autophagy

In very general terms, autophagy means "self-eating" at the subcellular level. There are different types of autophagy-related processes, but in regard to starvation two are most relevant: chaperone-mediated autophagy and macroautophagy. Chaperone-mediated autophagy involves the translocation of unfolded proteins directly across the lysosomal membrane (63). It is a secondary response to starvation in mammals, being induced after macroautophagy, and is not covered in this review. Macroautophagy (hereafter referred to as autophagy) is the primary response to nutrient limitation. During autophagy, cytoplasm is nonspecifically sequestered within a double-membrane cytosolic vesicle, an autophagosome, which fuses with the lysosome (the vacuole in yeast and plants) (**Figure 1**, see color insert). The fusion event releases the inner vesicle, now termed an autophagic body, into the lysosome lumen where it, along with the cytoplasmic cargo, is broken down by hydrolases. The resulting macromolecules are released back into the cytosol via permeases in the lysosome membrane, where they can be reused for anabolic or catabolic reactions (123).

Autophagy is unique as a degradative mechanism in that it has the capacity for sequestration of entire organelles. That is, unlike other degradative pathways such as chaperone-mediated autophagy or proteasomal degradation, autophagic breakdown of substrates is essentially not limited by steric considerations. In addition, the process of autophagy involves a topological rearrangement of the cytoplasm; the mechanism of sequestration moves the cargo from the cytoplasm into the lysosome lumen, the topological equivalent of the extracellular space. It is the special mechanism of sequestration, enwrapment within a double-membrane vesicle, which is able to move cargo intact across a membrane (**Figure 1**).

Selective Types of Autophagy

Autophagy is generally considered a nonselective degradation system; however, there are many examples of selective autophagy in both yeasts and higher eukaryotes. In yeast, even bulk autophagy may have some selective capacity, as the Ald6 protein was shown to be rapidly degraded in an autophagy-dependent manner compared with other cytosolic proteins, although the precise mechanism remains unknown (87). One of the clearest examples of selective autophagy is seen with the degradation of superfluous peroxisomes via pexophagy (15). When yeast grows on carbon sources that require peroxisome function, such as oleic acid or methanol, these organelles proliferate. If the cells are subsequently fed a preferred carbon source such as glucose, the peroxisomes are rapidly and specifically degraded. The tag on the peroxisome membrane that appears to allow for specific recognition appears to be Pex14 (7). The autophagy-related (Atg) components that are needed for pexophagy are mostly common with those needed for another type of selective autophagy, the cytoplasm-to-vacuole targeting (Cvt) pathway (24, 40). In contrast to other autophagic processes, the Cvt pathway is biosynthetic and is used for delivery of at least two resident hydrolases to the vacuole (45).

In mammals, p62/SQSTM1 seems to be a selective substrate for autophagy that is mediated by microtubule-associated protein 1 light chain 3 (LC3) binding (discussed below) (8). Although information of selectivity for other endogenous cytosolic proteins is very limited, pathogenic bacteria invading host cytosol appear to be enclosed selectively in a process termed xenophagy (81, 84). In the case of autophagic degradation of intracellular *Shigella* species, VirG on the bacteria might be the target protein that allows specific sequestration (84). It was proposed that Atg5 is involved in the recognition process, but the unique localization of Atg5 on the outer side of the autophagosome implies the presence of a more complicated mechanism.

Autophagic Machinery

The formation of the autophagosome is a complex process and is said to be de novo,

Autophagosome: the double-membrane cytosolic vesicle that sequesters cytoplasm during macroautophagy

Autophagic body: the single-membrane vesicle that is generated by fusion of the autophagosome with the lysosome

Pexophagy: a specific type of macroautophagy involving the targeted sequestration and degradation of peroxisomes

Atg: autophagy related

Microtubule-associated protein 1 light chain 3 (LC3): the mammalian homologue of yeast ubiquitin-like Atg8, which is present as a proteolytically processed, LC3-I (cytosolic), or lipidated, LC3-II (autophagosome-associated) form

Phagophore: the initial membrane structure that initiates the sequestration process during macroautophagy, also called the isolation membrane

Atg proteins: the protein machinery of the process of macroautophagy

involving a range of unique machinery. Autophagosome formation is de novo in that a budding process does not directly generate the autophagosome as occurs with transient transport vesicles that operate in the secretory pathway. Rather, the autophagosome is formed by expansion of a membrane core of unknown origin, termed the phagophore or isolation membrane. The protein machinery of autophagy participates primarily at the step of autophagosome formation.

The Atg proteins were first identified in yeasts, and there are currently 29 proteins that are specific to autophagy (38, 46, 108). These proteins function at the various steps of the process including induction, vesicle formation, and breakdown of the autophagic body. Additional proteins play a role during targeting of the autophagosome to, and fusion with, the vacuole, the yeast analogue of the lysosome, but these proteins are common to all pathways that deliver material to the lysosome/vacuole and are not considered Atg proteins. Many of the Atg proteins have clear homologues in higher eukaryotes and, in some cases the proteins have been shown to function heterologously, indicating that they are true orthologues. The functions of these proteins have been the focus of several reviews (45, 120, 124).

Almost all of the Atg proteins associate at least transiently with the preautophagosomal structure (PAS), which is thought to be the site for assembly of the autophagosome in yeast (111). Thus, the PAS is essentially composed of the phagophore, or its precursor, and its associated Atg proteins. The current view is that the phagophore represents the nucleation membrane for autophagosome biogenesis. Additional membrane is delivered to the phagophore; although the origin of this membrane is not definitely known, it appears to include the early secretory pathway (14, 18, 28, 94, 95) and, in yeast, the mitochondria (94). The Atg proteins may function in part by directing membrane to the phagophore as well as in causing it to form into the three-dimensional double-membrane sphere that will become an autophagosome. Autophagosome biogenesis is a structurally complex process because it is a very large vesicle, 300–900 nm diameter in yeast and even larger in mammalian cells, and it is not clear how the curvature is enforced upon the expanding membrane.

For the purposes of this review, we briefly highlight a few of the Atg proteins that are relevant in sections below. One of the most striking features of the autophagic machinery is the involvement of more than one-quarter of the Atg proteins in two interconnected processes of protein conjugation (85, 86). Atg8 (LC3 in mammals) and Atg12 are ubiquitin-like proteins. Atg8/LC3 is processed by the proteolytic removal of a C-terminal residue(s) through the action of Atg4 (also referred to as autophagins in mammals), exposing a glycine as the ultimate amino acid, whereas Atg12 is synthesized with the glycine exposed (22, 23, 33, 34, 41, 42, 61, 71). Both proteins are activated by Atg7, which is homologous with the ubiquitin-activating (E1) enzyme (39, 115, 127). The activated intermediates are transferred to ubiquitin-conjugating (E2) analogues, Atg3 and Atg10 (27, 75, 82, 107), respectively. Atg8/LC3 is then covalently attached to phosphatidylethanolamine (in mammalian cells the precursor form is termed LC3-I, and the lipidated species is termed LC3-II), causing it to become membrane-associated, whereas Atg12 covalently modifies Atg5 via an isopeptide linkage to an internal lysine of the latter. These types of reactions are clearly reminiscent of ubiquitination; however, Atg8/LC3 and Atg12 are not ubiquitin homologues, although these proteins have some structural similarity (19, 109, 110, 112).

The functions of Atg8/LC3 and Atg12 are not known, although the proteins in both conjugation systems are normally needed for autophagosome formation. Atg8/LC3 is the only Atg protein that remains associated with the completed autophagosome in mammalian cells, and thus serves as one of the few markers for autophagy (33). LC3 can also be found on the surface of autolysosomes, but at much lower levels than is seen with autophagosomes, because LC3-II on the outer surface of the autophagosome is deconjugated from phosphatidylethanolamine through a second cleavage event involving Atg4 (22, 34, 61, 114). Atg5 binds Atg16 noncovalently (69, 70), and the tetramerization of Atg16 results in the formation of a large complex (55, 69). These two protein conjugation systems are highly conserved from yeast to human (72).

Regulation

The in vivo regulation of autophagy is a very important topic; for example, to use autophagy therapeutically it will be critical to be able to finely regulate its induction because too high a level of autophagy can result in cell death. Autophagy occurs at a basal level in most or all cells, and it can be induced by a variety of conditions; however, many details of the regulatory process remain unclear. Regulation of autophagy has been extensively reviewed (1, 35, 36, 65, 76, 80), and we only briefly highlight this topic here. As a starvation response, autophagy is subject to control by a range of nutrients including nitrogen and carbon in yeast, and by amino acids and certain hormones such as insulin and glucagons in mammals. The autophagy-inhibitory effect of amino acids and insulin has been well established in cell culture and organ perfusion experiments (78). However, the blood amino acid concentration remains virtually unchanged or decreases only slightly during short-term starvation (10, 90, 105). On the other hand, insulin levels rise following a meal, causing the activation of plasma membrane insulin receptors. These receptors in turn activate downstream effectors such as the class I phosphatidylinositol 3-kinase, and Akt/protein kinase B, resulting in the eventual activation of mTor kinase, one of the primary negative regulators of autophagy; however, downstream effectors of mTor are largely unknown. In contrast, nutrient depletion results in mTor inhibition and activation of autophagy. The induction process also requires a class III phosphatidylinositol 3-kinase. There are many additional factors reported to affect autophagic activity (summarized in **Table 1**). Which of these are the critical factors under physiological conditions is not fully

Table 1 Factors/reagents that can regulate autophagosome formation

Stimulators
Extracellular
Glucagon
TNFα
Intracellular
Rapamycin
G_{i3}, GAIP, Erk1/2
Ecdysone
Death-associated protein kinase (DAPK)
Death-associated related protein kinase-1 (DRP-1)
Bacterial/viral infection
Protein aggregates
C2-ceramide
BNIP3
Anticancer agents
TRAIL
FADD
Lithium
ER stress
$p19^{ARF}$
p53, DRAM
UVRAG
Inhibitors
Extracellular
Amino acids
Insulin
Intracellular
Amino acids
3-methyladenine
Cycloheximide
Insulin signaling pathway—mTOR
Phosphatidylinositol 3-kinase inhibitors
Bcl-2
myo-inositol-1,4,5-triphosphate (IP_3)

These factors are classified based on the localization of their targets. For example, ecdysone is a *Drosophila* steroid hormone and binds its receptor inside cells. This table does not cover factors functioning at the autophagosome maturation step and autophagosome-lysosome fusion step.

understood. For example, the involvement of one of the mTor substrates, S6 kinase, is very controversial (48).

Methods for Monitoring Autophagy

A wide range of methods exist for monitoring autophagy in yeasts, and several approaches can be used in higher eukaryotes; these have been covered in various reviews (43, 47, 67). Here we briefly mention the methods that are applicable to mammalian cells. To understand the physiology of autophagy, it is essential to use quantitative diagnostic/monitoring methods. Classic methods include electron microscopy and the measurement of long-lived protein degradation or lysosomotropic reagent-sensitive degradation. Electron microscopy has been useful for following the morphology of autophagy due to the relatively unique size and double-membrane nature of the autophagosome; however, immunoelectron microscopy using anti-LC3 is necessary for unequivocal identification. Various degradation and/or sequestration assays can be used that rely on the uptake of endogenous or exogenously introduced cytosolic markers. The simplest of these is to monitor the degradation of long-lived radioactively labeled cytosolic proteins in the absence and presence of an inhibitor of lysosomal degradation to differentiate autophagy from cytosolic (e.g., proteasomal) degradation events. Alternatively, the measurement of autophagic lactolysis (i.e., the degradation of lactose) is a specific method for monitoring autophagic degradation because there is no degradative enzyme in the cytosol (47). Sequestration assays include the lysosomal uptake of raffinose or long-lived enzymes such as lactate dehydrogenase (measured in the presence of a lysosomal protease inhibitor) (47). Sequestration assays typically provide a more specific means of measuring autophagy; however, these require subcellular fractionation to purify the lysosome.

Additional methods for monitoring autophagosome formation, which rely on fluorescent microscopy or monitoring protein modifications, have been developed since the identification of the Atg proteins (47, 67). One such approach is to monitor the change in localization of LC3 that has been tagged with the green fluorescent protein (GFP) or a similar fluorophore. During autophagosome formation, LC3 is recruited from the cytosol to autophagosomes (33). Thus, the number of autophagosomes is easily estimated by counting the GFP-LC3 dots or ring-shaped structures, if they are large enough. Alternatively, the total dot area can be measured using computer software (e.g., Meta Morph Series, Molecular Device). This method has been applied to whole animals by generating GFP-LC3 transgenic mice (74). Possible pitfalls and limitations of this method are listed in **Table 2**. It should be noted that the (GFP-)LC3 protein itself is nonspecifically incorporated into protein aggregates independent of autophagy (54a). This is a serious problem if one would like to analyze whether protein aggregates can be engulfed by autophagosomes. Accordingly, other methods should be used at the same time for this purpose.

The other method of monitoring autophagy with LC3 is through immunoblotting of the endogenous protein. As indicated above, nascent LC3 is modified posttranslationally similar to yeast Atg8 (27, 42, 85). The two forms of LC3, LC3-I and LC3-II, are easily separated by SDS-PAGE; LC3-II migrates faster than LC3-I because of its extreme hydrophobicity (33). Consequently, immunoblotting of LC3 usually gives two bands: LC3-I (apparent mobility, 16 kD) and LC3-II (apparent mobility, 14 kD). The amount of LC3-II correlates well with the number of autophagosomes. It was recently found that the immunoreactivity of LC3-II is higher than that of LC3-I due to the conformational change produced by the conjugation to phosphatidylethanolamine (26, 34). Therefore, the amount of LC3-II on immunoblots is overestimated. Accordingly, the LC3-II/LC3-I ratio is not a good indicator of autophagy (**Table 2**). On the other hand, it is reasonable to compare the amounts of LC3-II between samples. One important caveat is that an increase in LC3-II levels can result from either the induction of or a block in autophagy; LC3-II that is localized on the autophagosome inner membrane is normally degraded by lysosomal hydrolases. Thus, to monitor the autophagic flux, it is necessary to measure the amount of LC3-II delivered to lysosomes by comparing LC3-II levels in the presence and absence of lysosomal protease inhibitors (114).

Table 2 Pitfalls in autophagy monitoring using LC3

Pitfalls	Solution
(GFP-)LC3 localization	
(GFP-)LC3 protein can be incorporated into protein aggregates or inclusion bodies in an autophagy-independent manner.	1. Conjugation-defective LC3 (the C-terminal glycine mutant, $LC3^{G120A}$) can be used as a negative control. 2. Immunoelectron microscopy if necessary.
Some structures with autofluorescent signal such as lipofuscin might be misrecognized.	1. True GFP-LC3 signals should not be detected with other fluorescence filter sets such as rhodamine, Cy5, and UV. 2. Nontransgenic control should be prepared.
Autophagy flux cannot be monitored because most (GFP-)LC3 is not present in autolysosomes.	Inhibitors of lysosomal enzymes may be used to inhibit (GFP-)LC3 degradation in lysosomes (50, 114).
LC3 immunoblotting	
LC3-II is more reactive to anti-LC3 antibody than LC3-I.	The amount of LC3-II among samples should be compared. The LC3-II/LC3-I ratio is not very meaningful.
Autophagy flux cannot be monitored because LC3-II is degraded in autolysosomes.	Inhibitors of lysosomal enzymes can be used to inhibit LC3-II degradation in lysosomes (50, 114).
The amount of LC3-II fluctuates even using the same cell line.	Strict controls should be prepared in each experiment. It is difficult to compare independently cultured cell lines.

CONTRIBUTION OF AUTOPHAGY TO INTRACELLULAR PROTEIN DEGRADATION

General Concepts of Protein Degradation

Intracellular proteins can be classified into two groups: short-lived proteins (half-life, 10–20 min) and long-lived proteins (25, 37). In hepatocytes, although less than 1% of the total proteins are short-lived, they contribute to as much as one-third of the total protein degradation because of their rapid turnover (37, 78). It is generally considered that most short-lived proteins are degraded by the ubiquitin-proteasome system, whereas most long-lived proteins are degraded in lysosomes via the autophagic pathway; however, this statement sometimes leads to a misunderstanding that autophagy selectively degrades long-lived proteins. Because more than 99% of intracellular proteins are long-lived (37), random sequestration by autophagosomes could provide a simple explanation for the above observation. Furthermore, short-lived proteins can also be degraded in lysosomes (4).

The diameter of mammalian autophagosomes is usually 0.5–1.5 micrometers. Therefore, the volume of each autophagosome represents less than 0.1% of the total cellular volume; however, as the half-life of autophagosomes is considered to be very short (approximately 10 min) (91, 102), the total degradative capacity of autophagy could be large. In perfused rat liver, the rate of protein degradation varies from 1.5%/h (basal) to 4.5%/h (accelerated by starvation) of total cellular protein (102). Similar rates were reported for isolated hepatocytes; 4%–5% of total protein was degraded under amino acid–free conditions (104). In fibroblasts, 3-methyladenine-sensitive degradation, which would account for autophagy, is estimated to be 0.5%–1%/h (16).

Although these degradation rates likely represent autophagy, the contribution of autophagy was demonstrated in a more specific manner using autophagy-deficient cells. The rate of autophagy in isolated hepatocytes could be estimated as about 2%/h by comparison between wild-type and Atg7-deficient hepatocytes (53). In Atg7-deficient hepatocytes, accelerated proteolysis under starvation conditions is abolished almost completely. Similarly, the contribution of autophagy in embryonic stem cells is estimated to be about 2%/h (73). These values might be underestimated, however, because some other degradation systems may be up-regulated when macroautophagy is defective. This type of cross-talk is clearly seen, for example, with the up-regulation of macroautophagy to partially compensate for defects in chaperone-mediated autophagy (62). In addition, the relative contribution of autophagy depends on the cell type. Under starvation conditions, autophagic degradation represents less than 1%/h in transformed fibroblasts (N. Mizushima, unpublished data) and about 1%/h in yeast (117).

In the following sections, we discuss the role of autophagy focusing on protein metabolism. Because of space limitations, the roles of autophagy in cell death, cancer, antigen presentation, killing of intracellular bacteria, support of viral replication, and pathogenesis of human diseases are not covered.

ROLE OF INDUCED AUTOPHAGY AS A STARVATION RESPONSE

Induction of Autophagy Following Starvation

Much attention has been paid to the role of autophagy during starvation because autophagy is drastically induced by nutrient limitation. The most striking demonstration of starvation-dependent induction was provided by yeast studies. Autophagy is induced in yeast cells most efficiently by nitrogen starvation and to a lesser extent by starvation of carbon sources, auxotrophic amino acids, or sulfate (113). When haploid yeast cells defective in autophagy are subjected to nitrogen starvation, most of them die within five days, which is much faster than occurs with wild-type cells (117). These observations clearly indicate that autophagic degradation of cytoplasm (self-eating) is critically important to maintain cell viability during nitrogen starvation.

Autophagy is also induced in mammalian cells cultured in various starvation media such as amino acid–free and serum-free media. Glucose starvation also can induce autophagy, but the effect is milder. Unlike yeast cells, it is very difficult to see phenotypic differences between wild-type and autophagy-defective cells cultured in vitro. As far as we have tested, there is no significant difference in sensitivity to stresses such as various nutrient starvation and endoplasmic reticulum (ER) stress (N. Mizushima, unpublished data); however, as discussed below, the role of induced autophagy was clearly demonstrated in whole animals.

Starvation Response in Whole Animals

Differential levels of autophagy in tissues. Although much attention has been paid to autophagy in liver, where the protein turnover rate is very high, autophagy occurs in almost all tissues. Autophagic activity is enhanced following starvation. This phenomenon was confirmed by studies with GFP-LC3 transgenic mice and by monitoring endogenous LC3. Active autophagosome formation was observed in skeletal muscle, liver, heart, exocrine glands such as pancreatic acinar cells and seminal gland cells, and podocytes in kidney after 24-h food withdrawal (74). Interestingly, autophagy is differentially regulated among organs. In most tissues, the autophagic activity reaches maximal levels within 24 h and then gradually decreases, whereas it is further accelerated even after 24 h in some tissues, such as the heart, and in slow-twitching muscles, such as the soleus. On the other hand, autophagy induction in liver seems to be quicker than in other tissues (A. Kuma & N. Mizushima, unpublished observation). This observation is consistent with earlier findings on total proteolysis (78). Some tissues show constitutively active autophagy. Thymic epithelial cells are the best example: autophagy actively occurs under nutrient-rich conditions (74) and even during embryogenesis (N. Mizushima, unpublished observation). In this case, autophagy might be involved in presentation of cytosolic antigens onto major histocompatibility complex (MHC) class II proteins for lymphocyte selection (79).

In contrast, autophagy is not observed in the brain even after 48-h food withdrawal. This might be because the brain is nutritionally protected under physiological conditions. For example, the brain can utilize nutrients such as glucose and ketone bodies supplied by the liver and other tissues. Nonetheless, neural cells retain autophagic ability, because high levels of autophagy (or accumulation of autophagosomes) are observed in other adverse conditions, such as cerebral ischemia (2) and neurodegeneration (51, 122, 126).

Autophagy in the neonate. Autophagy is also up-regulated during the early neonatal period in response to the nutrient limitations imposed by the sudden termination of the transplacental supply of nutrients (54). Although autophagy seems to be suppressed throughout the embryonic period, except in some tissues such as thymic epithelial cells (discussed above), autophagy is rapidly and extensively induced in various tissues soon after birth. In particular, the heart muscle, diaphragm, alveolar cells, and skin, but not the brain, display massive autophagy. The autophagic activity reaches the maximal level 3–6 h after birth, although the neonatal mice begin suckling before that time. The number of autophagic vacuoles gradually decreases to basal levels by day 1 or 2.

Physiological Significance of Starvation-Induced Autophagy

Autophagy in the liver. The studies described above suggest that induced autophagy is a fundamental response to adapt to starvation. However, in contrast to the well-established roles of carbohydrate and lipid catabolism, the contribution of proteolysis to nutrient and energy homeostasis is less clear. Analyses of *ATG* gene–deficient mice have provided valuable information along these lines (53, 54). Komatsu et al. (53) generated inducible liver-specific Atg7 knockout mice. As discussed, Atg7 is an ubiquitin-activating enzyme (E1)-like protein that catalyzes the first step of both Atg12—Atg5 conjugation and LC3—PE conjugation (85, 116). Mice homozygous for the *Atg7* flox allele ($Atg7^{flox/flox}$) were crossed with Mx1-Cre transgenic mice. In the resulting mice, exon 14 of the *Atg7* gene is excised by intraperitoneal injection of interferon γ or poly-inosinic acid-polycytidylic acid (pIpC). In wild-type mice, liver proteins in the cytosol and organelles such as mitochondria decrease to about 70% after one-day starvation, whereas the decrease is not significant in $Atg7^{flox/flox}$;Mx1 mice, suggesting that autophagy accounts for the majority of starvation-induced protein degradation in the liver (53).

Flox: a DNA segment utilizing repetitive sequences to facilitate directed gene removal by recombination mediated via Cre recombinase

Maintenance of amino acid pools in yeast. The contribution of autophagy in the maintenance of amino acid pools has been directly shown in yeast. When yeast cells are cultured in nitrogen-deficient media, autophagy is induced within one hour and reaches a maximal level by three hours (113). During the first two hours of starvation, the intracellular total amino acid level rapidly decreases (88). The amino acid pool is partially restored thereafter. Such restoration is not observed in *atg* mutants, clearly indicating that autophagy is critical for the maintenance of the cytosolic amino acid pool during starvation. Onodera & Ohsumi (88) further demonstrated that synthesis of total proteins as well as certain specific proteins whose expression is up-regulated in response to starvation was markedly inhibited in *atg* mutants under starvation conditions. Similarly, release of vacuolar amino acids derived from autophagic proteolysis via membrane permeases is the critical final step of autophagy (123). Thus, yeast cells utilize amino acids produced by enhanced autophagy for new protein synthesis, which would account, at least in part, for the loss of viability phenotype of starved *atg* mutants. The contribution of amino acids to energy production in yeast is considered less important than in mammals.

The role of autophagy in maintaining plasma amino acids in the newborn. Likewise, the role of autophagy has been examined in neonatal mice using *Atg5*$^{-/-}$ and *Atg7*$^{-/-}$ mice. As noted above, Atg5 is an acceptor molecule for the ubiquitin-like modifier, Atg12 (71, 72, 85). It has been already found that Atg5 and its proper modification with Atg12 are required for the elongation of the phagophore/isolation membrane (73). *Atg5*$^{-/-}$ and *Atg7*$^{-/-}$ mice are born at the expected Mendelian frequency, and they appear almost normal at birth (53, 54). These findings suggest that autophagy could be dispensable for mammalian embryogenesis, although many studies have suggested possible roles for autophagy in development and cell death in other species (59).

Despite the minimal abnormalities present at birth, most *Atg5*$^{-/-}$ and *Atg7*$^{-/-}$ neonates die within one day of delivery (53, 54; **Figure 2**, see color insert). The cause of death, however, is not straightforward. *Atg5*$^{-/-}$ and *Atg7*$^{-/-}$ neonates have a suckling defect of unknown etiology (probably due to neurological defects, as discussed below); however, the early death of the homozygous mice was not simply due to the suckling failure because the survival time of these knockout mice was still much shorter than that of wild-type mice when compared under nonsuckling conditions after cesarean delivery. The survival time of the knockout neonates could be delayed by forced milk feeding, suggesting that they suffer from a nutritional problem (54). Indeed, plasma amino acid concentrations of *Atg5*$^{-/-}$ and *Atg7*$^{-/-}$ neonates rapidly decrease after birth (53, 54). In particular, the plasma concentrations of essential amino acids and branched-chain amino acids (BCAAs) show large differences. A similar pattern is also observed for amino acid concentrations in various tissues such as liver, heart, and brain. Therefore, autophagy-defective neonates suffer from systemic amino acid insufficiency. Taken together, these studies emphasize the point that increased intracellular generation of amino acids by autophagy is a physiologically important starvation response.

Autophagic versus proteasomal contributions. Recently, the critical contribution of the ubiquitin-proteasome system to the maintenance of the intracellular amino acid pool also has been shown (119). Upon acute amino acid restriction up to 3 h, the amino acid supply mostly relies on proteasome function rather than autophagy. After prolonged starvation, however, amino acids are primarily generated by autophagy. Subsequently, chaperone-mediated autophagy may be induced as a secondary response (63). Therefore, the ubiquitin-proteasome system and autophagy differentially contribute to maintenance of the amino acid pool, dependent on nutrient conditions.

Use of autophagy-derived amino acids. How amino acids produced by autophagy during starvation are utilized in mammals remains to be determined. Although amino acids are not generally considered a good fuel source, such amino acids, particularly BCAA, can be used to generate energy. The activity of the branched-chain α-ketoacid dehydrogenase complex, which is the most important regulatory enzyme for BCAA catabolism, is up-regulated in starvation (21). In addition, in disease conditions such as liver cirrhosis, BCAA is reduced, probably due to

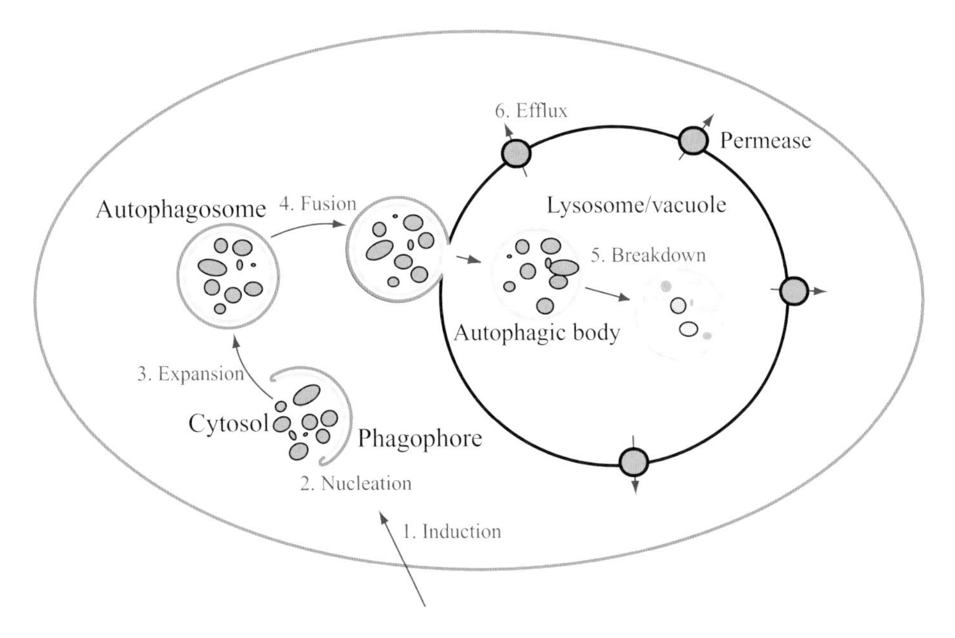

Figure 1

Schematic model of macroautophagy. Autophagy occurs at basal levels and can be induced (*1*) by certain environmental or intracellular cues. The process begins with the nucleation step (*2*) in which a membrane core of unknown origin, termed the phagophore or isolation membrane, sequesters a portion of cytoplasm. The phagophore expands (*3*), probably through the vesicle-mediated addition of membrane (not shown) to generate the double-membrane autophagosome. Upon completion, the autophagosome outer membrane fuses (*4*) with the lysosome, releasing the inner single-membrane vesicle. The autophagic body is broken down (*5*) by lysosomal hydrolases and the resulting macromolecules are released back into the cytosol via membrane permeases (*6*) for reuse in the cytosol in catabolic or anabolic reactions. The steps of cargo recognition and packaging needed for specific types of autophagy are not depicted. The numbers correspond to the individual steps in the figure.

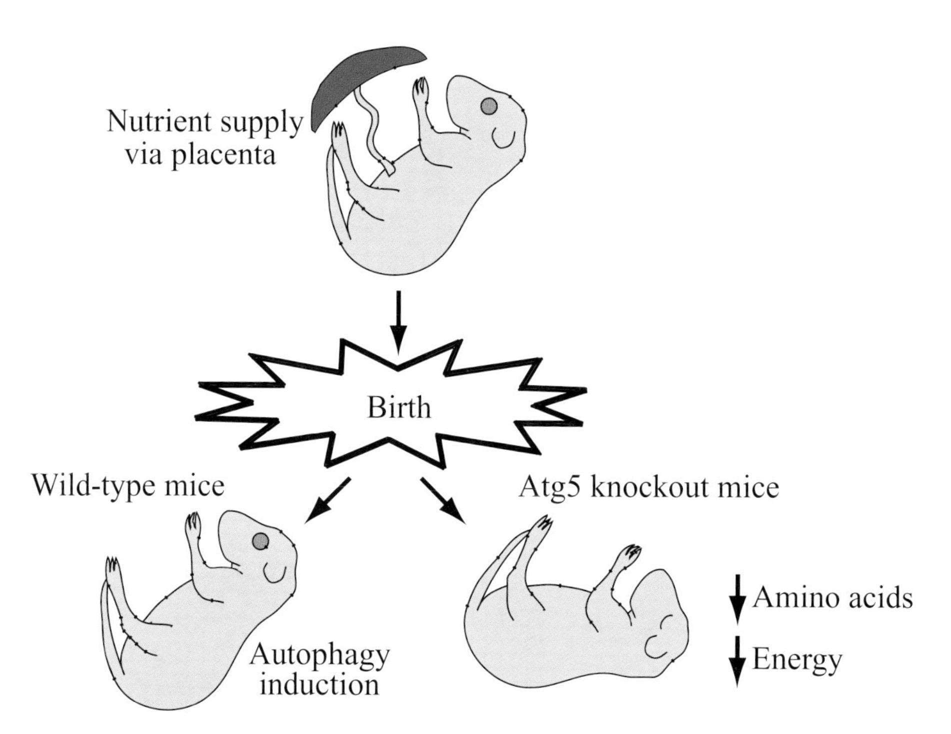

Figure 2

The role of autophagy during the early neonatal starvation period. Embryos receive a transplacental nutrient supply, but the supply becomes suddenly interrupted upon birth, leaving neonates to face severe starvation until the supply is restored through milk nutrients. Atg5 knockout neonates appear grossly normal at birth, but plasma and tissue amino acid levels decrease immediately and the newborns rapidly lose viability. In contrast, wild-type animals survive this unique kind of starvation by inducing autophagy, in addition to the use of carbohydrates and fat stocks.

enhanced consumption as an energy source (77). The preferential reduction of BCAA in *Atg5*$^{-/-}$ and *Atg7*$^{-/-}$ neonates may indicate an increase in BCAA consumption during this period. In addition, tissue energy levels estimated by the activity of AMP-activated protein kinase seem to be low in 10-h-fasting *Atg5*$^{-/-}$ mice, suggesting that neonates could use the amino acids produced by autophagy for energy homeostasis (54). The significance of amino acid production by autophagy in energy metabolism was also shown in an in vitro study. In an IL-3-dependent hematopoietic cell line established from *Bax*$^{-/-}$*Bak*$^{-/-}$ mice, amino acid availability from the media relies on IL-3 stimulation (60); however, these cells can maintain viability even after IL-3 withdrawal by up-regulating autophagy. RNAi-mediated inhibition of autophagy is lethal to these cells; however, the effect of autophagy inhibition can be overcome by the addition of methylpyruvate, a cell-permeable tricarboxylic acid cycle substrate. These results suggest that cultured cells use amino acids as an energy source. In addition to direct energy production, amino acids produced by autophagy can be used for gluconeogenesis and ketogenesis in the liver or for new protein synthesis required for the proper starvation response, as discussed above in yeast cells (88, 123).

Developmental steps related to nutrient limitation. Autophagy-defective mutants have been generated in various species. Thus far, a number of developmental defects have been reported in the mutants (59). In *Saccharomyces cerevisiae*, autophagy mutants are unable to sporulate (117). Autophagy mutants of *Dictyostelium discoideum* are defective in normal multicellular developmental processes such as aggregate formation and fruiting body formation (89). In *Drosophila melanogaster*, lethality from the third larval to pupal stages was reported in autophagy mutants (32, 103). Finally, dauer formation is abnormal in *Caenorhabditis elegans* autophagy mutants (66). As described above, *Atg5*$^{-/-}$ and *Atg7*$^{-/-}$ mice die soon after birth (53, 54). In contrast, mice deficient for Beclin 1, a mammalian homolog of Atg6/Vps30, die at about embryonic day 7.5 (93, 128). Beclin 1 is a subunit of the class III phosphatidylinositol 3-kinase and probably has multiple functions. Thus, the very early embryonic lethality could be explained by some additional roles beyond its function in autophagy. These phenotypes of loss of autophagy seem to be very divergent, but all of them are highly related to nutrient starvation. Therefore, these studies likely indicate the stages at which endogenous amino acid production by autophagy is critically important, probably for both energy metabolism and remodeling.

ROLE OF BASAL AUTOPHAGY IN INTRACELLULAR QUALITY CONTROL

Autophagy and Protein Quality Control

Basal autophagy as a homeostatic mechanism. Although autophagy is characteristically induced upon starvation, it occurs constitutively at low levels even under nutrient-rich conditions. Because yeast cells defective in autophagy do not show obvious abnormalities unless they are cultured under various starvation conditions (117), the role of basal autophagy has not been clarified in this system. However, recent mouse genetic studies have provided evidence that basal autophagy functions as an important quality-control system, particularly in hepatocytes and neural cells.

Liver-specific Atg7 knockout mice. The role of basal autophagy was first demonstrated in liver-specific knockout mice. As discussed above, liver-specific conditional Atg7 knockout (*Atg7*$^{flox/flox}$;Mx1) mice are defective in starvation-induced proteolysis. However, even if maintained in nutrient-rich conditions, *Atg7*$^{flox/flox}$;Mx1 mice develop various abnormalities in the liver (53). For example, these mice show hepatomegaly

20 days after gene targeting by pIpC injection. Some abnormal organelles such as deformed mitochondria and endoplasmic reticulum also accumulate in hepatocytes. Finally, *Atg7*$^{flox/flox}$;Mx1 mice at 90 days after pIpC injection show severe hepatomegaly with disorganized hepatic lobules, cell swelling, and cell death. Serum alanine aminotransferase and aspartate aminotransferase are significantly elevated at this stage. The most unexpected finding with these mice, however, is that many ubiquitin-positive aggregates are generated in hepatocytes (53).

Knockout embryos. Although phenotypic abnormality of *Atg5*$^{-/-}$ and *Atg7*$^{-/-}$ mice was minimal at birth, they showed some significant defects (53, 54). The body size of *Atg5*$^{-/-}$ and *Atg7*$^{-/-}$ neonates was slightly reduced and they displayed a suckling defect. Because embryos are not starved and autophagy seems to be maintained at low levels during embryogenesis, autophagy presumably plays a role other than starvation adaptation. Indeed, accumulation of protein aggregates is already detected in the liver of *Atg5*$^{-/-}$ neonates (20). However, systematic analysis of *Atg5*$^{-/-}$ neonates revealed that the importance of basal autophagy differs among cell and tissue types. Ubiquitin-positive aggregates accumulate vigorously only in hepatocytes, a subset of neurons, the anterior lobe of the pituitary gland, and the adrenal gland (20). As for the nervous system, aggregates are observed in large neurons of dorsal root ganglion (DRG), pons, spinal cord (ventral horn cells), hypothalamus, midbrain, and trigeminal ganglia. The neurons in DRG showed the most extensive accumulation of the inclusions; more than 10 aggregates were observed in a single cell slice. In contrast, very few aggregates are seen in skeletal muscle, heart, and kidney.

It is unclear why autophagy is so important in certain cell types. There was no apparent correlation between the level of basal autophagic activity and the extent of aggregate accumulation (A. Kuma & N. Mizushima, unpublished observation), and autophagic activity in the brain is very low in both embryos and adult mice (74). One possible explanation for cell-specific differences is that intracellular quality control is more important in nondividing, postmitotic cells than in rapidly dividing cells, in which abnormal constituents can be quickly diluted even if they are not degraded. In addition, endogenous aggregation-prone proteins may be more highly expressed in certain affected cell types. Another factor may be cell volume. Larger neurons, such as DRG neurons, tend to accumulate inclusion bodies more readily. These cells may contain greater quantities of proteins per cell that must be turned over through autophagy. Finally, autophagy may occur at higher rates than were previously determined in some cells due to an acceleration of autophagosome turnover (3).

Neural cell–specific Atg5 and Atg7 knockouts. The role of basal autophagy in the nervous system has been further analyzed in neural cell–specific Atg5 and Atg7 knockout mice (*Atg5*$^{flox/flox}$;*Nestin-Cre* mice and *Atg7*$^{flox/flox}$;*Nestin-Cre* mice). These mice are born normally but exhibit growth retardation. After three weeks, they develop progressive motor and behavioral deficits, including ataxic gait, impaired motor coordination, abnormal limb clasping reflexes, and systemic tremor (20, 52). Histological examination revealed the presence of degenerative changes such as partial loss of cerebellar Purkinje cells and cerebral pyramidal cells, and axonal swelling in various brain regions. There is a difference in survival rate between *Atg5*$^{flox/flox}$;*Nestin-Cre* mice and *Atg7*$^{flox/flox}$;*Nestin-Cre* mice. Most *Atg7*$^{flox/flox}$;*Nestin-Cre* mice die within three weeks, whereas only sporadic death is observed for *Atg5*$^{flox/flox}$;*Nestin-Cre* mice. This might be due to the difference in the number of backcrossings; the phenotype seems to be severe in the C57BL/6 background (T. Hara, M. Komatsu, & N. Mizushima, unpublished observation). Alternatively, Atg7 may have some functions other than autophagy because it is a common activating enzyme for mammalian Atg8 homologs such as γ-aminobutyric acid $(GABA)_A$-receptor-associated protein (121) and GATE-16 (99). Ubiquitin-positive protein aggregates extensively accumulated in the cytoplasm of neurons in many regions. Accumulation of aggregates is time-dependent because the distribution of aggregate-positive cells is more limited in autophagy-deficient neonates. Finally, aggregates do not accumulate in glial cells. The studies of Atg5 and Atg7 knockout mice indicate that autophagy is required to prevent neurodegeneration, even in the absence of disease-associated mutant proteins.

The mechanism underlying the accumulation of ubiquitin-positive aggregates is unknown. Loss of autophagy first leads to accumulation of diffuse ubiquitinated proteins in the cytoplasm and is followed by the generation of protein aggregates (20). Therefore, aggregate formation is likely a secondary result of a general protein turnover defect. This idea is in contrast with the hypothesis that autophagosomes specifically degrade inclusion bodies that might be continuously formed under normal conditions. It has been suggested that large aggregates themselves may not be pathogenic, whereas mutant proteins diffusely present in the cytosol could be the primary source of toxicity (5). Thus, continuous clearance of diffuse cytosolic proteins, not protein aggregates themselves, by basal autophagy is important for preventing the accumulation of abnormal proteins that can disrupt neural function.

In this scenario, accumulation of soluble ubiquitinated proteins could be interpreted as a secondary result of impaired protein turnover in the absence of autophagy. Turnover of most cytosolic proteins would be impaired, which provides more opportunities to be damaged or misfolded. In that situation, they have a greater chance to be both ubiquitinated and aggregated. This is consistent with the general agreement that autophagic sequestration is random and nonselective. However, there is yet another possibility that ubiquitinated proteins are recognized via the inner membrane of autophagosomes and thus are preferentially degraded. A number of studies suggest that ubiquitinated proteins are delivered to lysosomes (13, 56, 58, 101, 118). Recently, it was proposed that p62/SQSTM1 mediates the specific recognition of ubiquitinated aggregates by autophagosomes (8). p62/SQSTM1 has been reported to function in various processes such as in the IL-1/TNF signaling pathways toward NF-κB and MAPK9 that is involved in the RNAK-signaling pathway (100), protein kinase C-ζ signaling (92), oxidative stress response (29), and p56lck signaling (31). Because p62/SQSTM1 can bind both ubiquitin and LC3, it could function as an adaptor protein linking ubiquitinated proteins and autophagosomes (8). The p62/SQSTM1 protein is selectively degraded by the autophagy pathway: p62/SQSTM1 is extensively enriched in various autophagy-deficient cells and organs (122) (T. Hara, A. Kuma & N. Mizushima, unpublished observation; M. Komatsu, personal communication). However, it has not been determined how much this pathway contributes to the total degradation of ubiquitinated proteins under normal conditions. The p62/SQSTM1 mutation is associated with Paget disease of the bone in human (57), and p62 knockout mice develop mature-onset obesity (96). Because no apparent neurological abnormality is reported in these human and mouse models, abnormal protein metabolism in autophagy-defective neural cells would not be explained solely by a defect in the p62/SQSTM1-mediated ubiquitinated protein turnover. As almost all proteins in autophagosomes do not directly associate with the autophagosome membrane, selective substrate recognition would account, at most, for only a small fraction of total autophagic degradation.

Clearance of Intracellular Organelles

In contrast to the ubiquitin-proteasome system, autophagy (including microautophagy) can degrade not only proteins but also intracellular organelles such as mitochondria (44, 97, 113), peroxisomes (15), and endoplasmic reticulum (17). Some of these organelles seem to be selectively recognized by autophagy. More recently, the physiological importance of peroxisome degradation by autophagy was directly shown using *Atg7*$^{flox/flox}$;Mx1 mice (30). That study estimates that 70%–80% of peroxisomes induced by phthalate ester are degraded via autophagy during one week after secession of phthalate ester. Finally, even under steady state conditions, abnormal organelles were observed in autophagy-deficient hepatocytes (53). Taken together, these observations suggest that both basal autophagy and induced autophagy are important for control of number and quality of organelles.

Drastic degradation of organelles is also observed in the processes of lens and erythroid development. The lens fiber cells originate from lens epithelial cells. During this process, membrane-bound organelles within the epithelial cells are rapidly lost, which allows fiber cells to be transparent (6). Similarly, intracellular organelles are eliminated during erythroid cell maturation, and the possible involvement of autophagy has been suggested in these processes. More recently, it was reported that the degradation of nuclei of lens cells depends on DNase II-like acid DNase/DNase IIb (83), suggesting that chromatin degradation occurs in an acidic organelle, possibly in the lysosome. However, organelle degradation in lens and erythroid cells occurs normally in autophagy-deficient *Atg5*$^{-/-}$ mice (64). Therefore, a degradation system(s) other than autophagy appears to play a major role in organelle degradation during these processes.

CONCLUDING REMARKS

In this review, we have discussed the molecular mechanism and physiological role of autophagy in protein metabolism. Recent studies have demonstrated that autophagy has many physiological roles and that this process is more pleiotropic than ever expected. Because autophagy is one of the major degradation systems, all of the proposed roles of autophagy are presumably linked to the degradation of intracellular components. Three modes of autophagy, specific, induced nonspecific, and basal, are all critical for nutrient regulation and intracellular quality control/homeostasis. Further investigations into the mechanism of autophagy and the effects of autophagic dysfunction will likely continue to provide important insights into this complex but ubiquitous process.

SUMMARY POINTS

1. Autophagy occurs in all eukaryotes and is induced to higher levels in response to certain types of stress, particularly nutrient starvation.
2. The process of autophagy is typically nonspecific, but can involve specific targeting of cargo. The basic process involves the sequestration of cytoplasm within a double-membrane cytosolic vesicle, followed by delivery to, and degradation within, the lysosome.
3. The autophagosome has an essentially unlimited capacity for sequestering cargo, allowing for the degradation of large protein complexes and entire organelles.
4. Autophagy is involved in tumor suppression, preventing some types of neurodegeneration, and in removing pathogenic bacteria and viruses from host cells.
5. Autophagy occurs constitutively at basal levels, which is important for homeostatic purposes.

6. Induced autophagy is important for maintaining the appropriate amino acid levels for both protein synthesis and supplying energy during starvation.
7. Intracellular quality control is one function of autophagy, which can remove misfolded and aggregated proteins as well as damaged organelles before they become toxic to the cell.

FUTURE ISSUES

1. The regulation of autophagy needs to be better understood to allow its modulation for potential therapeutic purposes.
2. The interactions among, and functions of, the Atg proteins along with structural data from crystallographic studies will provide important information about mechanism and about ways to stimulate and/or inhibit autophagy.
3. Continued analyses with tissue-specific and temporally controlled autophagy genes will allow an assessment of the different roles of autophagy in the whole organism.

ACKNOWLEDGMENTS

This work was supported by Public Health Service Grant GM53396 from the National Institutes of Health (to DJK) and by a Grant-in-Aid from the Ministry of Education, Culture, Sports, Science and Technology of Japan, Kato Memorial Bioscience Foundation, and Toray Science Foundation (to NM). We apologize to those authors whose work could not be cited due to space limitations.

LITERATURE CITED

1. Abeliovich H. 2004. Regulation of autophagy by the target of rapamycin. In *Autophagy*, ed. DJ Klionsky, pp. 60–69. Georgetown, TX: Landes Biosci.
2. Adhami F, Liao G, Morozov YM, Schloemer A, Schmithorst VJ, et al. 2006. Cerebral ischemia-hypoxia induces intravascular coagulation and autophagy. *Am. J. Pathol.* 169:566–83
3. Adhami F, Schloemer A, Kuan CY. 2007. The roles of autophagy in cerebral ischemia. *Autophagy* 3:42–44
4. Ahlberg J, Berkenstam A, Henell F, Glaumann H. 1985. Degradation of short- and long-lived proteins in isolated rat liver lysosomes. Effects of pH, temperature, and proteolytic inhibitors. *J. Biol. Chem.* 260:5847–54
5. Arrasate M, Mitra S, Schweitzer ES, Segal MR, Finkbeiner S. 2004. Inclusion body formation reduces levels of mutant huntingtin and the risk of neuronal death. *Nature* 431:805–10
6. Bassnett S. 2002. Lens organelle degradation. *Exp. Eye Res.* 74:1–6
7. Bellu AR, Komori M, van der Klei IJ, Kiel JAKW, Veenhuis M. 2001. Peroxisome biogenesis and selective degradation converge at Pex14p. *J. Biol. Chem.* 276:44570–74

8. Bjørkøy G, Lamark T, Brech A, Outzen H, Perander M, et al. 2005. p62/SQSTM1 forms protein aggregates degraded by autophagy and has a protective effect on huntingtin-induced cell death. *J. Cell Biol.* 171:603–14
9. Cahill GF Jr. 1970. Starvation in man. *N. Engl. J. Med.* 282:668–75
10. Chikenji T, Elwyn DH, Kinney JM. 1983. Protein synthesis rates in rat muscle and skin based on Lysyl-tRNA radioactivity. *J. Surg. Res.* 34:68–82
11. Cuervo AM, Bergamini E, Brunk UT, Droge W, Ffrench M, Terman A. 2005. Autophagy and aging: the importance of maintaining "clean" cells. *Autophagy* 1:131–40
12. Debnath J, Baehrecke EH, Kroemer G. 2005. Does autophagy contribute to cell death? *Autophagy* 1:66–74
13. Doherty FJ, Osborn NU, Wassell JA, Heggie PE, Laszlo L, Mayer RJ. 1989. Ubiquitin-protein conjugates accumulate in the lysosomal system of fibroblasts treated with cysteine proteinase inhibitors. *Biochem. J.* 263:47–55
14. Dunn WA Jr. 1990. Studies on the mechanisms of autophagy: formation of the autophagic vacuole. *J. Cell Biol.* 110:1923–33
15. Dunn WA Jr, Cregg JM, Kiel JAKW, van der Klei IJ, Oku M, et al. 2005. Pexophagy: the selective autophagy of peroxisomes. *Autophagy* 1:75–83
16. Fuertes G, Martin De Llano JJ, Villarroya A, Rivett AJ, Knecht E. 2003. Changes in the proteolytic activities of proteasomes and lysosomes in human fibroblasts produced by serum withdrawal, amino-acid deprivation and confluent conditions. *Biochem. J.* 375:75–86
17. Hamasaki M, Noda T, Baba M, Ohsumi Y. 2005. Starvation triggers the delivery of the endoplasmic reticulum to the vacuole via autophagy in yeast. *Traffic* 6:56–65
18. Hamasaki M, Noda T, Ohsumi Y. 2003. The early secretory pathway contributes to autophagy in yeast. *Cell Struct. Funct.* 28:49–54
19. Hanada T, Ohsumi Y. 2005. Structure-function relationship of Atg12, a ubiquitin-like modifier essential for autophagy. *Autophagy* 1:110–18
20. Hara T, Nakamura K, Matsui M, Yamamoto A, Nakahara Y, et al. 2006. Suppression of basal autophagy in neural cells causes neurodegenerative disease in mice. *Nature* 441:885–89
21. Harris RA, Goodwin GW, Paxton R, Dexter P, Powell SM, et al. 1989. Nutritional and hormonal regulation of the activity state of hepatic branched-chain alpha-keto acid dehydrogenase complex. *Ann. NY Acad. Sci.* 573:306–13
22. Hemelaar J, Lelyveld VS, Kessler BM, Ploegh HL. 2003. A single protease, Apg4B, is specific for the autophagy-related ubiquitin-like proteins GATE-16, MAP1-LC3, GABARAP and Apg8L. *J. Biol. Chem.* 278:51841–50
23. Huang W-P, Scott SV, Kim J, Klionsky DJ. 2000. The itinerary of a vesicle component, Aut7p/Cvt5p, terminates in the yeast vacuole via the autophagy/Cvt pathways. *J. Biol. Chem.* 275:5845–51
24. Hutchins MU, Veenhuis M, Klionsky DJ. 1999. Peroxisome degradation in *Saccharomyces cerevisiae* is dependent on machinery of macroautophagy and the Cvt pathway. *J. Cell Sci.* 112:4079–87
25. Hutson NJ, Mortimore GE. 1982. Suppression of cytoplasmic protein uptake by lysosomes as the mechanism of protein regain in livers of starved-refed mice. *J. Biol. Chem.* 257:9548–54
26. Ichimura Y, Imamura Y, Emoto K, Umeda M, Noda T, Ohsumi Y. 2004. In vivo and in vitro reconstitution of Atg8 conjugation essential for autophagy. *J. Biol. Chem.* 279:40584–92

27. Ichimura Y, Kirisako T, Takao T, Satomi Y, Shimonishi Y, et al. 2000. A ubiquitin-like system mediates protein lipidation. *Nature* 408:488–92
28. Ishihara N, Hamasaki M, Yokota S, Suzuki K, Kamada Y, et al. 2001. Autophagosome requires specific early Sec proteins for its formation and NSF/SNARE for vacuolar fusion. *Mol. Biol. Cell* 12:3690–702
29. Ishii T, Yanagawa T, Kawane T, Yuki K, Seita J, et al. 1996. Murine peritoneal macrophages induce a novel 60-kDa protein with structural similarity to a tyrosine kinase p56lck-associated protein in response to oxidative stress. *Biochem. Biophys. Res. Commun.* 226:456–60
30. Iwata J, Ezaki J, Komatsu M, Yokota S, Ueno T, et al. 2006. Excess peroxisomes are degraded by autophagic machinery in mammals. *J. Biol. Chem.* 281:4035–41
31. Joung I, Strominger JL, Shin J. 1996. Molecular cloning of a phosphotyrosine-independent ligand of the p56lck SH2 domain. *Proc. Natl. Acad. Sci. USA* 93:5991–95
32. Juhasz G, Csikos G, Sinka R, Erdelyi M, Sass M. 2003. The *Drosophila* homolog of Aut1 is essential for autophagy and development. *FEBS Lett.* 543:154–58
33. Kabeya Y, Mizushima N, Ueno T, Yamamoto A, Kirisako T, et al. 2000. LC3, a mammalian homologue of yeast Apg8p, is localized in autophagosome membranes after processing. *EMBO J.* 19:5720–28
34. Kabeya Y, Mizushima N, Yamamoto A, Oshitani-Okamoto S, Ohsumi Y, Yoshimori T. 2004. LC3, GABARAP and GATE16 localize to autophagosomal membrane depending on form-II formation. *J. Cell Sci.* 117:2805–12
35. Kadowaki M, Kanazawa T. 2003. Amino acids as regulators of proteolysis. *J. Nutr.* 133:2052–56S
36. Kamada Y, Sekito T, Ohsumi Y. 2004. Autophagy in yeast: a TOR-mediated response to nutrient starvation. *Curr. Top. Microbiol. Immunol.* 279:73–84
37. Kato H, Takahashi S, Takenaka A, Funabiki R, Noguchi T, Naito H. 1989. Degradation of endogenous proteins and internalized asialofetuin in primary cultured hepatocytes of rats. *Int. J. Biochem.* 21:483–95
38. Kawamata T, Kamada Y, Suzuki K, Kuboshima N, Akimatsu H, et al. 2005. Characterization of a novel autophagy-specific gene, *ATG29*. *Biochem. Biophys. Res. Commun.* 338:1884–89
39. Kim J, Dalton VM, Eggerton KP, Scott SV, Klionsky DJ. 1999. Apg7p/Cvt2p is required for the cytoplasm-to-vacuole targeting, macroautophagy, and peroxisome degradation pathways. *Mol. Biol. Cell* 10:1337–51
40. Kim J, Klionsky DJ. 2000. Autophagy, cytoplasm-to-vacuole targeting pathway, and pexophagy in yeast and mammalian cells. *Annu. Rev. Biochem.* 69:303–42
41. Kirisako T, Baba M, Ishihara N, Miyazawa K, Ohsumi M, et al. 1999. Formation process of autophagosome is traced with Apg8/Aut7p in yeast. *J. Cell Biol.* 147:435–46
42. Kirisako T, Ichimura Y, Okada H, Kabeya Y, Mizushima N, et al. 2000. The reversible modification regulates the membrane-binding state of Apg8/Aut7 essential for autophagy and the cytoplasm to vacuole targeting pathway. *J. Cell Biol.* 151:263–76
43. Kirkegaard K, Taylor MP, Jackson WT. 2004. Cellular autophagy: surrender, avoidance and subversion by microorganisms. *Nat. Rev. Microbiol.* 2:301–14
44. Kissova I, Deffieu M, Manon S, Camougrand N. 2004. Uth1p is involved in the autophagic degradation of mitochondria. *J. Biol. Chem.* 279:39068–74
45. Klionsky DJ. 2005. The molecular machinery of autophagy: unanswered questions. *J. Cell Sci.* 118:7–18
46. Klionsky DJ, Cregg JM, Dunn WAJ, Emr SD, Sakai Y, et al. 2003. A unified nomenclature for yeast autophagy-related genes. *Dev. Cell* 5:539–45

47. Klionsky DJ, Cuervo AM, Seglen PO. 2007. Methods for monitoring autophagy from yeast to human. *Autophagy* 3:In press
48. Klionsky DJ, Meijer AJ, Codogno P, Neufeld TP, Scott RC. 2005. Autophagy and p70S6 kinase. *Autophagy* 1:59–61
49. Klionsky DJ, Ohsumi Y. 1999. Vacuolar import of proteins and organelles from the cytoplasm. *Annu. Rev. Cell Dev. Biol.* 15:1–32
50. Köchl R, Hu XW, Chan EYW, Tooze SA. 2006. Microtubules facilitate autophagosome formation and fusion of autophagosomes with endosomes. *Traffic* 7:129–45
51. Koike M, Shibata M, Waguri S, Yoshimura K, Tanida I, et al. 2005. Participation of autophagy in storage of lysosomes in neurons from mouse models of neuronal ceroid-lipofuscinoses (Batten disease). *Am. J. Pathol.* 167:1713–28
52. Komatsu M, Waguri S, Chiba T, Murata S, Iwata JI, et al. 2006. Loss of autophagy in the central nervous system causes neurodegeneration in mice. *Nature* 441:880–84
53. Komatsu M, Waguri S, Ueno T, Iwata J, Murata S, et al. 2005. Impairment of starvation-induced and constitutive autophagy in Atg7-deficient mice. *J. Cell Biol.* 169:425–34
54. Kuma A, Hatano M, Matsui M, Yamamoto A, Nakaya H, et al. 2004. The role of autophagy during the early neonatal starvation period. *Nature* 432:1032–36
54a. Kuma A, Matsui M, Mizushima N. 2007. LC3, an autophagosome marker, can be incorporated into protein aggregates independent of autophagy: caution in the interpretation of LC3 localization. *Autophagy* 3: In press
55. Kuma A, Mizushima N, Ishihara N, Ohsumi Y. 2002. Formation of the approximately 350-kDa Apg12-Apg5·Apg16 multimeric complex, mediated by Apg16 oligomerization, is essential for autophagy in yeast. *J. Biol. Chem.* 277:18619–25
56. Laszlo L, Doherty FJ, Osborn NU, Mayer RJ. 1990. Ubiquitinated protein conjugates are specifically enriched in the lysosomal system of fibroblasts. *FEBS Lett.* 261:365–68
57. Laurin N, Brown JP, Morissette J, Raymond V. 2002. Recurrent mutation of the gene encoding sequestosome 1 (SQSTM1/p62) in Paget disease of bone. *Am. J. Hum. Genet.* 70:1582–88
58. Lenk SE, Susan PP, Hickson I, Jasionowski T, Dunn WA Jr. 1999. Ubiquitinated aldolase B accumulates during starvation-induced lysosomal proteolysis. *J. Cell Physiol.* 178:17–27
59. Levine B, Klionsky DJ. 2004. Development by self-digestion: molecular mechanisms and biological functions of autophagy. *Dev. Cell* 6:463–77
60. Lum JJ, Bauer DE, Kong M, Harris MH, Li C, et al. 2005. Growth factor regulation of autophagy and cell survival in the absence of apoptosis. *Cell* 120:237–48
61. Marino G, Uria JA, Puente XS, Quesada V, Bordallo J, Lopez-Otin C. 2003. Human autophagins, a family of cysteine proteinases potentially implicated in cell degradation by autophagy. *J. Biol. Chem.* 278:3671–78
62. Massey AC, Kaushik S, Sovak G, Kiffin R, Cuervo AM. 2006. Consequences of the selective blockage of chaperone-mediated autophagy. *Proc. Natl. Acad. Sci. USA* 103:5805–10
63. Massey AC, Zhang C, Cuervo AM. 2006. Chaperone-mediated autophagy in aging and disease. *Curr. Top. Dev. Biol.* 73:205–35
64. Matsui M, Yamamoto A, Kuma A, Ohsumi Y, Mizushima N. 2006. Organelle degradation during the lens and erythroid differentiation is independent of autophagy. *Biochem. Biophys. Res. Commun.* 339:485–89
65. Meijer AJ, Codogno P. 2004. Regulation and role of autophagy in mammalian cells. *Int. J. Biochem. Cell Biol.* 36:2445–62

66. Melendez A, Tallóczy Z, Seaman M, Eskelinen E-L, Hall DH, Levine B. 2003. Autophagy genes are essential for dauer development and life-span extension in *C. elegans*. *Science* 301:1387–91
67. Mizushima N. 2004. Methods for monitoring autophagy. *Int. J. Biochem. Cell Biol.* 36:2491–502
68. Mizushima N. 2005. The pleiotropic role of autophagy: from protein metabolism to bactericide. *Cell Death Differ.* 12:1535–41
69. Mizushima N, Kuma A, Kobayashi Y, Yamamoto A, Matsubae M, et al. 2003. Mouse Apg16L, a novel WD-repeat protein, targets to the autophagic isolation membrane with the Apg12-Apg5 conjugate. *J. Cell Sci.* 116:1679–88
70. Mizushima N, Noda T, Ohsumi Y. 1999. Apg16p is required for the function of the Apg12p-Apg5p conjugate in the yeast autophagy pathway. *EMBO J.* 18:3888–96
71. Mizushima N, Noda T, Yoshimori T, Tanaka Y, Ishii T, et al. 1998. A protein conjugation system essential for autophagy. *Nature* 395:395–98
72. Mizushima N, Sugita H, Yoshimori T, Ohsumi Y. 1998. A new protein conjugation system in human. The counterpart of the yeast Apg12p conjugation system essential for autophagy. *J. Biol. Chem.* 273:33889–92
73. Mizushima N, Yamamoto A, Hatano M, Kobayashi Y, Kabeya Y, et al. 2001. Dissection of autophagosome formation using Apg5-deficient mouse embryonic stem cells. *J. Cell Biol.* 152:657–67
74. Mizushima N, Yamamoto A, Matsui M, Yoshimori T, Ohsumi Y. 2004. In vivo analysis of autophagy in response to nutrient starvation using transgenic mice expressing a fluorescent autophagosome marker. *Mol. Biol. Cell* 15:1101–11
75. Mizushima N, Yoshimori T, Ohsumi Y. 2002. Mouse Apg10 as an Apg12-conjugating enzyme: analysis by the conjugation-mediated yeast two-hybrid method. *FEBS Lett.* 532:450–54
76. Moller MTN, Samari HR, Holden L, Seglen PO. 2004. Regulation of mammalian autophagy by protein phosphorylation. In *Autophagy*, ed. DJ Klionsky, pp. 48–59. Georgetown, TX: Landes Biosci.
77. Moriwaki H, Miwa Y, Tajika M, Kato M, Fukushima H, Shiraki M. 2004. Branched-chain amino acids as a protein- and energy-source in liver cirrhosis. *Biochem. Biophys. Res. Commun.* 313:405–9
78. Mortimore GE, Poso AR. 1987. Intracellular protein catabolism and its control during nutrient deprivation and supply. *Annu. Rev. Nutr.* 7:539–64
79. Munz C. 2006. Autophagy and antigen presentation. *Cell Microbiol.* 8:891–98
80. Nair U, Klionsky DJ. 2005. Molecular mechanisms and regulation of specific and non-specific autophagy pathways in yeast. *J. Biol. Chem.* 280:41785–88
81. Nakagawa I, Amano A, Mizushima N, Yamamoto A, Yamaguchi H, et al. 2004. Autophagy defends cells against invading group A *Streptococcus*. *Science* 306:1037–40
82. Nemoto T, Tanida I, Tanida-Miyake E, Minematsu-Ikeguchi N, Yokota M, et al. 2003. The mouse APG10 homologue, an E2-like enzyme for Apg12p conjugation, facilitates MAP-LC3 modification. *J. Biol. Chem.* 278:39517–26
83. Nishimoto S, Kawane K, Watanabe-Fukunaga R, Fukuyama H, Ohsawa Y, et al. 2003. Nuclear cataract caused by a lack of DNA degradation in the mouse eye lens. *Nature* 424:1071–74
84. Ogawa M, Yoshimori T, Suzuki T, Sagara H, Mizushima N, Sasakawa C. 2005. Escape of intracellular *Shigella* from autophagy. *Science* 307:727–31
85. Ohsumi Y. 2001. Molecular dissection of autophagy: two ubiquitin-like systems. *Nat. Rev. Mol. Cell Biol.* 2:211–16

86. Ohsumi Y, Mizushima N. 2004. Two ubiquitin-like conjugation systems essential for autophagy. *Semin. Cell Dev. Biol.* 15:231–36
87. Onodera J, Ohsumi Y. 2004. Ald6p is a preferred target for autophagy in yeast, *Saccharomyces cerevisiae*. *J. Biol. Chem.* 279:16071–76
88. Onodera J, Ohsumi Y. 2005. Autophagy is required for maintenance of amino acid levels and protein synthesis under nitrogen starvation. *J. Biol. Chem.* 280:31582–86
89. Otto GP, Wu MY, Kazgan N, Anderson OR, Kessin RH. 2003. Macroautophagy is required for multicellular development of the social amoeba *Dictyostelium discoideum*. *J. Biol. Chem.* 278:17636–45
90. Palou A, Remesar X, Arola L, Herrera E, Alemany M. 1981. Metabolic effects of short-term food deprivation in the rat. *Horm. Metab. Res.* 13:326–30
91. Pfeifer U. 1978. Inhibition by insulin of the formation of autophagic vacuoles in rat liver. A morphometric approach to the kinetics of intracellular degradation by autophagy. *J. Cell Biol.* 78:152–67
92. Puls A, Schmidt S, Grawe F, Stabel S. 1997. Interaction of protein kinase Cζ with ZIP, a novel protein kinase C-binding protein. *Proc. Natl. Acad. Sci. USA* 94:6191–96
93. Qu X, Yu J, Bhagat G, Furuya N, Hibshoosh H, et al. 2003. Promotion of tumorigenesis by heterozygous disruption of the *beclin 1* autophagy gene. *J. Clin. Invest.* 112:1809–20
94. Reggiori F, Shintani T, Nair U, Klionsky DJ. 2005. Atg9 cycles between mitochondria and the pre-autophagosomal structure in yeasts. *Autophagy* 1:101–9
95. Reggiori F, Wang C-W, Nair U, Shintani T, Abeliovich H, Klionsky DJ. 2004. Early stages of the secretory pathway, but not endosomes, are required for Cvt vesicle and autophagosome assembly in *Saccharomyces cerevisiae*. *Mol. Biol. Cell* 15:2189–204
96. Rodriguez A, Duran A, Selloum M, Champy MF, Diez-Guerra FJ, et al. 2006. Mature-onset obesity and insulin resistance in mice deficient in the signaling adapter p62. *Cell Metab.* 3:211–22
97. Rodriguez-Enriquez S, Kim I, Currin RT, Lemasters JJ. 2006. Tracker dyes to probe mitochondrial autophagy (mitophagy) in rat hepatocytes. *Autophagy* 2:39–46
98. Rubinsztein DC, Difiglia M, Heintz N, Nixon RA, Qin ZH, et al. 2005. Autophagy and its possible roles in nervous system diseases, damage and repair. *Autophagy* 1:11–22
99. Sagiv Y, Legesse-Miller A, Porat A, Elazar Z. 2000. GATE-16, a membrane transport modulator, interacts with NSF and the Golgi v-SNARE GOS-28. *EMBO J.* 19:1494–504
100. Sanz L, Diaz-Meco MT, Nakano H, Moscat J. 2000. The atypical PKC-interacting protein p62 channels NF-κB activation by the IL-1-TRAF6 pathway. *EMBO J.* 19:1576–86
101. Schwartz AL, Ciechanover A, Brandt RA, Geuze HJ. 1988. Immunoelectron microscopic localization of ubiquitin in hepatoma cells. *EMBO J.* 7:2961–66
102. Schworer CM, Shiffer KA, Mortimore GE. 1981. Quantitative relationship between autophagy and proteolysis during graded amino acid deprivation in perfused rat liver. *J. Biol. Chem.* 256:7652–58
103. Scott RC, Schuldiner O, Neufeld TP. 2004. Role and regulation of starvation-induced autophagy in the *Drosophila* fat body. *Dev. Cell* 7:167–78
104. Seglen PO, Gordon PB. 1981. Vanadate inhibits protein degradation in isolated rat hepatocytes. *J. Biol. Chem.* 256:7699–701
105. Shenoy ST, Rogers QR. 1977. Effect of starvation on the charging levels of transfer ribonucleic acid and total acceptor capacity in rat liver. *Biochim. Biophys. Acta* 476:218–27
106. Shintani T, Klionsky DJ. 2004. Autophagy in health and disease: a double-edged sword. *Science* 306:990–95

107. Shintani T, Mizushima N, Ogawa Y, Matsuura A, Noda T, Ohsumi Y. 1999. Apg10p, a novel protein-conjugating enzyme essential for autophagy in yeast. *EMBO J.* 18:5234–41
108. Stasyk OV, Stasyk OG, Mathewson RD, Farre JC, Nazarko VY, et al. 2006. Atg28, a novel coiled-coil protein involved in autophagic degradation of peroxisomes in the methylotrophic yeast *Pichia pastoris*. *Autophagy* 2:30–38
109. Sugawara K, Suzuki NN, Fujioka Y, Mizushima N, Ohsumi Y, Inagaki F. 2003. Crystallization and preliminary X-ray analysis of LC3-I. *Acta Crystallogr. D Biol. Crystallogr.* 59:1464–65
110. Sugawara K, Suzuki NN, Fujioka Y, Mizushima N, Ohsumi Y, Inagaki F. 2004. The crystal structure of microtubule-associated protein light chain 3, a mammalian homologue of *Saccharomyces cerevisiae* Atg8. *Genes Cells* 9:611–18
111. Suzuki K, Kirisako T, Kamada Y, Mizushima N, Noda T, Ohsumi Y. 2001. The pre-autophagosomal structure organized by concerted functions of *APG* genes is essential for autophagosome formation. *EMBO J.* 20:5971–81
112. Suzuki NN, Yoshimoto K, Fujioka Y, Ohsumi Y, Inagaki F. 2005. The crystal structure of plant ATG12 and its biological implication in autophagy. *Autophagy* 1:119–26
113. Takeshige K, Baba M, Tsuboi S, Noda T, Ohsumi Y. 1992. Autophagy in yeast demonstrated with proteinase-deficient mutants and conditions for its induction. *J. Cell Biol.* 119:301–11
114. Tanida I, Minematsu-Ikeguchi N, Ueno T, Kominami E. 2005. Lysosomal turnover, but not a cellular level, of endogenous LC3 is a marker for autophagy. *Autophagy* 1:84–91
115. Tanida I, Mizushima N, Kiyooka M, Ohsumi M, Ueno T, et al. 1999. Apg7p/Cvt2p: a novel protein-activating enzyme essential for autophagy. *Mol. Biol. Cell* 10:1367–79
116. Tanida I, Tanida-Miyake E, Ueno T, Kominami E. 2001. The human homolog of *Saccharomyces cerevisiae* Apg7p is a protein-activating enzyme for multiple substrates including human Apg12p, GATE-16, GABARAP, and MAP-LC3. *J. Biol. Chem.* 276:1701–6
117. Tsukada M, Ohsumi Y. 1993. Isolation and characterization of autophagy-defective mutants of *Saccharomyces cerevisiae*. *FEBS Lett.* 333:169–74
118. Ueno T, Kominami E. 1991. Mechanism and regulation of lysosomal sequestration and proteolysis. *Biomed. Biochim. Acta* 50:365–71
119. Vabulas RM, Hartl FU. 2005. Protein synthesis upon acute nutrient restriction relies on proteasome function. *Science* 310:1960–63
120. Wang C-W, Klionsky DJ. 2003. The molecular mechanism of autophagy. *Mol. Med.* 9:65–76
121. Wang H, Bedford FK, Brandon NJ, Moss SJ, Olsen RW. 1999. $GABA_A$-receptor-associated protein links $GABA_A$ receptors and the cytoskeleton. *Nature* 397:69–72
122. Wang QJ, Ding Y, Kohtz S, Mizushima N, Cristea IM, et al. 2006. Induction of autophagy in axonal dystrophy and degeneration. *J. Neurosci.* 26:8057–68
123. Yang Z, Huang J, Geng J, Nair U, Klionsky DJ. 2006. Atg22 recycles amino acids to link the degradative and recycling functions of autophagy. *Mol. Biol. Cell.* 17:5094–104
124. Yorimitsu T, Klionsky DJ. 2005. Autophagy: molecular machinery for self-eating. *Cell Death Differ.* 12(Suppl. 2):1542–52
125. Young VR, Scrimshaw NS. 1971. The physiology of starvation. *Sci. Am.* 225:14–21
126. Yu WH, Cuervo AM, Kumar A, Peterhoff CM, Schmidt SD, et al. 2005. Macroautophagy—a novel β-amyloid (Aβ) peptide-generating pathway activated in Alzheimer's disease. *J. Cell Biol.* 171:87–98

127. Yuan W, Stromhaug PE, Dunn WA Jr. 1999. Glucose-induced autophagy of peroxisomes in *Pichia pastoris* requires a unique E1-like protein. *Mol. Biol. Cell* 10:1353–66
128. Yue Z, Jin S, Yang C, Levine AJ, Heintz N. 2003. Beclin 1, an autophagy gene essential for early embryonic development, is a haploinsufficient tumor suppressor. *Proc. Natl. Acad. Sci. USA* 100:15077–82

Metabolic Regulation and Function of Glutathione Peroxidase-1

Xin Gen Lei,[1] Wen-Hsing Cheng,[2] and James P. McClung[3]

[1] Department of Animal Science, Cornell University, Ithaca, New York 14853; email: XL20@Cornell.edu

[2] Laboratory of Molecular Gerontology, National Institute on Aging, National Institutes of Health, Baltimore, Maryland 21224, and Department of Nutrition and Food Science, University of Maryland, College Park, Maryland 20742

[3] Military Nutrition Division, U.S. Army Research Institute of Environmental Medicine, Natick, Massachusetts 01760

Annu. Rev. Nutr. 2007. 27:41–61

First published online as a Review in Advance on April 27, 2007

The *Annual Review of Nutrition* is online at http://nutr.annualreviews.org

This article's doi:
10.1146/annurev.nutr.27.061406.093716

0199-9885/07/0821-0041$20.00

Key Words

selenium, reactive oxygen species, reactive nitrogen species, signaling, chronic disease

Abstract

Glutathione peroxidase-1 (GPX1) represents the first identified mammalian selenoprotein, and our understanding in the metabolic regulation and function of this abundant selenoenzyme has greatly advanced during the past decade. Selenocysteine insertion sequence–associating factors, adenosine, and Abl and Arg tyrosine kinases are potent, Se-independent regulators of GPX1 gene, protein, and activity. Overwhelming evidences have been generated using the GPX1 knockout and transgenic mice for the in vivo protective role of GPX1 in coping with oxidative injury and death mediated by reactive oxygen species. However, GPX1 exerts an intriguing dual role in reactive nitrogen species (RNS)-related oxidative stress. Strikingly, knockout of GPX1 rendered mice resistant to toxicities of drugs including acetaminophen and kainic acid, known as RNS inducers. Intracellular and tissue levels of GPX1 activity affect apoptotic signaling pathway, protein kinase phosphorylation, and oxidant-mediated activation of NFκB. Data are accumulating to link alteration or abnormality of GPX1 expression to etiology of cancer, cardiovascular disease, neurodegeneration, autoimmune disease, and diabetes. Future research should focus on the mechanism of GPX1 in the pathogeneses and potential applications of GPX1 manipulation in the treatment of these disorders.

Contents

INTRODUCTION

Discovery of Glutathione Peroxidase-1 as a Selenoprotein

Glutathione peroxidase-1 (glutathione: H_2O_2 oxidoreductase, EC 1.11.1.9; GPX1) was initially discovered by Mills in 1957 as an erythrocyte enzyme that protects hemoglobin from oxidative breakdown (103). In the early 1970s, two groups demonstrated that GPX1 is a selenium (Se)-dependent enzyme (58, 121). Subsequently, selenocysteine (Sec) was identified as the moiety of Se in the GPX1 protein (21). Today, Sec is recognized as the twenty-first amino acid, despite similar structure to cysteine. Although Se may exist in mammalian proteins in other chemical forms, such as selenomethionine via a nonspecific replacement of sulfur in methionine and other Se-binding proteins that do not contain Sec (9), this essential trace element probably confers its metabolic functions mainly in the form of Sec in selenoproteins. A unique consensus Sec-insertion sequence (SECIS) in the mRNA of selenoproteins is required for the synthesis of Sec (12). Using this unique SECIS signature to search the published genome database, Gladyshev and coworkers have reported that there are 25 selenoproteins in humans (85).

GPX1: glutathione peroxidase-1

Se: selenium

Selenocysteine-insertion sequence (SECIS): unique mRNA stem loop structure associated with the incorporation of essential micronutrient selenium into selenium-containing proteins

Incorporation of Se into GPX1 and Other Selenoproteins

As discussed above, Se is incorporated into GPX1 and other selenoproteins in the form of Sec coded by UGA and directed by SECIS (12, 21, 125). This SECIS represents an mRNA stem loop structure and serves as a platform for the recruitment of specific translation elongation factors and Sec tRNA (designated as Sec-$tRNA^{[Ser]Sec}$). As such, $tRNA^{[Ser]Sec}$ decodes the UGA codon for the entire family of selenoproteins. Targeted disruption of this tRNA gene in mice leads to embryonic lethality (14). In bacteria, the SelB protein binds to SECIS and recruits Sec-tRNA$^{[Ser]Sec}$ (13, 48, 129). In eukaryotes, the mRNA-tRNA interaction is more complex, as the eukaryotic SECIS element is recognized by a protein complex containing SECIS-binding protein 2 (SBP2) and elongation factor EFSec (149). The most recent list of eukaryotic tRNA$^{[Ser]Sec}$-interacting proteins includes two selenophosphate synthetases, ribosomal protein L30, SECp43, and soluble liver antigen (22, 128, 145). It seems that the interaction between SBP2-binding protein and SECIS mobilizes EFsec and Sec-tRNA$^{[Ser]Sec}$ to the ribosome, while the binding of L30 protein to SECIS stimulates the completion of selenocysteine synthesis (22).

Enzyme Family of GPX1

In addition to GPX1, there are five other known GPX enzymes: GPX2–GPX6. Data from in vitro activity assays suggest that all members use GSH to catalyze the reduction of hydrogen peroxide and lipid peroxides. Whereas GPX1 is the most abundant selenoperoxidase and is ubiquitously expressed in almost all tissues (25, 26, 58, 121), GPX2 expression is most prominent in the gastrointestinal tract (30). Expression of GPX3 is greatest in the kidney, although this enzyme is expressed in various tissues and is secreted into extracellular fluids as a glycoprotein (135, 147). Different from other glutathione peroxidases, GPX4, or phospholipid hydroperoxide GPX, is not a tetramer, but rather a monomer, and is the only GPX enzyme that reduces phospholipid hydroperoxides (141). In addition, GPX4 contains a mitochondrial isoform that mediates the apoptotic response to oxidative stress (3, 112) and has a peroxidase-independent structural role after sperm maturation (142). Recently, GPX6 was identified as a selenoprotein in the human genome by homology search (85). However, GPX6 from rodents and GPX5 from both humans and rodents do not contain Sec or Se (85).

REGULATION OF GPX1 mRNA, PROTEIN, AND ACTIVITY EXPRESSION

Regulation by Se Supply

The expression of GPX1 mRNA, protein, and activity in tissues is more sensitive to dietary Se deficiency than other selenoperoxidases or selenoproteins (11). In fact, Se deficiency in rats results in a 90% loss of liver GPX1 mRNA and a 99% loss in GPX activity (122). In cells, Se deficiency results in a 60% reduction in GPX1 mRNA and a 93% loss in GPX1 activity (4). Nonsense codon-mediated decay seems to be the mechanism by which Se deficiency reduces the abundance of GPX1 mRNA, as the Sec codon reduces the abundance of cytoplasmic GPX1 mRNA by a translation-dependent mechanism under conditions of Se deprivation (106).

Injection of Se into deficient animals results in the rapid restoration of both GPX mRNA and activity (132). However, the Se-induced restoration of GPX1 activity seems to be saturable in a number of animal models and cell types (132, 133). Because of the sensitive and saturable nature of GPX1 activity in response to dietary Se, GPX1 has been used as a biomarker to assess body Se status or the nutritional requirement of Se. Furthermore, the low rank of GPX1 in the hierarchical partitioning of Se prompted the conception of the "GPX1 buffer" hypothesis (16, 131). Based on this hypothesis, GPX1 functions as a body storage form of Se, instead of as an important antioxidant enzyme, to release Se for maintaining the expression of essential selenoproteins in Se depletion and to take up Se for avoiding Se toxicity in Se repletion. However, two lines of solid evidence from GPX1 knockout or overexpressing mice do not support the GPX1 buffer hypothesis. First, alteration of GPX1 expression does not affect the mRNA or activity expression of other selenoproteins (25, 26). Second, knockout of GPX1 renders mice susceptible to severe acute oxidative stress, whereas overexpression of GPX1 confers extra protection against the insult (27).

Glutathione peroxidases: antioxidant enzymes that use glutathione as a substrate (reductant) to catalyze the breakdown of peroxides

Knockout (null): genetically delete or disrupt functional expression of selected single or multiple genes in animals

Overexpression: genetically elevate the functional expression of selected single or multiple genes above normal levels in animals

Regulation by SECIS-Associating Factors

Reactive oxygen species (ROS): oxygen-containing molecules that are more active than the triplet oxygen molecule present in the air and can cause oxidative stress

Pro-oxidants: compounds that induce formation of reactive oxygen species and reactive nitrogen species

Oxidant stress: exposure to reactive oxygen or nitrogen species and (or) the loss of balance between antioxidant defense and pro-oxidant or oxidant attack

The SECIS-associating factors may regulate selenoprotein expression in at least two ways. First, the intracellular location of SBP2 is shifted from the cytoplasm to the nucleus upon exposure to reactive oxygen species (ROS), suggesting a mechanism by which oxidative stress decreases selenoprotein expression (116). Consistently, tissue GPX1 protein and activity are decreased after administration of pro-oxidant paraquat to mice (24). Secondly, Se status modulates Sec-tRNA$^{[Ser]Sec}$ methylation at position 34 of this tRNA, and such modification alters Sec-tRNA$^{[Ser]Sec}$ secondary and tertiary structure (43). Mice engineered to express a mutant Sec-tRNA$^{[Ser]Sec}$ (Sec-tRNA$^{[Ser]Sec}$ i^6A^- transgenic mice) are unable to carry out this specific tRNA methylation, but expression of various selenoproteins in these animals is not equally affected (19). Selenoproteins such as GPX1 and GPX3, whose expression is highly responsive to Se deficiency, appear to require the tRNA methylation (2). In contrast, TR-1 and thioredoxin reductase-3 are less affected by Se deficiency, and their expression is independent of the tRNA methylation.

Adenosine-Dependent Activation of GPX1

Adenosine is a widely distributed molecule with a number of biological functions, including protection against myocardial ischemia/reperfusion injury (96). It has been hypothesized that adenosine may impart protection against ROS, as it attenuates oxidant-induced damage in cells (88) and animals (87). Because overexpression of GPX1 in mice is known to diminish tissue damage following myocardial ischemia/reperfusion (146), one recent study examined the ability of adenosine to affect GPX1 regulation. In that study, treatment of human primary pulmonary endothelial cells with adenosine in the presence of erythro-9-(2-hydroxy-3-nonyl)adenine (EHNA), an adenosine deaminase inhibitor, resulted in increased GPX1 mRNA levels, protein expression, and enzyme activity (151). The adenosine-driven induction of GPX1 expression was due to enhanced mRNA stability. The adenosine-driven induction of GPX1 conferred protection against ROS, as adenosine/EHNA-treated cells were resistant to hydrogen peroxide–induced oxidant stress. Meanwhile, inhibition of GPX1 pharmacologically or by siRNA diminished the protection by adenosine against ROS. These findings suggest that adenosine may be a potent, Se-independent regulator of GPX1 expression, and that the associated GPX1 activity change may exert important physiological functions.

Regulation Via c-Abl and Arg Tyrosine Kinases

The c-Abl and Arg nonreceptor tyrosine kinases represent another Se-independent regulator of GPX1 expression. The cytoplasmic forms of these kinases are activated in response to ROS and may be involved in the apoptotic response to oxidant stress (18). In fact, hydrogen peroxide–induced apoptosis is attenuated in cells deficient in c-Abl and Arg (18, 130). Because of the association between c-Abl and Arg and oxidant stress, one recent study explored the interactions between these proteins and GPX1 (17). In that study, it was determined that c-Abl and Arg associate with GPX1 in a yeast two-hybrid system and in 293 cells, and that the interaction is regulated by intracellular oxidant levels. Furthermore, it was demonstrated that GPX1 functions as a substrate for c-Abl- and Arg-mediated phosphorylation at Tyr-96, which induces GPX1 activity. Lastly, treatment of c-Abl- and Arg-deficient cells with hydrogen peroxide resulted in a greater apoptotic response as compared with wild-type cells, suggesting that the loss of GPX1 regulation by c-Abl and Arg results in increased sensitivity to ROS-induced apoptosis.

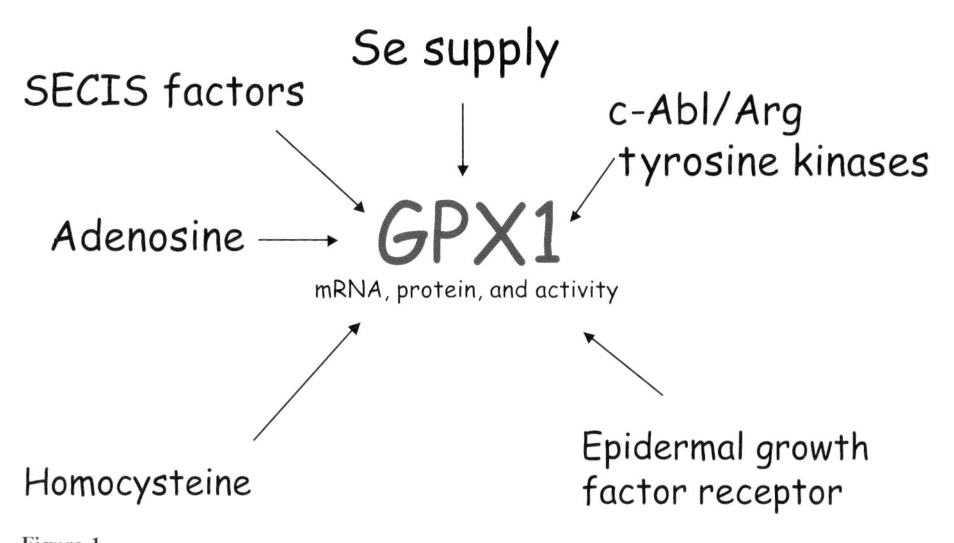

Figure 1

Regulators of GPX1 expression and activity.

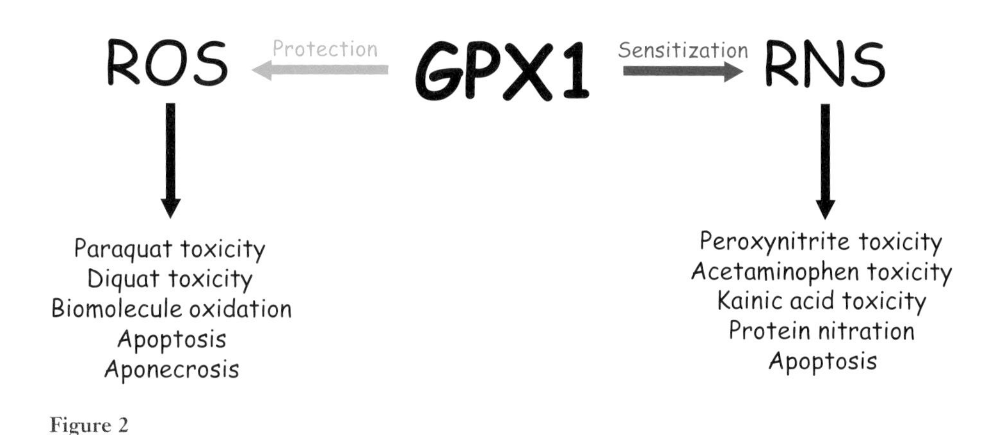

Figure 2

Dual roles of GPX1 in ROS- versus RNS-related oxidative stress.

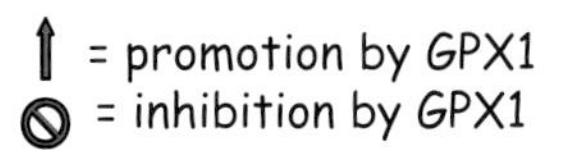

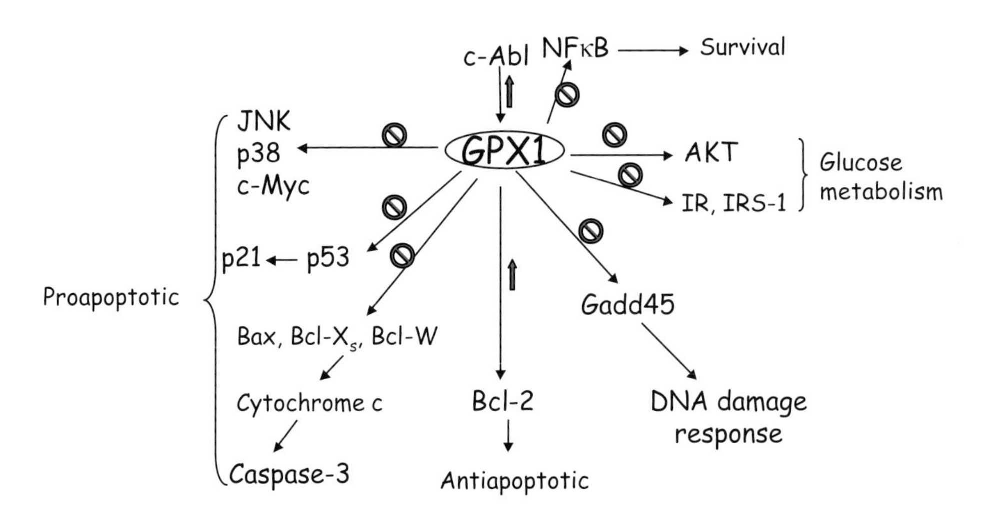

Figure 3

Roles of GPX1 in ROS-induced signal transduction; ↑ = promotion by GPX1; ⊘ = inhibition by GPX1.

Furthermore, recent studies have demonstrated that other factors, including epidermal growth factor receptor (50) and homocysteine (67), may participate in the regulation of GPX1. Factors that may participate in the regulation of GPX1 gene expression and enzyme activity are summarized in **Figure 1** (see color insert).

Altered Expression in Diseases

One recent report demonstrated that GPX1 expression was decreased by hyperhomocysteinemia (67), a risk factor for cardiovascular disease. In that study, homocysteine was shown to interfere with the SECIS readthrough such that GPX1 expression was reduced at the translational level. It has also been observed that GPX1 activity is diminished in lung cancers with GPX1 loss of heterozygosity (69), and GPX1 protein expression is decreased in T cells during HIV infection (64). Moreover, bone loss induced by estrogen deficiency has been shown to be associated with hydrogen peroxide formation and increased GPX1 expression (86).

ROLES OF GPX1 IN REDOX REGULATION

Protection Against ROS

Although in vitro cellular studies demonstrated that modulation of GPX1 activity expression by ectopic expression or antisense RNA down-regulation affected cell resistance to oxidative stress (104, 140), the most convincing evidence for the in vivo antioxidant role of GPX1 was attributed to the observation that GPX1-overexpressing [GPX1(+/+)] mice were more resistant, while GPX1 knockout mice [GPX1(−/−)] were more susceptible to paraquat-induced lethality than were wild-type mice (27). In fact, mouse survival time in these experiments was solely a function of tissue GPX1 activity. Furthermore, GPX1 was not only antioxidative, but also the mediator of body Se in protecting against such drastic, acute oxidative stress (24, 27). Its protection was conferred by preventing a collapse of redox status and attenuating oxidation of lipids, protein, NADPH, and NADH (24, 27). Meanwhile, the in vivo antioxidant role of GPX1 has been substantiated by a number of publications using independently developed GPX1(−/−) mouse lines and various ROS-inducing agents (41, 53, 59, 60).

The physiological essentiality of GPX1 protection against ROS-related stress depends upon Se status and the severity of the stress. After an injection of paraquat at a dose of 12.5 mg/kg, all Se-adequate mice, regardless of their GPX1 status, survived (28). Thus, GPX1 is not essential for Se-adequate mice to cope with moderate oxidant stress. However, even minute amounts of tissue GPX1 activity become important for the antioxidant defense in Se-deficient mice. Although the majority of Se-deficient wild-type and GPX1(−/−) mice died of the injection of paraquat at 12.5 mg/kg, a prior injection of Se (50 μg/kg as Na_2SeO_3) that restored only 4% of the normal GPX1 activity in wild-type mice resulted in significant reductions in mortality and severity of liver aponecrosis compared with Se-injected GPX1(−/−) mice. Liver injury was more apoptotic in GPX1(−/−) mice, but more necrotic in wild-type mice. The repletion of minute GPX1 activity in wild-type mice also attenuated activation of caspase-3 and c-Jun N-terminal kinase (JNK) and the expression of Bcl-X_s and GADD45 (28, 29).

Dual Roles Against Reactive Nitrogen Species

Although reactive nitrogen species (RNS) such as nitric oxide (NO), peroxynitrite (PN), and their reactive intermediates are produced constantly in aerobic metabolism, their distinct features are not often recognized from those of ROS. Nitric oxide is an uncharged lipophilic molecule that contains a single unpaired electron that causes it to be reactive with other molecules, including GSH.

GPX1(+/+): GPX1 overexpression

GPX1(−/−): GPX1 knockout

Reactive nitrogen species (RNS): highly reactive, nitrogen-containing molecules that can cause oxidative stress

PN: peroxynitrite

APAP: acetaminophen

SOD: superoxide dismutase

Release of NO by nitric oxide synthase (NOS) may result in the production of superoxide (76). When superoxide is produced in parallel with NO, the two react to form PN, which is highly cytotoxic (8) and is capable of oxidizing numerous biomolecules, including lipids, amino acids, and DNA (127). PN is especially harmful to proteins due to its ability to react with tyrosine residues to form 3-nitrotyrosine. This chemical modification, called protein nitration, may lock enzymes or proteins in an inactive form by preventing the phosphorylation of tyrosine residues (136).

Early in vitro studies suggested that the GPX1 enzyme and its mimetic ebselen catalyzed PN reduction and prevented tyrosine nitration in cell lysates (127). However, a recent study demonstrated a promotion, instead of a protecting, role of GPX1 in coping with the PN-induced cell death (61). In that study, primary hepatocytes isolated from GPX1(−/−) mice were more resistant than those from wild-type mice to PN-induced apoptosis, DNA fragmentation, cytochrome-c release, caspase activation, and cellular GSH depletion.

The promoting role of GPX1 in RNS-related stress and its metabolic relevance have been well illustrated in a number of animal studies with acetaminophen (APAP). As the vascular production of PN is induced by APAP overdose, PN formation has been suggested as a critical mediator of APAP-induced hepatotoxicity (81, 82, 102). Initially, Mirochnitchenko and coworkers (105) found that mice overexpressing GPX1 had reduced survival time and increased oxidant damage as compared with wild-type mice when both groups were treated with 450 mg of APAP/kg. Meanwhile, another group demonstrated that GPX1(−/−) mice were not more susceptible to an injection of 300 mg of APAP/kg, but had lower plasma alanine aminotransferase activity increases than did wild-type mice (81). Furthermore, double knockout of GPX1 and Cu,Zn-superoxide dismutase (SOD1) rendered primary hepatocytes (152) and mice (90) more resistant to APAP-induced toxicity than wild-type controls. In addition, the enhanced resistance of GPX1(−/−) mice to kainic acid–mediated mortality and seizures (75) represents another strong in vivo evidence for the promoting role of GPX1 in RNS-related stress, as kainic acid is a neurodegenerative drug that has been shown to induce PN formation in brain (117). Thus, GPX1 may play dual roles in coping with oxidative stress mediated by ROS versus RNS (**Figure 2**, see color insert).

ROLE OF GPX1 IN SIGNAL TRANSDUCTION

Apoptotic Signaling Pathway

Results from early studies suggested a role of GPX1 in hydrogen peroxide–induced apoptosis in bovine renal epithelial cells (79) and in murine myeloid progenitor cells (115). More directly, primary hepatocytes isolated from GPX1(−/−) mice were more susceptible to ROS-induced apoptosis, but were more resistant to RNS-induced apoptosis than cells from wild-type mice (61). After the treatment with each of the oxidants, cells of the two genotypes displayed completely opposite profiles including cell viability, DNA fragmentation, capase-3 activation, p21WAF1/CIP1, cytochrome C release, protein nitration, and the GSH/GSSG ratio. As mentioned above, repletion of minute amounts of GPX1 activity in liver of wild-type mice exerted a significant impact on paraquat-mediated activation of caspase-3, p53 stability, and expression of Bcl-X_s and GADD45 (28, 29). In addition, increased GPX1 activity was associated with the inhibition of apoptosis induced by growth factor withdrawal from pro-B-lymphocytes (70) or by c-Myc (115). Because levels of ROS were low in such condition, GPX1 likely modulated apoptosis caused by factors other than oxygen tension. In human endothelial cells, overexpression of GPX1 alone, in the absence of exogenous stress, resulted in a significant decrease in the expression of the proapoptotic Bax, whereas that of antiapoptotic

Bcl-2 remained unchanged (57). Primary myoblasts isolated from GPX1(−/−) mice in the absence of exogenous apoptotic stimuli consistently showed increased rates of apoptosis (89). Interestingly, primary hepatocytes isolated from GPX1(−/−) mice were more resistant to APAP-induced cell death due to an attenuation in APAP-induced GSH depletion (152).

Protein Kinase Phosphorylation

The p38 mitogen-activated protein kinase (MAPK) and JNK pathways impart essential roles in ROS-induced apoptosis (95, 114). Overexpression of GPX1 in mouse embryonic fibroblasts has been shown to prevent p38 MAPK phosphorylation at Thr-180/Tyr-182 under hypoxia that presumably induces oxidative stress (52). However, decomposing endogenous ROS by expression of GPX1 in GPX1-underexpressed MCF-7 cells did not affect p38 MAPK expression and phosphorylation (110). Also, GPX1 had no significant impact on p38 MAPK phosphorylation in mice and cells treated with paraquat or diquat (29, 61). Interestingly, low GPX1 activity (4% of the adequate level) in Se-deficient mice was sufficient to attenuate JNK phosphorylation at Thr-183/Tyr-185 mediated by a low dose of pro-oxidant (29). In addition, protein kinase B (also known as Akt) phosphorylation at Ser-308 was reduced in MCF-7 cells overexpressing GPX1 (110), or in GPX1(+/+) mice following an insulin challenge (99). Meanwhile, fibroblasts from GPX1(−/−) mice showed decreased Akt phosphorylation at Ser-473 upon stimulation with hydrogen peroxide (139).

Oxidant-Mediated Activation of NFκB

NFκB is a transcriptional factor involved in regulating cellular responses to a variety of environmental stressors (78). Overexpression of GPX1 has been implicated in the reduction of hydrogen peroxide–induced NFκB activation in MCF-7 cells (92, 93). Recent evidence has suggested that GPX1 and the c-Src tyrosine kinase likely function in the same process of IκBα phosphorylation that leads to NFκB activation in response to hypoxia (56). Strikingly, both GPX1 and catalase, but not Mn-SOD (SOD2) or SOD1, modulate IκBα phosphorylation, suggesting a difference between hydrogen peroxide and superoxide in the activation of NFκB. Conversely, NFκB activation was found to be elevated in GPX1(−/−) embryonic fibroblasts treated with hydrogen peroxide (139) or GPX1(−/−) brains after stroke (36).

The effect of GPX1 expression level on the NFκB pathway has clinical implications. For instance, bone resorption depends on osteoclasts that express high levels of GPX1 protein and require NFκB activation for cell development (86). The level of GPX1 activity may also affect pathogenesis involving COX-2 up-regulation, as Se-deficient macrophages show increased NFκB activation and subsequent COX-2 up-regulation (148). The signal pathways that involve GPX1 are summarized in **Figure 3** (see color insert).

ROLES OF GPX1 IN CANCER AND CHRONIC DISEASES

GPX1 Expression and Cancer

Cells from cancer patients often show defects in the regulation of proliferation, apoptosis, and senescence (40). Analysis of a long-term clinical trial concluded that daily supplementation with Se at a supranutritional dose (200 μg) resulted in significant reductions in mortality associated with total carcinomas as well as lung, prostate, and colon cancers (31, 32). It remains unclear as to how Se decreases cancer risk and whether GPX1 is involved in the action. It is also unclear whether the anticarcinogenic properties of Se are a result of pro-oxidant or antioxidant function (46, 113). The paradox is that Se compounds per se are known to initiate ROS-induced apoptosis in cancer cells, yet some selenoproteins attenuate ROS levels in the body (24, 113). In the Sec-tRNA$^{[Ser]Sec}$ i^6A^- transgenic mouse model, GPX1 is one of the selenoproteins that demonstrate reduced expression (19). Using this line of transgenic mice that has a preference for GPX1 suppression among all selenoproteins, azoxymethane treatment resulted in aberrant crypts in the colon as compared with wild-type mice.

Although GPX1 was unlikely to be the only selenoprotein involved, these results suggested the involvement of GPX1 in the chemoprevention imparted by dietary Se. However, this finding raises a question regarding GPX2 involvement, as its expression is primarily confined to the gastrointestinal system (30). This issue was partially addressed by a recent report showing that GPX1, instead of GPX2, was expressed in selective colon locations including lymphatic tissues (47). Using a TGF$^{\alpha}$/c-Myc mouse model of cancer, Novoselov et al. (113) suggested that both selenoproteins and Se compounds contributed to the inhibition of liver carcinogenesis, although it was unclear as to the relative contribution of GPX1 to this protection. On the other hand, GPX1 expression has been found to be decreased or repressed in estrogen receptor–positive breast cancer cells (54), in a mouse model for liver tumors, and in a prostate cancer cell line (63). It will be of great interest to discern whether GPX1 expression and the associated ROS changes are directly involved in the chemopreventive effects of dietary Se.

GPX1 Polymorphisms and Allelic Changes

In the 201 amino acid–containing GPX1 protein peptide, the single-nucleotide polymorphism (SNP) that alters particular amino acid sequences is associated with certain diseases. Moscow et al. (107) first reported an SNP within the GPX1 gene that resulted in either a proline (Pro) or leucine (Leu) at codon 198 in lung cancer specimens. This SNP has also been reported to be associated with bladder cancer (73). Although the SNP was later found in some breast cancer patients (72, 118), there is no consistent evidence to support an association between the GPX1 Pro198Leu polymorphism and susceptibility to breast cancer (1, 20, 34). Likewise, another GPX1 polymorphism GCG in exon 1 was not associated with prostate cancer risk (84). Nonetheless, analysis of breast and colorectal cancer DNA revealed that 36% to 42% of GPX1 genes showed loss of heterozygosity during tumor formation (71, 72). It seems that the GPX1 Pro198Leu SNP resulted in a decreased response of GPX1 catalytic activity to Se supplementation (72), suggesting that GPX1 activity may involve the regulation of carcinogenesis via modulation of ROS levels. Consistent with this notion, a recent report using samples from alcoholic patients with cirrhosis suggested that polymorphisms in GPX1 and Mn-SOD likely collaborated to regulate carcinogenesis in liver (134). Identification of additional GPX1 SNPs and systematic evaluation of their associations with cancer will help expand our ability to diagnose and treat GPX1-related cancers.

Cardiovascular Diseases

The GPX1 protein is expressed in blood vessels and has been implicated in cardiovascular disease (83). Atherosclerosis occurs predominantly at low sheer stress areas, and such stress has been shown to enhance GPX1 mRNA levels in cultured bovine aortic endothelial cells (137). An important association between GPX1 expression and plasma homocysteine levels has been documented (67). Elevated levels of homocysteine can increase levels of ROS, leading to endothelial injury in the pathogenesis of atherogenesis (66). In cultured bovine aortic endothelial cells, overexpression of GPX1 alleviated homocysteine-induced endothelial dysfunction (144), and the addition of homocysteine suppressed GPX1 expression at the translation level (67). Homocysteine likely interrupts the UGA read-through such that GPX1 expression is down-regulated. Moreover, a report using GPX1(−/−) mice suggested that GPX1 contributed to the protection of Se against myocarditis induced by a benign strain of coxsackievirus B3 that likely increased cellular oxidative stress (7). Taken together, these results suggest that GPX1 may protect against atherogenesis in vessels and virus-induced myocarditis by reducing ROS levels.

Neurodegenerative Diseases

Considerable evidence links GPX1 to the pathogenesis of neurodegenerative diseases, most likely through its peroxide-eliminating activity. GPX1 is known to localize primarily in glial cells (138), in which GPX1 activity is tenfold higher than in other brain regions (124). Moreover, there is an increase in GPX1 expression surrounding the damaged brain regions in Parkinson's disease patients (38). Ridet et al. (119) employed a lentivirus-based system delivering GPX1 to neuroblastoma cells in vitro, in which a twofold increase in GPX1 expression protected cells from 6-hydroxydopamine-induced neurotoxicity. Furthermore, the delivery of GPX1 to nigral dopaminergic neurons in vivo attenuated 6-hydroxydopamine toxicity in a mouse model of Parkinson's disease (119). Similarly, knockout of GPX1 rendered mouse neurons more susceptible to damage induced by neurotoxins such as malonate, 3-nitropropionic acid, and tetrahydropyridine (80, 150), whereas overexpression of GPX1 protected mice against neurotoxicity (10).

Furthermore, GPX1 may also play a role in Alzheimer's disease. Although amyloid β-peptide-induced oxidative stress has been implicated in the pathogenesis of this disease, cultured neurons from GPX1(−/−) mice are more susceptible to treatment of amyloid β-peptides (35), and overexpression of GPX1 in the PC12 pheochromocytoma cells or rat embryonic cultured cortical neurons renders these cells more resistant to the peptides (5). In stark contrast, in comparison with wild-type mice, knockout of GPX1 rendered mice more resistant to kainic acid–mediated mortality and seizures (75). As mentioned above, kainic acid is a neurodegenerative drug that induces PN formation in brain (117). It is likely that the roles of GPX1 in neurodegenerative diseases are case- or cause-specific.

Autoimmune Diseases

Low dietary Se intake has been suggested to correlate with a 20-fold increase in the risk of developing AIDS in HIV-infected individuals (6). Consistently, HIV-infected individuals have diminished total body Se content and GPX1 activity (51). Analysis of ^{75}Se-labeled human Jurkat T cells has revealed four ^{75}Se-containing proteins including GPX1, GPX4, TR1, and Sep15 (64). Based on the known function of these selenoproteins, we may speculate that Se imparts its function in the pathogenesis of AIDS via redox regulation. Similarly, a GPX protein from the *Molluscum contagiosum* virus (80% homology to human GPX1) conferred protection against hydrogen peroxide insult when expressed in HeLa cells (126). One possible mechanism is that GPX1 may protect HIV-infected individuals from loss of helper T cells by the prevention of oxidant-induced apoptosis.

Diabetes

DM: diabetes mellitus

Diabetes mellitus (DM) is a chronic state of glucose imbalance that affects 20 million Americans (39), and the prevalence will likely rise from 6% to more than 10% in the next decade (120). There are three forms of DM. Type I DM, or juvenile diabetes, is caused by an autoimmune inflammatory reaction affecting the β-cells in the pancreatic islet. Type II DM is characterized by an inability to utilize glucose in the presence of insulin, and is associated with weight gain and adiposity, hyperinsulinemia and insulin resistance, and impaired glucose tolerance (91). The third form of DM, gestational diabetes, occurs only during pregnancy and is associated with insulin resistance and, in extreme cases, β-cell insufficiency (77).

Antioxidant enzymes: proteins that catalyze reactions to suppress the formation of free radicals or to repair the oxidative damage. Free radicals are chemical species with unpaired electrons, in general reactive and attacking other molecules

Oxidant stress has been implicated in both the pathogenesis and complications associated with all three types of DM. In humans and animals with DM, persistent hyperglycemia results in the elevated production of ROS due to the direct autoxidation processes of glucose and the nonenzymatic glycation of proteins resulting in the formation of glucose-derived advanced glycosylation end products (15). Other mechanisms that may result in the formation of ROS during DM include metabolic stress due to weight gain and changes in energy metabolism, activation of RNS (33), activation of xanthine oxidase (42), increased expression of inflammatory mediators, and altered expression of antioxidant enzymes (101).

It is likely that ROS and RNS contribute to the destruction of the pancreatic β-cell during the pathogenesis of type I DM, as these cells express low levels of antioxidant enzymes, including GPX (65). Furthermore, significant reductions in erythrocyte GPX activity and total GSH content occur in young type I DM patients as compared with age-matched controls (44, 98). Although the specific roles of GPX1 in the pathogenesis of type I DM have not been identified, Se is known to protect against the destruction of pancreatic β-cells in streptozotocin-induced diabetic mice. Treatment of these mice with sodium selenite results in nearly complete attenuation of hyperglycemia, lipid peroxidation, and plasma GSH depletion (45, 100, 108).

Although human studies have not established a direct link between GPX1 activity and type II DM, recent studies have proposed a role for ROS and altered antioxidant enzyme expression in the development of disease (55, 120). Depletion of antioxidants is associated with the pathogenesis of type II DM, as reduced vitamin E and C status is a predictor of disease (123, 143), and patients with type II DM exhibit high SOD3 (extracellular), but low GPX3 activity (101).

Insulin resistance occurs during normal pregnancy and results in gestational diabetes when women become glucose intolerant (77). One recent study investigated the association of erythrocyte GPX1 activity with insulin resistance during pregnancy (23). Interestingly, erythrocyte GPX activity increased significantly during the course of normal pregnancy, and the activity was positively associated with fasting plasma insulin and glucose concentrations and incidence of insulin resistance. The authors concluded that enhanced maternal GPX1 activity might be a protective response to pregnancy-induced increases in ROS and that there might be a link between GPX activity, insulin resistance, and β-cell function.

Transgenic mice overexpressing GPX1 have been utilized in two recent studies involving glucose homeostasis and insulin function. The first study reported the development of insulin resistance and obesity in GPX1(+/+) as compared with age-matched wild-type mice (99). The GPX1(+/+) mice developed hyperglycemia, hyperinsulinemia, and elevated plasma leptin concentrations, as well as reduced phosphorylation of Akt (a kinase downstream of the insulin receptor) in both liver and muscle after insulin stimulation. It is possible that the increased GPX1 activity might interfere with insulin function by overquenching intracellular ROS that are required for insulin signaling. This finding is supported by a recent report that β-cell-specific overexpression of catalase and metallothionein in mice resulted in accelerated spontaneous diabetes and altered insulin signaling (94).

A second study utilized pancreatic islets isolated from GPX1(+/+) mice to study the effects of oxidant injury on glucose metabolism following grafting to STZ-treated wild-type mice (109). In that study, islets that were isolated from GPX1(+/+) mice were not protected from pro-oxidant-induced cell death in vitro; however, islets isolated from animals overexpressing both GPX1 and SOD (both SOD1 and SOD2) were protected. Furthermore, when islets from transgenic animals were grafted into streptozotocin-treated mice, overexpression with both GPX1 and SOD enzymes resulted in significantly improved control of blood glucose. However, overexpression of GPX1 alone had no significant effect.

Disruptions in insulin sensitivity often involve diminished signaling at the insulin receptor, which is a tyrosine kinase (49). The role of hydrogen peroxide and oxidant tone at the insulin receptor is controversial. Negative effects of hydrogen peroxide include the inhibition of insulin-induced tyrosine phosphorylation of the insulin receptor β subunit in NIH-B cells (68) and the inhibition of insulin-induced Akt phosphorylation in vascular smooth muscle cells (62). In contrast, early studies suggested that hydrogen peroxide could function as an insulin mimetic (37), and more recent reports suggest that insulin stimulation generates a burst of hydrogen peroxide in hepatoma and adipose cells that is associated with a reversible oxidative inhibition of overall cellular tyrosine phosphatase activity (97). Maintenance of tyrosine phosphatase activity is essential for the regulation of tyrosine phosphorylation in the insulin signaling cascade, and as such, insulin sensitivity. When considered in conjunction with the findings from GPX1(+/+) mice, it appears that the appropriate concentration of hydrogen peroxide is a key factor for insulin signaling. Likely, GPX1 plays a critical role in regulating the concentration of hydrogen peroxide through the enzyme-substrate reaction.

CONCLUSIONS AND PERSPECTIVES

Our understanding of GPX1 function and regulation has advanced significantly during the past ten years. Several new factors such as c-Abl and Arg tyrosine kinases and adenosine have been identified as Se-independent regulators of GPX1 expression. These identifications help explain responses of GPX1 gene expression and enzyme activity to changes other than Se supply in cells and tissues. It will be interesting to find out if and how these new regulators, as well as other regulators not yet identified, affect the functional coordination between GPX1 and other selenoproteins or antioxidant enzymes in various metabolic circumstances. The application of GPX1 knockout and transgenic mouse models has generated convincing evidence for the in vivo role of GPX1 in protecting against ROS-related oxidative stress. The physiological importance of that protection by GPX1 varies with severity of the employed stress and status of body Se. Strikingly, RNS-related oxidative stress is potentiated by GPX1. Knockout of GPX1 renders mice resistant to toxicities of RNS inducers acetaminophen and kainic acid. It will be scientifically fascinating and clinically important to determine how GPX1 exerts dual roles in coping with ROS and RNS. The illustration of GPX1 impact on signal transduction related to cell death, protein kinase phosphorylation, and oxidation allows us to unveil mechanisms of GPX1 functions at the cell biology level. Data from human studies and animal experiments increasingly show associations between alteration or abnormality of GPX1 expression and incidences of cancer, cardiovascular disease, neurodegeneration, autoimmune disease, and diabetes. Although it remains as a challenge to elucidate the mechanism of GPX1 in the pathogenesis of these common disorders, it will be helpful to develop novel tools and therapies to diagnose and treat these diseases through manipulation of GPX1 expression and function.

SUMMARY POINTS

1. Glutathione peroxidase-1 is the first identified and most abundant mammalian selenium-containing protein and has been considered a major intracellular antioxidant enzyme.

2. Although selenium serves as the primary regulator of GPX1 expression, selenocysteine-insertion sequence-associating factors, adenosine, c-Abl and Arg tyrosine kinase, homocysteine, and epidermal growth factor receptor may impart potent impacts on the levels of GPX1 mRNA, protein, and activity.
3. Application of GPX1-overexpressing or knockout mouse models has produced convincing evidence for the in vivo protection of GPX1 against oxidative injuries and mortality mediated by reactive oxygen species.
4. Knockout of GPX1 renders mice and their primary hepatocytes resistant to, whereas overexpression of GPX1 sensitizes mice to, oxidative injuries or death mediated by reactive nitrogen species.
5. GPX1 functions in cellular signaling pathways, including cell death and survival, protein kinase phosphorylation, and oxidant-mediated activation of NFκB.
6. Development of hyperglycemia, hyperinsulinemia, insulin resistance, and obesity in GPX1-overexpressing mice, along with the strong positive correlation between gestational diabetes and elevation of erythrocyte GPX1 activity in pregnant women, indicates the importance of maintaining normal GPX1 activity in regulating body glucose homeostasis.
7. Alteration or abnormality of GPX1 expression may be associated with etiology of a number of chronic diseases including cancer, cardiovascular disease, neurodegeneration, autoimmune disorder, and diabetes.
8. Future research should be focused on the molecular mechanisms of GPX1 in the development of chronic diseases and the potential application of GPX1 manipulation in treating the diseases.

ACKNOWLEDGMENTS

The GPX1-related research conducted in X.G. Lei's laboratory was supported in part by NIH grant DK53018. W.H. Cheng was supported in part by the Intramural Research Program of the NIH, National Institute on Aging. J.P. McClung was supported in part by the Military Nutrition Division, U.S. Army Research Institute of Environmental Medicine, Natick, Massachusetts. The opinions or assertions contained herein are the private views of the authors and are not to be construed as official or as reflecting the views of the U.S. Department of the Army or Department of Defense. Any citations of commercial organizations and trade names in this report do not constitute an official Department of the Army endorsement of approval of the products or services of these organizations.

LITERATURE CITED

1. Ahn J, Gammon MD, Santella RM, Gaudet MM, Britton JA, et al. 2005. No association between glutathione peroxidase Pro198Leu polymorphism and breast cancer risk. *Cancer Epidemiol. Biomarkers Prev.* 14:2459–61
2. Allan CB, Lacourciere GM, Stadtman TC. 1999. Responsiveness of selenoproteins to dietary selenium. *Annu. Rev. Nutr.* 19:1–16

3. Arai M, Imai H, Koumura T, Yoshida M, Emoto K, et al. 1999. Mitochondrial phospholipid hydroperoxide glutathione peroxidase plays a major role in preventing oxidative injury to cells. *J. Biol. Chem.* 274:4924–33
4. Baker RD, Baker SS, LaRosa K, Whitney C, Newburger PE. 1993. Selenium regulation of glutathione peroxidase in human hepatoma cell line Hep3B. *Arch. Biochem. Biophys.* 304:53–57
5. Barkats M, Millecamps S, Abrioux P, Geoffroy MC, Mallet J. 2000. Overexpression of glutathione peroxidase increases the resistance of neuronal cells to Abeta-mediated neurotoxicity. *J. Neurochem.* 75:1438–46
6. Baum MK, Shor-Posner G, Lai S, Zhang G, Lai H, et al. 1997. High risk of HIV-related mortality is associated with selenium deficiency. *J. Acquir. Immune Defic. Syndr. Hum. Retrovirol.* 15:370–74
7. Beck MA, Esworthy RS, Ho YS, Chu FF. 1998. Glutathione peroxidase protects mice from viral-induced myocarditis. *FASEB J.* 12:1143–49
8. Beckman JS, Koppenol WH. 1996. Nitric oxide, superoxide, and peroxynitrite: the good, the bad, and ugly. *Am. J. Physiol* 271:C1424–37
9. Behne D, Kyriakopoulos A. 2001. Mammalian selenium-containing proteins. *Annu. Rev. Nutr.* 21:453–73
10. Bensadoun JC, Mirochnitchenko O, Inouye M, Aebischer P, Zurn AD. 1998. Attenuation of 6-OHDA-induced neurotoxicity in glutathione peroxidase transgenic mice. *Eur. J. Neurosci.* 10:3231–36
11. Bermano G, Nicol F, Dyer JA, Sunde RA, Beckett GJ, et al. 1995. Tissue-specific regulation of selenoenzyme gene expression during selenium deficiency in rats. *Biochem. J.* 311(Pt. 2):425–30
12. **Berry MJ, Banu L, Chen YY, Mandel SJ, Kieffer JD, et al. 1991. Recognition of UGA as a selenocysteine codon in type I deiodinase requires sequences in the 3′-untranslated region. *Nature* 353:273–76**
13. Bock A. 2000. Biosynthesis of selenoproteins—an overview. *Biofactors* 11:77–78
14. Bosl MR, Takaku K, Oshima M, Nishimura S, Taketo MM. 1997. Early embryonic lethality caused by targeted disruption of the mouse selenocysteine tRNA gene (Trsp). *Proc. Natl. Acad. Sci. USA* 94:5531–34
15. Brownlee M, Cerami A, Vlassara H. 1988. Advanced glycosylation end products in tissue and the biochemical basis of diabetic complications. *N. Engl. J. Med.* 318:1315–21
16. Burk RF. 1991. Molecular biology of selenium with implications for its metabolism. *FASEB J.* 5:2274–79
17. Cao C, Leng Y, Huang W, Liu X, Kufe D. 2003. Glutathione peroxidase 1 is regulated by the c-Abl and Arg tyrosine kinases. *J. Biol. Chem.* 278:39609–14
18. Cao C, Ren X, Kharbanda S, Koleske A, Prasad KV, Kufe D. 2001. The ARG tyrosine kinase interacts with Siva-1 in the apoptotic response to oxidative stress. *J. Biol. Chem.* 276:11465–68
19. Carlson BA, Xu XM, Gladyshev VN, Hatfield DL. 2005. Selective rescue of selenoprotein expression in mice lacking a highly specialized methyl group in selenocysteine tRNA. *J. Biol. Chem.* 280:5542–48
20. Cebrian A, Pharoah PD, Ahmed S, Smith PL, Luccarini C, et al. 2006. Tagging single-nucleotide polymorphisms in antioxidant defense enzymes and susceptibility to breast cancer. *Cancer Res.* 66:1225–33
21. **Chambers I, Frampton J, Goldfarb P, Affara N, McBain W, Harrison PR. 1986. The structure of the mouse glutathione peroxidase gene: the selenocysteine in the active site is encoded by the "termination" codon, TGA. *EMBO J.* 5:1221–27**

12. Illustrates a stem-loop structure in the 3′-untranslated region of selenoprotein mRNA for translating the UGA codon into selenocysteine.

21. Reports the first cloning of GPX1 gene from mice, and unveils UGA that decodes selenocysteine.

22. Chavatte L, Brown BA, Driscoll DM. 2005. Ribosomal protein L30 is a component of the UGA-selenocysteine recoding machinery in eukaryotes. *Nat. Struct. Mol. Biol.* 12:408–16
23. Chen X, Scholl TO, Leskiw MJ, Donaldson MR, Stein TP. 2003. Association of glutathione peroxidase activity with insulin resistance and dietary fat intake during normal pregnancy. *J. Clin. Endocrinol. Metab.* 88:5963–68
24. Cheng W, Fu YX, Porres JM, Ross DA, Lei XG. 1999. Selenium-dependent cellular glutathione peroxidase protects mice against a pro-oxidant-induced oxidation of NADPH, NADH, lipids, and protein. *FASEB J.* 13:1467–75
25. Cheng WH, Combs GFJ, Lei XG. 1998. Knockout of cellular glutathione peroxidase affects selenium-dependent parameters similarly in mice fed adequate and excessive dietary selenium. *Biofactors* 7:311–21
26. Cheng WH, Ho YS, Ross DA, Valentine BA, Combs GF, Lei XG. 1997. Cellular glutathione peroxidase knockout mice express normal levels of selenium-dependent plasma and phospholipid hydroperoxide glutathione peroxidases in various tissues. *J. Nutr.* 127:1445–50
27. **Cheng WH, Ho YS, Valentine BA, Ross DA, Combs GFJ, Lei XG. 1998. Cellular glutathione peroxidase is the mediator of body selenium to protect against paraquat lethality in transgenic mice. *J. Nutr.* 128:1070–76**

27. First demonstration of GPX1 as an in vivo antioxidant enzyme against pro-oxidant-induced oxidative stress in mice.

28. Cheng WH, Quimby FW, Lei XG. 2003. Impacts of glutathione peroxidase-1 knockout on the protection by injected selenium against the pro-oxidant-induced liver aponecrosis and signaling in selenium-deficient mice. *Free Radic. Biol. Med.* 34:918–27
29. Cheng WH, Zheng X, Quimby FR, Roneker CA, Lei XG. 2003. Low levels of glutathione peroxidase 1 activity in selenium-deficient mouse liver affect c-Jun N-terminal kinase activation and p53 phosphorylation on Ser-15 in pro-oxidant-induced aponecrosis. *Biochem. J.* 370:927–34
30. Chu FF, Esworthy RS, Ho YS, Bermeister M, Swiderek K, Elliott RW. 1997. Expression and chromosomal mapping of mouse Gpx2 gene encoding the gastrointestinal form of glutathione peroxidase, GPX-GI. *Biomed. Environ. Sci.* 10:156–62
31. **Clark LC, Combs GFJ, Turnbull BW, Slate EH, Chalker DK, et al. 1996. Effects of selenium supplementation for cancer prevention in patients with carcinoma of the skin. A randomized controlled trial. Nutritional Prevention of Cancer Study Group. *JAMA* 276:1957–63**

31. Demonstrates that daily Se supplementation reduces mortality of lung, colon, and prostate cancer in humans.

32. Combs GF Jr. 2004. Status of selenium in prostate cancer prevention. *Br. J. Cancer* 91:195–99
33. Cosentino F, Hishikawa K, Katusic ZS, Luscher TF. 1997. High glucose increases nitric oxide synthase expression and superoxide anion generation in human aortic endothelial cells. *Circulation* 96:25–28
34. Cox DG, Hankinson SE, Kraft P, Hunter DJ. 2004. No association between GPX1 Pro198Leu and breast cancer risk. *Cancer Epidemiol. Biomarkers Prev.* 13:1821–22
35. Crack PJ, Cimdins K, Ali U, Hertzog PJ, Iannello RC. 2006. Lack of glutathione peroxidase-1 exacerbates αβ-mediated neurotoxicity in cortical neurons. *J. Neural Transm.* 113:645–57
36. Crack PJ, Taylor JM, Ali U, Mansell A, Hertzog PJ. 2006. Potential contribution of NF-κβ in neuronal cell death in the glutathione peroxidase-1 knockout mouse in response to ischemia-reperfusion injury. *Stroke* 37:1533–38
37. Czech MP, Lawrence JCJ, Lynn WS. 1974. Evidence for electron transfer reactions involved in the Cu^{2+}-dependent thiol activation of fat cell glucose utilization. *J. Biol. Chem.* 249:1001–6

38. Damier P, Hirsch EC, Zhang P, Agid Y, Javoy-Agid F. 1993. Glutathione peroxidase, glial cells and Parkinson's disease. *Neuroscience* 52:1–6
39. Davidson JA. 2006. Introductory remarks: diabetes care in America—"a sense of urgency." *Endocr. Pract.* 12(Suppl. 1):13–15
40. Dawson TM, Dawson VL. 2003. Molecular pathways of neurodegeneration in Parkinson's disease. *Science* 302:819–22
41. de Haan JB, Bladier C, Griffiths P, Kelner M, O'Shea RD, et al. 1998. Mice with a homozygous null mutation for the most abundant glutathione peroxidase, Gpx1, show increased susceptibility to the oxidative stress-inducing agents paraquat and hydrogen peroxide. *J. Biol. Chem.* 273:22528–36
42. Desco MC, Asensi M, Marquez R, Martinez-Valls J, Vento M, et al. 2002. Xanthine oxidase is involved in free radical production in type 1 diabetes: protection by allopurinol. *Diabetes* 51:1118–24
43. Diamond AM, Choi IS, Crain PF, Hashizume T, Pomerantz SC, et al. 1993. Dietary selenium affects methylation of the wobble nucleoside in the anticodon of selenocysteine tRNA([Ser]Sec). *J. Biol. Chem.* 268:14215–23
44. Dominguez C, Ruiz E, Gussinye M, Carrascosa A. 1998. Oxidative stress at onset and in early stages of type 1 diabetes in children and adolescents. *Diabetes Care* 21:1736–42
45. Douillet C, Bost M, Accominotti M, Borson-Chazot F, Ciavatti M. 1998. Effect of selenium and vitamin E supplements on tissue lipids, peroxides, and fatty acid distribution in experimental diabetes. *Lipids* 33:393–99
46. Drake EN. 2006. Cancer chemoprevention: selenium as a prooxidant, not an antioxidant. *Med. Hypotheses* 67:318–22
47. Drew JE, Farquharson AJ, Arthur JR, Morrice PC, Duthie GG. 2005. Novel sites of cytosolic glutathione peroxidase expression in colon. *FEBS Lett.* 579:6135–39
48. Driscoll DM, Copeland PR. 2003. Mechanism and regulation of selenoprotein synthesis? *Annu. Rev. Nutr.* 23:17–40
49. Dupont J, LeRoith D. 2001. Insulin and insulin-like growth factor I receptors: similarities and differences in signal transduction. *Horm. Res.* 55(Suppl. 2):22–26
50. Duval C, Auge N, Frisach MF, Casteilla L, Salvayre R, Negre-Salvayre A. 2002. Mitochondrial oxidative stress is modulated by oleic acid via an epidermal growth factor receptor-dependent activation of glutathione peroxidase. *Biochem. J.* 367:889–94
51. Dworkin BM. 1994. Selenium deficiency in HIV infection and the acquired immunodeficiency syndrome (AIDS). *Chem. Biol. Interact.* 91:181–86
52. Emerling BM, Platanias LC, Black E, Nebreda AR, Davis RJ, Chandel NS. 2005. Mitochondrial reactive oxygen species activation of p38 mitogen-activated protein kinase is required for hypoxia signaling. *Mol. Cell. Biol.* 25:4853–62
53. Esposito LA, Kokoszka JE, Waymire KG, Cottrell B, MacGregor GR, Wallace DC. 2000. Mitochondrial oxidative stress in mice lacking the glutathione peroxidase-1 gene. *Free Radic. Biol. Med.* 28:754–66
54. Esworthy RS, Baker MA, Chu FF. 1995. Expression of selenium-dependent glutathione peroxidase in human breast tumor cell lines. *Cancer Res.* 55:957–62
55. Evans JL, Goldfine ID, Maddux BA, Grodsky GM. 2002. Oxidative stress and stress-activated signaling pathways: a unifying hypothesis of type 2 diabetes. *Endocr. Rev.* 23:599–622
56. Fan C, Li Q, Ross D, Engelhardt JF. 2003. Tyrosine phosphorylation of Iκβ alpha activates NFκβ through a redox-regulated and c-Src-dependent mechanism following hypoxia/reoxygenation. *J. Biol. Chem.* 278:2072–80

57. Faucher K, Rabinovitch-Chable H, Cook-Moreau J, Barriere G, Sturtz F, Rigaud M. 2005. Overexpression of human GPX1 modifies Bax to Bcl-2 apoptotic ratio in human endothelial cells. *Mol. Cell Biochem.* 277:81–87

58. Flohe L, Gunzler WA, Schock HH. 1973. Glutathione peroxidase: a selenoenzyme. *FEBS Lett.* 32:132–34

58. Establishes that GPX1 is an Se-containing enzyme.

59. Fu Y, Cheng WH, Porres JM, Ross DA, Lei XG. 1999. Knockout of cellular glutathione peroxidase gene renders mice susceptible to diquat-induced oxidative stress. *Free Radic. Biol. Med.* 27:605–11

60. Fu Y, Cheng WH, Ross DA, Lei X. 1999. Cellular glutathione peroxidase protects mice against lethal oxidative stress induced by various doses of diquat. *Proc. Soc. Exp. Biol. Med.* 222:164–69

61. Fu Y, Sies H, Lei XG. 2001. Opposite roles of selenium-dependent glutathione peroxidase-1 in superoxide generator diquat- and peroxynitrite-induced apoptosis and signaling. *J. Biol. Chem.* 276:43004–9

61. Reports the opposite roles of GPX1 in coping with reactive oxygen species versus reactive nitrogen species–induced cell death and related signaling pathways.

62. Gardner CD, Eguchi S, Reynolds CM, Eguchi K, Frank GD, Motley ED. 2003. Hydrogen peroxide inhibits insulin signaling in vascular smooth muscle cells. *Exp. Biol. Med. (Maywood)* 228:836–42

63. Gladyshev VN, Factor VM, Housseau F, Hatfield DL. 1998. Contrasting patterns of regulation of the antioxidant selenoproteins, thioredoxin reductase, and glutathione peroxidase, in cancer cells. *Biochem. Biophys. Res. Commun.* 251:488–93

64. Gladyshev VN, Stadtman TC, Hatfield DL, Jeang KT. 1999. Levels of major selenoproteins in T cells decrease during HIV infection and low molecular mass selenium compounds increase. *Proc. Natl. Acad. Sci. USA* 96:835–39

65. Grankvist K, Marklund SL, Taljedal IB. 1981. CuZn-superoxide dismutase, Mn-superoxide dismutase, catalase and glutathione peroxidase in pancreatic islets and other tissues in the mouse. *Biochem. J.* 199:393–98

66. Handy DE, Loscalzo J. 2003. Homocysteine and atherothrombosis: diagnosis and treatment. *Curr. Atheroscler. Rep.* 5:276–83

67. Handy DE, Zhang Y, Loscalzo J. 2005. Homocysteine down-regulates cellular glutathione peroxidase (GPx1) by decreasing translation. *J. Biol. Chem.* 280:15518–25

68. Hansen LL, Ikeda Y, Olsen GS, Busch AK, Mosthaf L. 1999. Insulin signaling is inhibited by micromolar concentrations of H(2)O(2). Evidence for a role of H(2)O(2) in tumor necrosis factor alpha-mediated insulin resistance. *J. Biol. Chem.* 274:25078–84

69. Hardie LJ, Briggs JA, Davidson LA, Allan JM, King RF, et al. 2000. The effect of hOGG1 and glutathione peroxidase I genotypes and 3p chromosomal loss on 8-hydroxydeoxyguanosine levels in lung cancer. *Carcinogenesis* 21:167–72

70. Hockenbery DM, Oltvai ZN, Yin XM, Milliman CL, Korsmeyer SJ. 1993. Bcl-2 functions in an antioxidant pathway to prevent apoptosis. *Cell* 75:241–51

71. Hu Y, Benya RV, Carroll RE, Diamond AM. 2005. Allelic loss of the gene for the GPX1 selenium-containing protein is a common event in cancer. *J. Nutr.* 135:3021–24S

72. Hu YJ, Diamond AM. 2003. Role of glutathione peroxidase 1 in breast cancer: loss of heterozygosity and allelic differences in the response to selenium. *Cancer Res.* 63:3347–51

73. Ichimura Y, Habuchi T, Tsuchiya N, Wang L, Oyama C, et al. 2004. Increased risk of bladder cancer associated with a glutathione peroxidase 1 codon 198 variant. *J. Urol.* 172:728–32

74. Irons R, Carlson BA, Hatfield DL, Davis CD. 2006. Both selenoproteins and low molecular weight selenocompounds reduce colon cancer risk in mice with genetically impaired selenoprotein expression. *J. Nutr.* 136:1311–17

75. Jiang D, Akopian G, Ho YS, Walsh JP, Andersen JK. 2000. Chronic brain oxidation in a glutathione peroxidase knockout mouse model results in increased resistance to induced epileptic seizures. *Exp. Neurol.* 164:257–68

76. Juliet PA, Hayashi T, Iguchi A, Ignarro LJ. 2003. Concomitant production of nitric oxide and superoxide in human macrophages. *Biochem. Biophys. Res. Commun.* 310:367–70

77. Kaaja RJ, Greer IA. 2005. Manifestations of chronic disease during pregnancy. *JAMA* 294:2751–57

78. Karin M. 2006. Nuclear factor-κβ in cancer development and progression. *Nature* 441:431–36

79. Kayanoki Y, Fujii J, Islam KN, Suzuki K, Kawata S, et al. 1996. The protective role of glutathione peroxidase in apoptosis induced by reactive oxygen species. *J. Biochem. (Tokyo)* 119:817–22

80. Klivenyi P, Andreassen OA, Ferrante RJ, Dedeoglu A, Mueller G, et al. 2000. Mice deficient in cellular glutathione peroxidase show increased vulnerability to malonate, 3-nitropropionic acid, and 1-methyl-4-phenyl-1,2,5,6-tetrahydropyridine. *J. Neurosci.* 20:1–7

81. Knight TR, Ho YS, Farhood A, Jaeschke H. 2002. Peroxynitrite is a critical mediator of acetaminophen hepatotoxicity in murine livers: protection by glutathione. *J. Pharmacol. Exp. Ther.* 303:468–75

82. Knight TR, Kurtz A, Bajt ML, Hinson JA, Jaeschke H. 2001. Vascular and hepatocellular peroxynitrite formation during acetaminophen toxicity: role of mitochondrial oxidant stress. *Toxicol. Sci.* 62:212–20

83. Kobayashi S, Inoue N, Azumi H, Seno T, Hirata K, et al. 2002. Expressional changes of the vascular antioxidant system in atherosclerotic coronary arteries. *J. Atheroscler. Thromb.* 9:184–90

84. Kote-Jarai Z, Durocher F, Edwards SM, Hamoudi R, Jackson RA, et al. 2002. Association between the GCG polymorphism of the selenium dependent GPX1 gene and the risk of young onset prostate cancer. *Prostate Cancer Prostatic Dis.* 5:189–92

85. Kryukov GV, Castellano S, Novoselov SV, Lobanov AV, Zehtab O, et al. 2003. Characterization of mammalian selenoproteomes. *Science* 300:1439–43

86. Lean JM, Jagger CJ, Kirstein B, Fuller K, Chambers TJ. 2005. Hydrogen peroxide is essential for estrogen-deficiency bone loss and osteoclast formation. *Endocrinology* 146:728–35

87. Lee HT, Emala CW. 2001. Systemic adenosine given after ischemia protects renal function via A(2a) adenosine receptor activation. *Am. J. Kidney Dis.* 38:610–18

88. Lee HT, Emala CW. 2002. Adenosine attenuates oxidant injury in human proximal tubular cells via A(1) and A(2a) adenosine receptors. *Am. J. Physiol. Renal Physiol.* 282:F844–52

89. Lee S, Shin HS, Shireman PK, Vasilaki A, Van RH, Csete ME. 2006. Glutathione-peroxidase-1 null muscle progenitor cells are globally defective. *Free Radic. Biol. Med.* 41:1174–84

90. Lei XG, Zhu JH, McClung JP, Aregullin M, Roneker CA. 2006. Mice deficient in Cu,Zn-superoxide dismutase are resistant to acetaminophen toxicity. *Biochem. J.* 399(3):455–61

91. Leiter EH. 2002. Mice with targeted gene disruptions or gene insertions for diabetes research: problems, pitfalls, and potential solutions. *Diabetologia* 45:296–308

92. Li Q, Engelhardt JF. 2006. Interleukin-1β induction of NFκβ is partially regulated by H2O2-mediated activation of NFκβ-inducing kinase. *J. Biol. Chem.* 281:1495–505

93. Li Q, Sanlioglu S, Li S, Ritchie T, Oberley L, Engelhardt JF. 2001. GPx-1 gene delivery modulates NFκβ activation following diverse environmental injuries through a specific subunit of the IKK complex. *Antioxid. Redox Signal.* 3:415–32

75. Demonstrates that knockout of GPX1 actually protects mice from kainic acid–induced epileptic seizures and mortality.

85. Concludes that there are a total of 25 selenoproteins in the human genome by searching for SECIS in the entire genome.

94. Li X, Chen H, Epstein PN. 2006. Metallothionein and catalase sensitize to diabetes in nonobese diabetic mice: reactive oxygen species may have a protective role in pancreatic β-cells. *Diabetes* 55:1592–604
95. Lin A. 2003. Activation of the JNK signaling pathway: breaking the brake on apoptosis. *Bioessays* 25:17–24
96. Liu GS, Thornton J, Van Winkle DM, Stanley AW, Olsson RA, Downey JM. 1991. Protection against infarction afforded by preconditioning is mediated by A1 adenosine receptors in rabbit heart. *Circulation* 84:350–56
97. Mahadev K, Wu X, Zilbering A, Zhu L, Lawrence JT, Goldstein BJ. 2001. Hydrogen peroxide generated during cellular insulin stimulation is integral to activation of the distal insulin signaling cascade in 3T3-L1 adipocytes. *J. Biol. Chem.* 276:48662–69
98. Martin-Gallan P, Carrascosa A, Gussinye M, Dominguez C. 2003. Biomarkers of diabetes-associated oxidative stress and antioxidant status in young diabetic patients with or without subclinical complications. *Free Radic. Biol. Med.* 34:1563–74
99. **McClung JP, Roneker CA, Mu W, Lisk DJ, Langlais P, et al. 2004. Development of insulin resistance and obesity in mice overexpressing cellular glutathione peroxidase. *Proc. Natl. Acad. Sci. USA* 101:8852–57**

99. Presents physiological evidence that overexpression of GPX1 disturbs glucose metabolism in mice.

100. McNeill JH, Delgatty HL, Battell ML. 1991. Insulinlike effects of sodium selenate in streptozocin-induced diabetic rats. *Diabetes* 40:1675–78
101. Memisogullari R, Taysi S, Bakan E, Capoglu I. 2003. Antioxidant status and lipid peroxidation in type II diabetes mellitus. *Cell Biochem. Funct.* 21:291–96
102. Michael SL, Mayeux PR, Bucci TJ, Warbritton AR, Irwin LK, et al. 2001. Acetaminophen-induced hepatotoxicity in mice lacking inducible nitric oxide synthase activity. *Nitric Oxide* 5:432–41
103. Mills GC. 1957. Hemoglobin catabolism. I. Glutathione peroxidase, an erythrocyte enzyme which protects hemoglobin from oxidative breakdown. *J. Biol. Chem.* 229:189–97
104. Mirault ME, Tremblay A, Beaudoin N, Tremblay M. 1991. Overexpression of seleno-glutathione peroxidase by gene transfer enhances the resistance of T47D human breast cells to clastogenic oxidants. *J. Biol. Chem.* 266:20752–60
105. **Mirochnitchenko O, Weisbrot-Lefkowitz M, Reuhl K, Chen L, Yang C, Inouye M. 1999. Acetaminophen toxicity. Opposite effects of two forms of glutathione peroxidase. *J. Biol. Chem.* 274:10349–55**

105. Demonstrates that overexpression of GPX1 sensitizes mice to acetaminophen toxicity.

106. Moriarty PM, Reddy CC, Maquat LE. 1998. Selenium deficiency reduces the abundance of mRNA for Se-dependent glutathione peroxidase 1 by a UGA-dependent mechanism likely to be nonsense codon-mediated decay of cytoplasmic mRNA. *Mol. Cell. Biol.* 18:2932–39
107. Moscow JA, Schmidt L, Ingram DT, Gnarra J, Johnson B, Cowan KH. 1994. Loss of heterozygosity of the human cytosolic glutathione peroxidase I gene in lung cancer. *Carcinogenesis* 15:2769–73
108. Mukherjee B, Anbazhagan S, Roy A, Ghosh R, Chatterjee M. 1998. Novel implications of the potential role of selenium on antioxidant status in streptozotocin-induced diabetic mice. *Biomed. Pharmacother.* 52:89–95
109. Mysore TB, Shinkel TA, Collins J, Salvaris EJ, Fisicaro N, et al. 2005. Overexpression of glutathione peroxidase with two isoforms of superoxide dismutase protects mouse islets from oxidative injury and improves islet graft function. *Diabetes* 54:2109–16
110. Nasr MA, Fedele MJ, Esser K, Diamond AM. 2004. GPx-1 modulates Akt and P70S6K phosphorylation and Gadd45 levels in MCF-7 cells. *Free Radic. Biol. Med.* 37:187–95
111. National Research Council. 1989/1983. *Selenium Nutrition*. Washington, DC: Nat. Acad. Press

112. Nomura K, Imai H, Koumura T, Arai M, Nakagawa Y. 1999. Mitochondrial phospholipid hydroperoxide glutathione peroxidase suppresses apoptosis mediated by a mitochondrial death pathway. *J. Biol. Chem.* 274:29294–302
113. Novoselov SV, Calvisi DF, Labunskyy VM, Factor VM, Carlson BA, et al. 2005. Selenoprotein deficiency and high levels of selenium compounds can effectively inhibit hepatocarcinogenesis in transgenic mice. *Oncogene* 24:8003–11
114. Ono K, Han J. 2000. The p38 signal transduction pathway: activation and function. *Cell. Signal.* 12:1–13
115. Packham G, Ashmun RA, Cleveland JL. 1996. Cytokines suppress apoptosis independent of increases in reactive oxygen levels. *J. Immunol.* 156:2792–800
116. Papp LV, Lu J, Striebel F, Kennedy D, Holmgren A, Khanna KK. 2006. The redox state of SECIS binding protein 2 controls its localization and selenocysteine incorporation function. *Mol. Cell. Biol.* 26:4895–910
117. Parathath SR, Parathath S, Tsirka SE. 2006. Nitric oxide mediates neurodegeneration and breakdown of the blood-brain barrier in tPA-dependent excitotoxic injury in mice. *J. Cell Sci.* 119:339–49
118. Ravn-Haren G, Olsen A, Tjonneland A, Dragsted LO, Nexo BA, et al. 2006. Associations between GPX1 Pro198Leu polymorphism, erythrocyte GPX activity, alcohol consumption and breast cancer risk in a prospective cohort study. *Carcinogenesis* 27:820–25
119. Ridet JL, Bensadoun JC, Deglon N, Aebischer P, Zurn AD. 2006. Lentivirus-mediated expression of glutathione peroxidase: neuroprotection in murine models of Parkinson's disease. *Neurobiol. Dis.* 21:29–34
120. Rosen P, Nawroth PP, King G, Moller W, Tritschler HJ, Packer L. 2001. The role of oxidative stress in the onset and progression of diabetes and its complications: a summary of a Congress Series sponsored by UNESCO-MCBN, the American Diabetes Association and the German Diabetes Society. *Diabetes Metab. Res. Rev.* 17:189–212
121. Rotruck JT, Pope AL, Ganther HE, Swanson AB, Hafeman DG, Hoekstra WG. 1973. Selenium: biochemical role as a component of glutathione peroxidase. *Science* 179:588–90
122. Saedi MS, Smith CG, Frampton J, Chambers I, Harrison PR, Sunde RA. 1988. Effect of selenium status on mRNA levels for glutathione peroxidase in rat liver. *Biochem. Biophys. Res. Commun.* 153:855–61
123. Salonen JT, Nyyssonen K, Tuomainen TP, Maenpaa PH, Korpela H, et al. 1995. Increased risk of noninsulin-dependent diabetes mellitus at low plasma vitamin E concentrations: a four-year follow up study in men. *BMJ* 311:1124–27
124. Savolainen H. 1978. Superoxide dismutase and glutathione peroxidase activities in rat brain. *Res. Commun. Chem. Pathol. Pharmacol.* 21:173–76
125. Shen Q, Chu FF, Newburger PE. 1993. Sequences in the 3′-untranslated region of the human cellular glutathione peroxidase gene are necessary and sufficient for selenocysteine incorporation at the UGA codon. *J. Biol. Chem.* 268:11463–69
126. Shisler JL, Senkevich TG, Berry MJ, Moss B. 1998. Ultraviolet-induced cell death blocked by a selenoprotein from a human dermatotropic poxvirus. *Science* 279:102–5
127. Sies H, Sharov VS, Klotz LO, Briviba K. 1997. Glutathione peroxidase protects against peroxynitrite-mediated oxidations. A new function for selenoproteins as peroxynitrite reductase. *J. Biol. Chem.* 272:27812–17
128. Small-Howard A, Morozova N, Stoytcheva Z, Forry EP, Mansell JB, et al. 2006. Supramolecular complexes mediate selenocysteine incorporation in vivo. *Mol. Cell. Biol.* 26:2337–46

121. Establishes that GPX1 is an Se-containing enzyme.

122. Shows that dietary Se deficiency in rats resulted in dramatic reduction of liver GPX1 mRNA levels and provides evidence for the regulation of Se on GPX1 gene expression.

129. Stadtman TC. 1996. Selenocysteine. *Annu. Rev. Biochem.* 65:83–100
130. Sun X, Majumder P, Shioya H, Wu F, Kumar S, et al. 2000. Activation of the cytoplasmic c-Abl tyrosine kinase by reactive oxygen species. *J. Biol. Chem.* 275:17237–40
131. Sunde RA. 1994. Intracellular glutathione peroxidases-structures, regulation, and functions. In *Selenium in Biology and Human Health*, ed. RF Burk, 10:45–77. New York: Springer-Verlag
132. Sunde RA, Saedi MS, Knight SAB, Smith CG, Evanson JK. 1989. Regulation of expression of glutathione peroxidase by selenium. In *Selenium in Biology and Medicine*, ed. A Wendel, 4:8–13. Heidelberg: Springer-Verlag
133. Sunde RA, Thompson BM, Palm MD, Weiss SL, Thompson KM, Evenson JK. 1997. Selenium regulation of selenium-dependent glutathione peroxidases in animals and transfected CHO cells. *Biomed. Environ. Sci.* 10:346–55
134. Sutton A, Nahon P, Pessayre D, Rufat P, Poire A, et al. 2006. Genetic polymorphisms in antioxidant enzymes modulate hepatic iron accumulation and hepatocellular carcinoma development in patients with alcohol-induced cirrhosis. *Cancer Res.* 66:2844–52
135. Takahashi K, Avissar N, Whitin J, Cohen H. 1987. Purification and characterization of human plasma glutathione peroxidase: a selenoglycoprotein distinct from the known cellular enzyme. *Arch. Biochem. Biophys.* 256:677–86
136. Takakura K, Beckman JS, Millan-Crow LA, Crow JP. 1999. Rapid and irreversible inactivation of protein tyrosine phosphatases PTP1B, CD45, and LAR by peroxynitrite. *Arch. Biochem. Biophys.* 369:197–207
137. Takeshita S, Inoue N, Ueyama T, Kawashima S, Yokoyama M. 2000. Shear stress enhances glutathione peroxidase expression in endothelial cells. *Biochem. Biophys. Res. Commun.* 273:66–71
138. Takizawa S, Matsushima K, Shinohara Y, Ogawa S, Komatsu N, et al. 1994. Immunohistochemical localization of glutathione peroxidase in infarcted human brain. *J. Neurol. Sci.* 122:66–73
139. Taylor JM, Crack PJ, Gould JA, Ali U, Hertzog PJ, Iannello RC. 2004. Akt phosphorylation and NFκβ activation are counterregulated under conditions of oxidative stress. *Exp. Cell Res.* 300:463–75
140. Taylor SD, Davenport LD, Speranza MJ, Mullenbach GT, Lynch RE. 1993. Glutathione peroxidase protects cultured mammalian cells from the toxicity of adriamycin and paraquat. *Arch. Biochem. Biophys.* 305:600–5
141. Thomas JP, Maiorino M, Ursini F, Girotti AW. 1990. Protective action of phospholipid hydroperoxide glutathione peroxidase against membrane-damaging lipid peroxidation. In situ reduction of phospholipid and cholesterol hydroperoxides. *J. Biol. Chem.* 265:454–61
142. Ursini F, Heim S, Kiess M, Maiorino M, Roveri A, et al. 1999. Dual function of the selenoprotein PHGPx during sperm maturation. *Science* 285:1393–96
143. Vijayalingam S, Parthiban A, Shanmugasundaram KR, Mohan V. 1996. Abnormal antioxidant status in impaired glucose tolerance and noninsulin-dependent diabetes mellitus. *Diabet. Med.* 13:715–19
144. Weiss N, Zhang YY, Heydrick S, Bierl C, Loscalzo J. 2001. Overexpression of cellular glutathione peroxidase rescues homocyst(e)ine-induced endothelial dysfunction. *Proc. Natl. Acad. Sci. USA* 98:12503–8
145. Xu XM, Mix H, Carlson BA, Grabowski PJ, Gladyshev VN, et al. 2005. Evidence for direct roles of two additional factors, SECp43 and soluble liver antigen, in the selenoprotein synthesis machinery. *J. Biol. Chem.* 280:41568–75

146. Yoshida T, Watanabe M, Engelman DT, Engelman RM, Schley JA, et al. 1996. Transgenic mice overexpressing glutathione peroxidase are resistant to myocardial ischemia reperfusion injury. *J. Mol. Cell. Cardiol.* 28:1759–67
147. Yoshimura S, Watanabe K, Suemizu H, Onozawa T, Mizoguchi J, et al. 1991. Tissue specific expression of the plasma glutathione peroxidase gene in rat kidney. *J. Biochem. (Tokyo)* 109:918–23
148. Zamamiri-Davis F, Lu Y, Thompson JT, Prabhu KS, Reddy PV, et al. 2002. Nuclear factor-κβ mediates overexpression of cyclooxygenase-2 during activation of RAW 264.7 macrophages in selenium deficiency. *Free Radic. Biol. Med.* 32:890–97
149. Zavacki AM, Mansell JB, Chung M, Klimovitsky B, Harney JW, Berry MJ. 2003. Coupled tRNA(Sec)-dependent assembly of the selenocysteine decoding apparatus. *Mol. Cell* 11:773–81
150. Zhang J, Graham DG, Montine TJ, Ho YS. 2000. Enhanced N-methyl-4-phenyl-1,2,3,6-tetrahydropyridine toxicity in mice deficient in CuZn-superoxide dismutase or glutathione peroxidase. *J. Neuropathol. Exp. Neurol.* 59:53–61
151. Zhang Y, Handy DE, Loscalzo J. 2005. Adenosine-dependent induction of glutathione peroxidase 1 in human primary endothelial cells and protection against oxidative stress. *Circ. Res.* 96:831–37
152. **Zhu JH, Lei XG. 2006. Double null of selenium-glutathione peroxidase-1 and copper, zinc-superoxide dismutase enhances resistance of mouse primary hepatocytes to acetaminophen toxicity. *Exp. Biol. Med. (Maywood)* 231:545–52**

152. Demonstrates that double knockout of GPX1 and Cu,Zn-superoxide dismutase does not potentiate but actually enhances resistance of mouse primary hepatocytes to acetaminophen toxicity.

Mechanisms of Food Intake Repression in Indispensable Amino Acid Deficiency

Dorothy W. Gietzen,[1] Shuzhen Hao,[1] and Tracy G. Anthony[2]

[1]Department of Anatomy, Physiology and Cell Biology, School of Veterinary Medicine, University of California, Davis, California 95616; email: dwgietzen@ucdavis.edu, hao@ucdavis.edu

[2]Department of Biochemistry and Molecular Biology, Indiana University School of Medicine, Evansville, Indiana 47712; email: tganthon@iupui.edu

Annu. Rev. Nutr. 2007. 27:63–78

First published online as a Review in Advance on February 28, 2007

The *Annual Review of Nutrition* is online at http://nutr.annualreviews.org

This article's doi: 10.1146/annurev.nutr.27.061406.093726

0199-9885/07/0821-0063$20.00

Key Words

essential amino acids, anterior piriform cortex, GCN2, tRNA, amino acid transporters, signal transduction

Abstract

Animals reject diets that lead to indispensable amino acid (IAA) depletion or deficiency. This behavior is adaptive, as continued IAA depletion is incompatible with maintenance of protein synthesis and survival. Following rejection of the diet, animals begin foraging for a better IAA source and develop conditioned aversions to cues associated with the deficient diet. These responses require a sensory system to detect the IAA depletion and alert the appropriate neural circuitry for the behavior. The chemosensor for IAA deprivation is in the highly excitable anterior piriform cortex (APC) of the brain. Recently, the well-conserved general AA control non-derepressing system of yeast was discovered to be activated by IAA deprivation via uncharged tRNA in mammalian APC. This system provides the sensory limb of the mechanism for recognition of IAA depletion that leads to activation of the APC, diet rejection, and subsequent adaptive strategies.

Contents

Anterior piriform cortex (APC): located in the anterior ventro-lateral forebrain, the APC houses the chemosensor for IAA deficiency, also known as the area tempestas

INTRODUCTION

To survive, all organisms must maintain a full complement of the amino acids (AAs) that are the precursors for protein synthesis. Nearly half of the AAs present in protein cannot be synthesized or stored in metazoans because the genes for their synthesis were lost early in evolution (41); these are the essential or dietary indispensable amino acids (IAAs). The inability of incomplete proteins (i.e., those missing or having inadequate IAA balance in the food) to support human health was appreciated as early as the 1800s (14). For generalist herbivores and omnivores, rejection of an inadequate diet and selection (of a complete food or at least one containing a complementary IAA profile) must provide a full supply of IAA in a timely fashion or general protein synthesis is halted and degradation exceeds synthesis (62). The time course for repletion via complementation varies with the limiting IAA, but it is short. Degradation of protein in brain begins within 2 h in animals prefed a basal (6%–8% crude protein equivalent) diet and then provided a diet missing a single IAA (41, 78).

When animals are given an IAA-deficient or imbalanced diet, they fail to grow because they simply won't eat the diet. That the growth failure is due to rejection of the diet, rather than toxicity, was shown in the 1930s (33, 34, 41, 49, 50, 81, 94, 95).

The behavioral responses to differing IAA proportions in the diet have been well studied (3, 33, 34, 36, 37, 41, 49, 50, 65, 92, 94, 95). Rejection of a test diet and dietary choice in laboratory animals continue to be useful nutritional tools for evaluating protein quality and IAA balance.

BEHAVIORAL RESPONSES

Rejection of IAA-Deficient Food

The behavioral strategies for dealing with limiting amounts of IAA include meal termination, altered food choice, foraging for foods that will complement or correct the deficiency, development of a learned aversion to a deficient or imbalanced food in order to avoid that food in the future, and memory for the taste, smell, or place associated with repleting food (24, 28, 29, 33, 34, 40, 65–68, 84, 102). The first three of these strategies will help the animal obtain a complete meal only if they occur as a consequence of sensing the IAA deficiency within that meal. The last two are adaptive in the longer term and are associated with learning, subsequent to the sensing of the deficiency and termination of the meal.

Many of the parts are in place to complete the puzzle of how IAA deficiencies affect food intake. Neural links from the chemosensory brain area (anterior piriform cortex, APC) to the circuits for food intake and learning are known (1, 44) (see below). The brain circuits associated with the motor behaviors that control feeding have been reviewed (9, 13). Thoroughly documented models are available for "conditioned taste aversion" (24, 28, 29, 32–34, 40, 111) and "long-term potentiation" (28, 86), for the learned aversions and memory for place, respectively. Here we address the mechanisms that provide sensing of the IAA deficiency (36, 41, 48, 80) and activation of the neurons in the APC (36, 97–100).

Dietary Selection and Food Choice

The most parsimonious method of obtaining a balanced profile of IAA in the diet is available to carnivores, because each meal contains animal-source foods with all the IAA required for maintenance and growth. Where animal-source foods are not available, or there are cultural histories of famine or vegetarian cultural food preference, complementary nonanimal-source proteins, such as rice and beans, are used routinely by omnivores. These dietary practices in humans predate the discovery of IAA (41), and animals including birds, pigs, and rodents select appropriate complimentary proteins (41, 65). In rats, the threshold for sensing IAA, with a variety of limiting IAA, is in the range of 90–120 ppm (54, 55), showing exquisite sensitivity to IAA depletion. If rats are given even a limited choice, as with near-basal levels of lysine, the more adequate diet is chosen at lysine levels that do not decrease food intake (55). Therefore, given a choice, rats will switch diets rather than stop eating. Because they continue eating an alternative food, it is safe to assume that they are neither sick nor satiated. A constructive behavioral response is seen when animals reject the deficient food and, in the absence of another food source, begin foraging. This is seen as increased locomotor activity and digging in the food cup with increased spillage, and begins rapidly as well (65). With repletion, a rapid rate of eating continues to satiation, seen as the satiety sequence: a set of behaviors including grooming and sleep that correlate with the end of a normal meal (59).

IAA DEFICIENCY

Indispensable amino acid (IAA)–deficient diets are associated with increased seizure susceptibility in animals [reviewed in (98)]. It is clear that the highly sensitive APC is activated by acute IAA deficiency. Given the ongoing oscillatory activity of the APC (26), the excitatory effects of signaling systems such as CaMKII (100) and ERK (97, 99), and the paucity of inhibitory elements (23, 98, 105), the findings reviewed here may account for the potentiation of the APC in response to IAA deficiency. Some seizure disorders seem intractable and seizure patients may have occasional unexplained breakthrough seizures. Because the APC can be activated within the duration of a single IAA-deficient meal, these findings offer the novel suggestion that people who suffer from poorly controlled seizure disorders might be advised of the potential seizure risk from IAA-imbalanced meals. This important clinical question deserves further study.

The Time Course for Sensing IAA Deficiency

In the absence of a choice, rats stop eating an IAA-deficient meal before they are satiated, but not so quickly that the rejection could be on the basis of taste. In one Skinner box study, the fastest-responding rat stopped bar pressing for threonine-devoid pellets in 28 min (37). Using computerized online meal-pattern analysis and a threonine-devoid diet, Koehnle and colleagues found that 90% of the rats eating an IAA-deficient meal stopped eating in 20 min, whereas 50% of the control rats continued eating their balanced meal (66–68). These meal terminations are not due to satiety, as evidenced by the absence of the satiety sequence (24).

In a choice situation, the deficient diet was rejected in 15 to 30 min (37). Within five days of exposure to a lysine-deficient diet, groups of rats locate the bottle containing a bitter solution of lysine HCl among 15 bottles containing various solutions. As long as the rats remain lysine deficient, they continue to ingest enough lysine HCl solution to replete their lysine stores (83, 103, 104). Very soon

Conditioned taste aversion: single-trial long-term learning, associating malaise with a flavor, i.e., smell and/or taste, also known as bait shyness or the Garcia effect

CaMKII: calcium calmodulin dependent protein kinase II. The phosphorylated form, CaMKII-P, is the active form

tRNA: transfer ribonucleic acid

after the rats are given a diet containing adequate lysine, they switch their fluid intake to a preferred solution (83). These results replicate earlier studies with histidine HCl in solution (95). Similarly, rats rapidly increase their rate of eating within 30 min when switched from an IAA-deficient or imbalanced diet to a complete diet (94). Thus, the time to sensing IAA repletion is less than 30 min. The evidence is clear that the biochemical and neurobiological mechanisms for IAA sensing must be studied in the very short term, i.e., less than 30 min.

THE CHEMOSENSOR FOR IAA DEFICIENCY

The Anterior Piriform Cortex in the Brain

Evidence that the chemosensor for IAA deficiency is not in the gastrointestinal tract and does not involve the classical chemical senses of either taste or smell has been thoroughly reviewed (33–36, 41, 50, 94, 95). Rather, the involvement of the brain in responding to IAA depletion was first suggested by the finding that, after an IAA-imbalanced meal, the limiting IAA decreased in brain tissue as rapidly as it did in the plasma (90). Also, infusions of the limiting IAA reverse the feeding response to an IAA-imbalanced diet at a much lower concentration in the carotid artery than in the jugular vein (72). Using the classical brain-lesioning techniques that were state of the art in the 1960s, Leung and Rogers destroyed a series of brain areas associated with feeding and the food selection circuitry (33, 74, 95); the chemosensor for IAA depletion was found in the very rostral brain area called the anterior prepyriform cortex, now termed the anterior piriform cortex (APC) (73). Rats with lesions in the APC fail to reject IAA-deficient diets (73). Subsequently, this finding was replicated in the rat (87) and in the bird (25). Later microinjection and histochemical studies provided confirmatory results (10, 82, 96, 99).

THE MECHANISM

The question arising from the various behavioral observations was, "The responses are rapid and reliable, but how do the animals know the diet is deficient?" Several important transcriptional effects of AA depletion are known to occur in a matter of a few hours, and have been the subject of an excellent recent review (63). However, it is highly unlikely that gene transcription activates neuronal signaling within a half hour.

General Amino Acid–Control Pathway

The biochemical pathway in the APC that serves as the sensory limb in an IAA-detection system is conserved across eukaryotic species (48) and is activated within the requisite 20-min period for identification of the IAA sensor. The initial event, after ingestion of an IAA-imbalanced or -deficient diet, is a decrease in the concentration of the limiting IAA in the APC; the limiting IAA is decreased in APC tissue by 56% at 21 min (67) (**Figure 1**, see color insert).

In the earliest steps leading to the initiation of mRNA translation, AAs are acylated (charged) to transfer ribonucleic acid (tRNA) by their cognate amino acyl tRNA synthetases. Although the dispensable AAs are by definition continuously available, in IAA depletion, the cognate tRNA may be deacylated (uncharged). The abundance of deacylated tRNA in vivo is controversial because the Kms for the amino acyl synthetases are very low (101). Dennis and colleagues (19) reported no change in deacylated tRNA after AA deprivation in serum-starved, transformed HEK293 (kidney) cells. However, experimental differences such as timing (78) may affect the results. A deficient meal is rejected by 20 min after first introduction of the diet, so the initial signal must have occurred by 20 min if it is to relate to the signal for meal termination. Differences due to tissue source (e.g., kidney versus neuron) are highly likely as well;

even in neural tissue, the responsive cells are in a very restricted area of the APC, falling in a rostro-caudal segment of the ventrolateral forebrain extending less than 1 mm in layer II of the APC (99).

A role for uncharged tRNA in sensing IAA deficiency by animals was shown directly by microinjecting nmol amounts of tRNA synthetase inhibitors (amino alcohols) precisely into the rat APC and observing the behavioral response (36, 41, 48). Aminoalcohols inhibit their respective amino-acyl-tRNA synthetases, increasing the concentration of deacylated tRNA (45). The effects of L-amino alcohols are stereospecific, competitive, and selective for their respective AA (36, 41, 48). Injection of nmol amounts of L-threoninol or L-leucinol, but neither D-threoninol nor a dispensable AA, into the APC decreases food intake at 20 min, the same as eating an IAA-devoid diet. These are the reciprocal of studies in which nmols of the limiting IAA, microinjected into the APC, restore feeding of an IAA-deficient or -imbalanced diet (10, 82, 96).

The next step in the yeast GCN pathway is the activation of the GCN2 kinase (52), which dimerizes and autophosphorylates when uncharged tRNA binds to a nonselective histidine tRNA site (HisRS; 88, 110). When a threonine-devoid diet is fed to naïve mice lacking the gene encoding the GCN2 kinase (*GCN2*$^{-/-}$ mice), they continue eating this IAA-depleting diet (48) while naïve intact mice reject it. Maurin and colleagues (80) confirmed this finding in their report that mice having a brain-specific deletion of *GCN2* also fail to reject an IAA-deficient diet and apparently do not develop the usual learned aversion to the IAA-depleting diet. Thus, conditioned aversion to an IAA-depleting diet may also be affected in the knockout mice. Of course, if the animals don't recognize that there is something amiss with the diet, they are unlikely to develop an aversion to it. In accord with this, lesions of the hippocampus, an area involved in learning, interfere with learning in rats fed IAA-imbalanced diets; the expected conditioned taste aversion is delayed (71). Other brain areas associated with IAA deficiency and aversion learning have been studied with similar results (34).

The activated kinase, GCN2-P, phosphorylates the alpha subunit of eukaryotic initiation factor 2 (eIF2α) (20, 109), a pivotal factor in the control of the initiation of translation in protein synthesis (5, 6, 109). The intact mouse not only rejects a threonine-devoid diet, but also responds by increasing the phosphorylation of eIF2α in APC neurons (48, 80), as does the rat (42). In contrast, the *GCN2*$^{-/-}$ mice neither reject the diet nor phosphorylate eIF2α (36, 41, 48).

GCN2 has interactions with the target of rapamycin (TOR) and its mammalian form (mammalian target of rapamycin; mTOR) in several models (5, 15, 53, 58). Not all cell types regulate mTOR through charging levels of tRNA, as some are resistant to activation by amino alcohols (93). To our knowledge, mTOR, despite its role in sensing rich sources of leucine and other nutrients in brain (18), has not been shown to have a direct role in detection of IAA deficiency (36). Still, IAA depletion, by limiting the mTOR agonists, could reduce its activation via a number of different pathways (113). To address this question, Hao and colleagues (46, 85) injected rapamycin into the APC and saw no effect on intake either of a control (basal) or IAA-deficient (threonine-devoid) diet from 20 min to 21 h after diet introduction. Therefore, the feeding response to IAA deficiency in the rat is not sensitive to rapamycin. Still, a rapamycin-insensitive mTOR complex (mTORC2) could be involved in the APC's responses to IAA deficiency, as mTORC2 is associated with the cytoskeleton and an actin-binding protein, IMPACT, inhibits activation of GCN2 (91). As noted above, mTOR is activated in the hypothalamus by injections of leucine; the feeding result is an inhibition of food intake by 4 h (18). Because mTOR is activated by many nutrients and energy sources, including glucose

General amino acid nonderepressing kinase 2 (GCN2): the eIF2α kinase activated by deficiencies of IAA, via uncharged tRNA

GCN2$^{-/-}$ mice: transgenic mice lacking the gene for GCN2

eIF2α: eukaryotic initiation factor 2 alpha. The phosphorylated form, eIF2α-P, is activated by phosphorylation on the alpha subunit at serine 51

mTOR: mammalian target of rapamycin

mTORC1/2: mammalian target of rapamycin complexes 1 and 2

GABA: gamma amino butyric acid

eIF2α-P: blocks initiation of translation at the formation of the ternary complex

Methylated amino-isobutyric acid (MeAIB): the classical substrate and indicator of System A amino acid transporter activity

Sodium-dependent neutral amino acid transporter (SNAT): formerly called ATA, System A amino acid transporter

and ATP, but in some models it is unaffected by AA deprivation (19), mTOR seems unlikely to be activated by depletion of a single IAA. However, the absence of mTOR's kinase activities such as phosphorylation of ribosomal proteins (4) in IAA deficiency could initiate signaling in other pathways. Alternatively, because other IAAs are increased, at least relatively, when one is depleted as in IAA imbalanced or single-IAA-devoid diets, the imbalance could cause activation of mTOR and the resulting decrease in food intake. This question remains open inasmuch as a role for mTOR no longer can be ruled out by rapamycin insensitivity.

Taken together, the evidence suggests a clear pathway for the first four steps in the mechanism for sensing IAA deficiency in the APC (**Figure 1**). Several attractive hypotheses have the potential to explain step 5, neuronal depolarization. Still, the precise mechanism for activating APC neurons in IAA deficiency has not yet been determined.

Biochemical Events Downstream of eIF2α Phosphorylation

Excitability of the APC. As a member of the olfactory cortical system (43), the APC is continually being activated by each breath in the respiratory rhythm, apart from its role in olfaction (26). Although destruction of the APC abolishes the animal's ability to reject an IAA-deficient diet (73), olfactory bulbectomy does not (70), so the IAA sensor in the APC is not dependent on the sense of smell. Another aspect of the APC, in its role as the IAA chemosensor, is that this brain area has the lowest threshold of any area in the brain for chemical stimulation by GABAergic antagonists (21, 22, 31). Indeed, its alternative name is the area tempestas (23). Such sensitivity is likely because the APC contains a paucity of inhibitory elements (23) and recurrent excitatory circuitry (43). This combination of neuronal elements sets up the probability for easy activation of the APC (61). A variety of signaling pathways affected by eIF2α and related kinases in the responses to IAA deficiency could be involved in exciting this highly sensitive brain area.

Transporter activation. The effects of IAA limitation on AA transporters have been very well reviewed (16, 57, 63, 64, 76, 89). A role for AA sensing also has been proposed for a calcium receptor (17). Although this receptor responds stereospecifically to most of the standard L-AA that are used in protein synthesis, selectivity for any particular IAA cannot be assumed. The cationic AA transporters are inducible by limitation for any IAA and not by dispensable AA, but there is a delay of 2 h for induction and a dependence on phosphorylation of eIF2α, suggesting that synthesis of new transporters is involved (51). Such delays and dependence on eIF2α-P indicate that these transporters are downstream from IAA sensing, although they help remediate the IAA deficiency in response to other signals by importing limiting IAA into the cell.

The classical system A amino acid transporter family is sodium dependent and was defined using 2 (methyl-amino) isobutyric acid (MeAIB) (11, 51, 76, 89). Recent studies have cloned and renamed the System A transporters (formerly ATA) the sodium-dependent neutral amino acid transporters SNAT1, 2, and 4. Both SNAT1 and 2 are found in brain (76). The IAA-sensitive cells in APC are the glutamatergic pyramidal cells (61) and so may use either SNAT1 or 2 as their System A transporters. Although threonine is not the preferred substrate for either SNAT1 or SNAT2, it is carried by System A (2).

MeAIB-blockable transport of labeled threonine is activated within 10 min after exposing neuron-rich cultures from the IAA-sensitive APC to a threonine-devoid medium (11, 36, 41). This rapid activation is likely due to recruitment rather than gene expression (75). Consistent with this finding, the rapid MeAIB-sensitive uptake of threonine in threonine-deficient APC neurons is

Sensory Limb of the Response

Step 1: Limiting IAA is decreased in APC by 20 min after introduction of the deficient diet

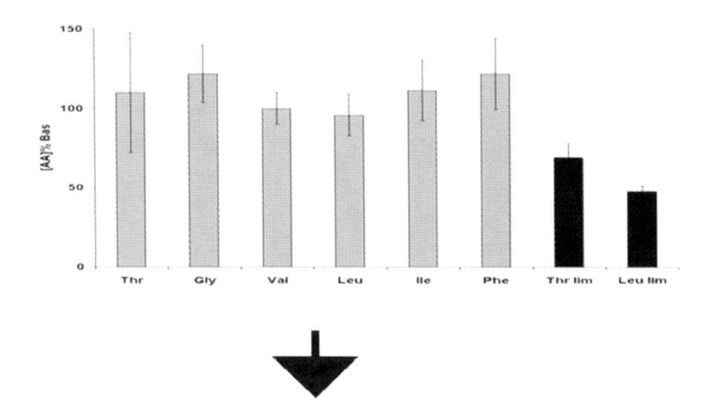

Step 2: Deacylated tRNA

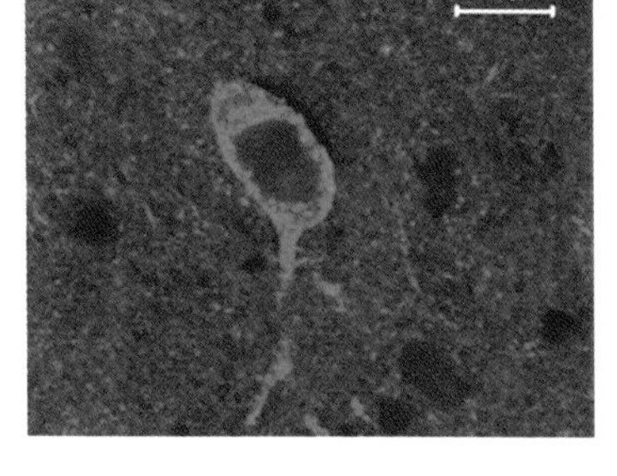

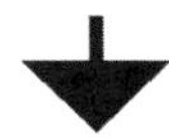

Step 3: Activated GCN2, an eIF2α kinase

Step 4: Phosphorylated eIF2α in APC pyramidal cells

Figure 1

The mechanisms underlying the sensory limb of the responses to dietary indispensable amino acid (IAA) deficiency are listed as steps 1–4. Bars in the top figure indicate the amino acid (AA) concentrations (common three-letter abbreviations on the *X* axis) of nonlimiting AAs (*blue*) or limiting IAA (*black*) in anterior piriform cortex (APC) tissue taken 20 min after introduction of a threonine- or leucine-devoid diet are given as a percent of control. *Black bars* show the decrease in the limiting IAA at 20 min after introduction of the appropriate IAA-deficient diet. Steps 2–4 describe the next three biochemical events, similar in yeast and in the rodent APC, after IAA depletion. (*Right*) Micrograph of a pyramidal cell from rat APC layer II showing increased fluorescence for eIF2alpha in the cytoplasm. The tissue was taken 20 min after introduction of a threonine-devoid meal (42).

Integration in the APC:
The Signaling Pathways

ERK1/2:
Activation in the
cytoplasm of the
primary cell
(20 min)

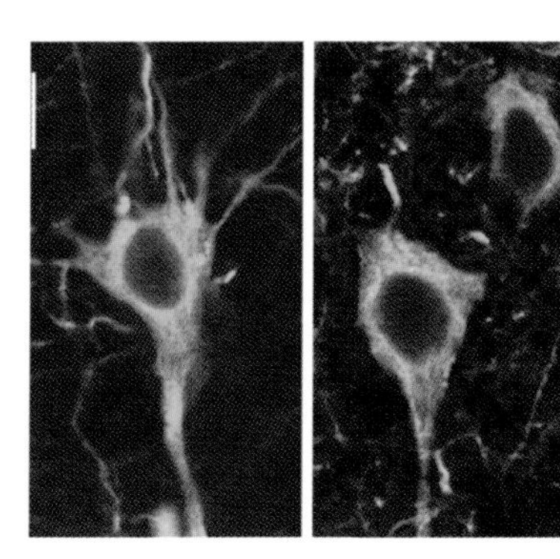

CaMKII:
Activation of
APC circuitry
(20 min)

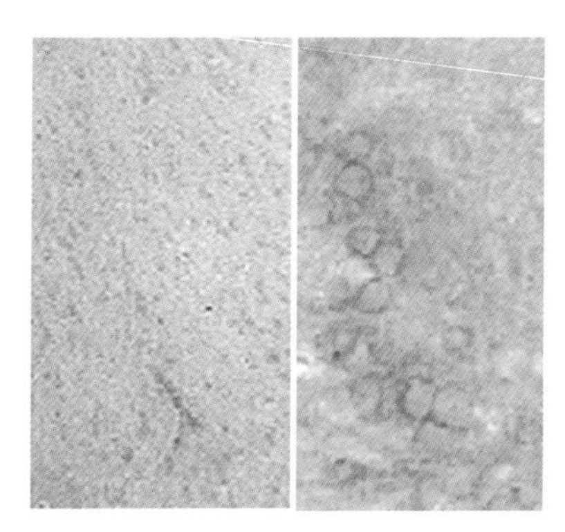

cFos:
Activation of
gene
expression
(later)

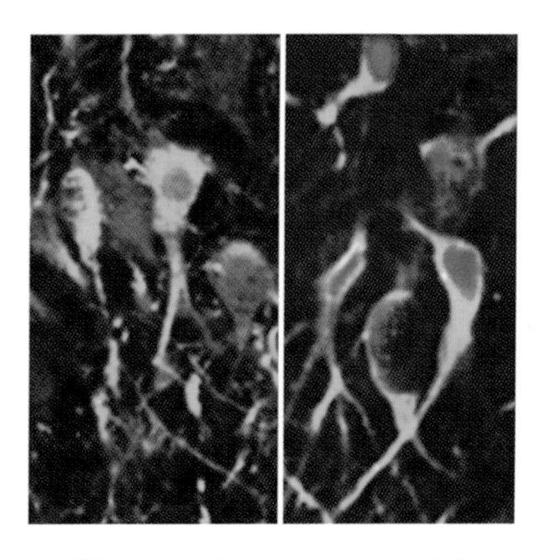

Control Devoid

Figure 2

See legend on next page

Figure 2

Integration in the anterior piriform cortex (APC). Examples of micrographs show signal transduction in the pyramidal cells of the APC. (*Top*) Phosphorylated extracellular signal-related kinase 1/2 (ERK1/2) in the cytoplasm. Green is a neuronal marker; red is a fluorescence-tagged antibody to ERK1/2. (*Middle*) Phosphorylated calcium calmodulin kinase II (CaMKII-P) in layer II of the APC. CaMKII-P is seen in many more neurons (*right panel*) than either ERK (**Figure 2**, *top*) or eIF2α-P (**Figure 1**, *bottom right*). (*Bottom*) The immediate early gene, c-Fos (red in nuclei), used here to show that 45 min after eating a threonine-devoid diet, gene expression can be seen. *Left panels*, control; *right panels*, devoid treatment.

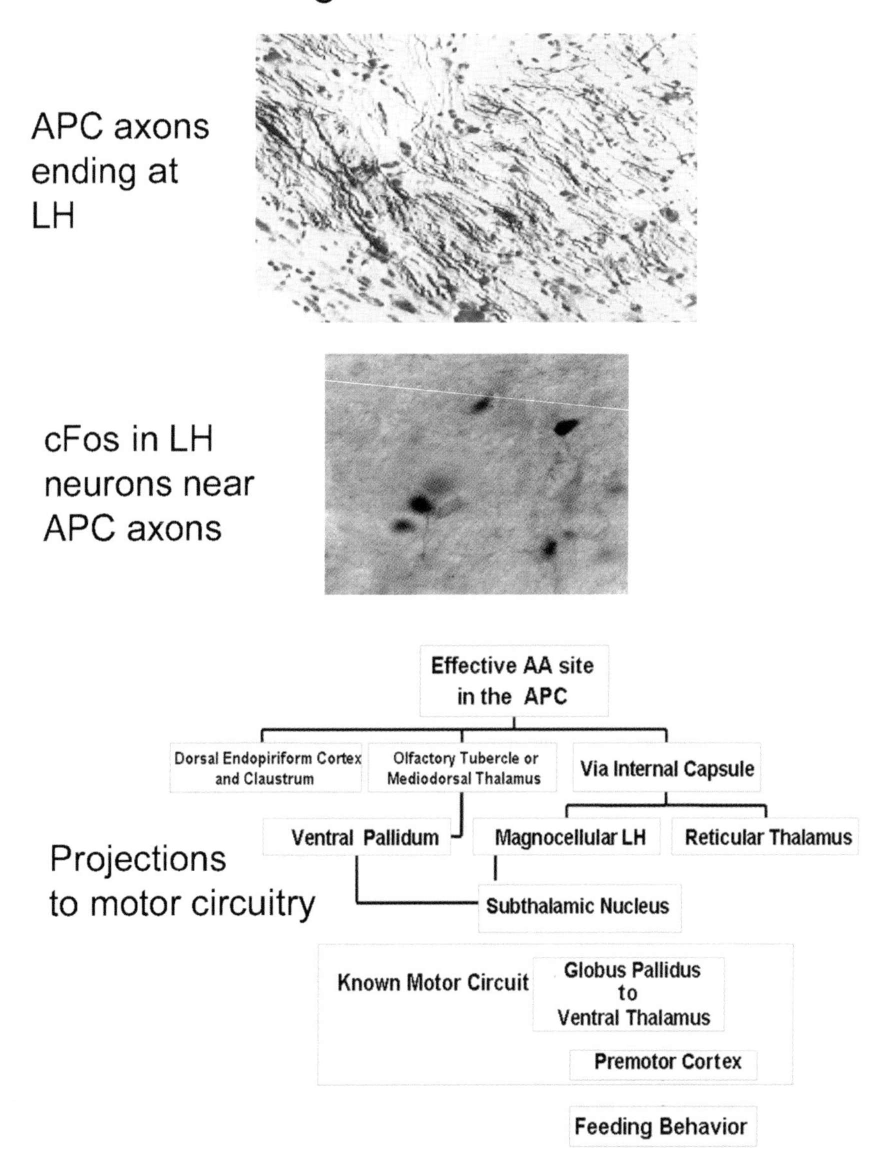

Figure 3

Representative data for output signaling from the anterior piriform cortex (APC). (*Top*) Dark lines extending from top left are biocytin-stained axons from APC neurons at their termination in the lateral hypothalamus. (*Middle*) Brown staining from upper right corner is of APC axons extending into the lateral hypothalamus and ending around or near c-Fos positive cells (*black*). (*Bottom*) Selected motor pathways traced from the APC after injections of the tract-tracing agent biocytin. Shown here are brain areas in known motor pathways where APC axon terminals were seen. AA, amino acid; LH, lateral hypothalamus.

dependent on phosphorylation for activation and movement to the membrane, placing it downstream of eIF2α-P (11). Increased translation of mRNA for SNAT2 in mouse embryonic fibroblasts deprived of IAA for 1 h also depends on phosphorylation of eIF2α (30). Of interest here, the increased intracellular sodium from cotransport by system A [either SNAT1 or SNAT2 (ATA1 or ATA2)] is electrogenic (2, 114), so it can depolarize a neuron, such as the glutamatergic output cells of the APC.

MAPK/ERK1/2 signaling. If the neurons of the APC are activated by increased intracellular sodium via the SNATs (11, 30), which require activation by eIF2α-P (30), then mitogen-activated protein kinase (MAPK)/ERK1/2 (27) should be involved as well. The cells colocalizing MAPK-P and eIF2α-P appear in a narrow (<1 mm) rostrocaudal segment of the cell body layer of the pyramidal output neurons of the APC (99). These MAPK-P + eIF2α-P-positive neurons may be the primary sensory cells that recognize IAA deficiency in the APC. In addition, the ERK1/2 signaling system is associated with neuronal excitation, giving another mechanism for excitation of signaling in the APC (97, 99). An APC neuron positive for ERK1/2 antibodies may be seen in **Figure 2** (see color insert).

Glutamatergic activity. Glutamate is the transmitter of the primary output cells of the APC (61). Releasable glutamate could be increased in the cells by transamination (56) of the IAAs that are in relative excess with the relative imbalance and that cannot be used for protein synthesis because translation is inhibited in the presence of eIF2α-P (4, 5, 109). Other sources of glutamatergic activity include the glutamate-glutamine cycle, which provides glutamate for neural transmission (56). Evidence supports the importance of glutamate α-amino-3-hydroxy-5-methyl-4-isoxazole propionate (AMPA) receptors in the behavioral and biochemical responses to IAA deficiency, secondary to the initial signal in the APC (39, 47, 100). When rats are injected with an AMPA receptor antagonist 1 h prior to receiving an IAA-deficient meal, they do not reject the meal, as do saline-injected rats (47). Therefore, metabolic activation of the glutamate output cells of the APC after ingestion of an IAA-deficient diet also has potential importance for signaling IAA depletion.

Intracellular calcium. In addition to sodium, ERK1/2, and glutamate, both intra- and extracellular sources of calcium are involved in the acute responses of the APC to IAA depletion. There are changes in intracellular calcium in the APC with changes in IAA but not dispensable AA (77), as well as increased phosphorylation of calcium calmodulin-dependent protein kinase II (CaMKII) in the cell body layer that houses the primary output neurons of the APC (100). CaMKII-P is a well-known indicator of increased intracellular calcium, and it is elevated within the 20 min window for the behavioral rejection of an IAA-depleting diet (**Figure 2**). CaMKII, among other functions, activates the glutamate AMPA receptor, GluR1, by phosphorylation in the postsynaptic density (106). Colocalization of CaMKII-P and the glutamate AMPA receptor subunit (GluR1) as GluR1-P in APC neurons, both already increased within 20 min after the introduction of an IAA-deficient diet, provides evidence for both calcium and glutamate in signaling IAA deficiency in the APC (100). CaMKII-P appears in far more APC cells than does eIF2α-P, and its increase in an IAA-depleted APC slice preparation depends on extracellular calcium (unpublished observation). Therefore, this phosphorylated kinase is likely to be in the postsynaptic (secondary) cells of the APC, which are activated in the positive feedback loop that characterizes the piriform cortex (43, 69) as well as in the primary chemosensory cells. The output signals are likely enhanced by such recruitment.

MAPK: mitogen-activated protein kinase; MAPK-P, the phosphorylated form

ERK1/2: extracellular signal-related kinase 1/2, a MAPK, active when phosphorylated

GABAergic signaling. Gamma amino butyric acid (GABA) is the primary source of inhibitory neurotransmission in the brain (79) and is crucially important in maintaining normal levels of neuronal activity in the APC (21, 22), providing damping of the recurrent excitatory circuitry. Agonists and antagonists of the GABAergic system injected into the APC of animals fed IAA-depleting diets have provided results correlating activity of the GABA system with food intake (105). This suggests that inhibitory transmission is associated with controlling the downstream effects of APC signaling, more directly involved in the food intake response, rather than with the chemosensory role of the APC. Recent results suggest that both the $GABA_A$ receptor and its associated potassium-chloride cotransporter are downregulated in the membranes of the APC 20 min after rats are offered a threonine-deficient meal (98). In addition, the β-3 subunit of the GABA receptor is downregulated at 2 h after an IAA-imbalanced meal (105). These proteins have short half-lives and require new translation for their continued presence in the membrane. In the presence of phosphorylated eIF2α, translation is blocked (4–6, 36, 41, 109), so the loss of rapidly turning-over membrane proteins, including GABA receptors, may be prolonged. The loss of GABAergic inhibition could be a major factor in exciting the APC (21, 22, 31, 98).

In sum, several downstream signaling pathways are candidates for an activating role in APC signaling of IAA deficiency. These include (*a*) sodium cotransport by System A transporters (11), dependent on ERK1/2 (27, 97, 99); (*b*) increased glutamate neurotransmission with either transamination or the glutamate-glutamine cycle, based on AA metabolism in the cells (56); (*c*) increased intracellular calcium from intracellular and extracellular sources (100); and (*d*) loss of GABAergic inhibition due to a rapid turnover of the protein and absence of new translation in the presence of eIF2α-P (48, 98, 109).

NEURAL CIRCUITRY AND INVOLVEMENT OF OTHER BRAIN AREAS

The APC is located in the anterior ventrolateral forebrain, and the neural circuitry associated with the feeding responses to IAA depletion has been reviewed elsewhere (34, 35, 65). Glutamatergic signaling originates in the APC, resulting from intracellular signals generated in response to IAA deficiency, such as those described above (34, 35, 39, 41). In addition to these activating systems, several neurotransmitters interact with glutamate in the APC, and inhibition of at least one receptor subtype each for serotonin, dopamine, norepinephrine, and for glutamate itself has been shown to reverse the feeding depression to IAA-deficient diets (34). This suggests that any inhibition of the glutamate output cells in the highly excitable APC will decrease signaling to food-intake-inhibitory systems and restore feeding. Taken together with the APC circuitry and oscillatory activity described above, one has a system that is poised for activation and is ideal for rapid responses to a dietary IAA deficiency.

Projections to Other Brain Areas

The APC has long been known to project to areas of the brain that are important for the control of food intake (1, 35, 44) (**Figure 3**, see color insert). Yet, several laboratories have indicated that other areas of the brain, particularly the hypothalamus (12, 83, 103, 104), are involved in the IAA response. The lateral hypothalamus is involved in the hyperphagia to 10% (moderately low) protein (112). The vagus projects AA-related information to the lateral hypothalamus (60). However, roles for the ventromedial hypothalamus and lateral hypothalamus (LH) as primary sensors of IAA deficiency were ruled out by the ablation studies of the 1970s (94). Data from Monda et al. (82) and Blevins et al. (12) suggest that the lateral hypothalamus acts secondarily, receiving signals generated in the APC (axons from the APC can be seen ending in the LH in **Figure 3**). The amygdala is important in the conditioned aversive responses, such as those for taste (33–35, 84, 95, 108). AA response elements have been studied in human hippocampal cells (63), where the much of the work on long-term potentiation is done. The most likely reconciliation of these data is that the sensing of IAA deficiency occurs in the APC and is signaled via its projections (12, 22, 35, 65, 82) to affect other brain areas, such as hypothalamic nuclei and hippocampus, or amygdala, for the feeding-motivational responses, and to motor circuits for motor acts associated with food intake, such as approach to the food cup, chewing, and swallowing (**Figure 3**).

The GCN2 Inhibitor IMPACT

Sattlegger, Castilho, and colleagues (91) have described an actin-binding protein, IMPACT, that is preferentially expressed in brain tissue and that inhibits the activation of the eIF2α kinase GCN2. The level of IMPACT is inversely correlated with the phosphorylation of eIF2α and is higher in several hypothalamic areas than in the APC (91). This could explain why the hypothalamus, which has classically been thought to house important feeding circuits (9, 13) and where mTOR responds to intra-third ventricular injections of leucine (18), has been so difficult to associate with the sensing of IAA deficiency (35, 38, 94). The paucity of the GCN2 inhibitor IMPACT in the APC is consistent with a role for GCN2 in the APC in sensing IAA deficiency (48, 80, 91).

After c-fos expression was seen in the dorsomedial hypothalamus when animals had eaten an IAA-imbalanced diet (107), this hypothalamic region was studied as well. Expression of c-fos in neuronal cell nuclei is an accepted tool for suggesting neuronal activation; micrographs showing nuclear c-fos may be seen in **Figures 1** and **3**. Cutting fibers running anteriorly from the dorsomedial hypothalamus increases intake of an IAA imbalanced diet for the entire first day, and the nucleus itself may be involved in the first 3 h of the responses (7, 8). It will be interesting to learn if IMPACT is expressed in the neurons of the dorsomedial hypothalamus.

CONCLUSIONS

The discovery of a role for the conserved GCN pathway in the APC sensing of IAA deficiency underscores the importance of AA homeostasis as crucial to survival in eukaryotes. It is likely that two separate systems function to sense increases (mTOR) or decreases (uncharged tRNA and GCN2) of IAA in the brain (36). The several signaling pathways activated by IAA deficiency downstream of eIF2α, combined with the excitable oscillating circuitry of the APC, finally yield potential mechanisms for activating the glutamatergic output cells of the APC, the chemosensor for IAA deficiency in the brain.

SUMMARY POINTS

1. Maintenance of indispensable amino acid (IAA) homeostasis is essential for protein synthesis and survival, requiring dietary selection in omnivores.
2. For appropriate dietary selection, sensing the depletion of an IAA is a crucial first step.
3. The brain area housing the IAA sensor is the anterior piriform cortex.
4. The mechanism of IAA sensing in the APC is the conserved general amino acid control pathway.

5. The four steps of the sensory mechanism are decreased IAA, increased deacylated tRNA, activation of GC nonderepressing kinase 2, and phosphorylation of eukaryotic initiation factor 2α, which binds to eIF2B and blocks initiation of translation.
6. The APC is highly excitable and has oscillatory activity coordinated with respiration.
7. Several signal transduction systems may be involved in potentiating the output cells of the APC.

FUTURE ISSUES

1. Which of the various possible mechanisms activate the output cells of the APC? Is there redundancy in the system, such that more than one signal transduction system is involved?
2. Where, precisely, among the various projection sites of the APC output cells, are the signals that cause inhibition of feeding received?
3. In spite of many years of work worldwide, the neural circuitry that controls feeding remains incompletely understood. Exactly how the motivation to eat is translated into actual food intake behavior needs to be explained.

ACKNOWLEDGMENTS

The authors appreciate the helpful comments of Drs. Beatriz Castilho and Evelyn Sattlegger about the manuscript. Financial support was provided by the NIH: NS 043210 and NS 33347 to DWG. Portions of this material, reviewed also in References 36 and 41, are used here with permission.

LITERATURE CITED

1. Aja SM. 1999. Efferent projections from the region of the anterior piriform cortex involved in aminoprivic feeding. In *Neural Transmitters and Neural Circuits Supporting Aminoprivic Feeding*, pp. 323–43. PhD thesis. Univ. Calif., Davis
2. Albers A, Bröer A, Wagner CA, Setiawan I, Lang PA. 2001. Na+ transport by the neural glutamine transporter ATA1. *Pflügers Arch.* 443:92–101
3. Anderson GH. 1977. Regulation of protein intake by plasma amino acids. In *Advances in Nutritional Research*, ed. HH Draper, 1:135–66. New York: Plenum
4. Anthony TG, Anthony JC, Yoshizawa F, Kimball SR, Jefferson LS. 2001. Oral administration of leucine stimulates ribosomal protein mRNA translation but not global rates of protein synthesis in the liver of rats. *J. Nutr.* 131:1171–76
5. Anthony TG, McDaniel BJ, Byerley RL, McGrath BC, Cavener DR, et al. 2004. Preservation of liver protein synthesis during dietary leucine deprivation occurs at the expense of skeletal muscle mass in mice deleted for eIF2 kinase GCN2. *J. Biol. Chem.* 279:36553–61
6. Anthony TG, Reiter AK, Anthony JC, Kimball SR, Jefferson LS. 2001. Deficiency of dietary EAA preferentially inhibits mRNA translation of ribosomal proteins in liver of meal-fed rats. *Am. J. Physiol.* 281:E430–39

7. Bellinger LL, Evans JF, Gietzen DW. 1998. Dorsomedial hypothalamic lesions alter intake of an imbalanced amino acid diet in rats. *J. Nutr.* 128:1213–17
8. Bellinger LL, Evans JF, Tillberg CM, Gietzen DW. 1999. Effects of dorsomedial hypothalamic nuclei lesions on intake of an imbalanced amino acid diet. *Am. J. Physiol.* 277:R250–62
9. Berthoud HR. 2002. Multiple neural systems controlling food intake and body weight. *Neurosci. Biobehav. Rev.* 26:393–428
10. Beverly JL, Gietzen DW, Rogers QR. 1990. Effect of dietary limiting amino acid in prepyriform cortex on food intake. *Am. J. Physiol.* 259:R709–15
11. Blais A, Huneau JF, Magrum LJ, Koehnle TJ, Sharp JW, et al. 2003. Threonine deprivation rapidly activates the system A amino acid transporter in primary cultures of rat neurons from the essential amino acid sensor in the anterior piriform cortex. *J. Nutr.* 133:2156–64
12. Blevins JE, Truong BG, Gietzen DW. 2004. NMDA receptor function within the anterior piriform cortex and lateral hypothalamus in rats on the control of intake of amino acid–deficient diets. *Brain Res.* 1019:124–44
13. Broberger C. 2005. Brain regulation of food intake and appetite: molecules and networks. *J. Intern. Med.* 258:301–27
14. Carpenter KJ. 2003. A short history of nutritional science: part 1 (1785–1885). *J. Nutr.* 133:638–45
15. Cherkasova VA, Hinnebusch AG. 2003. Translational control by TOR and TAP42 through dephosphorylation of eIF2α kinase GCN2. *Genes Dev.* 17:859–72
16. Christensen HN. 1990. Role of amino acid transport and countertransport in nutrition and metabolism. *Physiol. Rev.* 70:43–77
17. Conigrave AD, Quinn SJ, Brown EM. 2000. L-amino acid sensing by the extracellular Ca2+-sensing receptor. *Proc. Natl. Acad. Sci. USA* 97:4814–19
18. Cota D, Proulx K, Blake Smith KA, Kozma SC, Thomas G, et al. 2006. Hypothalamic mTOR signaling regulates food intake. *Science* 312:927–30
19. Dennis PB, Jaeschke A, Saitoh M, Fowler B, Kozma SC, et al. 2001. Mammalian TOR: a homeostatic ATP sensor. *Science* 294:1102–5
20. Dever TE. 2002. Gene-specific regulation by general translation factors. *Cell* 108:545–56
21. Doherty J, Gale K, Eagles DA. 2000. Evoked epileptiform discharges in the rat anterior piriform cortex: generation and local propagation. *Brain Res.* 861:77–87
22. Dybdal D, Gale K. 2000. Postural and anticonvulsant effects of inhibition of the rat subthalamic nucleus. *J. Neurosci.* 20:6728–33
23. **Ekstrand JJ, Domroese ME, Johnson DM, Feig SL, Knodel SM, et al. 2001. A new subdivision of anterior piriform cortex and associated deep nucleus with novel features of interest for olfaction and epilepsy. *J. Comp. Neurol.* 434:289–307**
24. Feurté S, Nicolaïdis S, Berridge KC. 2000. Conditioned taste aversion for a threonine-deficient diet in the rat: demonstration by the taste reactivity test. *Physiol. Behav.* 68:423–29
25. Firman JD, Kuenzel WJ. 1988. Neuroanatomical regions of the chick brain involved in monitoring amino acid deficient diets. *Brain Res. Bull.* 21:637–42
26. **Fontanini A, Bower JM. 2006. Slow-waves in the olfactory system: an olfactory perspective on cortical rhythms. *Trends Neurosci.* 29:429–37**
27. Franchi-Gazzola R, Visigalli R, Dall'Asta V, Gazzola GC. 1999. Adaptive increase of amino acid transport system A requires ERK1/2 activation. *J. Biol. Chem.* 274:28922–28
28. Fromentin G, Feurté S, Nicolaïdis S. 1998. Spatial cues are relevant for learned preference/aversion shifts due to amino-acid deficiencies. *Appetite* 30:223–34

23. Gives location and mechanism for activation of APC (ventro-rostral area) known as the area tempestas.

26. Reviews the importance of the olfactory cortex in setting the rate of brain rhythms.

29. Fromentin G, Gietzen DW, Nicolaïdis S. 1997. Aversion-preference patterns in amino acid– or protein-deficient rats: a comparison with previously reported responses to thiamin-deficient diets. *Br. J. Nutr.* 77:299–314
30. Gaccioli F, Huang CC, Wang C, Bevilacqua E, Franchi-Gazzola R. 2006. Amino acid starvation induces the SNAT2 neutral amino acid transporter by a mechanism that involves eukaryotic initiation factor 2α phosphorylation and cap-independent translation. *J. Biol. Chem.* 281:17929–40
31. Gale K. 1988. Progression and generalization of seizure discharge: anatomical and neurochemical substrates. *Epilepsia* 29:S15–34
32. **Garcia J, Kimeldorf DJ, Koelling RA. 1955. Conditioned aversion to saccharin resulting from exposure to gamma radiation. *Science* 122:157–58**
33. Gietzen DW. 1993. Neural mechanisms in the responses to amino acid deficiency. *J. Nutr.* 123:610–25
34. Gietzen DW. 2000. Amino acid recognition in the central nervous system. In *Neural and Metabolic Control of Macronutrient Intake*, ed. HR Berthoud, RJ Seeley, pp. 339–57. New York: CRC Press
35. Gietzen DW, Erecius LF, Rogers QR. 1998. Neurochemical changes after imbalanced diets suggest a brain circuit mediating anorectic responses to amino acid deficiency. *J. Nutr.* 128:71–81
36. Gietzen DW, Hao S, Anthony TG. 2007. Amino acid sensing mechanisms: the biochemistry and the behavior. In *Handbook of Neurochemistry and Molecular Neurobiology*, ed. A Lajtha, Vol. 20C-10. New York: Kluwer/Plenum
37. Gietzen DW, Leung PMB, Castonguay TW, Hartman WJ, Rogers QR. 1986. Time course of food intake and plasma and brain amino acid concentrations in rats fed amino acid–imbalanced or -deficient diets. In *Interactions of the Chemical Senses with Nutrition*, ed. MR Kare, JG Brand, pp. 415–59. Philadelphia, PA: Academic
38. Gietzen DW, Leung PMB, Rogers QR. 1989. Dietary amino acid imbalance and neurochemical changes in three hypothalamic areas. *Physiol. Behav.* 46:503–11
39. Gietzen DW, Magrum LJ. 2001. Molecular mechanisms involved in the anorexia of branched chain amino acid deficiency. *J. Nutr.* 131:851–55S
40. Gietzen DW, McArthur LH, Theisen JC, Rogers QR. 1992. Learned preference for the limiting amino acid in rats fed a threonine-deficient diet. *Physiol. Behav.* 51:909–14
41. Gietzen DW, Rogers QR. 2006. Nutritional homeostasis and indispensable amino acid sensing: a new solution to an old puzzle. *Trends Neurosci.* 29:91–99
42. Gietzen DW, Ross CM, Hao S, Sharp JW. 2004. Phosphorylation of eIF2α is involved in the signaling of indispensable amino acid deficiency in the anterior piriform cortex of the brain in rats. *J. Nutr.* 134:717–23
43. Haberly LB. 2001. Parallel-distributed processing in olfactory cortex: new insights from morphological and physiological analysis of neuronal circuitry. *Chem. Senses* 26:551–76
44. Haberly LB, Price JL. 1978. Association and commissural fiber systems of the olfactory cortex of the rat: 1. Systems originating in the piriform cortex and adjacent areas. *J. Comp. Neurol.* 178:711–40
45. Hansen BS, Vaughan MH, Wang LJ. 1972. Reversible inhibition by histidinol of protein synthesis in human cells at the activation of histidine. *J. Biol. Chem.* 247:3854–57
46. Hao S, Ross-Inta CM, Gietzen DW. 2006. Rapamysin independent responses to amino acid deficiency in the anterior piriform cortex. Manuscr. submitted
47. Hao S, Ross-Inta CM, Rudell JB, Sharp JW, Gietzen DW. 2005. The role of glutamate AMPA receptors in the recognition of amino acid deficiency in the anterior piriform cortex of rats. *FASEB J.* 20: #970.6 (Abstr.)

32. First description of "bait shyness," single-trial learning based on gastrointestinal distress.

48. Hao S, Sharp JW, Ross-Inta CM, McDaniel BJ, Anthony TG, et al. 2005. Uncharged tRNA and sensing of amino acid deficiency in mammalian piriform cortex. *Science* 307:1776–78
49. Harper AE. 1976. Protein and amino acids in the regulation of food intake. In *Hunger: Basic Mechanisms and Clinical Implications*, ed. D Novin, W Wyrwicka, G Bray, pp. 103–13. New York: Raven
50. Harper AE, Benevenga NJ, Wohlhueter RM. 1970. Effects of ingestion of disproportionate amounts of amino acids. *Physiol. Rev.* 50:428–58
51. Hatzoglou M, Fernandez J, Yaman I. 2004. Regulation of cationic amino acid transport: the story of the CAT-1 transporter. *Annu. Rev. Nutr.* 24:377–99
52. Hinnebusch AG. 2000. Mechanism and regulation of initiator methionyl-tRNA binding to ribosomes. In *Translational Control of Gene Expression*, ed. N Sonenberg, JWB Hershey, MB Matthews, pp. 185–243. New York: Cold Spring Harbor Lab. Press
53. Hinnebusch AG, Natarajan K. 2002. Gcn4p, a master regulator of gene expression, is controlled at multiple levels by diverse signals of starvation and stress. *Eukaryot. Cell* 1:22–32
54. Hrupka BJ, Lin Y, Gietzen DW, Rogers QR. 1997. Small changes in essential amino acid concentrations dictate diet selection in amino acid–deficient states. *J. Nutr.* 127:777–84
55. Hrupka BJ, Lin Y, Gietzen DW, Rogers QR. 1999. Lysine deficiency alters diet selection without depressing food intake in rats. *J. Nutr.* 129:424–30
56. Hutson SM, Lieth E, LaNoue KF. 2001. Function of leucine in excitatory neurotransmitter metabolism in the central nervous system. *J. Nutr.* 131:846–50S
57. Hyde R, Taylor PM, Hundal HS. 2003. Amino acid transporters: roles in amino acid sensing and signaling in animal cells. *Biochem. J.* 373:1–18
58. Iiboshi Y, Papst PJ, Kawasome H, Hosoi H, Abraham RT, et al. 1999. Amino acid–dependent control of p70s6k: involvement of tRNA aminoacylation in the regulation. *J. Biol. Chem.* 274:1092–99
59. Ishii Y, Blundell JE, Halford JC, Rodgers RJ. 2003. Palatability, food intake and the behavioural satiety sequence in male rats. *Physiol. Behav.* 80:37–47
60. Jeanningros R. 1984. Lateral hypothalamic responses to preabsorptive and postabsorptive signals related to amino acid ingestion. *J. Auton. Nerv. Syst.* 10:261–68
61. Jung MW, Larson J, Lynch G. 1990. Role of NMDA and non-NMDA receptors in synaptic transmission in rat piriform cortex. *Exp. Brain Res.* 82:451–55
62. Kadowaki M, Kanazawa T. 2003. Amino acids as regulators of proteolysis. *J. Nutr.* 133:2052–56S
63. Kilberg MS, Pan YX, Chen H. 2005. Nutritional control of gene expression: how mammalian cells respond to amino acid limitation. *Annu. Rev. Nutr.* 25:59–85
64. Kilberg MS, Stevens BR, Novak C. 1993. Recent advances in mammalian amino acid transport. *Annu. Rev. Nutr.* 13:137–65
65. Koehnle TJ, Gietzen DW. 2005. Modulation of feeding behavior by amino acid deficient diets; present findings and future directions. In *Nutritional Neuroscience*, ed. HR Lieberman, RB Kanarek, C Prasad, pp. 147–61. Boca Raton, FL: CRC Press
66. Koehnle TJ, Russell MC, Gietzen DW. 2003. Rats rapidly reject diets deficient in essential amino acids. *J. Nutr.* 133:2331–35
67. Koehnle TJ, Russell MC, Morin AS, Erecius L, Gietzen DW. 2004. Diets deficient in indispensable amino acids rapidly decrease the concentration of the limiting amino acid in the anterior piriform cortex of rats. *J. Nutr.* 134:2365–71

50. Provides a definitive review of the topic up to 1970.

54. Determined the threshold of sensitivity for detection of IAA deficiency.

63. Provides an excellent review of gene transcription in IAA deficiency.

68. Koehnle TJ, Stephens AL, Gietzen DW. 2004. Threonine imbalanced diet alters first meal microstructure in rats. *Physiol. Behav.* 81:15–21
69. Larson J, Jessen RE, Kim D, Fine AK, du Hoffmann J. 2005. Age-dependent and selective impairment of long-term potentiation in the anterior piriform cortex of mice lacking the fragile X mental retardation protein. *J. Neurosci.* 25:9460–69
70. Leung PMB, Larson DM, Rogers QR. 1972. Food intake and preference of olfactory bulbectomized rats fed amino acid imbalanced or deficient diets. *Physiol. Behav.* 9:553–57
71. Leung PMB, Rogers QR. 1979. Effects of hippocampal lesions on adaptive intake of diets with disproportionate amounts of amino acids. *Physiol. Behav.* 23:129–36
72. Leung PMB, Rogers QR. 1969. Food intake: regulation by plasma amino acid pattern. *Life Sci.* 8:1–9
73. **Leung PMB, Rogers QR. 1971. Importance of prepyriform cortex in food-intake response of rats to amino acids. *Am. J. Physiol.* 221:929–35**

73. Describes discovery of APC as an IAA chemosensor.

74. Leung PMB, Rogers QR. 1987. The effect of amino acids and protein on dietary choice. In *Umami: A Basic Taste*, ed. Y Kawamura, MR Kare, pp 565–610. New York: Marcel Decker
75. Ling R, Bridges CC, Sugawara M, Fujita T, Leibach FH, et al. 2001. Involvement of transporter recruitment as well as gene expression in the substrate-induced adaptive regulation of amino acid transport system A. *Biochim. Biophys. Acta* 1512:15–21
76. Mackenzie B, Erickson JD. 2004. Sodium-coupled neutral amino acid (system N/A) transporters of the SLC38 gene family. *Pflügers Arch.* 447:784–95
77. Magrum LJ, Hickman MA, Gietzen DW. 1999. Increased intracellular calcium in rat anterior piriform cortex in response to threonine after threonine deprivation. *J. Neurophysiol.* 81:1147–49
78. Magrum LJ, Teh PS, Kreiter MR, Hickman MA, Gietzen DW. 2002. Transfer ribonucleic acid charging in rat brain after consumption of amino acid–imbalanced diets. *Nutr. Neurosci.* 5:125–30
79. Manns ID, Alonso A, Jones BE. 2003. Rhythmically discharging basal forebrain units comprise cholinergic, GABAergic, and putative glutamatergic cells. *J. Neurophysiol.* 89:1057–66
80. Maurin AC, Jousse C, Averous J, Parry L, Bruhat A, et al. 2005. The GCN2 kinase biases feeding behavior to maintain amino acid homeostasis in omnivores. *Cell Metab.* 1:273–77
81. **McCoy RH, Meyer CE, Rose WC. 1935. Feeding experiments with mixtures of highly purified amino acids. VIII. Isolation and identification of a new essential amino acid. *J. Biol. Chem.* 112:283–302**

81. Describes discovery of final IAA, threonine.

82. Monda M, Sullo A, DeLuca V, Pellicano MP, Viggiano A. 1997. L-threonine injection into PPC modifies food intake, lateral hypothalamic activity, and sympathetic discharge. *Am. J. Physiol.* 273:R554–59
83. Mori M, Kawada T, Ono T, Torii K. 1991. Taste preference and protein nutrition and L-amino acid homeostasis in male Sprague-Dawley rats. *Physiol. Behav.* 49:987–95
84. Naito-Hoopes M, McArthur LH, Gietzen DW, Rogers QR. 1993. Learned preference and aversion for complete and isoleucine-devoid diets in the rat. *Physiol. Behav.* 53:485–94
85. Nemanic S, Ross CM, Hao S, Rudell JB, Gietzen DW. 2004. The effects of rapamycin injected into the anterior piriform cortex on food intake in rats. *FASEB J.* 19: #125.3 (Abstr.)
86. Nicoll RA, Schmitz D. 2005. Synaptic plasticity at hippocampal mossy fiber synapses. *Nat. Rev. Neurosci.* 6:863–76
87. Noda K, Chikamori K. 1976. Effect of ammonia via prepyriform cortex on regulation of food intake in the rat. *Am. J. Physiol.* 231:1263–66

88. Padyana AK, Qiu H, Roll-Mecak A, Hinnebusch AG, Burley SK. 2005. Structural basis for autoinhibition and mutational activation of eukaryotic initiation factor 2α protein kinase GCN2. *J. Biol. Chem.* 280:29289–99
89. Palacin M, Estevez R, Bertran J, Zorzano A. 1998. Molecular biology of mammalian plasma membrane amino acid transporters. *Physiol. Rev.* 78:969–1054
90. Peng Y, Tews JK, Harper AE. 1972. Amino acid imbalance, protein intake, and changes in rat brain and plasma amino acids. *Am. J. Physiol.* 222:314–21
91. Pereira CM, Sattlegger E, Jiang HY, Longo BM, Jaqueta CB, et al. 2005. IMPACT, a protein preferentially expressed in the mouse brain, binds GCN1 and inhibits GCN2 activation. *J. Biol. Chem.* 280:28316–23
92. Peters JC, Harper AE. 1984. Influence of dietary protein level on protein self-selection and plasma and brain amino acid concentrations. *Physiol. Behav.* 33:783–90
93. Pham PTT, Heydrick SJ, Fox HL, Kimball SR, Jefferson LS Jr, et al. 2000. Assessment of cell-signaling pathways in the regulation of mammalian target of rapamycin (mTOR) by amino acids in rat adipocytes. *J. Cell. Biochem.* 79:427–41
94. Rogers QR, Leung PMB. 1973. The influence of amino acids on the neuroregulation of food intake. *Fed. Proc.* 32:1709–19
95. Rogers QR, Leung PMB. 1977. The control of food intake: When and how are amino acids involved? In *The Chemical Senses and Nutrition*, ed. MR Kare, O Maller, pp. 213–49. New York: Academic
96. Russell MC, Koehnle TJ, Barrett JA, Blevins JE, Gietzen DW. 2003. The rapid anorectic response to a threonine imbalanced diet is decreased by injection of threonine into the anterior piriform cortex of rats. *Nutr. Neurosci.* 6:247–51
97. Sharp JW, Magrum LJ, Gietzen DW. 2002. Role of MAP kinase in signaling indispensable amino acid deficiency in the brain. *Brain Res. Mol. Brain Res.* 105:11–18
98. Sharp JW, Payne JA, Ross-Inta CM, Gietzen DW. 2006. Essential amino acid deficiency disinhibits the anterior piriform cortex. Manuscr. submitted
99. **Sharp JW, Ross-Inta CM, Hao S, Rudell JB, Gietzen DW. 2006. Co-localization of phosphorylated extracellular signal-related protein kinases 1/2 (ERK1/2) and phosphorylated eukaryotic initiation factor 2α (eIF2α) in response to a threonine-devoid diet. *J. Comp. Neurol.* 494:485–94**

99. Shows location of IAA chemosensory cells in APC.

100. Sharp JW, Ross CM, Koehnle TJ, Gietzen DW. 2004. Phosphorylation of Ca2+/calmodulin dependent protein kinase type II and the α-amino-3-hydroxy-5-methyl-4-isoxazole propionate (AMPA) receptor in response to a threonine-devoid diet. *Neuroscience* 126:1053–62
101. Shenoy ST, Rogers QR. 1978. Effect of dietary amino acids on transfer ribonucleic acid charging levels in rat liver. *J. Nutr.* 108:1412–21
102. Simson PC, Booth DA. 1973. Effect of CS-US interval on the conditioning of odour preferences by amino acid loads. *Physiol. Behav.* 11:801–8
103. Tabuchi E, Ono T, Nishijo H, Torii K. 1991. Amino acid and NaCl appetite, and LHA neuron responses of lysine-deficient rat. *Physiol. Behav.* 49:951–64
104. Torii K, Yokawa T, Tabuchi E, Hawkins RL, Mori M, et al. 1996. Recognition of deficient nutrient intake in the brain of rat with L-lysine deficiency monitored by functional magnetic resonance imaging, electrophysiologically and behaviorally. *Amino Acids* 10:73–81
105. Truong BG, Magrum LJ, Gietzen DW. 2002. GABA(A) and GABA(B) receptors in the anterior piriform cortex modulate feeding in rats. *Brain Res.* 924:1–9
106. Vinade L, Dosemeci A. 2000. Regulation of the phosphorylation state of the AMPA receptor GluR1 subunit in the postsynaptic density. *Cell Mol. Neurobiol.* 20:451–63

107. Wang Y, Cummings SL, Gietzen DW. 1996a. Temporal-spatial pattern of c-Fos expression in the rat brain in response to amino acid deficiency I: the initial recognition phase. *Mol. Brain Res.* 40:27–34
108. Wang Y, Cummings SL, Gietzen DW. 1996b. Temporal-spatial pattern of c-Fos expression in the rat brain in response to amino acid deficiency II: the learned aversion. *Mol. Brain Res.* 40:35–41
109. Wek RC, Jiang HY, Anthony TG. 2006. Coping with stress: eIF2 kinases and translational control. *Biochem. Soc. Trans.* 34:7–11
110. Wek SA, Zhu S, Wek RC. 1995. The histidyl-tRNA synthetase-related sequence in the eIF-2α protein kinase GCN2 interacts with tRNA and is required for activation in response to starvation for different amino acids. *Mol. Cell. Biol.* 15:4497–506
111. Welzl H, D'Adamo P, Lipp HP. 2001. Conditioned taste aversion as a learning and memory paradigm. *Behav. Brain Res.* 125:205–13
112. White BD, Du F, Higgenbotham DA. 2003. Low dietary protein is associated with an increase in food intake and a decrease in the in vitro release of radiolabeled glutamate and GABA from the lateral hypothalamus. *Nutr. Neurosci.* 6:361–67
113. Wullschleger S, Loewith R, Hall MN. 2006. TOR signaling in growth and metabolism. *Cell* 124:471–84
114. Yao D, Mackenzie B, Ming H, Varoqui H, Zhu H, et al. 2000. A novel System A isoform mediating Na+/neutral amino acid cotransport. *J. Biol. Chem.* 275:22790–97

Regulation of Lipolysis in Adipocytes

Robin E. Duncan, Maryam Ahmadian, Kathy Jaworski, Eszter Sarkadi-Nagy, and Hei Sook Sul

Department of Nutritional Sciences and Toxicology, University of California, Berkeley, California 94720; email: hsul@nature.berkeley.edu

Annu. Rev. Nutr. 2007. 27:79–101

First published online as a Review in Advance on February 21, 2007

The *Annual Review of Nutrition* is online at http://nutr.annualreviews.org

This article's doi: 10.1146/annurev.nutr.27.061406.093734

0199-9885/07/0821-0079$20.00

Key Words

adipocyte, lipolysis, triacylglyceride lipase, perilipin, desnutrin/ATGL, hormone-sensitive lipase

Abstract

Lipolysis of white adipose tissue triacylglycerol stores results in the liberation of glycerol and nonesterified fatty acids that are released into the vasculature for use by other organs as energy substrates. In response to changes in nutritional state, lipolysis rates are precisely regulated through hormonal and biochemical signals. These signals modulate the activity of lipolytic enzymes and accessory proteins, allowing for maximal responsiveness of adipose tissue to changes in energy requirements and availability. Recently, a number of novel adipocyte triacylglyceride lipases have been identified, including desnutrin/ATGL, greatly expanding our understanding of adipocyte lipolysis. We have also begun to better appreciate the role of a number of nonenzymatic proteins that are critical to triacylglyceride breakdown. This review provides an overview of key mediators of lipolysis and the regulation of this process by changes in nutritional status and nutrient intakes.

Contents

INTRODUCTION

WAT: white adipose tissue

White adipose tissue (WAT) triacylglycerol (TAG) is the major energy reserve in higher eukaryotes. This lipid pool is in a constant state of flux, resulting from a largely futile cycle of lipolysis and re-esterification (55). During times of energy deprivation, WAT undergoes a shift toward greater net rates of lipolysis, which can be defined as the hydrolysis of TAG to generate fatty acids (FAs) and glycerol that are released into the vasculature for use by other organs as energy substrates. Lipolysis proceeds in an orderly and regulated manner, with different enzymes acting at each step. TAG is hydrolyzed sequentially to form diacylglycerol (DAG), then monoacylglycerol (MAG), with the liberation of a FA at each step. MAG is hydrolyzed to release the final FA and glycerol. The storage of energy reserves as TAG, and the ability to rapidly mobilize these reserves as FA to fuel energy demands, represents a highly adapted metabolic response. The liberation of FA from TAG by adipocyte lipolysis is also important to supply substrate for hepatic synthesis of very-low-density lipoproteins (VLDLs). Circulating FAs are a major source of substrate for the hepatic production of TAG-rich lipoproteins (34, 80), and impairment of adipose tissue lipolysis inhibits VLDL synthesis (44, 94, 134).

Alterations in lipolysis are frequently associated with obesity, including an increase in basal rates of lipolysis that may contribute to the development of insulin resistance, as well as an impaired responsiveness to stimulated lipolysis (65, 102). Obesity is characterized primarily by an excess of WAT and an enlargement in adipocyte size that results from increased TAG storage. Obesity has become a prevalent health problem due to its close association with a number of disorders, including type 2 diabetes, hypertension, and atherosclerosis (133). Here, we review adipocyte lipolysis and the major nutritional determinants controlling this process. **Figure 1** (see color insert) provides an overview of the nutritional regulation of adipocyte lipolysis.

TRIACYLGLYCEROL HYDROLYSIS

Until recently, initiation of TAG hydrolysis in adipose tissue was believed to be controlled by hormone-sensitive lipase (HSL) (109). The generation of HSL-null mouse models, however, demonstrated clearly the existence of residual HSL-independent TAG lipase activity, suggesting the presence of previously unidentified adipocyte enzyme(s) with TAG hydrolase activity (44, 94, 134). In recent years, novel adipose tissue lipases have been identified and characterized. All are serine esterases that harbor a common structural element—the alpha/beta-hydrolase fold—and a conserved catalytic diad or triad that is composed of the G*X*S*X*G pentapeptide motif as well as an active aspartate or glutamate (D/E)GG tripeptide and an active histidine (H). Studies to determine the relative contribution of each enzyme to adipocyte lipolysis are ongoing.

Hormone-Sensitive Lipase

Adipose tissue HSL (E.C. 3.1.1.3) is an 84 kDa cytoplasmic protein with demonstrated activity against a wide variety of substrates including TAG, DAG, cholesteryl esters (CEs), and retinyl esters (51). Relative fatty acyl hydrolase activity of HSL in vitro is elevenfold greater against DAG than TAG, and twofold greater against CEs (51). HSL shows a preference for activity against fatty acids in the sn-1 or sn-3 position (99). Until recently, HSL was believed to be the primary enzyme responsible for virtually all TAG and DAG hydrolase activity in adipocytes, as well as neutral cholesteryl ester hydrolase (NCEH) activity. To address the functional role of HSL in vivo, several laboratories generated HSL-null mouse models (44, 94, 134). Although differences have been observed between these models, a great deal of insight has been gained regarding the relative contribution of HSL to adipocyte TAG hydrolysis. For instance, studies have demonstrated that although NCEH activity was indeed absent in HSL-null adipocytes, a substantial fraction of catecholamine stimulated lipolysis (90, 94), and most, if not all, basal lipolysis remained (30, 134). Moreover, the lipolytic response to extended fasting (>48 h) appeared to be normal in HSL-null mice that demonstrated adequate or even heightened mobilization and oxidation of FA (30). HSL-mediated lipolysis, however, did contribute an important component to adipose FA liberation. HSL-null mice displayed lower serum NEFA and TAG levels and reduced hepatic TAG storage, indicating that HSL-independent lipolysis was inadequate to maintain FA output from adipose tissue at levels that could meet normal demands for energy substrates and VLDL synthesis (45, 132).

Examination of the physiology of HSL-null mice offers additional insight into the relative importance of HSL in TAG hydrolysis in vivo. On a normal chow diet, HSL-null mice had body weights similar to wild-type mice (47), and adipocyte size was reportedly either similar or slightly larger (94)—a finding that is consistent with a role for HSL in adipocyte FA mobilization. However, WAT mass in these animals was either unchanged (94) or decreased in size (134). Furthermore, on a high-fat diet, HSL ablation was associated with a significant protective effect against the development of obesity (47). This result was unexpected, but could be explained by the finding that in the absence of HSL, adipocytes undergo a compensatory decrease in the re-esterification of FA that results in decreased resynthesis of TAG and increased liberation of FA to the vasculature (144). Although this compensatory response may have confounded measurement of the true contribution of HSL to adipose fatty acid mobilization, it is clear from a number of studies that HSL is not strictly required for the initiation of TAG hydrolysis. This fact is made even more evident by the finding that DAG, but not TAG, accumulated in adipocytes of HSL-null mice (44). The relative contribution of HSL to DAG lipolysis is further discussed below.

Desnutrin/Adipose Triglyceride Lipase

In 2004, using rat cDNA microarray analysis of adipocyte-specific genes, we identified and

TAG: triacylglyceride

FA: fatty acid

DAG: diacylglyceride

MAG: monoacylglyceride

Lipolysis: the hydrolysis of TAG to generate nonesterified fatty acids (FAs) and glycerol that are released into the vasculature for use by other organs as energy substrates

HSL: hormone-sensitive lipase

characterized a novel adipocyte TAG lipase that we called desnutrin (130). Desnutrin is a 54 kDa protein that contains an N-terminal patatin-like domain that is found in many plant acyl hydrolases and is characterized by a conserved serine in the G*X*S*X*G motif, an alpha/beta-hydrolase fold, a conserved aspartate belonging to the D*X*(G/A) motif, and a glycine-rich region (130). This same enzyme was subsequently identified by two other laboratories from database searches of proteins containing the conserved G*X*S*X*G pentapeptide motif and alpha/beta-hydrolase fold, and was named adipose triglyceride lipase (ATGL) (145) or iPLA2ζ (53, 145). Murine desnutrin/ATGL is found predominantly in adipose tissue, but it is also found at much lower levels in other tissues, notably cardiac and skeletal muscle and testis. When cells contain fat stores, such as differentiated 3T3-L1 cells (145) as well as HeLa cells grown in oleic acid–rich medium (115), desnutrin/ATGL is found both in the cytoplasm and tightly associated with the lipid droplet (115, 130, 145). In COS-7 cells that lack substantial lipid droplets, desnutrin/ATGL was found to be relatively homogenously distributed within the cytoplasm (130). Factors governing subcellular distribution of desnutrin/ATGL, including mechanisms by which the cytoplasmic enzyme accesses its substrate and potential translocation to the lipid droplet, remain to be determined.

ATGL: adipose triglyceride lipase

Several lines of evidence indicate that desnutrin/ATGL is a TAG-specific lipase. We have shown that overexpression of desnutrin/ATGL in COS-7 cells increased FFA release to the medium, decreasing intracellular stores of TAG without affecting intracellular phospholipid stores (130). A similar effect on TAG level has also been reported in 293HEK cells (62), while expression of desnutrin/ATGL in 3T3-L1 adipocytes has been shown to increase both glycerol and FA release (144). In vitro, TAG hydrolase activity has been demonstrated for the enzyme purified by expression in Sf9 insect cells and 293HEK cells as well as COS-7 cells (53, 130, 145). The specificity of desnutrin/ATGL for TAG has also been investigated. Zimmermann et al. (144) prepared cytosolic extracts from HepG2 cells infected with adenoviral-desnutrin/ATGL and incubated them with radiolabeled triolein and diolein substrates. They found significantly higher TAG lipase activity (approximately six- to tenfold higher) than DAG lipase activity, indicating a primary role for the enzyme in catalyzing the first, rate-limiting step in lipolysis. This finding was supported by work in COS-7 cells demonstrating a 21-fold increased accumulation of DAG in cells transfected with desnutrin/ATGL compared with HSL, as well as a modest increase in MAG levels (144). Extracts from COS-7 cells transiently expressing desnutrin/ATGL had activity against cholesteryl esters and retinyl esters that was comparable to control values (144), further demonstrating the specific role for desnutrin/ATGL in TAG hydrolysis.

Nutritional regulation of desnutrin/ATGL further supports a role for this enzyme in the mobilization of TAG stores in response to increased energy demand. We have shown that desnutrin/ATGL is induced by fasting in mice and is suppressed by refeeding (130). Regulation of desnutrin/ATGL mRNA by glucocorticoids may explain this, since dexamethasone was found to strongly upregulate the enzyme in a concentration- and dose-dependent manner in 3T3-L1 preadipocytes (130). We have also found that desnutrin/ATGL is downregulated in ob/ob and db/db mice, further supporting a role for the enzyme in fat breakdown and suggesting a possible contributory role in the development of obesity (130).

The relative importance of desnutrin/ATGL in lipolysis is illustrated by studies of gene ablation and functional loss of the enzyme. siRNA directed against desnutrin/ATGL has been shown to significantly decrease the release of glycerol and FA from

3T3-L1 adipocytes (144), indicating impaired lipolysis that was not compensated by the presence of other lipases. In support of this, treatment of cytosolic extracts from mouse WAT and BAT with desnutrin/ATGL antibodies decreased FA release by approximately two-thirds (144). This decrease was more pronounced when adipocytes from HSL-null mice were utilized, a finding that suggests cooperativity exists between the two enzymes, and indeed, a synergistic effect has been observed on lipolysis when cells are cotransfected with both desnutrin/ATGL and HSL (144). Achievement of optimal rates of lipolysis, therefore, likely requires the expression of both acyl hydrolases. Global loss of desnutrin/ATGL gene function in mice resulted in increased weight gain and a shift in favor of carbohydrate over fat as a primary fuel source during fasting, indicating that in vivo desnutrin/ATGL likely also functions in adipose tissue lipolysis (43). Surprisingly, however, WAT fat pad weights were elevated by only approximately twofold, which suggests that other TAG lipases may be present that could partially compensate for loss of desnutrin/ATGL. Also surprising was the finding that loss of desnutrin/ATGL was associated with premature death. This resulted from ectopic storage of fat in the heart, where cardiomyocyte TAG levels were found to have increased twentyfold by 12 weeks of age. Ectopic fat storage was also evident in other tissues. This effect was observed despite a more favorable plasma lipid profile and increased insulin sensitivity. Total lipase activity was dramatically reduced in several tissues, including WAT and BAT, but also cardiac muscle, skeletal muscle, testis, and liver. This finding highlights the potential metabolic importance of intracellular TAG hydrolysis in tissues other than adipose tissue and indicates that desnutrin/ATGL may play a critical role in the liberation of FA in multiple tissues. Generation of conditional knockout models lacking desnutrin/ATGL in individual tissues will be required to verify this hypothesis.

Triacylglycerol Hydrolases

Soni et al. (116) were the first group to report discovery of a novel TAG lipase that may contribute to non-HSL-mediated TAG lipolysis in adipocytes. Others have subsequently confirmed the presence of triacylglycerol hydrolase (TGH; carboxylesterase 3; EC 3.1.1.1) in adipose tissue (10). TGH is a 60 kDa microsomal lipase that contains a catalytic triad with an active site serine located in the G*X*S*X*G motif (68). TGH displays activity against long-, medium-, and short-chain TAGs and has also been reported to hydrolyze neutral cholesteryl esters (88), but it lacks phospholipase or acyl-CoA thioesterase activity (69). The enzyme is expressed predominantly in liver, where it functions in mobilization of intracellular TAG stores and likely plays a critical role in synthesis of TAG-rich very-low-density lipoproteins (VLDLs) (39).

TGH: triacylglyceride hydrolase

Recently, however, TGH has also been identified in other tissues, including kidney, heart, intestine, and adipose tissue (26). In 3T3-L1 cells, expression of TGH is upregulated tenfold upon differentiation of preadipocytes into adipocytes (25) due, at least in part, to transcriptional regulation by the adipogenic transcription factor C/EBPα (136). These findings suggest a functional role for TGH in the mature fat cell, and indeed, Soni and colleagues (116) have identified TGH as an adipocyte lipase using functional proteomics. In this study, they subjected infranatant and fat cake fractions prepared from mouse intra-abdominal WAT to oleic acid–linked agarose chromatography. One of the two major peaks of esterase activity eluted contained substantial lipase activity, and this fraction was also found to contain TGH. It is therefore likely that TGH contributes to adipose tissue lipolysis. However, additional molecular and genetic studies will be required to determine the relative contribution of this lipase to overall mobilization of FA from TAG in adipocytes.

Using a database search for serine esterases of the alpha/beta-hydrolase fold that also contain the G*X*S*X*G and His-Gly dipeptide motifs, Okazaki et al. (90) have uncovered a previously unannotated gene that is induced in 3T3-L1 cells during differentiation into adipocytes. This protein shares a high degree of sequence homology with TGH (>70%) as well as similar subcellular localization, and therefore was named TGH-2. Also similar to TGH, TGH-2 exhibits activity against mono- and tri- but not diolein, with a substantial preference for short-chain fatty acid TAG. TGH-2 was found to be expressed predominantly in liver but was also present in adipose tissue and kidney and was induced by fasting and inhibited by refeeding. Molecular studies utilizing siRNA directed against TGH-2 in 3T3-L1 adipocytes demonstrated a 10% decrease in isoproterenol-stimulated glycerol release, while TGH-2 overexpression was found to increase glycerol release by 20%. Further studies are required to determine the relative contribution of this novel lipase to basal lipolysis and to in vivo lipase activity in adipose tissue. However, these results suggest a role for TGH-2 in mobilization of stored TAG during times of increased energy demand.

Adiponutrin

Adiponutrin is a 45 kDa patatin domain–containing protein that is highly expressed primarily in adipose tissue (9). It shares a high degree of sequence homology with desnutrin, including positioning of the G*X*S*X*G and DGG active site motifs (9). Extracts from insect (53, 62) and mammalian cells (53, 62) transfected with adiponutrin possess functional TAG lipase activity that requires the active site serine (G*X*S*X*G motif) when assayed in vitro (62). However, overexpression of adiponutrin has no effect on TAG hydrolysis in 293 HEK cells, in contrast to desnutrin/ATGL and other patatin domain–containing proteins that increase TAG hydrolysis in these cells (62). Furthermore, unlike other known lipases, adiponutrin expression is dramatically upregulated in animals that have been refed following a fast, whereas adiponutrin mRNA is almost undetectable in fasted animals (9). Although desnutrin/ATGL mRNA is downregulated in obese rats (130), adiponutrin mRNA is induced 50-fold (9). This differential regulation of adiponutrin compared with other lipases suggests that in vivo this enzyme may serve a primary function other than lipolysis. In vitro, adiponutrin purified from insect cells has been shown also to have acyltransferase activity (53) consistent with an anabolic, rather than a catabolic, role in adipocyte metabolism. Clearly, additional work is required to clarify the role of this enzyme, if any, in adipocyte lipolysis.

GS2 and GS2-Like

GS2 was identified by Jenkins et al. (53) as a TAG lipase with a patatin homology domain that includes a combination of the G/A*X*G*XX*G and G*X*S*X*G motifs that are conserved in calcium-independent phospholipase A_2 family members. In vitro assay has demonstrated triolein hydrolase activity for GS2 that exceeded activities for adiponutrin or desnutrin (53). GS2 lipase activity has subsequently been confirmed in keratinocytes (35) and in 293 HEK cells overexpressing the enzyme (62). Overexpression of the related protein GS2-Like in HEK 293 cells also results in decreased TAG storage, which suggests a functional role for both of these proteins in lipolysis in vivo (62). GS2 transcripts have only been identified in humans (62). The relative contribution of GS2 and GS2-Like to lipolysis in white adipose tissue remains to be determined.

DIACYLGLYCEROL HYDROLYSIS

The second step of lipolysis involves the hydrolysis of DAG to yield MAG and a nonesterified fatty acid. This reaction occurs at a rate 10- to 30-fold higher than the hydrolysis of TAG, which is the initiating and rate-limiting

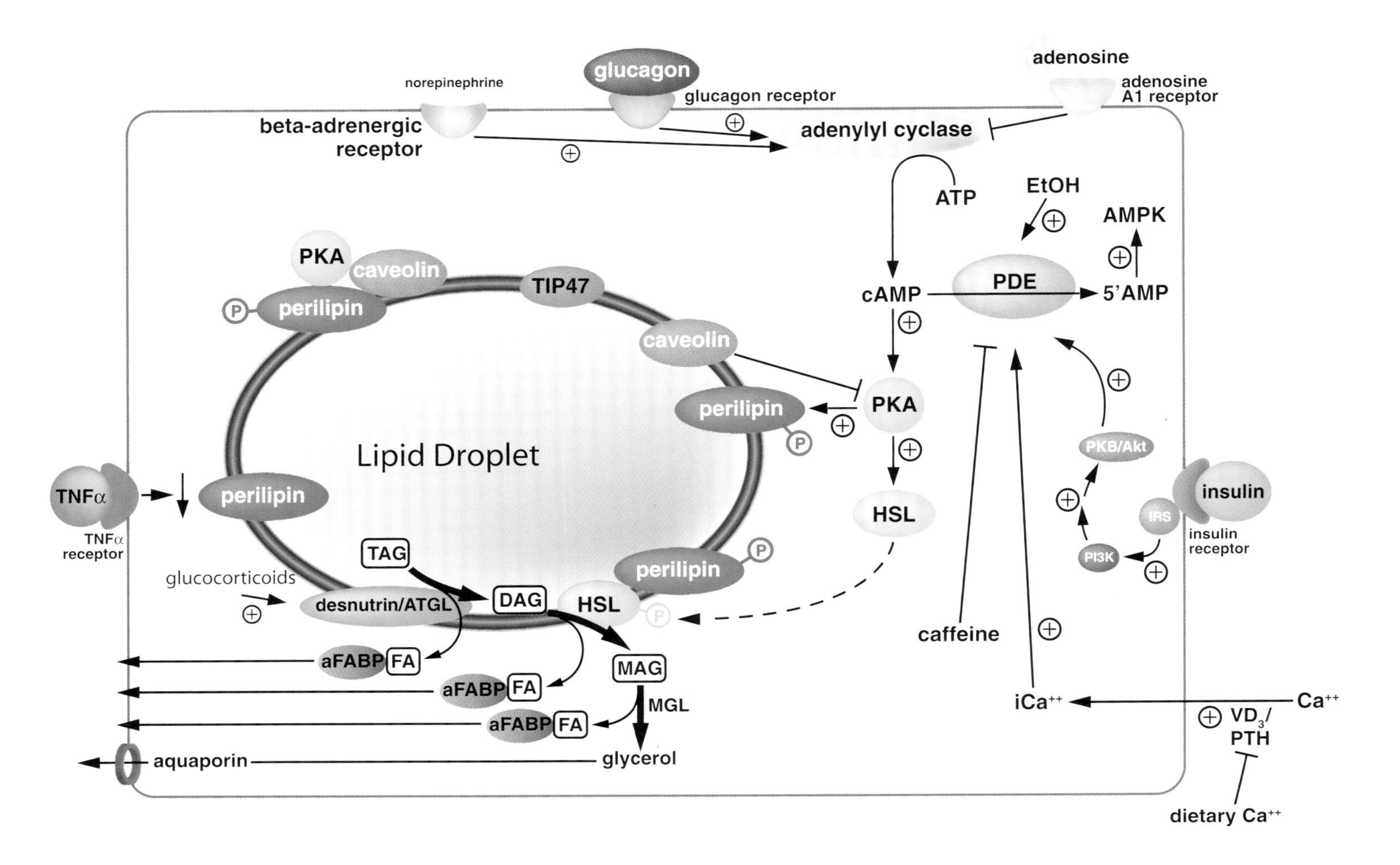

Figure 1

Regulation of adipocyte lipolysis.

step in lipolysis (40). To date, the only DAG lipase identified in adipocytes is HSL.

The maximum rate of hydrolysis of DAG by HSL in vitro is 11-fold greater than that of TAG (51). As described above, studies of murine models deficient in HSL have confirmed the importance of HSL for breakdown of DAG. While mice lacking adipose HSL can achieve near normal rates of TAG hydrolysis, these animals display severely blunted DAG lipase activity, and as a result, DAG accumulates in adipose tissues (44). Downregulation of the activity of a number of CoA-dependent acyltransferases has been reported in HSL-null mice, and it is believed to contribute to maintenance of normal weight in the face of complete ablation of this important lipolytic enzyme (144). The metabolic fate of accumulated DAG in adipocytes of HSL-null mice remains to be determined. Release of glycerol and fatty acids was normal or even elevated in fasted HSL-null mice, suggesting complete breakdown of TAG (94). Impaired re-esterification of DAG by acyltransferases could result in a normalized release of FA generated from the hydrolysis of TAG. Release of glycerol, however, would be impaired. Neither TGH nor ATGL/desnutrin has been shown to exhibit significant DAG lipase activity (90, 145). Results from HSL-null mouse models suggest, therefore, that adipocytes may harbor additional, less active DAG lipases, as well as TAG lipases.

MONOACYLGLYCEROL HYDROLYSIS

Monoglyceride lipase (MGL) is a 33 kDa hydrolase, purified 2500-fold from rat adipose tissue in 1975 by Tornqvist & Belfrage (129). In 1986, the respective roles of HSL and MGL in TAG hydrolysis were clarified when isolated HSL was found to hydrolyze acylglycerol with an accumulation of MAG in vitro, whereas glycerol release was blunted through selective removal of MGL by immunoprecipitation (31).

MGL hydrolyzes the 1(3) and 2-ester bonds of MAG at equal rates and exhibits no in vitro catalytic activity against DAG, TAG, or cholsteryl esters (57). MGL contains an alpha/beta-hydrolase fold, characteristic of known lipases (57). It is predicted to be composed of 302 amino acids (57). MGL is related to a number of microbial proteins that include esterases, lysophospholipases, and haloperoxidases (58). Two lipase motifs have been identified in the primary sequence: the active site serine motif G*X*S*X*G and the HG dipeptide (57). The catalytic triad of MGL is formed by Ser-122, Asp-239, and His-269. Mutating any of these three residues has been shown to completely abolish both the lipase and esterase activities of MGL (57).

MGL: monoglyceride lipase

ROLE OF LIPID DROPLET–ASSOCIATED PROTEINS IN LIPOLYSIS

Perilipin is the major protein found in association with lipid droplets in adipocytes (42). Analysis of lipid droplets from Chinese hamster ovary (CHO) cells by mass spectrometry has identified, in addition to perilipin, more than 40 structural and signaling proteins, as well as enzymes involved in lipid synthesis, storage, and utilization, suggesting that the lipid droplet should be considered a metabolic organelle rather than an inert storage site (70). Lipolysis requires that soluble lipases access the highly hydrophobic TAG substrate and that hydrophobic products of this reaction be removed. A number of cytosolic as well as lipid droplet–associated proteins are known to modulate rates of basal and/or stimulated lipolysis.

Perilipin

Perilipin A and B are isoforms of perilipin that arise from differential splicing (41). Perilipin A is the predominant isoform found in mature adipocytes, and it was among the earliest lipid droplet–associated proteins to be identified. As such, it has been studied extensively.

PKA: protein kinase A

cAMP: cyclic AMP

Much evidence supports a complex role for perilipin proteins in regulating both basal and stimulated adipocyte lipolysis.

Under unstimulated conditions, cell fractionation and confocal microscopy studies show that both desnutrin/ATGL (145) and a substantial proportion of HSL (up to 50% of cellular levels) are localized to the lipid droplet (84). The presence of perilipins A and B coating the lipid droplet is believed to function as a protective barrier that restricts access of TAG lipases to neutral lipid substrates in order to prevent unrestrained basal lipolysis (15). The physiologic and metabolic effects of perilipin ablation in mice support this idea. Perilipin-null mice have constitutively elevated basal lipolysis, resulting in a marked reduction in WAT mass and smaller adipocyte size (78, 106, 127). Perilipin-null mice also display a significant resistance to diet-induced obesity (78, 106, 127) that is explained, at least in part, by increased beta-oxidation of fatty acids, the products of lipolysis (106), following from a compensatory induction of genes involved in lipid and energy metabolism and a downregulation of genes involved in lipid biosynthesis (20). Ectopic expression of perilipin A, as expected, increases the storage of TAG by inhibiting hydrolysis (15, 127). 3T3-L1 preadipocytes transfected with perilipin A stored 6- to 30-fold more TAG than control 3T3-L1 cells, resulting from a 5-fold reduction in the rate of lipolysis (15). In CHO cells, perilipin A was found to inhibit TAG hydrolysis by 87% in cells maintained under unstimulated conditions (127). Although perilipin A clearly restrains the action of TAG lipases under basal conditions, this protein plays an entirely different role in stimulated adipocyte lipolysis.

Perilipin ablation is associated with near-maximal rates of lipolysis under basal conditions (78). However, loss of functional perilipin proteins also causes a dramatic attenuation of stimulated lipolytic activity (78, 127). As a target for protein kinase A (PKA; cAMP-dependent protein kinase)-mediated phosphorylation at up to six sites (Ser-81, Ser-223, Ser-277, Ser-434, Ser-492, and Ser-517), perilipin A is highly regulated by lipolytic stimuli that act through the beta-adrenergic receptor/adenylyl cyclase pathway (117, 125, 128, 140). Studies in CHO cells demonstrate that PKA-mediated phosphorylation of perilipin A alone is sufficient to increase lipolysis (126). Conversely, mutation of perilipin A phosphorylation sites blunts the contribution of this protein to stimulated lipolysis (84, 117). In adipocytes, the presence of perilipin proteins on the lipid droplet appears to be necessary for PKA-mediated stimulation of HSL translocation (84, 125). Although recent evidence indicates that these perilipins do not have to be phosphorylated in order to mediate translocation of HSL from the cytosol to the surface of the lipid droplet, phosphorylation does appear to be necessary for attainment of maximally stimulated lipolysis following PKA activation (84). PKA-dependent phosphorylation of perilipin A may facilitate interaction with HSL on the lipid droplet, thereby increasing activity of the enzyme (84). Coexpression of perilipin A and HSL in CHO cells results in a cooperative effect that produces a more rapidly accelerated lipolysis following PKA stimulation than is evident in cells that express either protein alone (125).

Perilipin A may also influence lipolysis by regulating the distribution and architecture of lipid droplets within adipocytes. Chronic stimulation of lipolysis in 3T3-L1 adipocytes causes the large perinuclear lipid droplets to fragment into many microlipid droplets coated with perilipin A (76). This dispersion is prevented by stable expression of perilipin A that has been mutated to prevent phosphorylation at serine 492 (76). Activation of perilipin A by PKA-mediated phosphorylation may, therefore, increase lipolysis by increasing the surface area of neutral lipid droplets accessible for attack by lipases (76, 85). Taken together, these studies indicate that perilipin expression and phosphorylation state are critical regulators of lipolysis in adipocytes. In nonadipocytes, the perilipin-related protein adipocyte differentiation-related protein/adipophilin replaces perilipin at the surface of neutral lipid storage droplets, although this protein is largely absent in mature adipocytes (13).

Adipose Fatty Acid–Binding Protein

Adipose fatty acid–binding protein (aFABP/ALBP/aP2) is a member of the cytosolic lipid-binding proteins that carry both fatty acids and retinoic acid in adipocytes (79). Maximal rates of lipolysis require the removal of fatty acids from the adipocyte in order to prevent accumulation of reaction products and feedback inhibition of lipases. aFABP/ALBP/aP2 is postulated to act as a molecular chaperone, facilitating the movement of fatty acids out of adipocytes following their liberation from cellular TAG stores by lipases (22). Studies of aFABP/ALBP/aP2 gene ablation in mice provide insight into the relative role of aFABP/ALBP/aP2 in lipolysis. Basal lipolysis has been reported to be decreased in aFABP/ALBP/aP2-null mice compared with wild-type littermates (22, 49), and stimulated lipolysis in adipocytes isolated from these mice has also been shown to be attenuated (22, 110). Consistent with a decrease in the rate of efflux of fatty acids, intracellular fatty acid levels have been found to be threefold higher in adipocytes from aFABP/ALBP/aP2 nulls compared with wild types (22). However, others have observed no difference in basal or stimulated rates of lipolysis in adipocytes isolated from aFABP/ALBP/aP2-null mice compared with wild-type littermates (110). In that study, a compensatory induction of keratinocyte lipid-binding protein was observed that was reported to overcome the functional effects of loss of adipocyte-specific aFABP/ALBP/aP2 (110). Intracellular lipid-binding proteins may be important regulators of lipolysis. Further work is required to discern the relative roles of these proteins in adipocyte lipolysis.

Caveolin-1

Caveolae and caveolar proteins are implicated in the regulation of multiple functions within cells (23, 93, 103). Caveolin-1 is found in particularly high abundance in adipose tissue, and it is strongly induced during the differentiation of 3T3-L1 fibroblasts to mature adipocytes (107). Although typically found in the caveolae of plasma membranes, proteomic analysis has demonstrated that in adipocytes caveolin-1 localizes to the lipid droplet as well (14, 23, 93, 103). A role for caveolin-1 in lipolysis has been suggested from studies of caveolin-1 null mice. These animals have markedly attenuated lipolytic activity in white adipose tissue (23) and fail to show the normal increase in serum nonesterified FA that is expected to occur in fasting, suggesting that caveolin-1 plays a role in activating lipolysis (24). Caveolin-1 knockout mice also fail to properly liberate fatty acids from TAG stores in brown adipose tissue in response to fasting, resulting in impaired thermogenesis (24). Regulation of cyclic AMP (cAMP)-mediated signal transduction may contribute to the effects of caveolin-1 on lipolysis (101). Caveolin-1 has been shown to directly interact with the catalytic subunit of PKA to inhibit cAMP-dependent signaling in vivo (101). In knockout mice, however, it has been shown that whereas PKA activity was greatly increased in the absence of caveolin-1, phosphorylation of perilipin was dramatically reduced (23). Activation of the β3-adrenergic receptor results in the formation of a ligand-induced complex between perilipin, caveolin-1, and the catalytic subunit of PKA in adipocytes (23). Caveolin-1, therefore, may facilitate PKA-mediated phosphorylation of perilipin, thereby contributing to increased stimulation of lipolysis.

CGI-58

Mutations in CGI-58 (Comparative Gene Identification 58), also known as ABHD5 (alpha/beta-hydrolase domain-containing protein 5) have been found to be the cause of a rare autosomal recessive disease called Chanarin-Dorfman syndrome (CDS) (67). CDS is characterized by excessive accumulation of TAG in the cells of many organs, and the clinical manifestations include ichthyosis, cataracts, ataxia, neurosensory hearing loss, and mental retardation (67). CGI-58 resembles lipases structurally; however, it lacks the conserved active site serine, which has been replaced by an asparagine (66). In 3T3-L1 adipocytes, CGI-58 is localized to the lipid droplet and has been shown to directly interact (139) and colocalize with perilipin A (121). However, when cells are treated with agents to promote lipolysis, it disperses off the lipid droplet (121). Recently, Lass et al. (66) demonstrated that CGI-58 stimulates in vitro lipolysis and is an activator of ATGL, but not HSL. When added to cytosolic extracts of mouse adipose tissue, CGI-58 stimulated lipolysis, while purified CGI-58 exhibited no lipase activity in vitro. Furthermore, they showed that mutant forms of CGI-58 fail to activate ATGL. Although CGI-58 appears to play a role in lipolysis, more studies are needed to elucidate the molecular mechanism of its activation of ATGL as well as its physiological role in living organisms.

Other Proteins Implicated in TAG Hydrolysis

Aquaporin 7 is a water- and glycerol-transporting protein expressed in the plasma membrane of adipocytes (46, 50, 75). Mice deficient in aquaporin 7 have impaired glycerol release in response to fasting and treatment with beta-adrenergic agonists, although FA release from adipocytes and plasma FFA levels are comparable to those observed in wild-type littermates (75). These animals develop age-associated obesity caused by an induction of glycerol kinase and increased storage of TAG (53).

Lipotransin was identified by yeast two-hybrid screening of a 3T3-L1 adipocyte cDNA library as an HSL-interacting protein (123). It is believed to function as a docking protein that mediates the hormonally induced translocation of HSL from cytoplasm to the lipid droplet (123).

TIP47 is a lipid droplet–associated PAT family protein of unknown function (36). TIP47 inhibits the hydrolysis of retinyl esters by GS2 and by HSL in human keratinocytes, suggesting that in adipocytes it may share a similar antilipolytic function with other PAT family proteins, such as perilipin or adipose differentiation-related protein/adipophilin (36).

NUTRITIONAL REGULATION OF LIPOLYSIS

Nutritional regulation of lipolysis occurs at multiple levels in response to changing metabolic conditions and nutrient intakes. Acute, rapid regulation of adipose tissue lipolysis occurs in order to maintain the supply of energy substrates during the postabsorptive state and to allow for efficient storage of excess fuels following a meal. Chronic exposure to extreme nutritional states, such as obesity or starvation, also induces metabolic adaptations that include changes in lipolysis. And, finally, a growing body of evidence indicates that exposure to specific metabolically active nutrients in the diet can also regulate lipolysis.

STIMULATION OF LIPOLYSIS DURING FASTING

Fasting acutely stimulates lipolysis, upregulating the serum concentration of fatty acids and glycerol that act as oxidative substrates to maintain energy requirements for other metabolic tissues. Catecholamines are the primary activators of fasting-induced lipolysis. The metabolic pathways through which these molecules act to stimulate TAG hydrolysis and FA release have been studied extensively and reviewed in detail (6, 17, 18, 29, 63, 64, and references contained therein).

The catecholamine norepinephrine binds beta-adrenergic receptors on the plasma membrane of adipocytes. These receptors are coupled with Gs-proteins that transmit a stimulatory signal to adenylyl cyclase to generate cyclic AMP (cAMP). cAMP binds PKA, causing the regulatory subunits to dissociate from the catalytically active subunits, resulting in increased activity of the enzyme (60).

PKA catalyzes the polyphosphorylation of HSL on multiple sites, including a nonactivating site (Ser-563) as well as two additional sites (Ser-659 and Ser-660) that cause activation and subsequent translocation of this lipase from the cytosol to the lipid droplet (4, 51, 120). As discussed above, PKA also phosphorylates perilipin on the lipid droplet, resulting in changes that enhance stimulated lipolysis, including movement of perilipin away from the lipid droplet (21), perilipin-mediated remodeling of lipid droplets that increases the surface area available for lipolytic attack (75), and perilipin-mediated activation of HSL activity at the surface of the lipid droplet (84, 125). Findings from studies in HSL-null mice suggest that catecholamine-stimulated lipolysis may also involve other TAG lipases. Treatment of adipocytes isolated from HSL-null mice with the beta-adrenergic agonist isoproterenol causes enhanced lipolysis, albeit at a blunted level compared with adipocytes from wild-type animals (91). This suggests that some or all of the newly discovered adipocyte TAG-lipases may be direct targets for PKA-mediated phosphorylation and activation, and indeed, Zimmerman et al. (145) have shown previously that desnutrin/ATGL is phosphorylated, although it was not a target for PKA. This also suggests that PKA may indirectly activate non-HSL-mediated TAG lipolysis. Perilipin expression alone has been shown to be sufficient to confer PKA-mediated lipolysis in CHO cells that lack HSL (126). Phosphorylation of perilipin by PKA may result in changes that increase the activity of multiple lipid droplet–associated lipases. Potential mechanisms include promoting access of soluble lipases to hydrophobic substrates, facilitating the formation of complexes between lipases and lipolysis-associated proteins, and stabilizing lipases at the surface of the lipid droplet. Further studies are required to elucidate the nature of PKA-mediated lipolysis in the absence of HSL.

Glucagon stimulates lipolysis in isolated mouse (48, 114) and human (96) adipocytes, independent of antagonistic effects on insulin action. Glucagon treatment causes an increase in adenylyl cyclase activity, resulting in an increase in intracellular adipocyte cAMP levels (95, 96). Gastric inhibitory polypeptide competes with glucagon for binding to the glucagon receptor and can inhibit glucagon-stimulated lipolysis in adipocytes, indicating that glucagon mediates lipolysis, at least in part, through direct activation of its receptor (27). Although glucagon action is primarily liver specific, glucagon receptors have been reported to be present in membranes of human adipose tissue (83), suggesting that direct action of glucagon likely plays an important role in regulating human, as well as rodent, lipolysis.

INHIBITION OF LIPOLYSIS DURING REFEEDING

Refeeding attenuates adipocyte lipolysis, primarily through the potent antilipolytic actions of insulin. This regulatory pathway has also been studied and reviewed extensively (6, 17, 18, 29, 63, and references contained therein). Rapid, acute regulation of lipolysis by insulin involves both cAMP-dependent and cAMP-independent mechanisms. cAMP-dependent suppression of lipolysis by insulin involves activation of phosphodiesterase 3B (63). Insulin binding causes autophosphorylation of its receptor, resulting in activation and subsequent tyrosine phosphorylation of insulin receptor substrates and binding of the p85 regulatory subunit of phosphatidyl inositol kinase-3 (PI3K). Activated PI3K autophosphorylates its inositol ring and the p85 regulatory subunit and p110 catalytic subunits,

PKB: protein kinase B

which is followed by phosphorylation and activation of protein kinase B/Akt (PKB/Akt). PKB/Akt phosphorylates and activates phosphodiesterase 3B, which degrades cAMP in adipocytes, releasing PKA from activation and decreasing lipolysis through a reduction in the phosphorylation-mediated activation of HSL and perilipin. cAMP-independent regulation of lipolysis by insulin involves the stimulation of protein phosphatase-1 through phosphorylation of its regulatory subunit (100). Activated protein phosphatase-1 rapidly dephosphorylates and deactivates HSL, causing a fall in the rate of lipolysis (73, 92, 100, 119, 143).

Insulin may also suppress lipolysis in 3T3-L1 adipocytes through downregulation of desnutrin/ATGL mRNA (59). In contrast, HSL mRNA expression is not regulated by short-term changes in nutritional status (124). In addition to inhibitory effects on the enzymes in TAG hydrolysis, insulin also decreases measurable rates of lipolysis (as indicated by the release of free fatty acids and glycerol from intact cells) by promoting the re-esterification of fatty acids (16). This serves to magnify the apparent suppression of TAG hydrolysis by insulin and the physiological effect of the hormone.

AMP-activated protein kinase (AMPK) as a master intracellular energy sensor is implicated in the regulation of both glucose and lipid metabolism (33, 86). Activation of AMPK in adipocytes by 5-aminoimidazole-4-carboxyamide-1-beta-D-ribofuranoside (AICAR) inhibits lipolysis (32, 33, 112). Infusion of obese Zucker rats as well as lean littermates with AICAR decreases plasma TAG and FA concentrations, as well as glycerol turnover (37), whereas mice lacking the AMPK-alpha2 subunit have been shown to have increased adiposity and weight gain (98, 131). Others have found, however, that AMPK activation may also play a role in the stimulation of maximal rates of lipolysis by cAMP (86). The molecular events and targets underlying regulation of lipolysis by AMPK are yet to be understood.

LIPOLYSIS IN OBESITY

Obesity is associated with an increase in basal lipolysis (102) but a decrease in catecholamine-stimulated lipolysis (65). Impaired sensitivity of adipocytes to insulin signaling, including the antilipolytic effects of this hormone, may contribute to enhanced basal lipolysis in obesity. Decreased insulin-mediated suppression of adipocyte lipolysis has been reported in obese rats (118) as well as in women with visceral obesity (3, 54), although several other studies in humans report that the antilipolytic effects of insulin are well conserved, even in subjects with highly impaired insulin-mediated glucose regulation (7, 8, 11, 52). In both obese and nonobese subjects, fasting and weight reduction cause a significant enhancement of sensitivity to the antilipolytic effects of insulin (7, 28, 71).

Overexpression of the leptin gene in adipocytes and increased circulating levels of leptin may also contribute to enhanced basal lipolysis in obesity (74). Treatment of adipocytes isolated from lean mice with leptin stimulates lipolytic activity (33). Treatment of adipocytes isolated from obese *ob/ob* mice that are deficient in leptin results in an even greater stimulation of lipolysis (33). Moreover, chronic (112) or acute (32) peripheral administration of leptin also stimulates adipose TAG hydrolysis in rats, resulting in a 9- to 16-fold increase in rates of lipolysis. Lipolytic actions of leptin are dependent on the leptin receptor, since obese *fa/fa* Zucker rats (112) and *db/db* mice (32) that have an inactivating mutation of the long form of the leptin receptor are resistant to leptin-induced lipolysis. Increased circulating leptin may also enhance lipolysis by counteracting the antilipolytic effects of insulin (86). Leptin impairs several metabolic effects of insulin, including the ability of the hormone to inhibit beta-adrenergic receptor-mediated lipolysis and PKA activation (86).

Beta-adrenergic receptor-stimulated lipolysis is impaired in obesity (65). Adipocytes from obese subjects have lower levels of adenylyl cyclase activity under hormone-stimulated conditions when compared with adipocytes from nonobese controls (77). Alterations in the adrenergic signaling pathways may contribute to this effect. Obesity is associated with a decreased lipolytic effect of catecholamines in adipose tissue (65). Adipocytes from obese Zucker rats have higher levels of antilipolytic α2 adrenoceptors compared with adipocytes from lean littermates (19). Conversely, adipocytes from obese mice express twofold lower levels of Gsα, a subunit of the GTP-binding protein through which beta-adrenergic receptors stimulate adenylyl cyclase (38). Post-receptor defects may also contribute to defects in hormone-stimulated lipolysis. The maximum lipolytic capacity has been shown to be reduced in adipocytes isolated from obese subjects compared with adipocytes from nonobese control subjects following stimulation with the phosphodiesterase-resistant cAMP analogue dibutyryl cAMP (65). This finding indicates impairment in the actions of cAMP downstream of effects of obesity on adrenergic receptor signaling, G-protein coupled activation of adenylyl cyclase, or cAMP levels. HSL and perilipin A are major targets for cAMP-dependent PKA activation. Decreased levels of HSL (65) and perilipin (135) in adipose tissue from obese subjects may contribute to the impairment of catecholamine-mediated lipolysis through a postreceptor defect. Weight reduction in obese subjects causes a substantial increase and normalization of sensitivity to catecholamine stimulation of lipolysis (77) without changing the number of β-adrenergic receptors (102).

Tumor necrosis factor-alpha (TNFα) production is increased in adipocytes from obese individuals and may contribute to enhanced basal lipolysis in obesity (97, 104, 105). This cytokine signals in an autocrine/paracrine manner through the TNFα receptor to activate the mitogen-activated protein kinases p44/42 and JNK that, in turn, downregulate perilipin mRNA and protein expression (104, 105). Studies with specific inhibitors of p44/42 and JNK support that the TNFα-mediated increase in lipolysis is largely attributed to a reduction in perilipin levels in adipocytes (104, 105), and lower levels of perilipin have been found in adipose tissues from obese subjects (135).

PTH: parathyroid hormone

VD_3: 1,25(OH)2 vitamin D_3

REGULATION OF ADIPOCYTE LIPOLYSIS BY DIETARY COMPOUNDS

Calcium

Higher intakes of calcium are associated with decreased adiposity and a reduced risk of obesity in a variety of epidemiological studies (108, and references therein). Moreover, calcium supplementation has been shown to aid in weight loss in obese humans consuming a calorie-deficient diet (142) and in calorie-restricted obese mice (111), and has also been reported to inhibit weight regain during refeeding in mice (122). Increased lipolysis is believed to contribute to these findings, and indeed, acute intakes of calcium have been reported to correlate significantly with fat oxidation in humans (82). Several studies have investigated the molecular mechanisms underlying potentiation of adipocyte lipolysis by dietary calcium. Increasing dietary calcium feedback inhibits the secretion of parathyroid hormone (PTH) and, subsequently, the activation of 25 hydroxycholecalciferol to 1,25 dihydroxycalciferol (vitamin D_3; VD_3) (87). Adipocytes are targets for the action of these hormones (141). PTH stimulates a dose-dependent rise in adipocyte intracellular calcium levels that is due to both increased influx and mobilization of intracellular stores (89). VD_3 has also been shown to elicit an increase in intracellular calcium levels (111). Increased intracellular calcium in human adipocytes inhibits lipolysis stimulated by the β-adrenergic receptor pathway (111, 138), resulting in decreased cAMP levels and reduced HSL phosphorylation (138). These effects appear to be mediated primarily through activation of phosphodiesterase 3B (138). Low dietary calcium intakes and increased circulating VD_3 may also have indirect inhibitory effects on adipocyte lipolysis by regulating the use of lipolytic substrates for energy metabolism (111, 122). Inverse regulation of intracellular calcium levels in adipocytes by calcitropic hormones may contribute to effects of dietary calcium on adiposity.

Caffeine

The lipolytic effects of caffeine and other methylxanthines derived from tea and coffee are well established and well characterized. These compounds stimulate lipolysis by increasing cellular levels of cAMP through two principal mechanisms. The first is antagonism of A1-adenosine receptors (72). These receptors predominate on differentiated mature adipocytes, where they inhibit adenylyl cyclase activity and suppress lipolysis (12). Antagonism of A1-receptors results in a derepression of adenylyl cyclase activity and increased lipolysis (72). Methylxanthines also inhibit phosphodiesterase activity, preventing the breakdown of cAMP and stimulating lipolysis in fat cells (2, 95). Caffeine ingestion increases lipid turnover (2) and the concentration of serum FFAs (5, 61). As such, high intakes of methylxanthines may also contribute to improved weight loss and weight maintenance through enhanced fat oxidation and thermogenesis (137).

Ethanol

Acute ethanol ingestion has antilipolytic effects that cause a significant fall in serum FFAs (1) and a decrease in whole-body lipid oxidation (113). Increased plasma acetate may contribute to this effect (1, 113). Chronic ethanol feeding in rats has been reported to suppress beta-adrenergic receptor-mediated lipolysis in adipocytes, likely through increased activation of phosphodiesterase 4 (56). This resulted in a decrease in beta-adrenergic receptor-stimulated PKA activation and decreased activating phosphorylation of perilipin A and HSL (56). Chronic ethanol consumption has also been reported to be associated with decreased PTH secretion, which may also contribute to increased lipolysis by decreasing intracellular calcium levels in adipocytes (81).

SUMMARY AND FUTURE DIRECTIONS

Adipocyte lipolysis is a complex process that is precisely controlled through integration of multiple and diverse hormonal and biochemical signals. Breakdown of this regulation may contribute to the development of obesity and associated pathologies. Many exciting advances have been made recently, including the discovery of major TAG lipases that contribute to in vivo adipocyte lipolysis. However, much remains to be elucidated regarding the in vivo functioning and relative contribution of these lipases to overall adipocyte lipolysis. As genetic mouse models of these enzymes are generated, our understanding of adipocyte lipolysis is likely to increase dramatically in the near future.

SUMMARY POINTS

1. Lipolysis is precisely regulated by multiple hormonal and biochemical signals that converge on adipocytes to regulate the function of lipases and nonenzymatic accessory proteins.
2. Hydrolysis of TAG is rate limiting in lipolysis and is catalyzed by one or more novel lipases that include desnutrin/ATGL and TGH.

3. Major regulators of lipolysis include the lipolytic activators glucagon and the catecholamines, and the antilipolytic agent insulin.
4. Dietary components may also regulate lipolysis. These include dietary calcium, ethanol, and caffeine.

FUTURE ISSUES

1. Generation of mice deficient in desnutrin/ATGL specifically in the adipose tissue will help to clarify the in vivo role of this lipase in adipose tissue lipolysis.
2. Genetic mouse models deficient in other TAG lipases will also be needed to determine their relative contribution to lipolysis.
3. The role of the energy sensor AMPK in mediating lipolysis remains unclear. Further work is required to resolve this issue.
4. Several dietary nutrients have been found to regulate lipolysis. Given the burden of chronic disease that is associated with obesity, discovery of dietary nutrients that stimulate lipolysis would be of great interest.

LITERATURE CITED

1. Abramson EA, Arky RA. 1968. Acute antilipolytic effects of ethyl alcohol and acetate in man. *J. Lab. Clin. Med.* 72:105–17
2. Acheson KJ, Gremaud G, Meirim I, Montigon F, Krebs Y, et al. 2004. Metabolic effects of caffeine in humans: lipid oxidation or futile cycling? *Am. J. Clin. Nutr.* 79:40–46
3. Albu JB, Curi M, Shur M, Murphy L, Matthews DE, Pi-Sunyer FX. 1999. Systemic resistance to the antilipolytic effect of insulin in black and white women with visceral obesity. *Am. J. Physiol.* 277:E551–60
4. Anthonsen MW, Ronnstrand L, Wernstedt C, Degerman E, Holm C. 1998. Identification of novel phosphorylation sites in hormone-sensitive lipase that are phosphorylated in response to isoproterenol and govern activation properties in vitro. *J. Biol. Chem.* 273:215–21
5. Arciero PJ, Gardner AW, Calles-Escandon J, Benowitz NL, Poehlman ET. 1995. Effects of caffeine ingestion on NE kinetics, fat oxidation, and energy expenditure in younger and older men. *Am. J. Physiol.* 268:E1192–98
6. Arner P. 2005. Human fat cell lipolysis: biochemistry, regulation and clinical role. *Best Pract. Res. Clin. Endocrinol. Metab.* 19:471–82
7. Arner P, Bolinder J, Engfeldt P, Hellmer J, Ostman J. 1984. Influence of obesity on the antilipolytic effect of insulin in isolated human fat cells obtained before and after glucose ingestion. *J. Clin. Invest.* 73:673–80
8. Arner P, Engfeldt P, Skarfors E, Lithell H, Bolinder J. 1987. Insulin receptor binding and metabolic effects of insulin in human subcutaneous adipose tissue in untreated noninsulin dependent diabetes mellitus. *Ups. J. Med. Sci.* 92:47–58
9. Baulande S, Lasnier F, Lucas M, Pairault J. 2001. Adiponutrin, a transmembrane protein corresponding to a novel dietary- and obesity-linked mRNA specifically expressed in the adipose lineage. *J. Biol. Chem.* 276:33336–44

10. Birner-Gruenberger R, Susani-Etzerodt H, Waldhuber M, Riesenhuber G, Schmidinger H, et al. 2005. The lipolytic proteome of mouse adipose tissue. *Mol. Cell. Proteomics* 4:1710–17
11. Bolinder J, Lithell H, Skarfors E, Arner P. 1986. Effects of obesity, hyperinsulinemia, and glucose intolerance on insulin action in adipose tissue of sixty-year-old men. *Diabetes* 35:282–90
12. Borglum JD, Vassaux G, Richelsen B, Gaillard D, Darimont C, et al. 1996. Changes in adenosine A1- and A2-receptor expression during adipose cell differentiation. *Mol. Cell. Endocrinol.* 117:17–25
13. Brasaemle DL, Barber T, Wolins NE, Serrero G, Blanchette-Mackie EJ, Londos C. 1997. Adipose differentiation-related protein is an ubiquitously expressed lipid storage droplet-associated protein. *J. Lipid Res.* 38:2249–63
14. Brasaemle DL, Dolios G, Shapiro L, Wang R. 2004. Proteomic analysis of proteins associated with lipid droplets of basal and lipolytically stimulated 3T3-L1 adipocytes. *J. Biol. Chem.* 279:46835–42
15. Brasaemle DL, Rubin B, Harten IA, Gruia-Gray J, Kimmel AR, Londos C. 2000. Perilipin A increases triacylglycerol storage by decreasing the rate of triacylglycerol hydrolysis. *J. Biol. Chem.* 275:38486–93
16. Campbell PJ, Carlson MG, Hill JO, Nurjhan N. 1992. Regulation of free fatty acid metabolism by insulin in humans: role of lipolysis and reesterification. *Am. J. Physiol.* 263:E1063–69
17. Carey GB. 1998. Mechanisms regulating adipocyte lipolysis. *Adv. Exp. Med. Biol.* 441:157–70
18. Carmen GY, Victor SM. 2006. Signalling mechanisms regulating lipolysis. *Cell Signal.* 18:401–8
19. Carpene C, Rebourcet MC, Guichard C, Lafontan M, Lavau M. 1990. Increased alpha 2-adrenergic binding sites and antilipolytic effect in adipocytes from genetically obese rats. *J. Lipid Res.* 31:811–19
20. Castro-Chavez F, Yechoor VK, Saha PK, Martinez-Botas J, Wooten EC, et al. 2003. Coordinated upregulation of oxidative pathways and downregulation of lipid biosynthesis underlie obesity resistance in perilipin knockout mice: a microarray gene expression profile. *Diabetes* 52:2666–74
21. Clifford GM, Londos C, Kraemer FB, Vernon RG, Yeaman SJ. 2000. Translocation of hormone-sensitive lipase and perilipin upon lipolytic stimulation of rat adipocytes. *J. Biol. Chem.* 275:5011–15
22. Coe NR, Simpson MA, Bernlohr DA. 1999. Targeted disruption of the adipocyte lipid-binding protein (aP2 protein) gene impairs fat cell lipolysis and increases cellular fatty acid levels. *J. Lipid Res.* 40:967–72
23. Cohen AW, Razani B, Schubert W, Williams TM, Wang XB, et al. 2004. Role of caveolin-1 in the modulation of lipolysis and lipid droplet formation. *Diabetes* 53:1261–70
24. Cohen AW, Schubert W, Brasaemle DL, Scherer PE, Lisanti MP. 2005. Caveolin-1 expression is essential for proper nonshivering thermogenesis in brown adipose tissue. *Diabetes* 54:679–86
25. Dolinsky VW, Gilham D, Hatch GM, Agellon LB, Lehner R, Vance DE. 2003. Regulation of triacylglycerol hydrolase expression by dietary fatty acids and peroxisomal proliferator-activated receptors. *Biochim. Biophys. Acta* 1635:20–28
26. Dolinsky VW, Sipione S, Lehner R, Vance DE. 2001. The cloning and expression of a murine triacylglycerol hydrolase cDNA and the structure of its corresponding gene. *Biochim. Biophys. Acta* 1532:162–72

27. Dupre J, Greenidge N, McDonald TJ, Ross SA, Rubinstein D. 1976. Inhibition of actions of glucagon in adipocytes by gastric inhibitory polypeptide. *Metabolism* 25:1197–99
28. Engfeldt P, Bolinder J, Ostman J, Arner P. 1985. Influence of fasting and refeeding on the antilipolytic effect of insulin in human fat cells obtained from obese subjects. *Diabetes* 34:1191–97
29. Fain JN, Garcija-Sainz JA. 1983. Adrenergic regulation of adipocyte metabolism. *J. Lipid Res.* 24:945–66
30. Fortier M, Wang SP, Mauriege P, Semache M, Mfuma L, et al. 2004. Hormone-sensitive lipase-independent adipocyte lipolysis during beta-adrenergic stimulation, fasting, and dietary fat loading. *Am. J. Physiol. Endocrinol. Metab.* 287:E282–88
31. Fredrikson G, Tornqvist H, Belfrage P. 1986. Hormone-sensitive lipase and monoacylglycerol lipase are both required for complete degradation of adipocyte triacylglycerol. *Biochim. Biophys. Acta* 876:288–93
32. Fruhbeck G, Aguado M, Gomez-Ambrosi J, Martinez JA. 1998. Lipolytic effect of in vivo leptin administration on adipocytes of lean and ob/ob mice, but not db/db mice. *Biochem. Biophys. Res. Commun.* 250:99–102
33. Fruhbeck G, Aguado M, Martinez JA. 1997. In vitro lipolytic effect of leptin on mouse adipocytes: evidence for a possible autocrine/paracrine role of leptin. *Biochem. Biophys. Res. Commun.* 240:590–94
34. Fukuda N, Ontko JA. 1984. Interactions between fatty acid synthesis, oxidation, and esterification in the production of triglyceride-rich lipoproteins by the liver. *J. Lipid Res.* 25:831–42
35. Gao JG, Simon M. 2005. Identification of a novel keratinocyte retinyl ester hydrolase as a transacylase and lipase. *J. Invest. Dermatol.* 124:1259–66
36. Gao JG, Simon M. 2006. Molecular screening for GS2 lipase regulators: inhibition of keratinocyte retinylester hydrolysis by TIP47. *J. Invest. Dermatol.* 126:2087–95
37. Gettys TW, Harkness PJ, Watson PM. 1996. The beta 3-adrenergic receptor inhibits insulin-stimulated leptin secretion from isolated rat adipocytes. *Endocrinology* 137:4054–57
38. Gettys TW, Ramkumar V, Uhing RJ, Seger L, Taylor IL. 1991. Alterations in mRNA levels, expression, and function of GTP-binding regulatory proteins in adipocytes from obese mice (C57BL/6J-ob/ob). *J. Biol. Chem.* 266:15949–55
39. Gilham D, Alam M, Gao W, Vance DE, Lehner R. 2005. Triacylglycerol hydrolase is localized to the endoplasmic reticulum by an unusual retrieval sequence where it participates in VLDL assembly without utilizing VLDL lipids as substrates. *Mol. Biol. Cell* 16:984–96
40. Giudicelli H, Combes-Pastre N, Boyer J. 1974. Lipolytic activity of adipose tissue. IV. The diacylglycerol lipase activity of human adipose tissue. *Biochim. Biophys. Acta* 369:25–33
41. Greenberg AG, Egan JJ, Wek SA, Moos MCJ, Londos C, Kimmel AR. 1993. Isolation of cDNAs of perilipins A and B: sequence and expression of lipid droplet–associated proteins of adipocytes. *Proc. Natl. Acad. Sci. USA* 90:12035–39
42. Greenberg AS, Egan JJ, Wek SA, Garty NB, Blanchette-Mackie EJ, Londos C. 1991. Perilipin, a major hormonally regulated adipocyte-specific phosphoprotein associated with the periphery of lipid storage droplets. *J. Biol. Chem.* 266:11341–46
43. Haemmerle G, Lass A, Zimmermann R, Gorkiewicz G, Meyer C, et al. 2006. Defective lipolysis and altered energy metabolism in mice lacking adipose triglyceride lipase. *Science* 312:734–37

44. Haemmerle G, Zimmermann R, Hayn M, Theussl C, Waeg G, et al. 2002. Hormone-sensitive lipase deficiency in mice causes diglyceride accumulation in adipose tissue, muscle, and testis. *J. Biol. Chem.* 277:4806–15
45. Haemmerle G, Zimmermann R, Strauss JG, Kratky D, Riederer M, et al. 2002. Hormone-sensitive lipase deficiency in mice changes the plasma lipid profile by affecting the tissue-specific expression pattern of lipoprotein lipase in adipose tissue and muscle. *J. Biol. Chem.* 277:12946–52
46. Hara-Chikuma M, Sohara E, Rai T, Ikawa M, Okabe M, et al. 2005. Progressive adipocyte hypertrophy in aquaporin-7-deficient mice: adipocyte glycerol permeability as a novel regulator of fat accumulation. *J. Biol. Chem.* 280:15493–96
47. Harada K, Shen WJ, Patel S, Natu V, Wang J, et al. 2003. Resistance to high-fat diet-induced obesity and altered expression of adipose-specific genes in HSL-deficient mice. *Am. J. Physiol. Endocrinol. Metab.* 285:E1182–95
48. Heckemeyer CM, Barker J, Duckworth WC, Solomon SS. 1983. Studies of the biological effect and degradation of glucagon in the rat perifused isolated adipose cell. *Endocrinology* 113:270–76
49. Hertzel AV, Smith LA, Berg AH, Cline GW, Shulman GI, et al. 2006. Lipid metabolism and adipokine levels in fatty acid-binding protein null and transgenic mice. *Am. J. Physiol. Endocrinol. Metab.* 290:E814–23
50. Hibuse T, Maeda N, Funahashi T, Yamamoto K, Nagasawa A, et al. 2005. Aquaporin 7 deficiency is associated with development of obesity through activation of adipose glycerol kinase. *Proc. Natl. Acad. Sci. USA* 102:10993–98
51. Holm C. 2003. Molecular mechanisms regulating hormone-sensitive lipase and lipolysis. *Biochem. Soc. Trans.* 31:1120–24
52. Howard BV, Klimes I, Vasquez B, Brady D, Nagulesparan M, Unger RH. 1984. The antilipolytic action of insulin in obese subjects with resistance to its glucoregulatory action. *J. Clin. Endocrinol. Metab.* 58:544–48
53. Jenkins CM, Mancuso DJ, Yan W, Sims HF, Gibson B, Gross RW. 2004. Identification, cloning, expression, and purification of three novel human calcium-independent phospholipase A2 family members possessing triacylglycerol lipase and acylglycerol transacylase activities. *J. Biol. Chem.* 279:48968–75
54. Johnson JA, Fried SK, Pi-Sunyer FX, Albu JB. 2001. Impaired insulin action in subcutaneous adipocytes from women with visceral obesity. *Am. J. Physiol. Endocrinol. Metab.* 280:E40–49
55. Kalderon B, Mayorek N, Berry E, Zevit N, Bar-Tana J. 2000. Fatty acid cycling in the fasting rat. *Am. J. Physiol. Endocrinol. Metab.* 279:E221–27
56. Kang L, Nagy LE. 2006. Chronic ethanol feeding suppresses beta-adrenergic receptor-stimulated lipolysis in adipocytes isolated from epididymal fat. *Endocrinology* 147:4330–38
57. Karlsson M, Contreras JA, Hellman U, Tornqvist H, Holm C. 1997. cDNA cloning, tissue distribution, and identification of the catalytic triad of monoglyceride lipase. Evolutionary relationship to esterases, lysophospholipases, and haloperoxidases. *J. Biol. Chem.* 272:27218–23
58. Karlsson M, Reue K, Xia YR, Lusis AJ, Langin D, et al. 2001. Exon-intron organization and chromosomal localization of the mouse monoglyceride lipase gene. *Gene* 272:11–18
59. Kershaw EE, Hamm JK, Verhagen LA, Peroni O, Katic M, Flier JS. 2006. Adipose triglyceride lipase: function, regulation by insulin, and comparison with adiponutrin. *Diabetes* 55:148–57
60. Kim C, Xuong NH, Taylor SS. 2005. Crystal structure of a complex between the catalytic and regulatory (RIalpha) subunits of PKA. *Science* 307:690–96

61. Kobayashi-Hattori K, Mogi A, Matsumoto Y, Takita T. 2005. Effect of caffeine on the body fat and lipid metabolism of rats fed on a high-fat diet. *Biosci. Biotechnol. Biochem.* 69:2219–23
62. Lake AC, Sun Y, Li JL, Kim JE, Johnson JW, et al. 2005. Expression, regulation, and triglyceride hydrolase activity of adiponutrin family members. *J. Lipid Res.* 46:2477–87
63. Langin D. 2006. Control of fatty acid and glycerol release in adipose tissue lipolysis. *C. R. Biol.* 329:598–607; discussion 653–55
64. Large V, Peroni O, Letexier D, Ray H, Beylot M. 2004. Metabolism of lipids in human white adipocyte. *Diabetes Metab.* 30:294–309
65. Large V, Reynisdottir S, Langin D, Fredby K, Klannemark M, et al. 1999. Decreased expression and function of adipocyte hormone-sensitive lipase in subcutaneous fat cells of obese subjects. *J. Lipid Res.* 40:2059–66
66. Lass A, Zimmermann R, Haemmerle G, Riederer M, Schoiswohl G, et al. 2006. Adipose triglyceride lipase-mediated lipolysis of cellular fat stores is activated by CGI-58 and defective in Chanarin-Dorfman syndrome. *Cell Metab.* 3:309–19
67. Lefevre C, Jobard F, Caux F, Bouadjar B, Karaduman A, et al. 2001. Mutations in CGI-58, the gene encoding a new protein of the esterase/lipase/thioesterase subfamily, in Chanarin-Dorfman syndrome. *Am. J. Hum. Genet.* 69:1002–12
68. Lehner R, Vance DE. 1999. Cloning and expression of a cDNA encoding a hepatic microsomal lipase that mobilizes stored triacylglycerol. *Biochem. J.* 343(Pt. 1):1–10
69. Lehner R, Verger R. 1997. Purification and characterization of a porcine liver microsomal triacylglycerol hydrolase. *Biochemistry* 36:1861–68
70. Liu P, Ying Y, Zhao Y, Mundy DI, Zhu M, Anderson RG. 2004. Chinese hamster ovary K2 cell lipid droplets appear to be metabolic organelles involved in membrane traffic. *J. Biol. Chem.* 279:3787–92
71. Lofgren P, Hoffstedt J, Naslund E, Wiren M, Arner P. 2005. Prospective and controlled studies of the actions of insulin and catecholamine in fat cells of obese women following weight reduction. *Diabetologia* 48:2334–42
72. Londos C, Cooper DM, Schlegel W, Rodbell M. 1978. Adenosine analogs inhibit adipocyte adenylate cyclase by a GTP-dependent process: basis for actions of adenosine and methylxanthines on cyclic AMP production and lipolysis. *Proc. Natl. Acad. Sci. USA* 75:5362–66
73. Londos C, Honnor RC, Dhillon GS. 1985. cAMP-dependent protein kinase and lipolysis in rat adipocytes. III. Multiple modes of insulin regulation of lipolysis and regulation of insulin responses by adenylate cyclase regulators. *J. Biol. Chem.* 260:15139–45
74. Lonnqvist F, Arner P, Nordfors L, Schalling M. 1995. Overexpression of the obese (ob) gene in adipose tissue of human obese subjects. *Nat. Med.* 1:950–53
75. Maeda N, Funahashi T, Hibuse T, Nagasawa A, Kishida K, et al. 2004. Adaptation to fasting by glycerol transport through aquaporin 7 in adipose tissue. *Proc. Natl. Acad. Sci. USA* 101:17801–6
76. Marcinkiewicz A, Gauthier D, Garcia A, Brasaemle DL. 2006. The phosphorylation of serine 492 of perilipin A directs lipid droplet fragmentation and dispersion. *J. Biol. Chem.* 281:11901–9
77. Martin LF, Klim CM, Vannucci SJ, Dixon LB, Landis JR, LaNoue KF. 1990. Alterations in adipocyte adenylate cyclase activity in morbidly obese and formerly morbidly obese humans. *Surgery* 108:228–34; discussion 234–35
78. Martinez-Botas J, Anderson JB, Tessier D, Lapillonne A, Chang BH, et al. 2000. Absence of perilipin results in leanness and reverses obesity in Lepr(db/db) mice. *Nat. Genet.* 26:474–79

79. Matarese V, Bernlohr DA. 1988. Purification of murine adipocyte lipid-binding protein. Characterization as a fatty acid- and retinoic acid-binding protein. *J. Biol. Chem.* 263:14544–51
80. Mayes PA, Topping DL. 1974. Regulation of hepatic lipogenesis by plasma free fatty acids: simultaneous studies on lipoprotein secretion, cholesterol synthesis, ketogenesis and gluconeogenesis. *Biochem. J.* 140:111–14
81. McCarty MF, Thomas CA. 2003. PTH excess may promote weight gain by impeding catecholamine-induced lipolysis—implications for the impact of calcium, vitamin D, and alcohol on body weight. *Med. Hypotheses* 61:535–42
82. Melanson EL, Sharp TA, Schneider J, Donahoo WT, Grunwald GK, Hill JO. 2003. Relation between calcium intake and fat oxidation in adult humans. *Int. J. Obes. Relat. Metab. Disord.* 27:196–203
83. Merida E, Delgado E, Molina LM, Villanueva-Penacarrillo ML, Valverde I. 1993. Presence of glucagon and glucagon-like peptide-1-(7-36)amide receptors in solubilized membranes of human adipose tissue. *J. Clin. Endocrinol. Metab.* 77:1654–57
84. Miyoshi H, Souza SC, Zhang HH, Strissel KJ, Christoffolete MA, et al. 2006. Perilipin promotes hormone-sensitive lipase-mediated adipocyte lipolysis via phosphorylation-dependent and -independent mechanisms. *J. Biol. Chem.* 281:15837–44
85. Moore HP, Silver RB, Mottillo EP, Bernlohr DA, Granneman JG. 2005. Perilipin targets a novel pool of lipid droplets for lipolytic attack by hormone-sensitive lipase. *J. Biol. Chem.* 280:43109–20
86. Muller G, Ertl J, Gerl M, Preibisch G. 1997. Leptin impairs metabolic actions of insulin in isolated rat adipocytes. *J. Biol. Chem.* 272:10585–93
87. Murray RK, Granner DK, Mayes PA, Rodwell VW. 2000. *Harper's Biochemistry*. Stamford, CT: Appleton & Lange. 927 pp.
88. Natarajan R, Ghosh S, Grogan W. 1996. Catalytic properties of the purified rat hepatic cytosolic cholesteryl ester hydrolase. *Biochem. Biophys. Res. Commun.* 225:413–19
89. Ni Z, Smogorzewski M, Massry SG. 1994. Effects of parathyroid hormone on cytosolic calcium of rat adipocytes. *Endocrinology* 135:1837–44
90. Okazaki H, Igarashi M, Nishi M, Tajima M, Sekiya M, et al. 2006. Identification of a novel member of the carboxylesterase family that hydrolyzes triacylglycerol: a potential role in adipocyte lipolysis. *Diabetes* 55:2091–97
91. Okazaki H, Osuga J, Tamura Y, Yahagi N, Tomita S, et al. 2002. Lipolysis in the absence of hormone-sensitive lipase: evidence for a common mechanism regulating distinct lipases. *Diabetes* 51:3368–75
92. Olsson H, Belfrage P. 1987. The regulatory and basal phosphorylation sites of hormone-sensitive lipase are dephosphorylated by protein phosphatase-1, 2A and 2C but not by protein phosphatase-2B. *Eur. J. Biochem.* 168:399–405
93. Ostermeyer AG, Paci JM, Zeng Y, Lublin DM, Munro S, Brown DA. 2001. Accumulation of caveolin in the endoplasmic reticulum redirects the protein to lipid storage droplets. *J. Cell Biol.* 152:1071–78
94. Osuga J, Ishibashi S, Oka T, Yagyu H, Tozawa R, et al. 2000. Targeted disruption of hormone-sensitive lipase results in male sterility and adipocyte hypertrophy, but not in obesity. *Proc. Natl. Acad. Sci. USA* 97:787–92
95. Peers DG, Davies JI. 1971. Significance of the caffeine-like effect of various purines, pyrimidines and derivatives on adipose-tissue phosphodiesterase. *Biochem. J.* 124:P8–9
96. Perea A, Clemente F, Martinell J, Villanueva-Penacarrillo ML, Valverde I. 1995. Physiological effect of glucagon in human isolated adipocytes. *Horm. Metab. Res.* 27:372–75

97. Prins JB, Niesler CU, Winterford CM, Bright NA, Siddle K, et al. 1997. Tumor necrosis factor-alpha induces apoptosis of human adipose cells. *Diabetes* 46:1939–44
98. Qian H, Hausman GJ, Compton MM, Azain MJ, Hartzell DL, Baile CA. 1998. Leptin regulation of peroxisome proliferator-activated receptor-gamma, tumor necrosis factor, and uncoupling protein-2 expression in adipose tissues. *Biochem. Biophys. Res. Commun.* 246:660–67
99. Raclot T, Leray C, Bach AC, Groscolas R. 1995. The selective mobilization of fatty acids is not based on their positional distribution in white-fat-cell triacylglycerols. *Biochem. J.* 311(Pt. 3):911–16
100. Ragolia L, Begum N. 1998. Protein phosphatase-1 and insulin action. *Mol. Cell. Biochem.* 182:49–58
101. Razani B, Rubin CS, Lisanti MP. 1999. Regulation of cAMP-mediated signal transduction via interaction of caveolins with the catalytic subunit of protein kinase A. *J. Biol. Chem.* 274:26353–60
102. Reynisdottir S, Langin D, Carlstrom K, Holm C, Rossner S, Arner P. 1995. Effects of weight reduction on the regulation of lipolysis in adipocytes of women with upper-body obesity. *Clin. Sci. (Lond.)* 89:421–29
103. Robenek MJ, Severs NJ, Schlattmann K, Plenz G, Zimmer KP, et al. 2004. Lipids partition caveolin-1 from ER membranes into lipid droplets: updating the model of lipid droplet biogenesis. *FASEB J.* 18:866–68
104. Ryden M, Arvidsson E, Blomqvist L, Perbeck L, Dicker A, Arner P. 2004. Targets for TNF-alpha-induced lipolysis in human adipocytes. *Biochem. Biophys. Res. Commun.* 318:168–75
105. Ryden M, Dicker A, van Harmelen V, Hauner H, Brunnberg M, et al. 2002. Mapping of early signaling events in tumor necrosis factor alpha–mediated lipolysis in human fat cells. *J. Biol. Chem.* 277:1085–91
106. Saha PK, Kojima H, Martinez-Botas J, Sunehag AL, Chan L. 2004. Metabolic adaptations in the absence of perilipin: increased beta-oxidation and decreased hepatic glucose production associated with peripheral insulin resistance but normal glucose tolerance in perilipin-null mice. *J. Biol. Chem.* 279:35150–58
107. Scherer PE, Lisanti MP, Baldini G, Sargiacomo M, Mastick CC, Lodish HF. 1994. Induction of caveolin during adipogenesis and association of GLUT4 with caveolin-rich vesicles. *J. Cell Biol.* 127:1233–43
108. Schrager S. 2005. Dietary calcium intake and obesity. *J. Am. Board Fam. Pract.* 18:205–10
109. Schwartz JP, Jungas RL. 1971. Studies on the hormone-sensitive lipase of adipose tissue. *J. Lipid Res.* 12:553–62
110. Shaughnessy S, Smith ER, Kodukula S, Storch J, Fried SK. 2000. Adipocyte metabolism in adipocyte fatty acid binding protein knockout mice (aP2-/-) after short-term high-fat feeding: functional compensation by the keratinocyte [correction of keritinocyte] fatty acid binding protein. *Diabetes* 49:904–11
111. Shi H, Dirienzo D, Zemel MB. 2001. Effects of dietary calcium on adipocyte lipid metabolism and body weight regulation in energy-restricted aP2-agouti transgenic mice. *FASEB J.* 15:291–93
112. Siegrist-Kaiser CA, Pauli V, Juge-Aubry CE, Boss O, Pernin A, et al. 1997. Direct effects of leptin on brown and white adipose tissue. *J. Clin. Invest.* 100:2858–64
113. Siler SQ, Neese RA, Hellerstein MK. 1999. De novo lipogenesis, lipid kinetics, and whole-body lipid balances in humans after acute alcohol consumption. *Am. J. Clin. Nutr.* 70:928–36

114. Slavin BG, Ong JM, Kern PA. 1994. Hormonal regulation of hormone-sensitive lipase activity and mRNA levels in isolated rat adipocytes. *J. Lipid Res.* 35:1535–41
115. Smirnova E, Goldberg EB, Makarova KS, Lin L, Brown WJ, Jackson CL. 2006. ATGL has a key role in lipid droplet/adiposome degradation in mammalian cells. *EMBO Rep.* 7:106–13
116. Soni KG, Lehner R, Metalnikov P, O'Donnell P, Semache M, et al. 2004. Carboxylesterase 3 (EC 3.1.1.1) is a major adipocyte lipase. *J. Biol. Chem.* 279:40683–89
117. Souza SC, Muliro KV, Liscum L, Lien P, Yamamoto MT, et al. 2002. Modulation of hormone-sensitive lipase and protein kinase A-mediated lipolysis by perilipin A in an adenoviral reconstituted system. *J. Biol. Chem.* 277:8267–72
118. Stevens J, Green MH, Kaiser DL, Pohl SL. 1981. Insulin resistance in adipocytes from fed and fasted obese rats: dissociation of two insulin actions. *Mol. Cell. Biochem.* 37:177–83
119. Stralfors P, Honnor RC. 1989. Insulin-induced dephosphorylation of hormone-sensitive lipase. Correlation with lipolysis and cAMP-dependent protein kinase activity. *Eur. J. Biochem.* 182:379–85
120. Su CL, Sztalryd C, Contreras JA, Holm C, Kimmel AR, Londos C. 2003. Mutational analysis of the hormone-sensitive lipase translocation reaction in adipocytes. *J. Biol. Chem.* 278:43615–19
121. Subramanian V, Rothenberg A, Gomez C, Cohen AW, Garcia A, et al. 2004. Perilipin A mediates the reversible binding of CGI-58 to lipid droplets in 3T3-L1 adipocytes. *J. Biol. Chem.* 279:42062–71
122. Sun X, Zemel MB. 2004. Calcium and dairy products inhibit weight and fat regain during ad libitum consumption following energy restriction in aP2-agouti transgenic mice. *J. Nutr.* 134:3054–60
123. Syu LJ, Saltiel AR. 1999. Lipotransin: a novel docking protein for hormone-sensitive lipase. *Mol. Cell* 4:109–15
124. Sztalryd C, Kraemer FB. 1994. Regulation of hormone-sensitive lipase during fasting. *Am. J. Physiol.* 266:E179–85
125. Sztalryd C, Xu G, Dorward H, Tansey JT, Contreras JA, et al. 2003. Perilipin A is essential for the translocation of hormone-sensitive lipase during lipolytic activation. *J. Cell Biol.* 161:1093–103
126. Tansey JT, Huml AM, Vogt R, Davis KE, Jones JM, et al. 2003. Functional studies on native and mutated forms of perilipins: a role in protein kinase A-mediated lipolysis of triacylglycerols. *J. Biol. Chem.* 278:8401–6
127. Tansey JT, Sztalryd C, Gruia-Gray J, Roush DL, Zee JV, et al. 2001. Perilipin ablation results in a lean mouse with aberrant adipocyte lipolysis, enhanced leptin production, and resistance to diet-induced obesity. *Proc. Natl. Acad. Sci. USA* 98:6494–99
128. Tansey JT, Sztalryd C, Hlavin EM, Kimmel AR, Londos C. 2004. The central role of perilipin A in lipid metabolism and adipocyte lipolysis. *IUBMB Life* 56:379–85
129. Tornqvist H, Belfrage P. 1976. Purification and some properties of a monoacylglycerol-hydrolyzing enzyme of rat adipose tissue. *J. Biol. Chem.* 251:813–19
130. Villena JA, Roy S, Sarkadi-Nagy E, Kim KH, Sul HS. 2004. Desnutrin, an adipocyte gene encoding a novel patatin domain-containing protein, is induced by fasting and glucocorticoids: Ectopic expression of desnutrin increases triglyceride hydrolysis. *J. Biol. Chem.* 279:47066–75
131. Villena JA, Viollet B, Andreelli F, Kahn A, Vaulont S, Sul HS. 2004. Induced adiposity and adipocyte hypertrophy in mice lacking the AMP-activated protein kinase-alpha2 subunit. *Diabetes* 53:2242–49

132. Voshol PJ, Haemmerle G, Ouwens DM, Zimmermann R, Zechner R, et al. 2003. Increased hepatic insulin sensitivity together with decreased hepatic triglyceride stores in hormone-sensitive lipase-deficient mice. *Endocrinology* 144:3456–62
133. Walley AJ, Blakemore AI, Froguel P. 2006. Genetics of obesity and the prediction of risk for health. *Hum. Mol. Genet.* 15(Suppl. 2):R124–30
134. Wang SP, Laurin N, Himms-Hagen J, Rudnicki MA, Levy E, et al. 2001. The adipose tissue phenotype of hormone-sensitive lipase deficiency in mice. *Obes. Res.* 9:119–28
135. Wang Y, Sullivan S, Trujillo M, Lee MJ, Schneider SH, et al. 2003. Perilipin expression in human adipose tissues: effects of severe obesity, gender, and depot. *Obes. Res.* 11:930–36
136. Wei E, Lehner R, Vance DE. 2005. C/EBPalpha activates the transcription of triacylglycerol hydrolase in 3T3-L1 adipocytes. *Biochem. J.* 388:959–66
137. Westerterp-Plantenga MS, Lejeune MP, Kovacs EM. 2005. Body weight loss and weight maintenance in relation to habitual caffeine intake and green tea supplementation. *Obes. Res.* 13:1195–204
138. Xue B, Greenberg AG, Kraemer FB, Zemel MB. 2001. Mechanism of intracellular calcium ([Ca2+]i) inhibition of lipolysis in human adipocytes. *FASEB J.* 15:2527–29
139. Yamaguchi T, Omatsu N, Matsushita S, Osumi T. 2004. CGI-58 interacts with perilipin and is localized to lipid droplets. Possible involvement of CGI-58 mislocalization in Chanarin-Dorfman syndrome. *J. Biol. Chem.* 279:30490–97
140. Yamaguchi T, Omatsu N, Omukae A, Osumi T. 2006. Analysis of interaction partners for perilipin and ADRP on lipid droplets. *Mol. Cell. Biochem.* 284:167–73
141. Zemel MB. 2002. Regulation of adiposity and obesity risk by dietary calcium: mechanisms and implications. *J. Am. Coll. Nutr.* 21:146–51S
142. Zemel MB, Thompson W, Milstead A, Morris K, Campbell P. 2004. Calcium and dairy acceleration of weight and fat loss during energy restriction in obese adults. *Obes. Res.* 12:582–90
143. Zhang J, Hupfeld CJ, Taylor SS, Olefsky JM, Tsien RY. 2005. Insulin disrupts beta-adrenergic signaling to protein kinase A in adipocytes. *Nature* 437:569–73
144. Zimmermann R, Haemmerle G, Wagner EM, Strauss JG, Kratky D, Zechner R. 2003. Decreased fatty acid esterification compensates for the reduced lipolytic activity in hormone-sensitive lipase-deficient white adipose tissue. *J. Lipid Res.* 44:2089–99
145. Zimmermann R, Strauss JG, Haemmerle G, Schoiswohl G, Birner-Gruenberger R, et al. 2004. Fat mobilization in adipose tissue is promoted by adipose triglyceride lipase. *Science* 306:1383–86

Association of Maternal Obesity Before Conception with Poor Lactation Performance

Kathleen Maher Rasmussen

Division of Nutritional Sciences, Cornell University, Ithaca, New York 14853;
email: kmr5@cornell.edu

Annu. Rev. Nutr. 2007. 27:103–21

First published online as a Review in Advance on March 6, 2007

The *Annual Review of Nutrition* is online at http://nutr.annualreviews.org

This article's doi:
10.1146/annurev.nutr.27.061406.093738

0199-9885/07/0821-0103$20.00

Key Words

breastfeeding, mammary gland, lactogenesis, prolactin, gestational weight gain, pregnancy, adipose tissue

Abstract

The objective of this review is to evaluate the evidence for a link between maternal obesity and poor lactation performance. In non-human species, excess maternal fatness is deleterious for lactation and also for maternal health and survival. These effects occur during pregnancy and as milk production is beginning. They may result in poor growth and survival of the young. In women, there is a negative association between maternal obesity and the initiation as well as the continuation of breastfeeding. This appears to be derived from biological as well as sociocultural factors that are still poorly understood. Excessive gestational weight gain, complications of pregnancy and delivery, and the condition of the infant at birth may also contribute to this association. Given the increasingly high rates of obesity among women of reproductive age worldwide and the importance of breastfeeding for infant health, further study of this association is essential.

Contents

INTRODUCTION

Although it has been understood for some time that excess fatness contributes to poor health outcomes as well as to reduced milk production in dairy cows, it has only recently become evident that excess fatness may also be disadvantageous for lactation in women. The objective of this review is to evaluate the evidence for a link between maternal obesity and poor lactation performance. Much new information is available since this subject was last reviewed (81, 82). Data from production and experimental species are used to provide biological plausibility and information about potential mechanisms for this association. Data from women, which are primarily from observational epidemiologic studies, are used to establish that this association exists in women and to generate hypotheses about the additional factors that might also contribute to it.

The underlying conceptual model is complex (**Figure 1**, see color insert). Excess maternal adiposity may interfere with successful lactation by several different routes. Excess maternal adiposity may interfere with the development of the mammary glands at various times (before conception, during pregnancy, and during lactation, depending on the species). Along with hormonal and metabolic abnormalities associated with excess maternal adiposity, these developmental problems contribute to a delay in the onset of copious milk secretion (secretory activation or lactogenesis II) and, thus, to early cessation of lactation (**Figure 1*A***). Excess maternal adiposity may also lead to complications of pregnancy (such as preterm birth or cesarean section that themselves are associated with reduced success in lactation), the birth of a large baby who may be treated in ways that are not optimal for successful breastfeeding, and physical conditions (such as large breasts) that make proper breastfeeding more difficult (**Figure 1*B***). Several of these factors themselves lead to a delay in lactogenesis II and to early cessation of breastfeeding. Finally, excess maternal adiposity is negatively associated with the choice to breastfeed at all. This choice is modified by a variety of sociodemographic and psychosocial factors. These factors also modify the duration of breastfeeding among women who have chosen to breastfeed as do the physiological and mechanical factors previously associated with difficulties in establishing breastfeeding (**Figure 1*C***). In this review, these various possibilities are explored in turn.

BIOLOGICAL BASIS FOR AN ASSOCIATION BETWEEN MATERNAL OVERFATNESS AND MILK PRODUCTION

Production Species

In dairy cows, "high body condition" or excess fatness is associated with the development of "fat cow syndrome," which is characterized by "depression, anorexia, ketonuria, marked decrease in [milk] production ..." as well as other problems (66). These "overconditioned" cows experience an excessive depression of appetite after calving and, as a result, an even more negative energy balance than that of normally conditioned animals. Metabolic changes at this time include a reduction in Krebs cycle capacity as well as the inhibition of fatty acid synthesis and oxidation (68). This leads to an excess of nonesterified fatty acids in the blood, an amount that is more than the liver can process. This produces a build-up of triacylglycerols in the liver and, eventually, fatty liver (97). Animals may die from this condition (63, 66).

Although the negative energy balance that begins after delivery may precipitate the death of overconditioned dairy cows, poor milk production may have additional, earlier origins. It has long been known that "mammary development [is] incomplete in cows raised on a high feeding level" (102). "High feeding" (usually a high energy intake, but other dietary components may also be fed in excess) affects development of the mammary gland differently at various stages in the life of the dairy cow. Increased growth has no effect on development of the mammary gland before the calf weighs 90 kg, but between that weight and puberty, high feeding leads to reduced growth of the mammary gland and also reduced milk yield (102). After puberty and during pregnancy, high feeding does not affect mammary development (102), which is complete at calving (102). The negative effects of high feeding on mammary development appear to be driven by the energy, not the protein, component of the diet offered (11).

In the dairy cow, high feeding disproportionately increases the mass of the mammary stroma, a matrix of connective and adipose tissue, but inhibits growth of the parenchyma, which consists of epithelial cells (107). Sejrsen and coworkers (102) have investigated whether growth hormone, which is required for mammary gland development during puberty in the dairy cow and is affected by feeding level, might be involved. Based on the results of several experiments, they concluded that the "reduced sensitivity of the mammary tissue to IGF-I is the most logical explanation for the reduced mammary growth due to high feeding level" (102). More recently, they and others (107) have considered the additional hypothesis that leptin, which rises in response to high feeding, might be an important mediating factor. Although Thorn et al. (107) were able to show that leptin synthesis is increased in heifers fed at a high plane of nutrition, they also showed that leptin did not act directly on mammary epithelial cells. Thus, the exact cause of the inhibition of the growth of the mammary parenchyma with high feeding in dairy cows remains unknown.

Although there is no recognized "fat pig syndrome," some attention has been given to the association between nutritional status and the success of lactation in this species, with findings similar to those in dairy cows. Pigs that were overfed during pregnancy and, thus, were too fat at farrowing ate significantly less and had significantly higher concentrations of nonesterified fatty acids in their plasma during lactation than controls of normal fatness (89). In this same experiment, the milk production of the overfat sows was 10% and 15% lower than that of the control animals at 2 and 4 wk of lactation, respectively (88). The authors speculated that the poorer milk production of the overfat animals may have resulted from poor mammary development during pregnancy. There is support for this possibility because increased dietary energy was detrimental to the development of secretory tissue in the mammary gland in another experiment in which gilts were overfed during the last quarter of pregnancy and during lactation (112). In this study, mammary parenchymal weight as well as DNA, RNA, and protein concentrations in the parenchyma were significantly lower in the overfed than in normally fed animals; this was not the case in the mammary stroma (112).

There is one report (109) of an association between overnutrition and an indicator of lactation performance in sheep. In this study, ewes were overfed after breeding, and at parturition, were 20 kg heavier and produced significantly less colostrum. In horses, there is a positive association between condition score, a measure of body fatness (36), and reproductive performance, including success in lactation (20, 35). Although there did not appear to be reproductive difficulties among the relatively few obese mares studied, researchers have noted that there is "no reproductive advantage" to keeping animals in this condition and that it can be "economically prohibitive" (32).

In summary, it is not surprising that the association between maternal overfatness and milk production has been most thoroughly studied in the dairy cow, where the economic consequences of this association are the greatest. Poor milk production results from the metabolic sequelae of especially severe negative energy balance among so-called fat cows. Poor milk production may also result from impaired development of the mammary gland when overfeeding occurs before puberty in dairy cows. In pigs, poor milk production results from impaired development of the mammary gland when overfeeding occurs during pregnancy. The mechanism by which excess body fatness impairs the development of the mammary gland in these species has not yet been determined.

Experimental Species

Nearly all of the research on obesity and lactational performance in experimental species has been carried out in rodents, particularly rats, and has used either "cafeteria" feeding or high-fat diets to produce obesity before breeding. In cafeteria feeding, rats are offered a selection of high-fat snack items. As a result, the composition of the diet differs from rat to rat and the diet consumed may or may not provide adequate protein. With a high-fat diet, each rat consumes a diet of the same composition, which can be constructed to provide adequate dietary protein for animals at all life stages. Although it is easier to know what the rat has consumed and also to meet the relatively high protein requirements for lactation in rats with a high-fat diet than with cafeteria feeding, results obtained using these two approaches are concordant so they are considered together. Genetically obese rats and mice generally are infertile and, thus, not suitable for studying the association between obesity and lactation. Obese rats are significantly heavier and fatter than are their nonobese counterparts, but there is no cut-off point—as there is for human beings—for declaring a rat to be "obese." Studies in rodents have provided data to support many of the elements of the underlying conceptual framework for this review (82).

Development of the mammary glands. In a study of mice fed a high-fat diet for 2 mo before conception, Flint et al. (28) found that they were heavier throughout the reproductive period than controls, with heavier mammary glands during pregnancy and immediately after parturition. This difference in mammary gland weight was no longer evident at mid-lactation because adipose tissue had been mobilized from the mammary glands of the obese animals. There was no difference between the obese and control animals in the DNA content or the total amount of parenchymal tissue in the mammary glands during this experiment. The ductal structures had invaded the entire mammary fat pad in both obese and control animals. However, there were a number of abnormal aspects of the mammary glands of the obese mice, such as abnormal side branching of the ductules and abnormal alveolar development at mid-pregnancy. Taken together, these findings suggest that the problem caused by obesity is not one of growth or proliferation of epithelial tissue in the mammary gland but rather one of development or differentiation of the alveoli (28).

The growth and development of the parenchyma of the mammary gland is regulated by both systemic and local factors, and the mammary fat pad is central to this regulation (42). The mammary fat pad is a matrix of adipose and connective tissue that can mediate hormone action and synthesize compounds that regulate growth. Whether the excess fat that is deposited in the mammary gland as the animal becomes obese influences the development or differentiation of the gland is unknown at present. However, it is known that the lipids (or their derivatives) stored in the adipose tissue that is part of the fat pad could influence the growth of mammary epithelial cells (42). Thus, the results of Flint et al. (28) suggest that additional attention to the role of the mammary fat pad in obesity could prove to be informative.

Complications of pregnancy. In both rats (94, 95, 103, 110) and mice (28), a lower proportion of obese animals conceive and, among those that do become pregnant, obese animals deliver fewer pups in each litter and have lower pup survival than controls (84). Even with fewer pups in the litters, mean weight at birth for pups born to obese dams is either not different (94, 96, 103) or even less (19, 28)—not more—than those of normal-weight dams, as might be expected from excess maternal adiposity and lower litter number.

Metabolic conditions postpartum. Rodents dramatically increase their food and energy intakes during lactation. Surprisingly, obesity dampens these increases in rats (95, 96). This may be because heat production in the lactating rat is already maximal (30) and obesity exacerbates the animal's problem with heat disposal. Body weight (94, 96) and carcass fat (82) decrease substantially from late pregnancy to mid-lactation, but remain higher in obese rats in mid-lactation than in control animals. As was the case for the dairy cow, obese rats may develop fatty livers (1). In the single study in mice (28), obese animals decreased their food intake more than controls around the time of parturition, but remained heavier than controls throughout the remainder of lactation. Although these obese mice lost more parametrial fat than controls during lactation, they still had more fat in this depot in mid-lactation.

The transition from pregnancy to lactation is associated with numerous metabolic changes that permit the nursing animal to direct the substrates that are needed for milk production to the mammary gland. For example, concentrations of plasma insulin decrease while those of prolactin increase between day 20 of pregnancy and day 3 of lactation (87). These changes also occur in obese animals, but they are significantly reduced (103). Agius et al. (1) observed that by 6–10 d postpartum, blood concentrations of glucose and ketone bodies were higher in obese than in control animals. This combination may have contributed to the remarkably reduced rate of fatty acid synthesis that they observed in mammary tissue in the obese rats (1). Similar observations have been made in mice (28). In the experiment of Agius et al. (1), the obese rats also developed fatty livers, which the investigators attributed to increased mobilization of fat from their excessive amount of adipose tissue. This greater mobilization of adipose tissue during lactation in rats fed a high-fat diet has been confirmed by others (105).

Progress of lactation. In both rats and mice, obesity causes an initial impairment in milk production. This may result in the death of the litter because the pups may receive no milk at all in the first day of life (103). Alternatively, the milk volume may be low but still sufficient for the pups to survive, and then may increase over the next few days (28). Both of these findings suggest that obesity interferes with lactogenesis.

In their photomicrographs, Flint et al. (28) have provided visual evidence of impaired lactogenesis in mice: Lipid droplets remained within the alveolar cells of the obese animals but had moved to the lumen of the ductules of the controls at day 1 of lactation. Impaired lactogenesis is consistent with the observation of impaired alveolar development in these animals (28). Moreover, Flint et al. (28) also documented changes in mRNA expression that were consistent with a decrease in milk secretion at this time. On day 1 of lactation, the expression of major milk proteins—α-lactalbumin, β-casein, and whey acid protein—was reduced as was the expression of acetyl-CoA carboxylase, which indicates that the de novo synthesis of fatty acids in the mammary gland was also reduced (28).

Both milk production and composition are affected by obesity in rats. Obese animals produce less milk than controls (91). This is also seen in animals fed high-fat diets only during lactation who are not yet "obese," and is thought to result from ketosis in the dams (30). The milk of the obese rats contains a lower concentration of protein (93) and a higher concentration of fat (73, 92, 93) than that of control animals. The fatty acid composition of the milk reflects the diet fed to produce obesity and, thus, also the composition of the animals' adipose tissue (92, 93). The effects of these simultaneous changes in milk volume and composition have been inconsistent, with investigators reporting lower (94) or higher (5, 73, 96) pup weights at weaning among those nursed by obese dams compared with control animals.

In the single report in mice (28), the expression of α-lactalbumin and acetyl-CoA carboxylase remained depressed on day 10 of lactation. These changes in expression were associated with lower concentrations of protein and higher concentrations of fat in the milk of the obese dams. The litters nursed by obese dams grew less well than did those nursed by controls on the first day of life, but their growth was equivalent thereafter (28).

In one report in rats, maternal obesity was accompanied by changes in maternal behavior. Pups born to obese rat dams "were observed in contact with their mothers, but not suckling, and they were being licked more frequently than pups of control mothers" (110). From this single report, it is difficult to know how important changes in maternal behavior might be, but it may be fruitful to explore this possibility further.

Amelioration of the effects of obesity on lactation. Studies in experimental species also provide information about whether changes in diet during lactation can ameliorate the effects of pre-existing obesity on lactation. In these studies, the type of high-fat diet that was used to induce maternal obesity before conception appeared to matter. When rats fed a cafeteria diet were switched to a closed-formula, low-fat rat diet at delivery, they lost more weight during lactation than those who continued to be fed the cafeteria diet. Their pups also grew poorly (96) in spite of the fact that the milk energy concentration did not differ between these two groups of dams. Milk production was not measured in this experiment (93). In contrast, when rats fed an open-formula, high-fat diet were switched to an open-formula, low-fat diet, they lost less weight during lactation than those that continued to be fed the high-fat diet. In addition, the litters of the animals that switched diets grew better than the litters of those that continued to be fed the high-fat diet (87). Thus, the higher milk volume in the dams that were switched to the low-fat diet appeared to have compensated for lower milk lactose and lipid concentrations (87) to permit better growth of the pups.

In summary, the findings in production and experimental species are consistent: Consumption of a diet that is sufficient to cause excess maternal fatness is deleterious for lactation. In production species, excess maternal fatness is also deleterious for maternal health and survival. In experimental species, the deleterious effects of excess fatness occur during pregnancy and immediately after giving birth (when milk production is just beginning) and may be accompanied by poor growth and survival of the litter.

STUDIES IN LACTATING WOMEN

Development of the Mammary Glands

To date, the possibility that obesity might directly affect the development of the human mammary gland at any stage has not been studied in women. More generally, "little is known about the development of the normal human mammary gland" (43). The

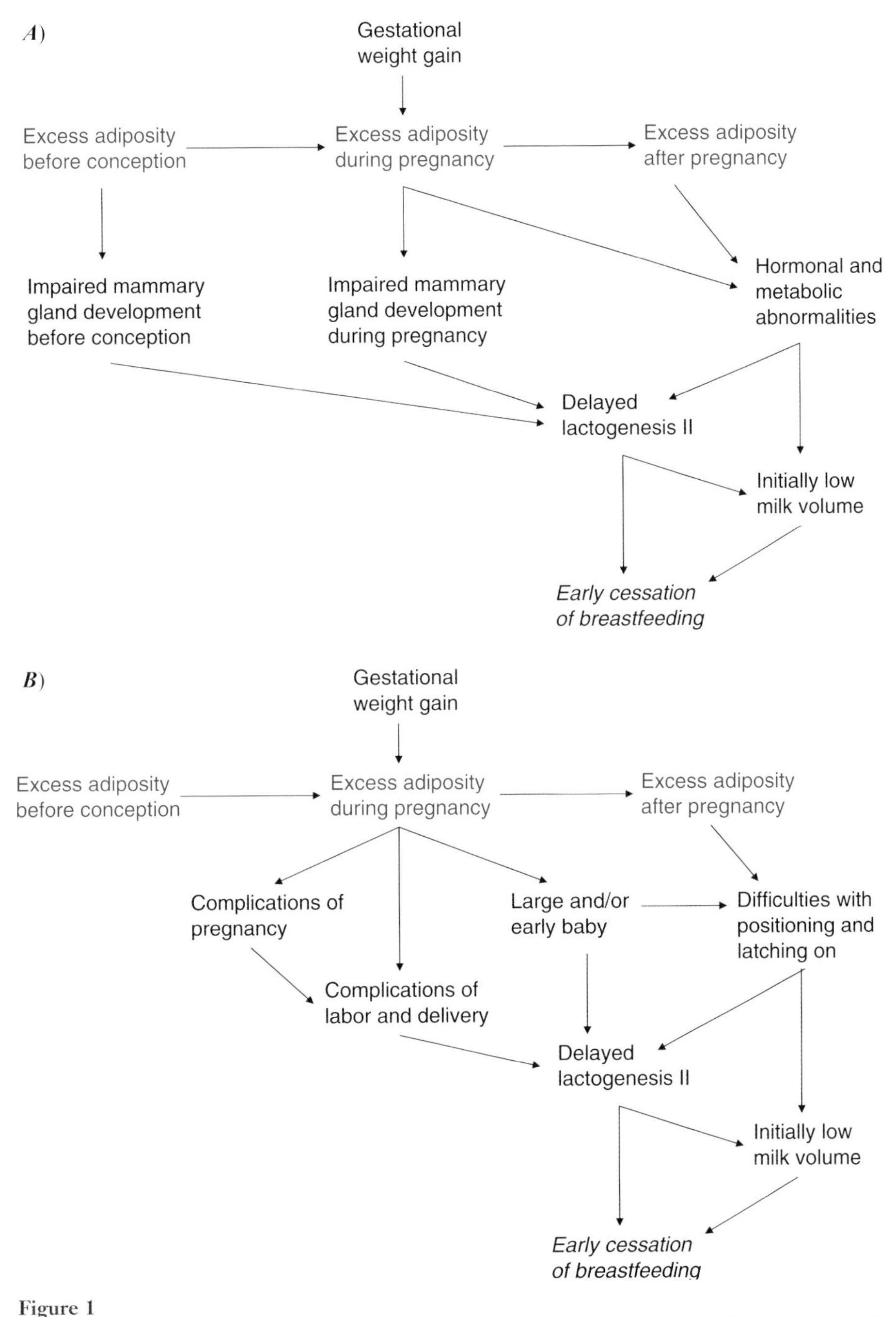

Figure 1

Possible pathways by which maternal obesity could lead to early cessation of breastfeeding. (*A*) Biological factors related to mammary gland development as well as physiological factors in the postpartum period. (*B*) Medical factors in pregnancy and mechanical and physiological factors in the postpartum period. (*C*) Modification of the choice to breastfeed and to continue to breastfeed by sociodemographic and psychosocial factors as well as mechanical and physiological difficulties with establishing breastfeeding.

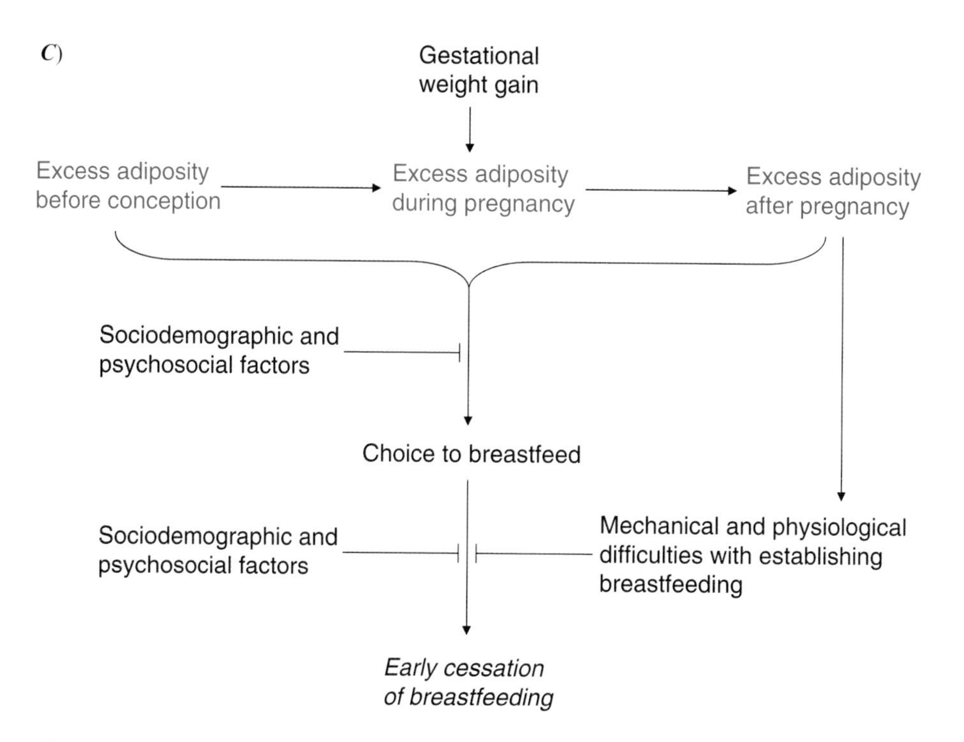

Figure 1

(Continued)

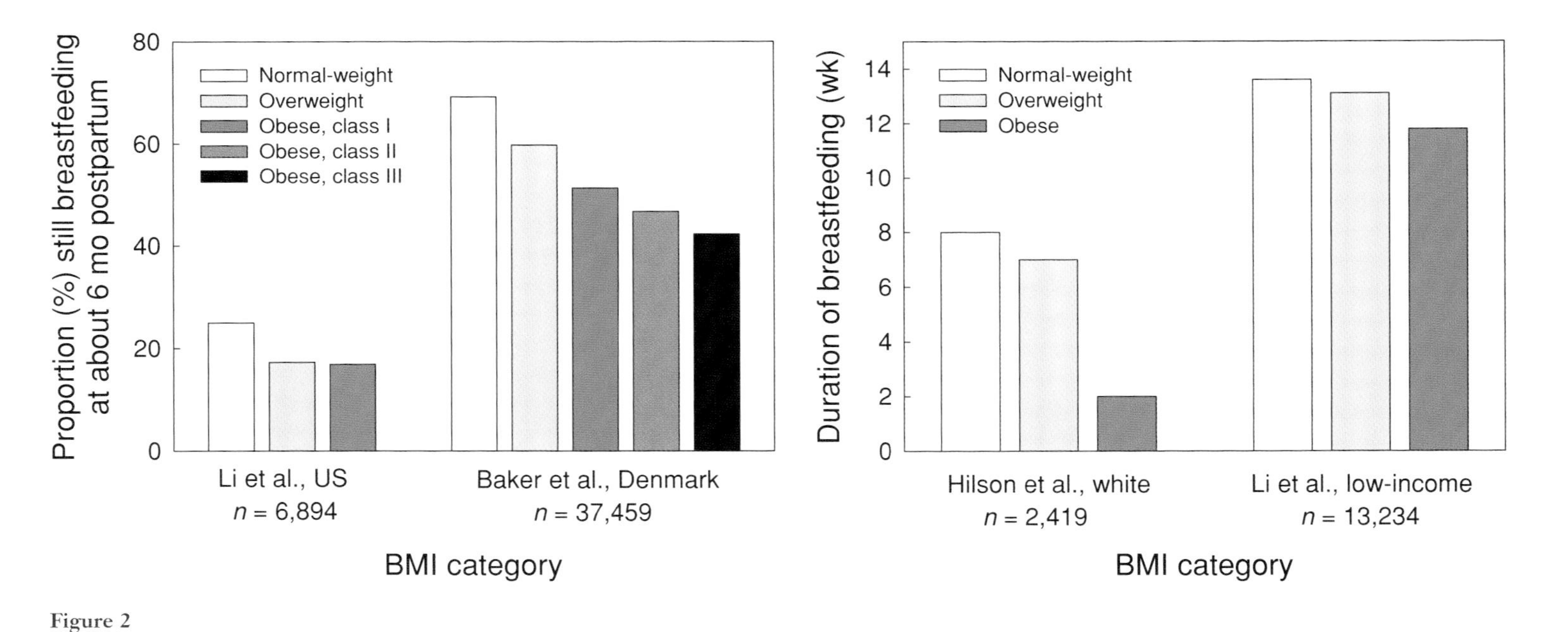

Figure 2

Association between maternal prepregnant body mass index (BMI) and the proportion of women still breastfeeding at 6 mo postpartum (*left panel*) and the duration of breastfeeding (*right panel*). The data of Li et al. (57) are from a nationally representative sample of American women, Hilson et al. (40) are from white women living in a rural area, and Li et al. (56) are from low-income women; all used the Institute of Medicine's categories (47) for overweight (26.1–29.0 kg/m^2) and obesity (>29 kg/m2). The data of Baker et al. (6) are from a national sample of Danish women and used the World Health Organization criteria (113) for overweight (BMI 25.0–29.9 kg/m^2) and obesity (BMI >30 kg/m^2).

development and function of the mammary gland are controlled by both reproductive and metabolic hormones (70). Moreover, adipose tissue should be considered an endocrine organ (65) (although perhaps only a "feeble" one at the whole-body level) (18). Thus, evaluating this link is warranted. The data from mice suggest that obesity affects development of the mammary gland during periods of morphological change and cellular differentiation (28). Thus, it reasonable to expect that obesity might act during similar periods in women. After puberty, these periods are during the menstrual cycle and, particularly, pregnancy (43). This expectation is in accord with the long-recognized positive association between increase in breast size during pregnancy (reflecting an increase in parenchymal breast tissue) and milk production early in lactation (44).

Women who are obese at conception can be assumed to have been so for some time. As a result, they could have experienced effects of their obesity on the proliferation and differentiation of the mammary parenchymal tissue that occur during each menstrual cycle (43). However, this possibility has not yet been evaluated.

Changes in their breasts are among the earliest signs of pregnancy that women notice. Proliferation of mammary gland tissue "begins very early after conception and is maximal during the first trimester of pregnancy, significant during the middle trimester, and moderate in the final trimester of gestation" (45). In early pregnancy, there is proliferation of the distal epithelial elements of the ductal tree in addition to an increase in the number of ductules. These changes increase the secretory potential of the gland. In later pregnancy, proliferation is less but the epithelial cells grow and the alveoli become distended as secretory material accumulates (45). The timing and pattern of mammary gland development suggest that being too fat at conception is likely to be important for later readiness to secrete milk. These findings also suggest that women who are of normal weight at conception but who subsequently gained excess adipose tissue during pregnancy could also compromise their readiness to secrete milk. As described below, this is what we and others have observed.

Obese women have excess adipose tissue in their breasts as well as in fat depots elsewhere in their bodies. Thus effects on lactation of excess fat in each of these locations should be considered, but to date have not been studied separately. In human beings, epithelial cells are not in direct contact with adipocytes in the mammary fat pad, rather "they are continuously ensheathed by multiple layers of connective tissue and fibroblasts" (42). Nonetheless, "epithelial cells grow within a depot of adipose tissue enriched with lipid and its derivatives" (42). Data from experimental species establish clearly that "fat cells and fibroblasts of the mammary gland are potentially capable of exerting a regulatory influence on the growth potential of the epithelium" (45). Recently a proteomic analysis of the adipose tissue in the human mammary gland was conducted using biopsy samples from women being treated for breast cancer. The tissue used for this analysis was collected at a site far from the tumor. These investigators found that a wide variety of cytokines (leptin, TNF-α, and components of the caspase cascade) as well as estrogen receptors and growth factors were present there (15). Estrogen receptors have previously been observed in autopsy samples of mammary gland tissue from normal women (7). The implications of this environment of adipose tissue for the development of human mammary epithelial cells are only beginning to be understood (71). The effects of obesity in amplifying or modifying this environment have not yet been explored.

Moreover, the behavior of adipose tissue itself changes as obesity becomes more severe, with macroscopic and histologic changes occurring in the tissue as well as changes in the secretion of endocrine and paracrine factors, among others (18). This suggests that as obesity becomes more severe so too might the

BMI: body mass index

effects of obesity on pregnancy and lactation. As described below, this is what we and others have observed.

An important issue is whether the hormonal and metabolic characteristics of obesity have the capacity to influence the next two major stages of mammary gland development after the proliferative stage of early pregnancy. The first stage is secretory differentiation, which begins in mid-pregnancy; this is the period (also called lactogenesis I) during which "the gland becomes competent to secrete milk" (69). The second stage is secretory activation, which occurs after birth, when milk secretion actually begins (also called lactogenesis II).

Compared with normal-weight women, obese women exhibit many differences in circulating concentrations of hormones and metabolites [see (4) for a review]. Among asymptomatic, eumenorrheic women, obesity is associated with accelerated androgen metabolism but normal plasma steroid values, an "extremely enlarged body steroid pool," and insulin resistance (4). The increase in estrogen values that is associated with obesity is still much less than basal estrogen values in premenopausal women (4). In addition, obese individuals respond differently to standard challenges to hormone secretion. For example, the response of prolactin to insulin hypoglycemia and stimulation by thyrotropin-releasing hormone may be reduced in obese compared with normal-weight individuals (13, 50).

There is some debate in the literature about whether basal prolactin concentrations in obese individuals are higher (13, 49), lower (78), or not different (51) from those of lean controls. The recent work of Kok et al. (49) may provide some explanation for these inconsistent findings. They showed that the daily release of prolactin was more highly correlated with visceral fat mass than body mass index [BMI, weight/(height^2)] among obese women. In contrast, there is no debate about the reduction in the release of prolactin in response to various standard stimuli (hypoglycemia, thyrotropin-releasing hormone, etc.) that occurs among obese individuals compared to lean controls (13, 50, 51). The interaction of prolactin with adipose tissue in nonlactating individuals is complex. Prolactin binds to receptors on the adipocyte and affects lipid metabolism by inhibiting lipoprotein lipase and suppressing fatty acid synthetase. It also inhibits the secretion of adiponectin and IL-6 and, depending on the conditions, may increase or stimulate leptin (8). In addition, prolactin is produced by adipose tissue in the breast as well as in subcutaneous and visceral fat depots (8, 114). Thus, prolactin may have an autocrine/paracrine role in both of these tissues (8).

In contrast to the detailed information available in the mouse (37, 69), among women the "hormonal regulation of lactogenesis [I] is poorly understood" (70). At this point, it is clear that prolactin is involved in secretory differentiation in women, although other hormones may also be involved, including progesterone and placental lactogen (69). Prolactin is stimulated by the increasing concentrations of estrogen that also occur at this time (70). In many species, a variety of paracrine factors are also involved in secretory differentiation (69), but their potential role has not been studied in women.

Compared to secretory differentiation, the control of secretory activation after delivery is much better understood in women. Initially, the plasma concentration of progesterone must fall while that of prolactin must remain high. It is still unclear whether the increase in glucocorticoid concentration that occurs around parturition is also a trigger for lactation (69). After the third or fourth day postpartum, milk removal is also required for the continuation of copious milk secretion (72). In women, the infant's demand controls the rate of milk secretion during the remainder of lactation (69). Prolactin "is required for maintenance of all alveolar cell processes associated with milk secretion as well as cell survival" (69)—even though its concentration is poorly correlated with milk volume. This is because prolactin is secreted in a pulsatile fashion in response to infant suckling and the amount released is a function of both the interval between feeds and the time after delivery (106).

Both estrogen and progesterone values fall rapidly in the first week after parturition (46, 60). Our small study provided no evidence that this pattern of change differed between normal-weight and overweight/obese women (85). However, there were too few subjects in this investigation to determine if values for these two hormones differed between normal-weight and heavier women.

We proposed that the reduction in release of prolactin in response to stimulus that has been observed among obese individuals might extend to the prolactin response to infant suckling (85). If true, this would help to explain why obesity is associated with a shorter duration of breastfeeding. We observed no difference between normal-weight and overweight/obese lactating women in basal prolactin values at 2 or 7 d postpartum. However, the prolactin response to suckling (the difference between basal and postsuckling values of prolactin, adjusted for confounding factors) was significantly lower in the overweight/obese women than in the normal-weight comparison group at both of these times (85). These times bracket the period of secretory activation and coincide with the period during which many overweight/obese women cease breastfeeding.

As is the case for nonlactating women (34), leptin values are correlated with maternal adiposity and BMI among normal-weight lactating women (12, 67, 100). As a result, it is not surprising that leptin values differ between normal-weight and overweight/obese lactating women (85). In addition to being produced in adipose tissue, leptin is produced by the placenta (62). As a result, plasma leptin values fall rapidly following the delivery of the placenta (33, 62, 67, 100). An inverse relationship between leptin and prolactin values has been observed in normal-weight lactating women (12, 67), although the consequences of this association remain unexplored. Leptin also appears in human milk in amounts that reflect maternal adiposity (41, 108). The leptin in human milk appears to be derived both from maternal plasma as well as from mammary epithelial cells, but its functional significance for maternal health or milk production is unknown (104).

Another adipocytocine, adiponectin, also appears in human milk (10, 59). Its concentration in milk is much lower than its concentration in serum. In serum, adiponectin is positively associated with BMI but, in milk, the opposite is true (59). Whether the adiponectin in human milk is produced locally in the mammary gland or comes from the blood is unknown at present. As was the case for leptin, its functional significance is not understood but merits further study as both of these adipocytokines are regulated by prolactin (3, 8).

In summary, although the possibility exists that maternal obesity affects the development of the mammary glands before and during pregnancy as well as early in the postpartum period, direct evidence for this is quite limited in women. Although plasma hormone values change in response to obesity, the evidence to show that such changes are important for the success of breastfeeding is also quite limited. The finding that the prolactin response to suckling is blunted in obese women is intriguing and provides support for there being a biological basis for an association between maternal obesity and the duration of breastfeeding. However, additional factors are likely to be involved, so further study of these factors is also warranted.

Complications of Pregnancy

Women who are obese at the time of conception have an excess risk of suffering from many complications during pregnancy and at delivery. This association has been known for many years and has been reviewed elsewhere [see, for example, (2, 23, 31, 83)]. Recently it has received additional attention from researchers with access to exceptionally large datasets covering all deliveries in a large region (101) or country (14). Sebire et al. (101), for example, studied 287,213 women who delivered in the North West Thames Region (which includes London) from 1989 to 1997. Compared to normal-weight women (BMI 20–< 25 kg/m^2), those who were obese (BMI $\geq$ 30 kg/m^2) at the time of conception were significantly more likely to experience gestational diabetes and preeclampsia during pregnancy and were less likely to become anemic during this period (101). These obese women were more likely to experience induction of labor and cesarean section (emergency or elective) as well as infection and hemorrhage after delivery (101). Using national data from Sweden (805,275 pregnancies that occurred from 1992 to 2001), Cedergren (14) found that the risk of these same complications of pregnancy and delivery increased with the severity of obesity. Some similar associations have been observed in large samples of American births (24, 111).

The complications of pregnancy are important because several of them, including cesarean section, are known to interfere with establishing breastfeeding. Cesarean section is now more common than ever (occurring in 27.5% of deliveries in the United States in 2003) (58) and is a more difficult procedure with more postpartum complications in obese than normal-weight women (2). Women who have undergone a cesarean delivery have a longer recovery postpartum than do women who have not had this procedure and also put their babies to the breast later to suckle for the first time (16). Moreover, there is some evidence that undergoing a cesarean section may interfere with ever putting the newborn to the breast (77). The mechanism by which having a cesarean section leads to no breastfeeding or shorter breastfeeding has not been established, although both the delay in initially putting the baby to the breast, which by itself is associated with shorter breastfeeding (99), or a delay in the onset of secretory activation (lactogenesis II) (22, 26) may be contributing factors. However, cesarean section has not uniformly been associated with a delay in lactogenesis II (54, 76).

Condition of the Infant at Birth

The condition of babies born to obese women may also be compromised. For example, Sebire et al. (101) found that the babies of obese women were more likely to be born after 42 weeks of gestation, be stillborn, have a birthweight >90th percentile, be in poor condition at birth, and be admitted to the special care nursery than were babies of normal-weight women. Correspondingly, the babies of obese women were also less likely than were those of normal-weight women to be born before 32 weeks of gestation, to have a birthweight <5th percentile, and to be breastfed. In studies in Denmark and Sweden that also included large samples, researchers have observed that the fetuses and infants of obese women were more likely to die before or after 28 weeks of gestation or in the neonatal period (17, 52, 74). As maternal obesity becomes more severe, so too do the problems experienced by the infants born to these women. Cedergren (14) observed that the risk of preterm birth, stillbirth, and death within 7 d of delivery as well as shoulder dystocia and being large-for-gestational age rose progressively with the severity of maternal obesity.

Babies who are macrosomic (usually defined as having a birthweight >4000 g) or who are large (>90th percentile) for their gestational age are more likely to be in poor condition at birth (e.g., low APGAR score, admitted to the special care nursery, etc.), but they are not less likely to be breastfed (48). It is often routine practice to take blood samples from large-for-gestational age babies to screen them for neonatal hypoglycemia (C.L. Kjolhede & R.J. Schanler 2005, personal communication). Babies whose blood glucose values are too low are then given a dextrose-water solution or infant formula until their blood glucose values normalize. This practice is contrary to expert recommendations (55) and may make it more difficult to establish breastfeeding (9, 61, 64). Moreover, these babies can also be difficult to feed because of their size and their likelihood of having been delivered somewhat early to make birth easier. A more complete description of the infants of obese women and the challenges they present for breastfeeding is provided elsewhere (83). Although the unique needs of infants of diabetic mothers have been well characterized, the needs of infants born to nondiabetic, obese mothers have not. Inasmuch as the proportion of pregnant women who are obese has increased, it is time for further study of the needs of their babies, with particular attention to improving the success of breastfeeding.

In summary, obese women may experience complications during pregnancy and at delivery that affect their health and lead to difficulties in establishing breastfeeding. Similarly, infants born to these women may themselves have problems in the early neonatal period that make it more difficult to establish breastfeeding. These challenges are above and beyond those that might be related to inadequate development of the mammary glands during pregnancy.

Progress of Lactation

In production and experimental species, the progress of lactation is largely determined by biological factors; social, demographic, and psychological factors are not involved. Among women, the evidence discussed above supports the concept that at least one of the ways that obesity affects lactation in women may be through a biological pathway, the prolactin response to suckling (85). Obese women also may experience other kinds of challenges that act through more proximal biological pathways. In addition to the condition of the mother and baby at birth, these include difficulty in positioning the infant because of their overall body shape and size as well as difficulty with latching on because of the size of their breasts, areolas, and nipples. Infants who are poorly positioned or latched on can create nipple pain for the mother—a stress that is a disincentive to continue breastfeeding—and may fail to elicit an adequate prolactin response to suckling (16). Such factors are associated with delayed lactogenesis (16, 21), but whether they have a specific role in lactation failure among obese women has not been studied directly. In our recent study, some health care providers who work with lactating women reported that they thought that large breasts were more of a problem than obesity itself (86). Investigators have reported that obesity is not associated with breast size before pregnancy (79), and it has long been known that it is the increase in breast size during pregnancy that predicts milk production (44). Thus, the scientific evidence on this point is quite limited, but what is available does not support the viewpoint that breast size is more important than obesity in determining the progress of breastfeeding.

Among those women who ever gave their infants a chance to suckle, we found that obese white women living in a rural area (38) and obese Hispanic women living in an urban area (53) were more likely to fail to initiate breastfeeding (defined as continuing to breastfeed through the time of hospital discharge) than normal-weight women. This was not true of the black women living in an urban area whom we also studied (53). Among the women in the Danish National Birth Cohort, there was a dose-response relationship between maternal prepregnant BMI and the risk of early cessation of breastfeeding (6). Given the social support for breastfeeding that exists in Denmark, this is compelling evidence that a biological mechanism may underlie this association.

Among both white and Hispanic women we studied (38, 53), many obese women ceased to breastfeed their babies within the first days after delivery. This may be because overweight or obese women experience a delay in the timing of lactogenesis II (22, 39), which may result from the reduced prolactin response to suckling that we have observed in such women (85). These findings are concordant with the possibility that obese women may have difficulty with positioning their newborns and with proper latching on. The clear implication of these results is that obese women may benefit from extra support for breastfeeding in the immediate postpartum period (85).

Much more information is available about the duration of breastfeeding than its initiation (**Figure 2**, see color insert). Ferris et al. (27) noted a "tendency" for heavier women not to have continued breastfeeding beyond 10 wk. Rutishauser & Carlin (98) observed that, among primiparous Australian women who had breastfed their infants for at least 14 d, being heavier (BMI >26 kg/m^2) at this time was a risk factor for early cessation of breastfeeding. Obesity was also associated with shortened breastfeeding in a national sample of Australian women who provided information by recall (25) as well as in a sample of 1601 Italian women (90) who were interviewed within a month of delivery and followed for 12 months. In two other recent studies from Australia, high prepregnant BMI was also associated with reduced duration of breastfeeding (29, 75). Maternal obesity was associated with a shortened duration of breastfeeding (56) or with a lower proportion of women still breastfeeding at 6 and 12 mo postpartum (57) in large samples of American women. From a review of medical records, we evaluated the duration of exclusive and any breastfeeding separately in our studies of women in upstate New York. Both of these outcomes were negatively affected by maternal obesity among white (38) and Hispanic (53) but not black (53) women. The reason for this difference is unknown but may result from differences in commitment to breastfeeding or to differences in the effect of obesity in black compared to white women (53). In national samples (56, 57), black women breastfeed for much shorter periods than white women, but the association of obesity with their duration of breastfeeding has not been reported.

It is possible that maternal prepregnant BMI is an inadequate proxy for maternal adiposity, not only because BMI itself is an imperfect measure of adiposity but also because maternal adiposity changes substantially during pregnancy in response to maternal weight gain. Li et al. (56) found that the duration of any breastfeeding was indeed shorter among women who gained more than the amount recommended by the Institute of Medicine for their prepregnant BMI, but this did not modify the negative association of prepregnant BMI with the duration of any breastfeeding. For their analysis, they used a large sample of low-income American women from the pediatric and pregnancy surveillance systems. In our sample of 2783 white women from rural New York State, we also observed an additive relationship between maternal prepregnant BMI and category of gestational weight gain on the initiation of breastfeeding as well as both the duration of exclusive and any breastfeeding (40). In contrast, we found no independent association between gestational weight gain and the risk of early termination of breastfeeding in a much larger sample of women from the Danish National Birth Cohort when prepregnant BMI was also in the regression model (6). This was likely because prepregnant BMI and gestational weight gain were negatively associated in this sample. Taken together, these conflicting findings don't permit us to resolve if the additional adipose tissue that is gained during pregnancy, whether deposited in the breast or elsewhere (as this cannot be determined from the available data), interferes with lactation in some important way. The mechanism by which excessive gestational weight gain could contribute to lactation failure is unknown at present, but it is reasonable to conclude from the timing of this additional weight gain that it might particularly affect the development changes in the mammary gland that occur during pregnancy. Until this possible relationship is more fully understood, it is reasonable to continue to counsel women to gain an appropriate—not an excessive—amount of weight during pregnancy.

Unlike production and experimental species, however, social, demographic, and psychological factors are also likely to be important determinants of the duration of breastfeeding among women. Inasmuch as they represent possible targets for interventions to improve the success of obese women at breastfeeding, they merit attention. In the United States, overall support for breastfeeding is relatively low and the lack of any or adequate maternity leave are barriers to breastfeeding for all women (80). This creates a culture in which it is acceptable—even expected—for women to feed their babies infant formula instead of human milk. It also makes it socially acceptable for women not to breastfeed at all and, for women who are experiencing difficulties with breastfeeding, to supplement with infant formula or cease breastfeeding entirely. In this cultural context, motivation and self-efficacy for breastfeeding, attitudes toward body size and shape, and social support for breastfeeding—among other related factors—take on additional importance. The important issue here is whether these kinds of social factors affect obese women differentially. Only limited data are available with which to investigate this possibility.

One socially—not biologically—determined aspect of breastfeeding is the choice to do so at all. In nationally representative data collected as part of the National Health and Nutrition Examination Survey (57), only 44.8% of obese women ever breastfed their babies compared with 58.1% of normal-weight women. In a large sample of low-income women drawn from the pediatric and pregnancy surveillance data in the United States (57), the picture was more complicated as there was an interaction between prepregnant BMI and gestational weight gain. In this sample (56), obese women, regardless of their weight gain, were less likely to choose to breastfeed than the reference group, normal-weight women who gained appropriately. In our data, in contrast, obese women were as likely as were normal-weight women to ever put their babies to the breast (38). Thus, the available data suggest that there is both complexity and controversy about whether maternal prepregnant BMI is associated with the choice to breastfeed.

In the studies of obesity as a determinant of the initiation and continuation of breastfeeding cited above, analyses were adjusted for the various social and demographic determinants of breastfeeding. As a result, these studies provide no information about the separate role of these factors with respect to the success or failure of breastfeeding. We have investigated this possibility in more detail in a study of 151 women who were enrolled during pregnancy (39). Obese women planned to breastfeed for a shorter period and were less satisfied with their appearance than were normal-weight women, but other psychosocial characteristics, such as behavioral beliefs and knowledge about breastfeeding, exposure to models for breastfeeding, as well as maternal confidence and support for breastfeeding, did not differ between obese and normal-weight women. Some of these factors attenuated but did not eliminate the relationship between obesity and the duration of breastfeeding.

In summary, it is possible that maternal obesity affects development of the mammary glands before and during pregnancy as well as early in lactation, but evidence to support or refute this proposition is lacking. However, evidence is available to confirm an association between maternal obesity and the initiation as well as the continuation of breastfeeding in nearly all of the population groups that have been studied. This association appears to be derived from biological as well as sociocultural factors that are as yet poorly defined and understood. The deleterious effects of maternal obesity and excessive gestational weight gain on complications of pregnancy and delivery as well as the condition of the infant at birth may also contribute to this association.

CONCLUSIONS

There is clear evidence of an association between maternal obesity and lactation failure in production and experimental species as well as in women. A number of biological factors have been identified that contribute to this association. In women, sociocultural, demographic, and psychosocial factors may also be important. Given the high rate of obesity among women of reproductive age around the world and the central importance of breastfeeding for infant health, interventions are needed to address this challenge. Many interventions are possible—from the provision of more adequate maternity leave, to assistance to women to help them to conceive at a healthy weight and gain weight appropriately during pregnancy, to additional assistance with breastfeeding in the early postpartum period, among other possibilities.

LITERATURE CITED

1. Agius L, Rolls BJ, Rowe EA, Williamson DF. 1983. Obese rats develop hyperketonemia and fatty liver during lactation. *Int. J. Obes.* 7:447–52
2. Andreasen KR, Andersen ML, Schantz AL. 2004. Obesity and pregnancy. *Acta Obstet. Gynecol. Scand.* 83:1022–29
3. Asai-Sato M, Okamoto M, Endo M, Yoshida H, Murase M, et al. 2006. Hypoadiponectinemia in lean lactating women: prolactin inhibits adiponectin secretion from human adipocytes. *Endocrinol. J.* 53:555–62
4. Azziz R. 1989. Reproductive endocrinologic alterations in female asymptomatic obesity. *Fertil. Steril.* 52:703–25
5. Baker JL. 2003. *Maternal obesity, infant feeding methods and infant growth*. PhD dissert. Ithaca, NY: Cornell Univ.
6. Baker JL, Michaelsen KF, Sørensen TIA, Rasmussen KM. 2007. High prepregnant body mass index is associated with early termination of full and any breastfeeding among Danish women. Manuscr. submitted
7. Bartow SA. 1998. Use of the autopsy to study ontogeny and expression of the estrogen receptor gene in human breast. *J. Mammary Gland Biol. Neoplasia* 3:37–48
8. Ben-Jonathan N, Hugo ER, Brandebourg TD, LaPensee CR. 2006. Focus on prolactin as a metabolic hormone. *Trends Endocrinol. Metab.* 17:110–16
9. Bloomquist HK, Jonsbo F, Serenius F, Persson LÅ. 1994. Supplementary feeding in the maternity ward shortens the duration of breast feeding. *Acta Pædiatr.* 83:1122–26
10. Bonský J, Karpíšek M, Bronská M, Pechová M, Jancíkova B, et al. 2006. Adiponectin, adipocyte fatty acid binding protein, and epidermal fatty acid binding protein: proteins newly identified in human breast milk. *Clin. Chem.* 52:1763–70
11. Brown EG, VandeHaar MJ, Daniels KM, Liesman JS, Chapin LT, et al. 2005. Effect of increasing energy and protein intake on mammary development of heifer calves. *J. Dairy Sci.* 88:595–603
12. Butte NF, Hopkinson JM, Nicolson MA. 1997. Leptin in human reproduction: serum leptin levels in pregnant and lactating women. *J. Clin. Endocrinol. Metab.* 82:585–89
13. Cavagnini F, Maraschini C, Pinto M, Dubini A, Polli EE. 1981. Impaired prolactin secretion in obese patients. *J. Endocrinol. Invest.* 4:149–53
14. Cedergren MI. 2004. Maternal morbid obesity and the risk of adverse pregnancy outcome. *Obstet. Gynecol.* 103:219–24
15. Celis JE, Moreira JMA, Cabezón T, Gromov P, Friis E, et al. 2005. Identification of extracellular and intracellular signaling components of the mammary adipose tissue and its interstitial fluid in high risk breast cancer patients. *Mol. Cell. Proteomics* 4:492–522
16. Chen DC, Nommsen-Rivers L, Dewey KG, Lönnerdal B. 1998. Stress during labor and delivery and early lactation performance. *Am. J. Clin. Nutr.* 68:335–44

17. Cnattingius S, Bergström R, Lipworth L, Kramer MS. 1998. Prepregnancy weight and the risk of adverse pregnancy outcomes. *New Engl. J. Med.* 338:147–52
18. Coppack SW. 2005. Adipose tissue changes in obesity. *Biochem. Soc. Trans.* 33:1049–52
19. Crane SS, Wojtowycz MA, Dye TD, Aubry RH, Artal R. 1997. Association between pre-pregnancy obesity and the risk of cesarean delivery. *Obstet. Gynecol.* 89:213–16
20. Davison KE, Potter GD, Greene LW, Evans JW, McMullan WC. 1991. Lactation and reproductive performance of mares fed added dietary fat during late gestation and early lactation. *J. Equine Vet. Sci.* 11:111–15
21. Dewey KG. 2001. Maternal and fetal stress are associated with impaired lactogenesis in humans. *J. Nutr.* 131:3012–15S
22. Dewey KG, Nommsen-Rivers LA, Heinig MJ, Cohen RJ. 2003. Risk factors for suboptimal infant breastfeeding behavior, delayed onset of lactation, and excess neonatal weight loss. *Pediatrics* 112:607–19
23. Dietl J. 2005. Maternal obesity and complications during pregnancy. *J. Perinat. Med.* 33:100–5
24. Dietz PM, Callaghan WM, Morrow B, Cogswell ME. 2005. Population-based assessment of the risk of primary cesarean delivery due to excess prepregnancy weight among nulliparous women delivering term infants. *Matern. Child Health* 9:237–44
25. Donath SM, Amir LH. 2000. Does maternal obesity adversely affect breastfeeding initiation and duration? *J. Paediatr. Child Health* 36:482–86
26. Evans KC, Evans RG, Royal R, Esterman AJ, James SL. 2003. Effect of caesarean section on breast milk transfer to the normal term newborn over the first week of life. *Arch. Dis. Child Fetal Neonatal Ed.* 88:F380–82
27. Ferris AM, McCabe LT, Allen LH, Pelto GH. 1987. Biological and sociocultural determinants of successful lactation among women in eastern Connecticut. *J. Am. Dietet. Assoc.* 87:316–21
28. Flint DJ, Travers MT, Barber MC, Binart N, Kelly PA. 2005. Diet-induced obesity impairs mammary development and lactogenesis in murine mammary gland. *Am. J. Physiol. Endocrinol. Metab.* 288:e1179–87
29. Forster DA, McLachlan HL, Lumley J. 2006. Factors associated with breastfeeding at six months postpartum in a group of Australian women. *Int. Breastfeeding J.* 1:18
30. Friggens NC, Hay DEF, Oldham JD. 1993. Interactions between major nutrients in the diet and the lactational performance of rats. *Br. J. Nutr.* 69:59–71
31. Galtier-Dereure F, Boegner C, Bringer J. 2000. Obesity and pregnancy: complications and cost. *Am. J. Clin. Nutr.* 71(Suppl.):1242–48S
32. Gibbs PG, Davison KE. 2006. *Nutritional Management of Pregnant and Lactating Mares.* Equine Sci. Prog., Dept. Animal Sci., Texas A&M Univ., College Station, TX
33. Hardie L, Trayhurn P, Abramovich P, Fowler P. 1997. Circulating leptin in women: a longitudinal study in the menstrual cycle and during pregnancy. *Clin. Endocrinol.* 47:101–6
34. Havel PJ, Kasim-Karakas S, Meuller W, Johnson PR, Gingerich RL, Stern JS. 1996. Relationship of plasma leptin to plasma insulin and adiposity in normal weight and overweight women: effects of dietary fat content and sustained weight loss. *J. Clin. Endocrinol. Metab.* 81:4406–13
35. Henneke DR, Potter GD, Kreider JL. 1984. Body condition during pregnancy and lactation and reproductive efficiency of mares. *Theriogenology* 21:897–909
36. Henneke DR, Potter GD, Kreider JL, Yeates BF. 1993. Relationship between condition score, physical measurements and body fat percentage in mares. *Equine Vet. J.* 15:371–72
37. Hennighausen L, Robinson GW. 2005. Information networks in the mammary gland. *Nat. Rev. Mol. Cell. Biol.* 6:715–25

38. Hilson JA, Rasmussen KM, Kjolhede CL. 1997. Maternal obesity and breastfeeding success in a rural population of white women. *Am. J. Clin. Nutr.* 66:1371–78
39. Hilson JA, Rasmussen KM, Kjolhede CL. 2004. High prepregnant body mass index is associated with poor lactation outcomes among white, rural women independent of psychosocial and demographic correlates. *J. Hum. Lact.* 20:18–29
40. Hilson JA, Rasmussen KM, Kjolhede CL. 2006. Excessive weight gain during pregnancy is associated with earlier termination of breast-feeding among white women. *J. Nutr.* 136:1–7
41. Houseknecht KL, McGuire MK, Portocarrero CP, McGuire MA, Beerman K. 1997. Leptin is present in human milk and is related to maternal plasma leptin concentration and adiposity. *Biochem. Biophys. Res. Comm.* 240:742–47
42. Hovey RC, McFadden TB, Akers RM. 1999. Regulation of mammary gland growth and morphogenesis by the mammary fat pad: a species comparison. *J. Mammary Gland Biol. Neoplasia* 4:53–68
43. Hovey RC, Trott JF, Vonderhaar BK. 2002. Establishing a framework for the functional mammary gland: from endocrinology to morphology. *J. Mammary Gland Biol. Neoplasia* 7:17–38
44. Hytten FE. 1954. Clinical and chemical studies in human lactation. VI. The functional capacity of the breast. *Br. Med. J.* i:912–15
45. Imagawa W, Yang J, Guzman R, Nandi S. 1994. Control of mammary gland development. In *The Physiology of Reproduction*, ed. E Knobil, JD Neill, pp. 1033–63. New York: Raven
46. Ingram JC, Woolridge MW, Greenwood RJ, McGrath L. 1999. Maternal predictors of early breast milk output. *Acta Pœdiatr.* 88:493–99
47. Inst. Med. (Subcomm. Nutr. Status Weight Gain During Pregnancy and Dietary Intake and Nutr. Suppl. During Pregnancy, Comm. Nutr. Status During Pregnancy Lact., Food Nutr. Board). 1990. *Nutrition During Pregnancy: Part I, Weight Gain; Part II, Nutrient Supplements*. Washington, DC: Natl. Acad. Press
48. Jolly MC, Sebire NJ, Harris JP, Regan L, Robinson S. 2003. Risk factors for macrosomia and its clinical consequences: a study of 350,311 pregnancies. *Eur. J. Obstet. Gynecol. Reprod. Biol.* 111:9–14
49. Kok P, Roelfsema F, Frölich M, Meinders AE, Pijl H. 2004. Prolactin release is enhanced in proportion to excess visceral fat in obese women. *J. Clin. Endocrinol. Metab.* 89:4445–49
50. Kopelman PG. 2000. Physiopathology of prolactin secretion in obesity. *Int. J. Obes.* 24(Suppl. 2):S104–8
51. Kopelman PG, White N, Pilkington TRE, Jeffcoat SL. 1979. Impaired hypothalamic control of prolactin secretion in massive obesity. *Lancet* i:747–49
52. Kristensen J, Vestergaard M, Wisborg K, Kesmodel U, Secher NJ. 2005. Pre-pregnancy weight and the risk of stillbirth and neonatal death. *Br. J. Obstet. Gynœcol.* 112:403–8
53. Kugyelka JG, Rasmussen KM, Frongillo EAJ. 2004. Maternal obesity negatively affects breastfeeding success among Hispanic but not Black women. *J. Nutr.* 134:1746–53
54. Kulski JK, Smith M, Hartmann PE. 1981. Normal and caesarian section delivery and the initiation of lactation in women. *Aust. J. Exp. Biol. Med. Sci.* 59:405–12
55. Lawrence RA, Lawrence RM. 2005. *Breastfeeding: A Guide for the Medical Profession*. Philadelphia, PA: Elsevier Mosby
56. Li R, Jewell S, Grummer-Strawn LM. 2003. Maternal obesity and breast-feeding practices. *Am. J. Clin. Nutr.* 77:931–36
57. Li R, Ogden C, Ballew C, Gillespie C, Grummer-Strawn LM. 2002. Prevalence of exclusive breastfeeding among US infants: the Third National Health and Nutrition Examination Survey (Phase II, 1991–1994). *Am. J. Public Health* 92:1107–10

58. Martin JA, Hamilton BE, Sutton PD, Ventura SJ, Menacker F, Munson ML. 2005. Births: final data for 2003. *Nat. Vital Stat. Rep.* 54:1–116
59. Martin LJ, Woo JG, Geraghty SR, Altaye M, Davidson BS, et al. 2006. Adiponectin is present in human milk and is associated with maternal factors. *Am. J. Clin. Nutr.* 83:1111
60. Martin RH, Glass MR, Chapman C, Wilson GD, Woods KL. 1980. Human alpha-lactalbumin and hormonal factors in pregnancy and lactation. *Clin. Endocrinol. (Oxf.)* 13:223–30
61. Martin-Calama J, Buñuel J, Valero MT, Labay M, Lasarte JJ, et al. 1997. The effect of feeding glucose water to breastfeeding newborns on weight, body temperature, blood glucose and breastfeeding duration. *J. Hum. Lact.* 13:209–13
62. Mazusaki H, Ogawa Y, Sagawa N, Hosoda K, Matsumoto T, et al. 1997. Nonadipose tissue production of leptin: leptin as a novel placenta-derived hormone in humans. *Nat. Med.* 3:1029–33
63. McCormack J. 1978. Fat-cow syndrome and its complications. *Vet. Med. Small Anim. Clin.* 73:1057–60
64. Michaelsen KF, Larsen PS, Thomsen BL, Samuelsen G. 1984. The Copenhagen cohort study on infant nutrition and growth: duration of breast feeding and influencing factors. *Acta Pœdiatr.* 83:565–71
65. Mohamed-Ali V, Pinkney JH, Coppack SW. 1998. Adipose tissue as an endocrine and paracrine organ. *Int. J. Obes. Relat. Metab. Disord.* 22:1145–58
66. Morrow DA. 1976. Fat cow syndrome. *J. Dairy Sci.* 59:1625–29
67. Mukherjea R, Castonguay TW, Douglass LW, Moser-Veillon P. 1999. Elevated leptin concentrations in pregnancy and lactation: possible role as a modulator of substrate utilization. *Life Sci.* 65:1183–93
68. Murondoti A, Jorritsma R, Beynen AC, Wensing T, Geelen MJH. 2004. Unrestricted feed intake during the dry period impairs the postpartum oxidation and synthesis of fatty acids in the liver of dairy cows. *J. Dairy Sci.* 87:672–79
69. Neville MC. 2006. Lactation and its hormonal control. In *Knobil and Neill's Physiology of Reproduction*, ed. JD Neill, 2:2993–3054. Amsterdam: Elsevier
70. Neville MC, McFadden TB, Forsyth I. 2002. Hormonal regulation of mammary differentiation and milk secretion. *J. Mammary Gland Biol. Neoplasia* 7:49–66
71. Neville MC, Medina D, Monks J, Hovey RC. 1998. The mammary fat pad. *J. Mammary Gland Biol. Neoplasia* 3:109–16
72. Neville MC, Morton S. 2001. Physiology and endocrine changes underlying human lactogenesis II. *J. Nutr.* 131:3005–8S
73. Nicholas KR, Hartmann PE. 1990. Milk secretion in the rat: progressive changes in milk composition during lactation and weaning and the effect of diet. *Comp. Biochem. Physiol.* 98A:535–42
74. Nohr EA, Bech BH, Davies MJ, Frydenberg M, Henriksen TB, Olsen J. 2005. Prepregnancy obesity and fetal death: a study within the Danish National Birth Cohort. *Obstet. Gynecol.* 106:250–59
75. Oddy WH, Li J, Landsborough L, Kendall GE, Henderson S, Downie J. 2006. The association of maternal overweight and obesity with breastfeeding duration. *J. Pediatr.* 149:185–91
76. Patel RR, Liebling RE, Murphy DJ. 2003. Effect of operative delivery in the second stage of labor on breastfeeding success. *Birth* 30:255–60
77. Pérez-Escamilla R, Maulén-Radovan I, Dewey KG. 1996. The association between cesarean delivery and breast-feeding outcomes among Mexican Women. *Am. J. Public Health* 86:832–36

78. Pijl H, Koppeschaar HPF, Willekens FLA, Frolich M, Meinders AE. 1993. The influence of serotonergic neurotransmission on pituitary hormone release in obese and non-obese females. *Acta Endocrinol.* 128:319–24
79. Pisacane A, Continisio P. 2004. On behalf of the Italian Working Group on Breastfeeding. Breastfeeding and perceived changes in the appearance of the breasts: a retrospective study. *Acta Pœdiatr.* 93:1346–48
80. Raju TNK. 2005. Continued barriers for breast-feeding in public and the workplace. *J. Pediatr.* 148:677–79
81. Rasmussen KM. 1992. The influence of maternal nutrition on lactation. *Annu. Rev. Nutr.* 12:103–17
82. Rasmussen KM. 1998. Effects of under- and overnutrition on lactation in laboratory rats. *J. Nutr.* 128:390–93S
83. Rasmussen KM. 2007. Maternal obesity and the outcome of breastfeeding. In *Textbook of Human Lactation*, ed. TW Hale, PE Hartmann. Amarillo, TX: Hale Publ. In press
84. Rasmussen KM, Hilson JA, Kjolhede CL. 2001. Obesity may impair lactogenesis II. *J. Nutr.* 131:3009–11S
85. Rasmussen KM, Kjolhede CL. 2004. Prepregnant overweight and obesity diminish the prolactin response to suckling in the first week postpartum. *Pediatrics* 113:e465–71
86. Rasmussen KM, Lee VE, Ledkovsky TB, Kjolhede CL. 2006. A description of lactation counseling practices that are used with obese mothers. *J. Hum. Lact.* 22:322–27
87. Rasmussen KM, Wallace MH, Gournis E. 2001. A low-fat diet but not food restriction improves lactational performance in obese rats. In *Bioactive Substances in Human Milk*, ed. DS Newberg, pp. 101–5. New York: Kluwer Acad./Plenum
88. Revell DK, Williams IH, Mullan BP, Ranford JL, Smits RJ. 1998a. Body composition at farrowing and nutrition during lactation affect the performance of primiparious sows: II. Milk composition, milk yield, and pig growth. *J. Anim. Sci.* 76:1738–43
89. Revell DK, Williams IH, Mullan BP, Ranford JL, Smits RJ. 1998b. Body composition at farrowing and nutrition during lactation affect the performance of primiparous sows: I. Voluntary feed intake, weight loss, and plasma metabolites. *J. Anim. Sci.* 76:1729–37
90. Riva E, Banderali G, Agostini C, Silano M, Radaelli G, Giovannini M. 1999. Factors associated with initiation and duration of breastfeeding in Italy. *Acta Pœdiatr.* 88:411–15
91. Rolls BA, Barley JB, Gurr MI. 1983. The influence of dietary obesity on milk production in the rat. *Proc. Nutr. Soc.* 42:83A (Abstr.)
92. Rolls BA, Edwards-Webb JD, Gurr MI. 1981. The influence of dietary obesity on milk composition in the rat. *Proc. Nutr. Soc.* 40:66A (Abstr.)
93. Rolls BA, Gurr MI, van Duijvenvoode PM, Rolls BJ, Rowe EA. 1986. Lactation in lean and obese rats: effect of cafeteria feeding and of dietary obesity on milk composition. *Physiol. Behav.* 38:185–90
94. Rolls BJ, Rowe EA. 1982. Pregnancy and lactation in the obese rat: effects on maternal and pup weights. *Physiol. Behav.* 28:393–400
95. Rolls BJ, Rowe EA, Fahrbach SE, Agius L, Williamson DF. 1980. Obesity and high energy diets reduce survival and growth of rat pups. *Proc. Nutr. Soc.* 39:51A (Abstr.)
96. Rolls BJ, van Duijvenvoode PM, Rowe EA. 1984. Effects of diet and obesity on body weight regulation during pregnancy and lactation in the rat. *Physiol. Behav.* 32:161–68
97. Rukkwansuk T, Wensing T, Geelen MJH. 1999. Effect of overfeeding during the dry period on the rate of esterification in adipose tissue of dairy cows during the periparturient period. *J. Dairy Sci.* 82:1164–69
98. Rutishauser IHE, Carlin JB. 1992. Body mass index and duration of breast feeding: a survival analysis during the first six months of life. *J. Epidemiol. Comm. Health* 46:559–65

99. Salariya EM, Easton PM, Cater JI. 1978. Duration of breast-feeding after early initiation and frequent feeding. *Lancet* ii:1141–43
100. Schubring C, Englaro P, Siebler T, Blum WF, Demirakca T, et al. 1998. Longitudinal analysis of maternal serum leptin levels during pregnancy, at birth, and up to six weeks after birth: relation to body mass index, skinfolds, sex steroids and umbilical cord blood leptin levels. *Horm. Res.* 50:276–83
101. Sebire NJ, Jolly M, Harris JP, Wadsworth J, Joffe M, et al. 2001. Maternal obesity and pregnancy outcome: a study of 287,213 pregnancies in London. *Int. J. Obes. Relat. Metab. Disord.* 25:1175–82
102. Sejrsen K, Purup S, Vestergaard M, Foldager J. 2000. High body weight gain and reduced bovine mammary growth: physiological basis and implications for milk yield potential. *Domest. Anim. Endocrin.* 19:93–104
103. Shaw MA, Rasmussen KM, Myers TR. 1997. Consumption of a high-fat diet impairs reproductive performance in Sprague-Dawley rats. *J. Nutr.* 127:64–69
104. Smith-Kirwin SM, O'Connor DM, Johnston J, de Lancey E, Hassink SG, Funange VL. 1998. Leptin expression in human mammary epithelial cells and breast milk. *J. Clin. Endocrinol. Metab.* 83:1810–13
105. Steingrimsdottir L, Brasel JA, Greenwood MRC. 1980. Diet, pregnancy, and lactation: effects on adipose tissue, lipoprotein lipase, and fat cell size. *Metabolism* 29:837–41
106. Tay CCK, Glasier AF, McNeilly AS. 1996. Twenty-four hour patterns of prolactin secretion during lactation and the relationship to suckling and the resumption of fertility in breastfeeding women. *Hum. Reprod.* 11s:950–55
107. Thorn SR, Purup S, Cohick WS, Vestergaard M, Sejrsen K, Boisclair YR. 2006. Leptin does not act directly on mammary epithelial cells in prepubertal dairy heifers. *J. Dairy Sci.* 89:1467–77
108. Uysal FK, Önal EE, Aral YZ, Adam B, Dilmen U, Ardiçolu Y. 2002. Breast milk leptin: its relationship to maternal and infant adiposity. *Clin. Nutr.* 21:157–60
109. Wallace JM, Milne JS, Aitken RP. 2005. The effect of overnourishing singleton-bearing adult ewes on nutrient partitioning to the gravid uterus. *Br. J. Nutr.* 94:533–39
110. Wehmer F, Bertino M, Jen KLC. 1979. The effects of high fat diet on reproduction in female rats. *Behav. Neural Biol.* 27:120–24
111. Weiss JL, Malone FD, Emig D, Ball RH, Nyberg DA, et al. 2004. Obesity, obstetric complications and cesarean delivery rate—a population-based screening study. *Am. J. Obstet. Gynecol.* 190:1091–97
112. Weldon WC, Thulin AJ, MacDougald OA, Johnston LJ, Miller ER, Tucker HA. 1991. Effects of increased dietary energy and protein intake during late gestation on mammary development in gilts. *J. Anim. Sci.* 69:194–200
113. World Health Org. 1998. *Obesity: Preventing and Managing the Global Epidemic*. Geneva: WHO
114. Zinger M, McFarland M, Ben-Jonathan N. 2003. Prolactin expression and secretion by human breast glandular and adipose tissue explants. *J. Clin. Endocrinol. Metab.* 88:689–96

Evolution of Infant and Young Child Feeding: Implications for Contemporary Public Health

Daniel W. Sellen

Departments of Anthropology, Nutritional Sciences and Public Health Sciences, University of Toronto, Ontario, M5S 3G3 Canada; email: dan.sellen@utoronto.ca

Annu. Rev. Nutr. 2007. 27:123–48

First published online as a Review in Advance on March 15, 2007

The *Annual Review of Nutrition* is online at http://nutr.annualreviews.org

This article's doi:
10.1146/annurev.nutr.25.050304.092557

0199-9885/07/0821-0123$20.00

Key Words

lactation, breastfeeding, weaning, adaptation, primates, phylogeny

Abstract

Evolutionary anthropological and ethnographic studies are used to develop a general conceptual framework for understanding prehistoric, historic, and contemporary variation in human lactation and complementary feeding patterns. Comparison of similarities and differences in human and nonhuman primate lactation biology suggests humans have evolved an unusually flexible strategy for feeding young. Several lines of indirect evidence are consistent with a hypothesis that complementary feeding evolved as a facultative strategy that provided a unique adaptation for resolving tradeoffs between maternal costs of lactation and risk of poor infant outcomes. This evolved flexibility may have been adaptive in the environments in which humans evolved, but it creates potential for mismatch between optimal and actual feeding practices in many contemporary populations.

Contents

INTRODUCTION

Complementary foods: nutritionally rich and relatively sterile combinations of foods acquired and processed by caregivers and fed to breastfed infants and toddlers after about six months of age

Two observations about the patterns of infant and young child feeding (IYCF) in contemporary human societies are puzzling for nutritionists and anthropologists, respectively. First, the proportion of newborns that breastfeed exclusively for six months, receive timely and appropriate complementary foods, and continue to breastfeed into their third year is small, even though overwhelming evidence suggests such a pattern is optimal for most healthy, term infants (including low-birth-weight infants born at >37 weeks gestation). Second, humans tend to wean their babies significantly earlier than most other apes do, even though children depend on others for subsistence much longer than do the offspring of any other mammal (172). This article reviews zoological, anthropological, and nutritional data that suggest these two apparently paradoxical observations are evolutionarily linked. It summarizes recent conclusions about the unique characteristics of human life history and discusses how they may be related to unique characteristics of human lactation biology. It briefly reviews data on variation in lactation patterns among nonhuman patterns and data on variation in IYCF among preindustrial human societies and ancient populations. The aim is to provide an evolutionary perspective on why optimal IYCF is so rare and difficult to promote in modern human societies that are far removed from the original conditions shaping human adaptation.

COEVOLUTION OF LIFE HISTORY AND LACTATION BIOLOGY

It is possible to distinguish the evolutionarily derived features of human life history (44) and lactation biology from those that are shared with other mammals by using the comparative methods of zoology and drawing on physiological and epidemiological data that signal an evolved, optimal pattern of human IYCF.

VARIATION AMONG MAMMALS

Mammals vary in age at weaning, as well as in many other characteristics that together describe their life history (109), such as age at first reproduction, gestation length, interbirth intervals, and age at death. Much of this variation is linked to more or less species-typical patterns of growth and development, and is associated with variation in body size, demography, sociality, and ecology (36, 39, 153, 171,

187). Evolutionary theory suggests life history variation is an adaptive response to natural selection within physiological, ecological, and social constraints (37, 38, 44, 74, 186, 216).

Lactation probably evolved between 210 and 190 million years ago (mya) (20, 41, 91, 127, 145, 147) and prior to the origin of another defining characteristic of mammals, specialized hair and fur (143). Lactation probably evolved initially as an adaptation to transfer immune factors to offspring (99) and later as an adaptation to make efficient use of maternal body fat and other stored nutrients in feeding offspring and spacing births (45, 178, 179).

Significant diversity exists in the species-specific characteristics of lactation biology and their relation to life history (29, 91, 98, 152). Milk immune components (82), milk energy density (169), milk yield (168, 185), relative milk energy yield (152), and milk composition (79) vary among species with disease risk, body size, litter size and mass, maternal diet, maternal use of body stores, suckling patterns, and care behavior. This diversity reflects phylogenetic differences in the selective response to shifts in disease ecology, foraging opportunities, and constraints on growth and development. **Table 1** summarizes some key trends linking variation in lactation biology and life history across mammals.

Table 1 Key trends linking variation in lactation biology and life history across mammals

1. Marsupials commonly overlap lactation with gestation of younger offspring, whereas most placental species do not.
2. The period between first solid food consumption and weaning is long in species with single, precocial young, and provisioning may occur, whereas first solid food is usually eaten near weaning in polytokous species with altricial young (98).
3. Milk energy concentration decreases with maternal and neonatal size.
4. Milk fat and protein concentration are positively correlated, and both are negatively correlated with sugar, which is associated with suckling frequency.
5. Milk energy output at peak lactation scales with basal metabolic rate according to Kleiber's Law.

Nevertheless, all surviving mammals retain lactation as a key adaptation that contributes to the organization of life history characteristics (88). Four basic functions of lactation present as plesiomorphies are summarized in **Table 2**. Also highly conserved are similar mechanisms of lactogenesis (67, 89), mammary development (32), immunological activity (82), milk transport proteins (158), and metabolic adaptation during lactation (228).

SIMILARITIES AMONG NONHUMAN PRIMATES

More is known about the range of life history variation observed among nonhuman primates and hominids (40, 80, 92, 93, 140, 141, 176, 211–214, 227) than about variation in primate lactation biology (204, 242).

Life history: the temporal organization of major biological events over the lifetime of individuals. Life history theory aims to explain why life cycles vary among species and individuals

Lactation: the ability to secrete immunologically active and nutritious milk from ventral epidermal glands; a defining characteristic of mammals

Life History

Recent work suggests the common ancestor of primates weighed between 1 and 15 g and therefore had high metabolic, reproductive, and predation rates, and that body size remained below 50 g during the early Eocene primate radiations (78). Extant primates, however, range in size by an order of magnitude (92). Compared with other mammals, they are characterized by a slow life history and low postnatal growth rates (40, 92, 93). The few available data on variation in primate lactation biology suggest all species share common adaptations to meet infant nutritional needs conditioned by this characteristically slow life history.

Table 2 Basic functions of lactation present in all extant mammal species

1. Transfer protective functions of fully developed immune system across generations.
2. Optimize litter size to allow titration of maternal investment across sib sets.
3. Facilitate efficient reproduction in unpredictable environments lacking special foods for young.
4. Increase behavioral flexibility and opportunities for learning.

Milk Composition

Most previous reviews conclude that the gross composition of milk does not vary widely across nonhuman primate species with differences in body size, reproductive rates, patterns of maternal care, or other life history characteristics (32, 57, 69, 117, 173, 180). A single recent study reports variation in milk protein within a species in relation to parasitic infection (108). Primates are unusual among mammals because the milk they produce is lower in volume, more dilute, lower in energy, fat, and protein, and higher in lactose than would be predicted by body size (152), and because length of lactation is relatively long and always exceeds that of gestation (91).

It has long been hypothesized that these shared characteristics of primate milk coevolved with low reproductive rates and slow life histories relative to body size (15, 138, 167). Thus, a lower protein concentration of primate milks coevolved with slower growth rates (168, 169); lower fat concentration coevolved with the behavioral ecology of continuous infant carrying (which facilitates frequent suckling and is unusual in any other order of mammals) (15, 152, 170, 220); and a relatively high lactose content coevolved with the lower fat storage in adult females and low fat content of milk, and may also be linked to faster rates of postnatal brain growth. There is, however, no evidence that levels of long-chain polyunsaturated fatty acids (LCPUFAs) increase among primates with rates of postnatal brain growth (192).

Weaning: the termination of suckling. Weaning is a uniquely mammalian life history marker that may or may not be preceded by a period of feeding on other foods in addition to mother's milk

Plesiomorphies: shared primitive characteristics no older than the last common ancestor of a phylogenetic group of organisms

Exclusive suckling: a life history phase during which a juvenile mammal derives all nutrients from maternal milk. It is often referred to as "infancy" in nonhuman mammals

Transitional feeding: a life history phase during which nutrition is derived from a combination of maternal milk and other foods foraged by the infant, its parents, or others. It is poorly described for most primates

Juvenile Feeding Ecology

One correlate of a relatively slow life history is the relatively slow development and early maturation of the gastrointestinal tract in primates (195). This means that there is little clustering of gut maturational changes around the species-typical age at birth and age at weaning. Primates are therefore able to begin consuming milk even if born preterm and are generally viable from about 70% of the length of gestation without intensive neonatal care.

Nevertheless, from a nutritional perspective, nonhuman primate postnatal life can be divided into three phases (exclusive suckling, transitional feeding, and weanling) separated by two key life history markers (first consumption of solid food and weaning) that can be used to define two life history variables (age at first solid food and age at weaning) that increase with body size. Thus, nonhuman primates conform to a generalized mammalian pattern linking life history to feeding ecology (**Figure 1**). Juvenile daily intake of energy and specific nutrients increases from birth and is entirely due to greater milk intake during exclusive suckling. After weaning, further increase in total intake occurs by means of independent foraging or maternal provisioning.

Transitional Feeding

Variation in transitional feeding has yet to be fully described and explained and may be substantial both within and between species (136–138). There are few data with which to assess the length of transitional feeding in primates or the relative nutritional contribution of milk versus foraged foods (205). It has been hypothesized that relative length of transitional feeding is inversely related to adult diet quality (205), but available data are insufficient properly to test this. In the absence of good observational data it has been generally assumed that nonhuman primate infants wean relatively abruptly and begin to forage on foods similar to those selected by the mother, processing them largely for themselves. However, the transition to weaning is a gradual process in at least one ape, the orangutan (226), and possibly chimpanzees (165). Similarly, although it is commonly assumed that parental provisioning of juveniles is rare or absent in most species (75, 114, 122), there is limited evidence that it occurs in apes (166).

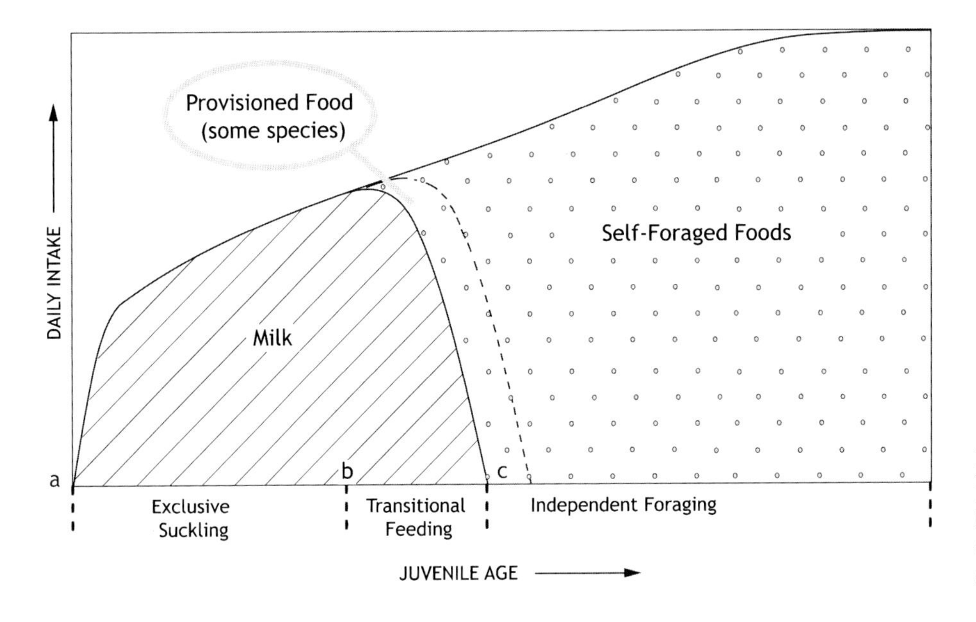

Figure 1

Key nutrition-related life history phases and markers for a generalized mammal.

Weaning

Last suckling is very difficult to observe directly in the wild, but captive data indicate that nonhuman primate weaning age is scaled to other life history traits, such as gestation length (92), birth weight (133, p. 245; 139), and adult weight (40), and developmental events such as age at molar eruption (193, 211, 212). However, such traits do not reliably predict age at weaning for all primate species, suggesting that age at weaning is labile. Studies of nonhuman primate behavioral ecology suggest that weaning age is plastic in most species and sensitive to ecological factors that constrain maternal ability to meet the increasing energy needs of growing offspring and the ability of infants to survive without mother's milk (4, 5, 136, 137, 139).

Infant Requirements

Few data are available on age-specific changes in energy requirements of nonhuman primates, of the total energy costs of growth and maintenance during infancy, or of the proportion met by milk consumed. Observation of ad libitum intakes among several captive large bodied cercopithecine species yields estimates of average infant energy requirements in the range 0.837–1.255 MJ/kg/d (160, 163). Such intakes are likely to differ from either average requirements or usual intakes in the wild, however. A study of free-living yearling baboons (*Papio cynocephalus*) estimated minimum total energy requirements for growth and maintenance at 0.871 MJ/d, or 0.383 MJ/kg/d (8).

It is difficult to identify studies that estimate the concentration of key nutrients such as vitamin A, vitamin D, iodine, calcium, and essential LCPUFAs in the milk of nonhuman primates (180). At present few conclusions can be drawn for any species about how milk nutrient content varies with maternal diet or about the extent to which exclusive suckling and milk consumption during transitional feeding satisfy age-specific nutrient requirements. Although evolved associations between feeding ecology and milk composition might be predicted across species, the data are too scant to test nutritional ecological hypotheses. For example, it is not known whether primate species that are nocturnal or obligatory carnivores (such as tarsiers) secrete milk richer in vitamin D levels in their milk as they are (no sun exposure) and are similar to felids. The milk of diurnal monkeys and apes is not reported as a rich source of vitamin D, and it is currently assumed that this is because endogenous synthesis satisfies requirement.

Weanling: a life history phase during which a recently weaned juvenile mammal must forage for itself and subsist on foods similar or identical to those selected by adults

Synapomorphic: evolutionarily derived or specialized characteristics shared only by one phylogenetic group of organisms

Maternal Costs

Relatively little is known about the reproductive ecology of wild nonhuman primate mothers. Evidence that they can accommodate the costs of protecting their infants against fluctuations in milk volume and composition when conditions are adverse is scant (57).

It is also unclear to what extent nonhuman primates share a capacity for maternal accommodation of lactation performance in response to moderate decreases in maternal energy or nutrient intakes. Free-living yearling baboons are estimated to consume 2.251 MJ/d, of which approximately 40% (0.900 MJ/d) comes from milk, suggesting their mothers bear the cost of minimal energy requirement (8).

Available data indicate that lactation places a significant metabolic demand on mothers and that limited mechanisms exist to accommodate this (6, 7, 57, 86, 135). Field observations of several species indicate that lactating females increase their intake of high-energy foods (27), overall food energy (196, 215), and time allocated to foraging (4, 58), particularly when forage quality is poor (59). Indirect evidence from captive studies suggests that in some species, energetic costs of lactation are accommodated by energy-sparing adaptations, physiological adaptations (17, 191), reductions in physical activity (17, 87), and shared care of infants (219, 242). No studies have shown conclusively that lactating nonhuman primate mothers are able to reduce the daily costs of milk production using fat stored during pregnancy.

Maternal Reproductive Ecology

Among wild great apes, female reproductive biology seems designed to avoid conception under food stress rather than to protect mothers from nutritional deficiency during lactation. Lactation, nutritional intake, energy expenditure, and net energy balance appear to be key influences on fecundity (16, 164). Field observations indicate conception is more likely to occur during periods of positive maternal energy balance because food availability is so unpredictable that conception cannot be timed so that birth will occur during periods of highest food availability (122).

DERIVED CHARACTERISTICS OF HUMANS

Table 3 summarizes some key differences in life history parameters among the great ape species, using values obtained for wild apes and hunter-gatherers with natural fertility. **Table 4** summarizes the shared and derived characteristics of human lactation biology.

Life History

There has been considerable debate about whether and why human life history differs from the typical primate pattern (25, 28, 77, 97, 105, 107, 119, 148, 229, 230, 239). A consensus has recently emerged that, in comparison to other primates, humans have evolved four distinctive life history traits: slow maturation, long lifespans with slow aging, postmenopausal longevity, and weaning before independent feeding (95).

Although not the largest living ape, humans have the slowest life history. This is evidenced by a markedly later age at maturity (marked by age at first birth), a longer period of nutritionally "independent" growth between weaning and maturity, longer maximum lifespan, and longer potential adult lifespan. Not all aspects of human life history are slowed, however. Duration of gestation is similar for all living ape species despite appreciable variation in size at maturity.

Healthy human neonates are relatively large for gestational age and relative to maternal body size, indicating faster fetal growth rates. Estimates of human weaning age and relative weaning weight are at the short end of the range for great apes.

Most striking, human birth interval is exceptionally short, both in absolute time and relative to body size. Average birth intervals rarely exceed four years in human populations without effective technological means of controlling fertility (232). In marked contrast, half of all randomly selected closed birth intervals exceed four, five, and eight years in wild gorillas, chimpanzees, and orangutans, respectively (75). Since fertility ends at similar ages in human and chimpanzee females, the "species-typical" rate of human reproduction is higher (25).

Milk Composition

A recent review (205) suggested that humans have retained a number of features of lactation biology that are plesiomorphic with mammals and synapomorphic with nonhuman primates. These shared characteristics include the four basic functions of lactation, similar spectra for the immune components of milk (82), and similar features of gross milk composition (22, 115, 117, 161, 167, 173). These design similarities are likely linked to recurring patterns of pathogen exposure, dietary ecology, and constraints on growth and development that shaped the adaptive radiation of primates. They must have been present in our last common ancestor with apes (which lived approximately 6–7 mya) and in all subsequent hominid species including those ancestral to humans (i.e., various members of the genera *Ardipithecus*, *Australopithecus*, and *Homo*).

Thus, all evidence suggests that the basic composition of human milk, its basic functions in the infant, and its mechanism of secretion and delivery remained unchanged during seven million years of human evolution. This is striking given that during this period there occurred a shift to bipedal locomotion, radical dental and cranial adaptations to a more omnivorous diet, a large increase in brain size, a doubling of adult body size, an even larger increase in the length of the juvenile period

Table 3 Phylogenetic relationships of great ape species and average values for selected life history parameters (adapted from sources cited in Reference 193)

	Estimated time of divergence from hominid lineage, mya	Adult female weight (range), kg	Gestation length, years	Birth interval, years	Age at weaning, years	Age at first birth, years	Maximum lifespan, years	Period of independent growth, years	Potential adult lifespan, years	Neonate weight/ maternal weight, %	Weaning weight/ maternal weight, %
Human, *Homo sapiens*	–	47.0 (38–56)	0.7	3.7	2.8	19.5	85.0	16.7	65.5	5.9	0.21
Chimpanzee, *Pan troglodytes*	5–7	35.0 (25–45)	0.6	5.5	4.5	13.3	53.4	8.8	40.1	5.4	0.27
Bonobo *Pan paniscus*	5–7	33.0 (27–39)	0.7	6.3	–	14.2	50.0	–	35.8	4.2	
Gorilla, *Gorilla gorilla*	6–8	84.5 (71–98)	0.7	4.4	2.8	10.0	54.0	7.2	44.0	2.3	0.21
Orangutan, *Pongo pygmaeus* and *Pongo abelii*	12–15	36.0	0.7	8.1	7.0	15.6	58.7	8.6	43.1	4.3	0.28

Table 4 Summary of shared and derived characteristics of human lactation biology

	Plesiomorphic Shared with other mammals	Symplesiomorphic Shared with other primates	Apomorphic Unique to humans
Postnatal immune defense	X		
Optimal postnatal nutrition	X		
Fertility regulation	X		
Developmental window for learning	X		
A period of exclusive lactation yields optimal benefits to mothers and offspring	X		
Low protein and fat and high lactose milk content		X	
Frequent suckling, high cost of infant carrying		X	
Slow infant growth		X	
A period of transitional feeding yields optimal benefits to mothers and offspring		?	
Age at weaning highly labile relative to other life history traits		?	
Complementary feeding			X
Increased plasticity in length of lactation relative to body size			X
Reduced infant energy needs			?
Significant buffering of lactation by fat storage in pregnancy			?

and of total lifespan, a shortening of birth intervals, and an increase in female postreproductive lifespan.

Juvenile Feeding Ecology

Current international recommendations (49–51, 55, 234, 237) based on clinical and epidemiological data (31, 49, 52, 125) provide a compelling model for the evolved pattern of human IYCF practices because they are predictive of optimal growth and development of healthy newborn humans in favorable environments (76, 202, 204). By this reasoning, the evolved template for human IYCF includes (*a*) initiation of breastfeeding within an hour of birth; (*b*) a period of exclusive breastfeeding followed by introduction of nutrient-rich and pathogen-poor complementary foods at about six months of infant age; (*c*) introduction of high-quality family foods, usually prepared from a variety of raw sources using some form of processing, heat treatment, and mixing; (*d*) continued breastfeeding at least until the third year; and (*e*) a package of "responsive caregiving" throughout the period of nutritional dependency but particularly during the transition to complementary feeding. This evolved human pattern is based on what is optimal for the child in terms of clinical outcomes and is schematized in **Figure 2**. Comparison of **Figures 1** and **2** suggests that important apomorphic features of human lactation biology include (*a*) complementary feeding and (*b*) early and flexible weaning (i.e., increased plasticity in the length of lactation).

Apomorphic features: derived characteristics that are not shared with an organism's ancestors and therefore are likely to be specialized and recent adaptations

Family foods: raw foods and combinations of foods collected, processed, and shared by older juveniles and adults and consumed by older members of the family

Complementary Feeding

The most remarkable change is the human use of complementary foods, which is unique among mammals (122) and results in a pattern of transitional feeding that appears to be fundamentally different from that of other primates.

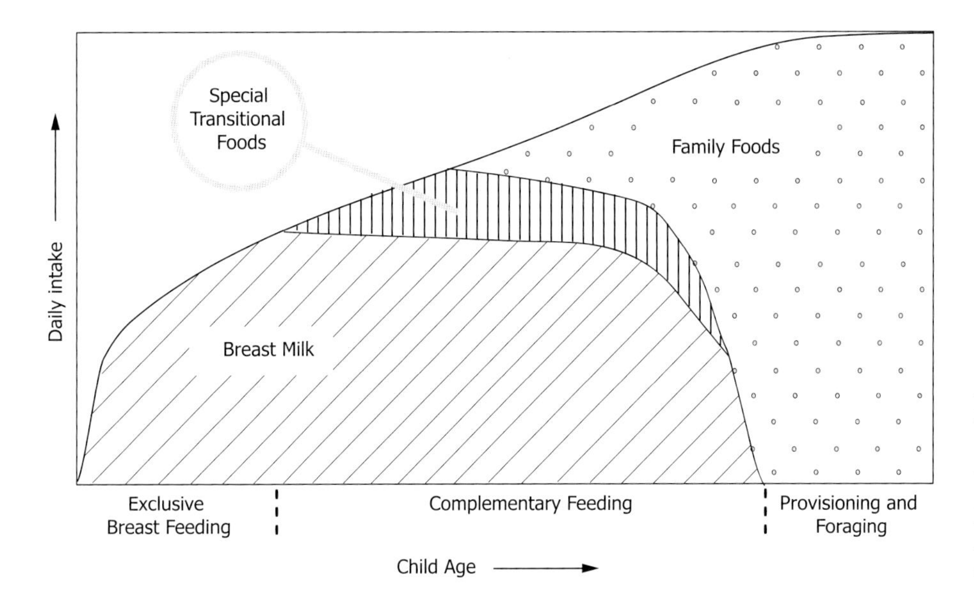

Figure 2

Key nutrition-related life history phases and markers for humans, optimal for infants and young children.

Overwhelming clinical and epidemiological evidence demonstrates that infants have not evolved to make efficient use of other foods before six months (53, 54, 126) and may suffer deficits and increased morbidity if not exclusively breastfed (42, 125). A wealth of data on the trajectory of infant development of feeding competency and changes in the nutritional needs of growing infants in relation to maternal milk supply supports the hypothesis that humans evolved to begin consuming complementary foods at approximately six months of age (205).

After approximately six months of age, complementary and family foods (235) increasingly contribute to the diet (131), as chewing (210, 211, 217), tasting (14, 47, 142), and digestive (134, 194) competencies develop. Frequency of suckling and volume of milk consumed do not necessarily diminish after six months in healthy babies, and the complementary feeding phase continues at least until the third year of life, during which breast milk remains an important, relatively sterile source of nutrients and immune protection.

Ethnographic evidence from preindustrial societies indicates that the duration of exclusive breastfeeding is extremely variable (201). Some indicators suggest that the age-related pattern for introduction of complementary foods in preindustrial societies concords loosely with the current clinical recommendations for normal, healthy children (203). The modal age of introduction of liquid and solid foods in a sample of published ethnographic reports was six months, suggesting a sizeable proportion of infants in these populations may have been exclusively breastfed for six months.

Early and Flexible Weaning

Humans are the only primates that wean juveniles before they can forage independently (94). The targeting and sharing of high-yield, nutrient-dense foods that entail high acquisition and processing costs is a specialization of human foragers (18), as is the use of heat treatments and combination of raw foods in "cuisine" (43, 240). We are also unusual in the extent to which we recruit and distribute help among conspecifics, including young child feeding and care (23, 221). Thus, weaning marks a shift to allo-caregiver support, not feeding independence.

Given the potential flexibility and observed variation in weaning age, it is difficult to conclude that humans have evolved a species-specific, global optimum weaning age. The clinical model suggests that there is no upper age limit at which breastfeeding ceases to be of some benefit to children (66, 151). Current international recommendations are based on evidence that infants benefit from breastfeeding into the third year (238). Continued breastfeeding must have remained a strongly selected component of ancestral maternal strategies because of its powerful anti-infective properties (100, 128, 157) and nutritional or physiological benefits to infants (19, 46) and mothers (10, 129, 223, 224).

The degree of flexibility in age at weaning is unusual among primates and probably a distinctive, derived characteristic. The diversity in human breastfeeding and complementary feeding patterns has long been a focus of lactation researchers (91). The duration of human lactation, if initiated at all, ranges from a few hours to more than five years in recent and contemporary societies (48, 121, 201, 202, 218). This spans most of the range observed for all other species of mammal (90). Ethnographic evidence from recent and contemporary foraging populations indicates that human weaning age is extremely variable within and between groups and that the process of weaning could be gradual (73, 123) or (less commonly) abrupt (71, 72). Humans also wean over a wide range of infant sizes; even among hunter-gatherers human infants are weaned after relatively smaller postnatal weight gain (11).

Nevertheless, some indicators suggest that the age-related pattern for termination of breastfeeding concords with the current clinical recommendations for normal, healthy children. It is estimated that breastfeeding beyond two years was the norm in between 75% (162) and 83% (12) of small-scale societies and that the modal age at weaning was approximately 30 months (201, 203). This suggests a sizeable proportion of infants in these populations may have been partially breastfed for more than two years, a pattern known to be optimal for growth and development. Rigorously collected data from hunter-gatherer populations suggest mean weaning age of 2.8 years (9). Even if we accept that the latest reliable estimate of modal age of weaning reported [four years among the !Kung (124)] is an indication of a species-typical value, it is well below the five to seven years predicted for primates with our life history parameters (48).

Archaeologists and skeletal biologists have made recent progress in developing approaches to estimating the timing of the trophic shifts associated with complementary feeding and weaning. Their studies use isotopic ratios in bony remains from juvenile and adult skeletons (21, 60, 197–200) and estimate childhood diet from tooth enamel recovered from adult remains (102, 120, 159). Results of such studies show that children in past populations often shifted to solid foods before two years of age while continuing to breastfeed.

Infant Energy Requirements

Cumulative energy requirements for male babies average 374.2 MJ between birth and 6 months and 959.4 MJ between birth and 12 months (data recalculated from data in Reference 34). Depending on age and sex, estimated mean total energy requirements for growth and maintenance in the first year range between 0.351 and 0.372 MJ/kg/d (1.347 and 3.519 MJ/d). These estimates are regarded as universally valid because healthy infants from different geographic areas show relative uniformity of growth, behavior, and physical activity (33, 76). They fall below the estimates for free-living yearling baboons (8) and well below those for captive large-bodied cercopithecines (160, 163). Thus, although comparative data are scant, human infants appear to have low energy requirements in comparison with other primates. This is likely due to comparatively slower growth.

Maternal Energy Cost

Human peak milk volume corresponds to a mean infant energy intake of 2.87 MJ/d

(183), which is well in excess of healthy infant requirements in the first six months. The crude energetic costs of human lactation estimated from measurements of daily milk intake among predominantly breastfed infants observed for two years postpartum is ~1686 MJ, more than half of which is borne in the first year of infant life (recalculated from data in Reference 183). This corresponds to a mean daily additional cost of approximately 2.3 MJ/d [actually 2.7 MJ/d in the first six months (183)]. Thus, the daily cost of lactation is potentially high (~25%–30%) in a mother compared with average total energy expenditure for a moderately active nonpregnant, nonlactating woman of average size (calculated from equations in Reference 70). However, two mechanisms allow mothers to accommodate the cost of lactation, both of which appear to be derived for humans relative to our nonhuman primate ancestors.

First, depletion of the maternal fat laid down before and during pregnancy has the potential to subsidize lactation by ~118.6 MJ (0.325 MJ/d) in the first year. Fat storage demands the largest proportion (~71%) of additional energy needed to sustain a healthy pregnancy in nonchronically energy-deficient women (62, 132, 183). Nevertheless, reductions in basal metabolic rates and physical activity (61, 183) ensure that for many women average daily costs of pregnancy (~0.7 MJ/d) are low (~8%) in relation to the usual dietary energy intakes and requirements of healthy nonpregnant, nonlactating women (~8.78 MJ/d). In favorable conditions, the average woman begins lactation with approximately 125 MJ of additional fat accumulated during pregnancy.

Second, feeding of nursing infants using safe and nutritionally adequate complementary foods can result in maternal energy savings of almost 1.8 MJ/d in the first year.

Together, healthy fat depletion and complementary feeding reduce the actual cost of lactation estimated to satisfy infant and young child needs for two years by 1023.6 MJ, or almost 61%. On a daily basis this reduces the net additional costs from ~2.3 MJ/d to ~0.9 MJ/d. For many women, this represents between 10% and 20% of usual total energy expenditure. Healthy people unconstrained in their access to food or choice of activities can comfortably increase energy intake, decrease physical activity, or both to accommodate increases in daily energy requirement of up to 30%. Despite these adaptations, however, the average daily energetic cost of human lactation is potentially higher than that of pregnancy (~2.3 MJ/d versus ~0.7 MJ/d).

One corollary is that human lactation performance is well buffered from fluctuations in maternal condition and nutrient supply (3, 112, 113, 181, 189). Aerobic exercise and gradual weight loss have no adverse impact on milk volume or composition, infant milk intake, infant growth, or other metabolic parameters (56, 144, 154, 155). A single intervention study has suggested that milk production can be improved by maternal food supplementation during exclusive lactation (83). However, most studies suggest lactation is rarely compromised even when mothers are multiparous, marginally undernourished, engaged in high levels of physical activity, and lose weight and fat with age and by season (1, 30, 146, 182, 184, 231).

Maternal Reproductive Ecology

Lactation, nutritional intake, energy expenditure, and net energy balance are the key influences on fecundity among humans (64, 65, 233). Reproductive endocrinology responds adaptively to maternal nutrient flux and behavioral ecology to schedule reproductive effort across the life span. Flexibility in weaning age reflects an evolved maternal capacity to vary reproduction in relation to ecology (23, 35, 63), the availability of alternate caregivers (110, 123, 150), and other environmental and social factors affecting the costs and benefits of weaning to mothers and infants (156). It has been hypothesized that the maternal cost of reproduction has likely been reduced in humans by the increased availability of help from older offspring [linked to the evolution of long childhood (24, 26)] and grandparents and other elders [linked to the evolution of greater longevity and vigorous postreproductive lifespan in females (96, 174)]. Observation in contemporary human societies shows lactation behavior is sensitive to maternal workload and the availability of cooperative childcare and feeding (13, 203). Weaning age is later among foragers than among subsistence herders and farmers (207), among whom women often do more of the kind of work that separates them from their infants for extended periods.

DEMOGRAPHIC IMPLICATIONS

The early age at weaning suggests that ancestral humans evolved an unusual capacity to reduce the length of exclusive and transitional feeding without increasing mortality. In humans, an inverse relationship between birth interval and child survival is mediated by breastfeeding (149, 209, 236). Birth intervals below two years are risky for older sibs. Nevertheless, as a species we are particularly good at keeping young alive in a peculiarly wide range of habitats. Infant and weanling survival is much greater among human foragers [60%–70% (103, 130)] than among apes [25%–50% (106, 107, 121)], and greater still in nonindustrial herding and farming economies (103, 104, 118, 164, 206). These simple demographic differences, which are based in part on differences in juvenile feeding ecology, have had enormous impact. The human population now exceeds six billion, whereas total populations of great ape species are estimated in the low thousands (122).

Shortened birth interval is currently regarded by anthropologists as one of the most evolutionarily significant human deviations from the expected pattern of great ape life history (75, 121, 122, 193, 204). Among our female ancestors, shortening of the periods of exclusive lactation or transitional feeding, or both, likely reduced birth intervals (by accelerating the return of ovarian cycling) and may have improved subsequent birth outcomes (by reducing maternal depletion). Shortened birth spacing would have increased maternal fitness only if it did not increase offspring mortality. Reduced juvenile mortality could be achieved only if many of the nutritional components of breast milk were provided by other kinds of foods or if infant development were accelerated so that the period of nutritional dependency was shortened (68, 85, 175).

IMPLICATIONS FOR CONTEMPORARY PUBLIC HEALTH

Despite burgeoning biomedical (81) and anthropological (225) research on human lactation in recent decades, few scholars have asked broader evolutionary questions about which characteristics of human lactation biology reflect evolutionarily conserved design features and which aspects, if any, reflect a distinctively human phenotype (204, 241). An evolutionary perspective provides insight into why contemporary patterns of IYCF often deviate from the optimal pattern indicated by clinical and epidemiological evidence. Human mothers are physiologically and behaviorally adapted to exercise more choice in the patterns and duration of full and partial breastfeeding than do other primates.

The evolution of the use of complementary foods to facilitate physiologically appropriate early weaning relative to other species has created potential for physiologically inappropriate early weaning and introduction of foods that are not complementary for breastfed infants. One recent and powerful manifestation of this potential is the development and widespread use of commercial infant formulas that meet some of the nutritional needs but none of the immunological needs of infants.

Contemporary human caregivers tend to titrate breastfeeding, complementary feeding, and child care in response to shifts in

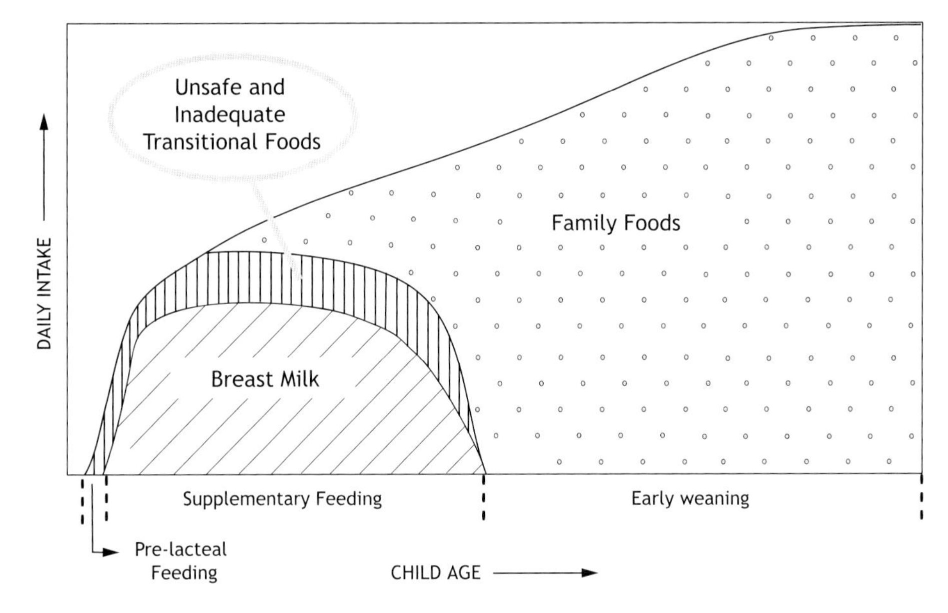

Figure 3

Commonly observed pattern of infant and young child feeding, not optimal for child outcomes.

ecology, subsistence, and social environment. Across cultures, underlying attitudes and values about child feeding are often broadly concordant with optimal practice, but focus more explicitly on tradeoffs between infant/child and maternal/caregiver needs. More often missing are the material conditions conducive for optimal breastfeeding and complementary feeding. Mismatch between optimal and actual infant feeding practices in contemporary populations is widespread and presents a major public health challenge (111, 188, 208, 222). Common practices such as discarding of colostrum (84, 190), use of prelacteal feeds (2, 177), reduced breast milk intake due to early introduction of formula and other substances, and early weaning (101) are associated with infant illness and death (116). These suboptimal practices are schematized in **Figure 3**.

CONCLUSION

Unlike other species, the life histories of mammals have coevolved with the special adaptive advantages and physiological demands of lactation biology. This review has suggested that human patterns of lactation and complementary feeding are intimately linked with the evolution of a distinctive set of human life history variables. Complementary feeding and fat storage in pregnancy probably evolved in the past 5–7 million years as unique and important human adaptations that together reduce the energetic and opportunity costs of lactation for mothers and the potential fitness costs of relatively early transitional feeding and weaning for infants and young children. The human lactation span is comparatively short. The lower bound for safe complementary feeding has been set at around six months for normal-term and preterm babies by constraints on the evolution of physiological factors such as the growth and maturation of infant systems affecting immune, feeding, and digestive competency. The upper bound for safe weaning has been set above two years of infant age by similar constraints, but the evolution of complementary feeding, together with many other distinctively human evolutionary changes, has introduced enormous behavioral flexibility in maternal response to social and ecological constraints.

This evolutionary perspective provides insight into why, in today's world, young child feeding practices are clinically suboptimal for most children and their mothers, and why many people in both rich and poor societies fail to adopt recommended feeding practices. Understanding the ultimate evolutionary causes of human variability in young child feeding can provide insights on the proximate causes of patterns of breastfeeding and complementary feeding that subsequently lead to poor health outcomes for mothers and babies. Such insight may help in the design of interventions to promote improved infant feeding practices.

SUMMARY POINTS

1. Human use of highly processed, nutrient-rich, complementary foods is hypothesized as unique among primates.
2. Complementary feeding is an evolutionarily derived (i.e. apomorphic) species characteristic that coevolved with changes in life history and physiology that reduce the maternal costs of lactation and with distinctive patterns of human foraging, parenting, social behavior, growth, and development.
3. The evolution of complementary feeding occurred because it made exclusive lactation relatively shorter and reduced birth intervals without increasing maternal or infant mortality.
4. Behavioral and physiological shifts during the evolution of complementary feeding enabled human infants to survive without breast milk at a relatively younger age and at a smaller size than infant apes.
5. Contemporary public health challenges arising from this evolutionary history include a strong behavioral tendency among humans to reduce the length of exclusive breastfeeding beyond the lower bounds consistent with optimal infant outcomes.

FUTURE ISSUES

The following issues have not yet been resolved:

1. The extent of behavioral and physiological variation in the timing and dietary impact of transitional feeding in nonhuman primates and its socioecological correlates (such as quality of adult diet).
2. The absolute timing of steps in the evolution of complementary feeding and the relation of these steps to other key derived human characteristics (such as the origins and maintenance of bipedal locomotion, increased brain size, reduced sexual dimorphism, tool use, food sharing, cooking, and allo-parenting).
3. How humans evolved to overcome the physiological and psychosocial challenges to successful establishment of exclusive breastfeeding that are observed in contemporary populations.
4. How humans evolved to meet the complex challenge of introducing appropriate complementary foods in a timely manner while satisfying other demands on caregivers.
5. How human lactation biology evolved to protect low-birth-weight and premature infants, and to reduce the risks of maternal-to-child transmission of pathogens.

LINK

http://www.who.int/child-adolescent-health/NUTRITION/infant.htm

ACKNOWLEDGMENTS

Support for the author's work was furnished by the Canada Research Chairs Program (CRC), the Canadian Institutes of Health Research (CIHR), and the Canadian Foundation for Innovation (CFI).

LITERATURE CITED

1. Adair LS, Pollitt E, Mueller WH. 1983. Maternal anthropometric changes during pregnancy and lactation in a rural Taiwanese population. *Hum. Biol.* 55:771–87
2. Akuse RM, Obinya EA. 2002. Why healthcare workers give prelacteal feeds. *Eur. J. Clin. Nutr.* 56:729–34
3. Allen LH. 1994. Maternal micronutrient malnutrition: effects on breast milk and infant nutrition, and priorities for intervention. *SCN News* 11:21–24
4. Altmann J. 1980. *Baboon Mothers and Infants.* Cambridge, MA: Harvard Univ. Press
5. Altmann J, Alberts SC. 2003. Variability in reproductive success viewed from a life-history perspective in baboons. *Am. J. Hum. Biol.* 14:401–9
6. Altmann J, Altmann SA, Hausfater G. 1978. Primate infant's effects on mother's future reproduction. *Science* 201:1028–30
7. Altmann J, Samuels A. 1992. Costs of maternal care: infant carrying in baboons. *Behav. Ecol. Sociobiol.* 29:391–98
8. Altmann SA. 1998. *Foraging for Survival: Yearling Baboons in Africa.* Chicago: Chicago Univ. Press. 609 pp.
9. Alvarez HP. 2000. Grandmother hypothesis and primate life histories. *Am. J. Phys. Anthropol.* 113:435–50
10. Am. Dietet. Assoc. 2005. *Position of the American Dietetic Association: Promoting and Supporting Breastfeeding.* Chicago/Washington, DC: Am. Dietet. Assoc.
11. Ball HL, Hill CM. 1996. Reevaluating "twin infanticide." *Curr. Anthropol.* 37:856–63
12. Barry H III, Paxson LM. 1971. Infancy and early childhood: cross-cultural codes 2. *Ethnology* 10:466–508
13. Baumslag N, Michels DL. 1995. *Milk, Money, and Madness: The Culture and Politics of Breastfeeding.* Westport, London: Bergin & Garvey. 256 pp.
14. Beauchamp GK, Cowart BL. 1987. Development of sweet taste. In *Sweetness*, ed. J Dobbing, pp. 127–38. Berlin: Springer-Verlag
15. Ben Shaul DM. 1962. The composition of the milk of wild animals. *Int. Zool. Yearbook* 4:333–42
16. Bentley GR. 1999. Aping our ancestors: comparative aspects of reproductive ecology. *Evol. Anthropol.* 7:175–85
17. Bercovitch FB. 1987. Female weight and reproductive condition in a population of olive baboons (*Papio anubis*). *Am. J. Primat.* 12:189–95
18. Bird DW. 2001. Human foraging strategies: human diet and food practices. In *Encyclopedia of Evolution*, ed. M Pagel. New York: Oxford Univ. Press
19. Black RF, Bhatia J. 1998. The biochemistry of human milk. In *The Science of Breastfeeding*, ed. RF Black, L Jarman, JB Simpson, pp. 103–52. Boston, MA: Jones & Bartlett

20. Blackburn DG. 1993. Lactation: historical patterns and potential for manipulation. *J. Dairy Sci.* 46:3195–212
21. Blakely RJ. 1989. Bone strontium in pregnant and lactating females form archaeological samples. *Am. J. Phys. Anthropol.* 80:173–85
22. Blaxter KL. 1961. Lactation and growth of the young. In *Milk: The Mammary Gland and Its Secretion*, ed. SK Kon, AT Cowie, pp. 305–61. London: Academic
23. Blurton Jones N. 2002. The lives of hunter-gatherer children: effects of parental behavior and parental reproductive strategy. In *Juvenile Primates: Life History, Development, and Behavior*, ed. ME Pereira, LA Fairbanks, pp. 309–26. New York: Oxford Univ. Press. 2nd ed.
24. Blurton Jones N. 2005. Introduction: Why does childhood exist? See Ref. 104a, pp. 105–8
25. Blurton Jones N, Hawkes K, O'Connell JF. 1999. Some current ideas about the evolution of the human life history. In *Comparative Primate Socioecology*, ed. PC Lee, pp. 140–66. London: Cambridge Univ. Press
26. Bock J, Sellen DW. 2002. Childhood and the evolution of the human life course: an introduction. *Hum. Nat.: An Interdiscipl. J.* 13:153–59
27. Boinski S. 1988. Sex differences in the foraging beahvior of squirrel monkeys in a seasonal habitat. *Behav. Ecol. Sociobiol.* 32:177–86
28. Bribiescas RG. 2001. Reproductive ecology and life history of the human male. *Yearbook Phys. Anthropol.* 44:148–76
29. Bronson FH. 1989. *Mammalian Reproductive Biology*. Chicago: Chicago Univ. Press
30. Brown KH, Akhtar NA, Robertson AD, Ahmed MG. 1986. Lactational capacity of marginally nourished mothers: relationships between maternal nutritional status and quantity and proximate composition of milk. *Pediatrics* 78:909–19
31. Brown KH, Dewey KG, Allen L. 1998. *Complementary Feeding of Young Children in Developing Countries: A Review of Current Scientific Knowledge*. Geneva: World Health Org. 178 pp.
32. Buss DH. 1971. Mammary glands and lactation. In *Comparative Reproduction of Nonhuman Primates*, ed. ESE Hafez, pp. 315–33. Springfield, IL: Thomas
33. Butte NF. 1996. Energy requirements of infants. *Eur. J. Clin. Nutr.* 50:S24–36
34. Butte NF, Henry CJK, Torun B. 1996. Report of the working group on energy requirements of infants, children and adolescents. *Eur. J. Clin. Nutr.* 50:S188–89
35. Caro TM, Sellen DW. 1990. On the reproductive advantages of fat in women. *Ethol. Sociobiol.* 11:51–66
36. Charnov EL. 1991. Evolution of life history variation among female mammals. *Proc. Natl. Acad. Sci. USA* 88:1134–37
37. Charnov EL. 1993. *Life History Invariants: Some Explorations of Symmetry in Evolutionary Ecology*. London: Oxford Univ. Press
38. Charnov EL. 1997. Trade-off-invariant rules for evolutionarily stable life histories. *Nature* 387:393–94
39. Charnov EL. 2001. Evolution of mammal life histories. *Evol. Ecol. Res.* 3:521–35
40. Charnov EL, Berrigan D. 1993. Why do female primates have such long lifespans and so few babies? Or life in the slow lane. *Evol. Anthropol.* 1:191–94
41. Cifelli RL, Rowe TB, Luckett WP, Banta J, Reyes R, Howes RI. 1996. Fossil evidence for the origin of the marsupial pattern of tooth replacement. *Nature* 379:715–18
42. Cohen R, Brown KH, Canahuati J, Rivera LL, Dewey KG. 1994. Effects of age of introduction of complementary foods on infant breast milk intake, total energy intake, and growth: a randomised intervention study in Honduras. *Lancet* 344:288–93

43. Conklin-Brittain N, Wrangham R, Smith CC. 2002. A two-stage model of increased dietary quality in early hominid evolution: the role of fiber. In *Human Diet: Perspectives on Its Origin and Evolution*, ed. PS Ungar, MF Teaford, pp. 61–67. Westport, CT: Greenwood
44. Daan S, Tinbergen JM. 1997. Adaptation of life histories. In *Behavioral Ecology: An Evolutionary Approach*, ed. JR Krebs, NB Davies, pp. 311–33. Oxford: Blackwell Sci.
45. Dall SRX, Boyd IL. 2004. Evolution of mammals: Lactation helps mothers to cope with unreliable food supplies. *Proc. R. Soc. Lond. B Biol. Sci.* 271:2049–57
46. Dept. Health Human Serv. Off. Women's Health. 2003. Benefits of breastfeeding. *Nutr. Clin. Care* 6:125–31
47. Desor JA, Bauchamp GK. 1987. Longitudinal changes in sweet preference in humans. *Physiol. Behav.* 39:639–41
48. Dettwyler KA. 2004. When to wean: biological versus cultural perspectives. *Clin. Obstetr. Gynecol.* 47:712–23
49. Dewey K. 2003. *Guiding Principles for Complementary Feeding of the Breastfed Child.* Geneva: World Health Org.
50. Dewey K. 2005. *Guiding Principles for Feeding Nonbreastfed Children 6–24 Months of Age.* Geneva: World Health Org.
51. Dewey KG. 2002. *Guiding Principles for Complementary Feeding of the Breast Fed Child.* Geneva: Pan Am. Health Org./World Health Org. 37 pp.
52. Dewey KG, Brown KH. 2003. Update on technical issues concerning complementary feeding of young children in developing countries and implications for intervention programs. *Food Nutr. Bull.* 24:5–28
53. Dewey KG, Cohen RJ, Brown KH, Rivera LL. 1999. Age of introduction of complementary foods and growth of term, low-birth-weight, breast-fed infants: a randomized intervention study in Honduras. *Am. J. Clin. Nutr.* 69:679–86
54. Dewey KG, Cohen RJ, Brown KH, Rivera LL. 2001. Effects of exclusive breastfeeding for four versus six months on maternal nutritional status and infant motor development: results of two randomized trials in Honduras. *J. Nutr.* 131:262–67
55. Dewey KG, Cohen RJ, Rollins NC. 2004. Feeding of nonbreastfed children from 6 to 24 months of age in developing countries. *Food Nutr. Bull.* 25:377–402
56. Dewey KG, Lovelady CA, Nommsen LA, McCrory MA, Lönnerdal B. 1994. A randomized study of the effects of aerobic exercise by lactating women on breastmilk volume and composition. *New Engl. J. Med.* 330:449–53
57. Dufour DL, Sauther ML. 2002. Comparative and evolutionary dimensions of the energetics of human pregnancy and lactation. *Am. J. Hum. Biol.* 14:584–602
58. Dunbar RIM, Dunbar P. 1988. Maternal time budgets of gelada baboons. *Anim. Behav.* 36:970–80
59. Dunbar RIM, Hannah-Stewart L, Dunbar P. 2002. Forage quality and the costs of lactation for female gelada baboons. *Anim. Behav.* 64:801–5
60. Dupras TL, Schwarcz HP, Fairgrieve SI. 2001. Infant feeding and weaning practices in Roman Egypt. *Am. J. Phys. Anthropol.* 115:204–12
61. Durnin JV, McKillop FM, Grant S, Fitzgerald G. 1985. Is nutritional status endangered by virtually no extra intake during pregnancy? *Lancet* 2:823–25
62. Durnin JV. 1987. Energy requirements of pregnancy: an integration of the longitudinal data from the five-country study. *Lancet* 2:1131
63. Ellison PT. 1994. Advances in human reproductive ecology. *Annu. Rev. Anthropol.* 23:255–75

64. Ellison PT. 2001. *On Fertile Ground: A Natural History of Human Reproduction*. Cambridge, MA: Harvard Univ. Press
65. Ellison PT. 2003. Energetics and reproductive effort. *Am. J. Hum. Biol.* 15:342–51
66. Fewtrell MS. 2003. The long-term benefits of having been breast-fed. *Curr. Paediatr.* 14:97–103
67. Fleet IR, Goode JA, Hamon MH, Laurie MS, Linzell JL, Peaker M. 1975. Secretory activity of goat mammary glands during pregnancy and the onset of lactation. *J. Physiol.* 251:763–73
68. Foley R. 1995. Evolution and adaptive significance of hominid behavior. In *Motherhood in Human and Nonhuman Primates*, ed. CR Pryce, RD Martin, SD, pp. 27–36. Basel, Switz.: Karger
69. Fomon SJ. 1986. Breast-feeding and evolution. *J. Am. Dietary Assoc.* 86:317–18
70. Food Nutr. Board. 1989. Energy. In *Recommended Dietary Allowances*, ed. National Research Council, pp. 24–38. Washington, DC: Natl. Acad. Press
71. Ford CS. 1945. *A Comparative Study of Human Reproduction*. New Haven, CT: Yale Univ. Press
72. Fouts HN, Hewlett BS, Lamb ME. 2005. Parent-offspring weaning conflicts among the Bofi farmers and foragers of central Africa. *Curr. Anthropol.* 46:29–50
73. Fouts HN, Lamb ME. 2005. Weanling emotional patterns among the Bofi foragers of Central Africa: the role of maternal availability. See Ref. 104a, pp. 309–21
74. Futuyma DJ. 1998. The evolution of life histories. In *Evolutionary Biology*, pp. 561–78. Sunderland, MA: Sinauer
75. Galdikas BMF, Wood JW. 1990. Birth spacing patterns in humans and apes. *Am. J. Phys. Anthropol.* 83:185–91
76. Garza C. 2006. New growth standards for the 21st century: a prescriptive approach. *Nutr. Rev.* 64:S72–91
77. Geary DC. 2002. Sexual selection and human life history. *Adv. Child Dev. Behav.* 30:41–101
78. Gebo DL. 2004. A shrew-sized origin for primates. *Phys. Anthropol.* 47:40–62
79. Gittleman JL, Thompson SD. 1988. Energy allocation in mammalian reproduction. *Am. Zool.* 28:863–75
80. Godfrey KM, Samonds KE, Jungers WL, Sutherland MR. 2001. Teeth, brains, and primate life histories. *Am. J. Phys. Anthropol.* 114:192–214
81. Goldman AS. 2001. Breastfeeding lessons from the past century. *Pediatr. Clin. North Am.* 48:xxiii–xxv
82. Goldman AS, Chheda S, Garofalo R. 1998. Evolution of immunologic functions of the mammary gland and the postnatal development of immunity. *Pediatr. Res.* 43:155–62
83. Gonzalez-Cossio T, Habicht JP, Rasmussen KM, Delgado HL. 1998. Impact of food supplementation during lactation on infant breast-milk intake and on the proportion of infants exclusively breast-fed. *J. Nutr.* 128:1692–702
84. Gunnlaugsson G, Einarsdottir J. 1993. Colostrum and ideas about bad milk—a case-study from Guinea-Bissau. *Soc. Sci. Med.* 36:283–88
85. Hammel EA. 1996. Demographic constraints on population growth of early humans. *Hum. Nat.* 7:217–55
86. Harcourt AH. 1987. Dominance and fertility among female primates. *J. Zool. Lond.* 213:471–87
87. Harrison MJS. 1983. Age and sex differences in the diet and feeding strategies of the green monkey, *Cercopithecus sabaeus*. *Anim. Behav.* 31:969–77

88. Hartmann P, Morgan S, Arthur P. 1986. Milk letdown and the concentration of fat in breast milk. In *Human Lactation 2: Maternal and Environmental Factors*, ed. M Hamosh, AS Goldman, pp. 275–81. New York: Plenum
89. Hartmann PE. 1973. Changes in the composition and yield of the mammary secretion of cows during the initiation of lactation. *Endocrinology* 59:231–47
90. Hartmann PE, Arthur PG. 1986. Assessment of lactation performance in women. In *Human Lactation 2: Maternal and Environmental Factors*, ed. M Hamosh, AS Goldman, pp. 215–30. New York: Plenum
91. Hartmann PE, Rattigan S, Prosser CG, Saint L, Arthur PG. 1984. Human lactation: back to nature. In *Physiological Strategies in Lacation*, ed. M Peaker, RG Vernon, CH Knight, pp. 337–68. London: Academic
92. Harvey PH, Clutton-Brock TH. 1985. Life history variation in primates. *Evolution* 39:559–81
93. Harvey PH, Martin RD, Clutton-Brock TH. 1987. Life histories in comparative perspective. In *Primate Societies*, ed. BB Smuts, DL Cheney, RM Seyfarth, RW Wrangham, TT Struhsaker, pp. 181–96. Chicago: Univ. Chicago Press
94. Hawkes K. 2006. Life history and the evolution of the human lineage: some ideas and findings. See Ref. 97, pp. 45–94
95. Hawkes K. 2006. Slow life histories and human evolution. See Ref. 97, pp. 95–126
96. Hawkes K, O'Connell JF, Blurton Jones NG, Alvarez H, Charnov EL. 1998. Grandmothering, menopause, and the evolution of human life histories. *Proc. Natl. Acad. Sci. USA* 95:1336–39
97. Hawkes K, Paine RL, eds. 2006. *The Evolution of Human Life History*. Santa Fe, NM: School Am. Res. Press
98. Hayssen V. 1993. Empirical and theoretical constraints on the evolution of lactation. *J. Dairy Sci.* 76:3213–33
99. Hayssen VD, Blackburn DG. 1985. Alpha-lactalbumin and the evolution of lactation. *Evolution* 39:1147–49
100. Heinig MJ. 2001. Host defense benefits of breastfeeding for the infant: effect of breastfeeding duration and exclusivity. *Pediatr. Clin. North Am.* 48:105–23
101. Heinig MJ, Nommsen LA, Peerson JM, Lonnerdal B, Dewey KG. 1993. Intake and growth of breast-fed and formula-fed infants in relation to the timing of introduction of complementary foods: the DARLING study. *Acta Paediatr.* 82:999–1006
102. Herring DA, Saunders SR, Katzenberg MA. 1998. Investigating the weaning process in past populations. *Am. J. Phys. Anthropol.* 105:425–39
103. Hewlett BS. 1991. Demography and childcare in preindustrial societies. *J. Anthropol. Res.* 47:1–37
104a. Hewlett BS, Lamb ME. 2005. *Hunter-Gatherer Childhoods: Evolutionary, Developmental, and Cultural Perspectives*. Piscataway, NJ: Aldine Trans.
104. Hewlett BS. 2005. Introduction: Who cares for hunter-gatherer children? See Ref. 104a, pp. 175–76
105. Hill K. 1993. Life history theory and evolutionary anthropology. *Evol. Anthropol.* 2:78–88
106. Hill K, Hurtado AM. 1995. *Ache Life History: The Ecology and Demography of a Foraging People*. New York: Aldine de Gruyter
107. Hill K, Kaplan H. 1999. Life history traits in humans: theory and empirical studies. *Annu. Rev. Anthropol.* 28:397–430
108. Hinde K. 2006. Milk composition varies in relation to the presence and abundance of *Balantidium coli* in the mother in captive rhesus macaques (*Macaca mulatta*). *Am. J. Primatol.* 69:1–10

109. Horn HS. 1978. Optimal tactics of reproduction and life history. In *Behavioral Ecology: An Evolutionary Approach*, ed. JR Krebs, NB Davies, pp. 272–94. Oxford: Blackwell Sci.
110. Hrdy S. 1999. *Mother Nature: A History of Mothers, Infants and Natural Selection*. New York: Pantheon. 944 pp.
111. Huffman SL, Martin LH. 1994. First feedings: optimal feeding of infants and toddlers. *Nutr. Res.* 14:127–59
112. Inst. Med. (U.S.) Subcomm. Nutr. During Lactation. 1991. Milk composition. In *Nutrition During Lactation*, pp. 113–52. Washington, DC: Natl. Acad. Sci.
113. Inst. Med. (U.S.) Subcomm. Nutr. During Lactation. 1991. Milk volume. In *Nutrition During Lactation*, pp. 80–112. Washington, DC: Natl. Acad. Sci.
114. Janson CH, Van Schaik CP. 2002. Ecological risk aversion in juvenile primates: Slow and steady wins the race. In *Juvenile Primates: Life History, Development and Behavior*, ed. ME Pereira, LA Fairbanks, pp. 56–76. New York: Oxford Univ. Press. 2nd ed.
115. Jenness R. 1974. Biosynthesis and composition of milk. *J. Invest. Dermatol.* 63:109–18
116. Jones G, Steketee RW, Black RE, Bhutta ZA, Morris SS, Bellagio Child Suriv. Study Group. 2003. How many child deaths can we prevent this year? *Lancet* 362:65–71
117. Kanazawa AT, Miyazawa T, Hirono H, Hayashi M, Fujimoto K. 1991. Possible essentiality of docosahexaenoic acid in Japanese monkey neonates: occurrence in colostrum and low biosynthetic capacity in neonate brains. *Lipids* 26:53–57
118. Kaplan H, Hill K, Hurtado AM, Lancaster J. 2001. The embodied capital theory of human evolution. In *Reproductive Ecology and Human Evolution*, ed. PT Ellison, pp. 293–317. New York: Aldine de Gruyter
119. Kaplan H, Hill K, Lancaster J, Hurtado AM. 2000. A theory of human life history evolution: diet, intelligence, and longevity. *Evol. Anthropol.* 9:156–84
120. Katzenberg MA, Herring DA, Saunders SR. 1996. Weaning and infant mortality: evaluating the skeletal evidence. *Yearbook Phys. Anthropol.* 39:177–99
121. Kennedy GE. 2005. From the ape's dilemma to the weanling's dilemma: early weaning and its evolutionary context. *J. Hum. Evol.* 48:123–45
122. Knott CD. 2001. Female reproductive ecology of the apes: implications for human evolution. In *Reproductive Ecology and Human Evolution*, ed. PT Ellison, pp. 429–63. New York: Aldine de Gruyter
123. Konner M. 2005. Hunter-gatherer infancy and childhood: The !Kung and others. See Ref. 104a, pp. 19–64
124. Konner MJ. 1977. Infancy among the Kalahari Desert San. In *Culture and Infancy*, ed. PH Leiderman, SR Tulkin, A Rosenfeld, pp. 69–109. New York: Academic
125. Kramer M, Kakuma R. 2002. The optimal duration of exclusive breastfeeding: a systematic review. *Cochrane Database System. Rev.* 1. **http://www.update-software.com/Abstracts/ab003517.htm**
126. Kramer MS, Guo T, Platt RW, Sevkovskaya Z, Dzikovich I, et al. 2003. Infant growth and health outcomes associated with 3 compared with 6 mo of exclusive breastfeeding. *Am. J. Clin. Nutr.* 78:291–95
127. Kumar S, Hedges B. 1998. A molecular timescale for vertebrate evolution. *Nature* 392:917–20
128. Labbok M, Clark D, Goldman A. 2005. Breastfeeding: maintaining an irreplaceable immunological resource. *Breastfeeding Rev.* 13:15–22
129. Labbok MH. 2001. Effects of breastfeeding on the mother. *Pediatr. Clin. North Am.* 48:143–58
130. Lamb ME, Hewlett BS. 2005. Reflections on hunter-gatherer childhoods. See Ref. 104a, pp. 407–15

131. Lartey A, Manu A, Brown KH, Peerson JM, Dewey KG. 1999. A randomized, community-based trial of the effects of improved, centrally processed complementary foods on growth and micronutrient status of Ghanaian infants from 6 to 12 mo of age. *Am. J. Clin. Nutr.* 70:391–404
132. Lawrence M, Lawrence F, Coward WA, Cole TJ, Whitehead RG. 1987. Energy requirements of pregnancy in the Gambia. *Lancet* 2:1072
133. Lawrence RA. 1989. *Breastfeeding: A Guide for the Medical Profession*. St. Louis, MO: Mosby
134. Lee MF, Krasinski SD. 1998. Human adult-onset lactase decline: an update. *Nutr. News* 56:1–8
135. Lee PC. 1987. Nutrition, fertility and maternal investment in primates. *J. Zool. Lond.* 213:409–22
136. Lee PC. 1996. The meanings of weaning: growth, lactation, and life history. *Evol. Anthropol.* 5:87–96
137. Lee PC. 1999. Comparative ecology of postnatal growth and weaning among haplorhine primates. In *Comparative Primate Socioecology*, ed. PC Lee, pp. 111–39. London: Cambridge Univ. Press
138. Lee PC, Bowman JE. 1995. Influence of ecology and energetics on primate mothers and infants. In *Motherhood in Human and Nonhuman Primates*, ed. CR Pryce, RD Martin, D Skuse, pp. 47–58. Basel, Switz.: Karger
139. Lee PC, Majluf P, Gordon IJ. 1991. Growth, weaning and maternal investment from a comparative perspective. *J. Zool.* 225:99–114
140. Leigh SR, Blomquist G. 2007. Life history. In *Primates in Perspective*, ed. CJ Campbell, A Fuentes, KC MacKinnon, M Panger, SK Beader, pp. 396–407. Oxford, UK: Oxford Univ. Press
141. Leigh SR, Shea BT. 1996. Ontogeny of body size variation in African apes. *Am. J. Phys. Anthropol.* 99:43–65
142. Liem DG, Mennella JA. 2003. Heightened sour preferences during childhood. *Chem. Senses* 28:173–80
143. Long A. 1972. Two hypotheses on the origin of lactation. *Am. Natural.* 106:141–44
144. Lovelady CA, Lönnerdal B, Dewey KG. 1990. Lactation performance of exercising women. *Am. J. Clin. Nutr.* 52:103–9
145. Luckett WP. 1993. An ontogenetic assessment of dental homologies in therian mammals. In *Mammal Phylogeny, Vol. 1: Mesozoic Differentiation, Multituberculates, Monotremes, Early Therians, and Marsupials*, ed. FS Szalay, MJ Novacek, MC McKenna, pp. 182–204. New York: Springer
146. Lunn PG. 1985. Maternal nutrition and lactational infertility: the baby in the driving seat. In *Maternal Nutrition and Lactational Infertility*, ed. J Dobbing, pp. 41–64. Vevey/New York: Nestlé Nutr./Raven
147. Luo ZX, Crompton AW, Sun AL. 2002. A new mammal form from the early Jurassic and evolution of mammalian characteristics. *Science* 292:1535–40
148. Mace R. 2000. Review: evolutionary ecology of human life history. *Anim. Behav.* 59:1–10
149. Manda SOM. 1999. Birth intervals, breastfeeding and determinants of childhood mortality in Malawi. *Soc. Sci. Med.* 48:301–12
150. Marlowe FW. 2005. Who tends Hadza children? See Ref. 104a, pp. 177–90
151. Marquis GS, Habicht J. 2000. Breastfeeding and stunting among toddlers in Peru. In *Short and Long Term Effects of Breast Feeding on Child Health*, ed. B Koletzko, KF Michaelsen, O Hernell, pp. 163–72. New York: Kluwer Acad./Plenum

152. Martin RD. 1984. Scaling effects and adaptive strategies in mammalian lactation. *Symposia Zool. Soc. Lond.* 51:87–117
153. Martin RD, MacLarnon AM. 1985. Gestation period, neonatal size and maternal investment in placental mammals. *Nature* 313:220–23
154. McCrory MA. 2000. Aerobic exercise during lactation: safe, healthful, and compatible. *J. Hum. Lactat.* 16:95–98
155. McCrory MA. 2001. Does dieting during lactation put infant growth at risk? *Nutr. Rev.* 59:18–27
156. McDade TW, Worthman CM. 1998. The weanling's dilemma reconsidered: a biocultural analysis of breastfeeding ecology. *J. Dev. Behav. Pediatr.* 19:286–99
157. McGuire E. 2005. *An Exploration of How Mother's Milk Protects the Infant*. East Malvern, Victoria, Australia: Austral. Breastfeed. Assoc. Lactat. Resource Cent.
158. Messer M, Weiss AS, Shaw DC, Westerman M. 1998. Evolution of the monotremes: phylogenetic relationship to marsupials and eutherians, and estimation of divergence dates based on α-lactalbumin amino acid sequences. *J. Mammalian Evol.* 5:95–105
159. Moggi-Cecchi J, Pacciani E, Pinto-Cisneros J. 1994. Enamel hypoplasia and age at weaning in nineteenth century Florence, Italy. *Am. J. Phys. Anthropol.* 93:299–306
160. Natl. Acad. Sci. 1989. *Nutrition and Diarrheal Diseases Control in Developing Countries*. Washington, DC: Natl. Acad. Press. 14 pp.
161. Natl. Res. Counc. Natl. Acad. Sci. 2003. *Nutrient Requirements of Nonhuman Primates, Table 9–4*. Washington, DC: Natl. Acad. Press. 286 pp.
162. Nelson EAS, Yu LM, Williams S, Int. Child Care Pract. Study Group. 2005. International Child Care Practices study: breastfeeding and pacifier use. *J. Hum. Lactat.* 21:289–95
163. Nicolosi RJ, Hunt RD. 1979. Dietary allowances for nutrients in nonhuman primates. In *Primates in Nutritional Research*, ed. KC Hayes, pp. 11–37. New York: Academic
164. Nishida T, Corp N, Hamai M, Hasegawa T, Hiraiwa-Hasegawa M, et al. 2003. Demography, female life history, and reproductive profiles among the chimpanzees of Mahale. *Am. J. Primatol.* 59:99–121
165. Nishida T, Ohigashi H, Koshimizu K. 2000. Tastes of chimpanzee plant foods. *Curr. Anthropol.* 41:431–38
166. Nishida T, Turner LA. 1996. Food transfer between mother and infant chimpanzees of the Mahale Mountains National Park, Tanzania. *Int. J. Primatol.* 17(6):947–68
167. Oftedal OT. 1984a. Body size and reproductive strategy as correlates of milk energy output in lactating mammals. *Acta Zool. Fennica* 171:183–86
168. Oftedal OT. 1984b. Milk composition, milk yield and energy output at peak lactation: a comparative review. *Symposia Zool. Soc. Lond.* 51:33–85
169. Oftedal OT. 1986. Milk intake in relation to body size. In *The Breastfed Infant: A Model for Performance*, ed. LJ Filer Jr, SJ Fomon, pp. 44–47. Columbus: Ross Lab.
170. Oftedal OT, Iverson SJ. 1987. Hydrogen isotope methodology for measurement of milk intake and energetics of growth in suckling young. In *Marine Mammal Energetics*, ed. AC Huntley, DP Costa, GAJ Worthy, MA Castellini, pp. 67–96. Lawrence, KS: Allen
171. Pagel MD, Harvey PH. 1993. Evolution of the juvenile period in mammals. In *Juvenile Primates: Life History, Development, and Behavior*, ed. ME Pereira, LA Fairbanks, pp. 528–37. New York: Oxford Univ. Press
172. Paine RR, Hawkes K. 2006. Introduction. See Ref. 97, pp. 3–16
173. Patino EM, Borda JT. 1997. The composition of primate's milks and its importance in selecting formulas for hand rearing. *Lab. Primate Newsl.* 36:8–9

174. Peccei J. 2001. A critique of the Grandmother Hypothesis: old and new? *Am. J. Hum. Biol.* 13:434–52
175. Pennington RL. 1996. Causes of early human population growth. *Am. J. Phys. Anthropol.* 99:259–74
176. Pereira ME, Fairbanks LA, eds. 2002. *Juvenile Primates: Life History, Development, and Behavior*. Chicago: Univ. Chicago Press
177. Pérez-Escamilla R, Segura-Millán S, Canahuati J, Allen H. 1996. Prelacteal feedings are negatively associated with breast-feeding outcomes in Honduras. *J. Nutr.* 126:2765–73
178. Pond CM. 1984. Physiological and ecological importance of energy storage in the evolution of lactation: evidence for a common pattern of anatomical organization of adipose tissue in mammals. *Symposia Zool. Soc. Lond.* 51:1–31
179. Pond CM. 1997. The biological origins of adipose tissue in humans. In *The Evolving Female*, ed. ME Morbeck, A Galloway, AL Zihlman, pp. 47–162. Princeton, NJ: Princeton Univ. Press
180. Power ML, Oftedal OT, Tardif SD. 2002. Does the milk of callitrichid monkeys differ from that of larger anthropoids? *Am. J. Primatol.* 56:117–27
181. Prentice A. 1986. The effect of maternal parity on lactational performance in a rural African community. In *Human Lactation 2: Maternal and Environmental Factors*, ed. M Hamosh, AS Goldman, pp. 165–73. New York: Plenum
182. Prentice A, Paul A, Prentice A, Black A, Cole T, Whitehead R. 1986. Cross-cultural differences in lactational performance. In *Human Lactation 2: Maternal and Environmental Factors*, ed. M Hamosh, AS Goldman, pp. 13–43. New York: Plenum
183. Prentice A, Spaaij C, Goldberg G, Poppitt S, van Raaij J, et al. 1996. Energy requirements of pregnant and lactating women. *Eur. J. Clin. Nutr.* 50:S82–111
184. Prentice A, Whitehead R, Roberts S, Paul A. 1981. Long-term energy balance in childbearing Gambian women. *Am. J. Clin. Nutr.* 34:2790–99
185. Prentice AM, Prentice A. 1988. Energy costs of lactation. *Annu. Rev. Nutr.* 8:63–79
186. Promislow D. 2003. Mate choice, sexual conflct, and evolution of senescence. *Behav. Genet.* 33:191–201
187. Promislow DE, Harvey PH. 1990. Living fast and dying young: a comparative analysis of life-history variation among mammals. *J. Zool. Lond.* 220:417–37
188. Quandt S. 1985. Biological and behavioral predictors of exclusive breastfeeding duration. *Med. Anthropol.* 9(2):139–51
189. Rasmussen KM. 1992. The influence of maternal nutrition on lactation. *Annu. Rev. Nutr.* 12:103–17
190. Rizvi N. 1993. Issues surrounding the promotion of colostrum feeding in rural Bangladesh. *Ecol. Food Nutr.* 30:27–38
191. Roberts SB, Cole TJ, Coward WA. 1985. Lactational performance in relation to energy intake in the baboon. *Am. J. Clin. Nutr.* 41:1270–76
192. Robson SL. 2004. Breast milk, diet, and large human brains. *Curr. Anthropol.* 45:419–24
193. Robson SL, van Schaik CP, Hawkes K. 2006. The derived features of human life history. See Ref. 97, pp. 17–44
194. Sahi T, Isokoski M, Jussila J, Launiala K. 1972. Lactose malabsorption in Finnish children of school age. *Acta Paediatr. Scand.* 61:11–16
195. Sangild PT. 2006. Gut responses to enteral nutrition in preterm infants and animals. *Exp. Biol. Med.* 231:1–16
196. Sauther ML. 1994. Changes in the use of wild plant foods in free-ranging ring-tailed lemurs during pregnancy and lactation: some implications for human foraging strategies.

In *Eating on the Wild Side: The Pharmacologic, Ecologic and Social Implications of Using Noncultigens*, ed. NL Etkin, pp. 240–46. Tucson: Univ. Arizona Press

197. Schurr MR. 1997. Stable nitrogen isotopes as evidence for the age of weaning at the Angel site: a comparison of isotopic and demographic measures of weaning age. *J. Archaeol. Sci.* 24:919–27
198. Schurr MR. 1998. Using stable nitrogen-isotopes to study weaning behavior in past populations. *World Archaeol.* 30:327–42
199. Schurr MR, Powell ML. 2005. The role of changing childhood diets in the prehistoric evolution of food production: an isotopic assessment. *Am. J. Phys. Anthropol.* 126:278–94
200. Schwarcz HP, Wright LE. 1998. Stable carbon and oxygen isotopes in human tooth enamel: identifying breastfeeding and weaning in prehistory. *Am. J. Phys. Anthropol.* 106:1–18
201. Sellen DW. 2001a. Comparison of infant feeding patterns reported for nonindustrial populations with current recommendations. *J. Nutr.* 131:2707–15
202. Sellen DW. 2001b. Of what use is an evolutionary anthropology of weaning? *Hum. Nat. Interdiscip. J.* 12:1–7
203. Sellen DW. 2001c. Weaning, complementary feeding, and maternal decision making in a rural east African pastoral population. *J. Hum. Lactat.* 17:233–44
204. Sellen DW. 2006b. Lactation, complementary feeding and human life history. See Ref. 97, pp. 155–97
205. Sellen DW. 2007. Evolution of human lactation and complementary feeding: implications for understanding contemporary cross-cultural variation. *Adv. Exper. Med. Biol.* In press
206. Sellen DW, Mace R. 1999. A phylogenetic analysis of the relationship between subadult mortality and mode of subsistence. *J. Biosoc. Sci.* 31:1–16
207. Sellen DW, Smay DB. 2001. Relationship between subsistence and age at weaning in "preindustrial societies." *Hum. Nat. Interdiscip. J.* 12:47–87
208. Sellen DW. Sub-optimal breast feeding practices: ethnographic approaches to building "baby friendly" communities. *Adv. Exper. Med. Biol.* 503:223–32
209. Shahidullah M. 1994. Breast-feeding and child survival in Matlab, Bangladesh. *J. Biosoc. Sci.* 26:143–54
210. Sheppard JJ, Mysak ED. 1984. Ontogeny of infantile oral reflexes and emerging chewing. *Child Dev.* 55:831–43
211. Smith BH. 1991. Dental development and the evolution of life history in Hominidae. *Am. J. Phys. Anthropol.* 86:157–74
212. Smith BH. 1992. Life history and the evolution of human maturation. *Evol. Anthropol.* 1:134–42
213. Smith BH, Crummett TL, Brandt KL. 1994. Ages of eruption of primate teeth: a compendium for aging individuals and comparing life histories. *Yearbook Phys. Anthropol.* 37:177–231
214. Smith RJ, Jungers WL. 1997. Body mass in comparative primatology. *J. Hum. Evol.* 32:523–59
215. Stacey PB. 1986. Group size and foraging efficiency in yellow baboons. *Behav. Ecol. Sociobiol.* 18:175–87
216. Stearns SC. 1992. *The Evolution of Life Histories*. Oxford: Oxford Univ. Press
217. Stevenson RD, Allaire JH. 1991. The development of normal feeding and swallowing. *Pediatr. Clin. North Am.* 38:1439–53
218. Sugarman M, Kendall-Tackett K. 1995. Weaning ages in a sample of American women who practice extended breastfeeding. *Clin. Pediatr.* 34:642–47

219. Tardif SD, Harrison ML, Simek MA. 1993. Communal infant care in marmosets and tamarins: relation to energetics, ecology, and social organization. In *Marmosets and Tamarins: Systematics, Behavior, and Ecology*, ed. AB Rylands, pp. 220–34. New York: Oxford Univ. Press
220. Tilden CD, Oftedal OT. 1997. Milk composition reflects pattern of maternal care in prosimian primates. *Am. J. Primatol.* 41:195–211
221. Trevathan WR, McKenna JJ. 1994. Evolutionary environments of human birth and infancy: insights to apply to contemporary life. *Child. Environ.* 11:88–104
222. Underwood BA, Hofvander Y. 1982. Appropriate timing for complementary feeding of the breast-fed infant. *Acta Paediatr. Scand.* S294:5–32
223. U.S. Breastfeeding Comm. 2002a. *Benefits of Breastfeeding*. Raleigh, NC: U.S. Breastfeeding Comm.
224. U.S. Breastfeeding Comm. 2002b. *Economic Benefits of Breastfeeding*. Raleigh, NC: U.S. Breastfeeding Comm.
225. van Esterik P. 2002. Contemporary trends in infant feeding research. *Annu. Rev. Anthropol.* 31:257–78
226. van Noordwijk MA, van Schaik CP. 2005. Development of ecological competence in Sumatran orangutans. *Am. J. Phys. Anthropol.* 127:79–94
227. van Schaik CP, Barrickman N, Bastian ML, Krakauer EB, van Noordwijk MA. 2006. Primate life histories and the role of brains. See Ref. 97, pp. 127–54
228. Vernon RG, Flint DJ. 1984. Adipose tissue: metabolic adaptation during lactation. *Symposia Zool. Soc. Lond.* 51:119–45
229. Walker R, Gurven M, Migliano A, Chagnon N, Djurovic G, et al. 2006. Growth rates, developmental markers, and life histories in 20 small-scale societies. *Am. J. Hum. Biol.* 18:295–311
230. Walker R, Hill K, Burger O, Hurtado AM. 2006. Life in the slow lane revisited: ontogenetic separation between chimpanzees and humans. *Am. J. Phys. Anthropol.* 129:577–83
231. Winkvist A, Jalil F, Habicht JP, Rasmussen KM. 1994. Maternal energy depletion is buffered among malnourished women in Punjab, Pakistan. *J. Nutr.* 124:2376–85
232. Wood JW. 1990. Fertility in anthropological populations. *Annu. Rev. Anthropol.* 19:211–42
233. Wood JW. 1994. *Dynamics of Human Reproduction: Biology, Biometry, Demography*. New York: Aldine de Gruyter
234. World Health Org. 1979. *Joint WHO/UNICEF Meeting on Infant and Young Child Feeding: Statement and Recommendations*. Geneva: World Health Org.
235. World Health Org. 2000a. *Complementary Feeding: Family Foods for Breast Fed Children*. Geneva: World Health Org.
236. World Health Org. 2000b. Effects of breastfeeding on infant and child mortality due to infectious diseases in less developed countries: a pooled analysis. *Lancet* 355:451–55
237. World Health Org. 2001. Global strategy for infant and young child feeding: the optimal duration of exclusive breastfeeding. *Rep. A54/INF.DOC./4*. Geneva: World Health Org.
238. World Health Org., U.N. Children's Fund. 2003. *Global Strategy for Infant and Young Child Feeding*. Geneva: World Health Org.
239. Worthman CM, Kuzara J. 2005. Life history and the early origins of health differentials. *Am. J. Hum. Biol.* 17:95–112

240. Wrangham R, Jones JH, Laden G, Pilbeam D, Conklin-Brittain N. 1999. The raw and the stolen: cooking and the ecology of human origins. *Curr. Anthropol.* 40:567–94
241. Wray J. 1991. Breast-feeding: an international and historical review. In *Infant and Child Nutrition Worldwide: Issues and Perspectives*, ed. F Falkner, pp. 62–117. Boca Raton, FL: CRC Press
242. Wright P. 1990. Patterns of paternal care in primates. *Int. J. Primat.* 11:89–102

Regional Fat Deposition as a Factor in FFA Metabolism

Susanne B. Votruba and Michael D. Jensen

Endocrine Research Unit, Division of Endocrinology, Metabolism and Nutrition, Mayo Clinic, Rochester, Minnesota 55905; email: jensen@mayo.edu

Annu. Rev. Nutr. 2007. 27:149–63

The *Annual Review of Nutrition* is online at http://nutr.annualreviews.org

This article's doi:
10.1146/annurev.nutr.27.061406.093754

0199-9885/07/0821-0149$20.00

Key Words

body fat distribution, obesity, body composition, isotope dilution techniques

Abstract

Humans have a large variability in body fat distribution, which has tremendous implications for metabolic health. Obese individuals with an upper-body-fat distribution have increased health complications such as dyslipidemia, hypertension, insulin resistance, and type 2 diabetes in comparison with lower-body-obese individuals. Additionally, females have more body fat, a greater proportion of fat in their lower body, and much less visceral fat than do lean males at the same body mass index. The reasons for these differences in body fat distribution have not been clearly identified but could be important. Herein we review what has been learned about regional differences in triglyceride storage capacity and lipolysis as they relate to the causes and consequences of regional fat accumulation. Both sex and site differences in regional fat storage have been described. In contrast, with the exception of variations between men and women in the contribution of visceral adipose tissue to hepatic FFA delivery, most studies have failed to show important sex differences in regional lipolysis in vivo.

Contents

DEXA: dual-energy X-ray absorptiometry

CT: computed tomography

INTRODUCTION

Importance of Regional Fat Distribution

The large variability in human body fat distribution has tremendous implications for metabolic health. Obese individuals with an upper-body-fat distribution have increased health complications such as dyslipidemia, hypertension, insulin resistance, and type 2 diabetes in comparison with lower-body-obese individuals (47). Additionally, females have more body fat, a greater proportion of fat in their lower body, and much less visceral fat than do lean males at the same body mass index. The reasons for these differences in body fat distribution have not been clearly identified but could be important. Regional differences in triglyceride storage capacity (71) and/or lipolysis (101) have been proposed as determining regional fat accumulation, and in vitro studies of regional adipocytes have suggested both mechanisms may be operative. Sex differences in regional storage capacity of meal triglycerides have been reported previously (77, 93, 99). Additionally, investigators attempting to find variations in regional lipolysis in vivo (36, 63) have been unable to document important sex differences in this regard.

POTENTIAL ROLE OF MEAL FAT UPTAKE AND REGIONAL BODY FAT DISTRIBUTION

Methodology

In order to quantitatively measure meal fat uptake, it is also necessary to accurately and reliably measure regional body fat distribution. Many methods of assessing total body fat are available today, each with their limitations. Skinfold thickness is the cheapest and most accessible measurement of body fat, but the accuracy and reproducibility is highly variable depending on the skill of the individual taking the measurements. Underwater weighing and bioelectrical impedance (34) analysis can also be used to determine total body fatness, but regional body fat distribution is not readily attainable. Dual-energy X-ray absorptiometry (DEXA), which has historically been used for measurement of bone mineral density, has become the most widely used and accepted means for determining total and regional fat-free and fat mass (102). Computer software can be used to analyze DEXA scans for upper- and lower-body fat/fat-free mass, but no distinction can be made between subcutaneous and visceral fat. For this, computed tomography (CT) scans can be used to obtain abdominal slices that can be examined, in combination with DEXA, to determine visceral fat content (39). Being able to accurately measure regional fatness allows further study of the uptake of fatty acids into fat and the release of fatty acid from fat in the context of the regional fat content.

Meal fatty acids labeled with stable (^{13}C and ^{2}H) and radioactive (^{14}C and ^{3}H) isotopes have been used in clinical research to monitor the fate of dietary fat (17, 42, 50, 77, 81, 93, 95, 103). In particular, carbon isotopes have a long history of use. When ^{13}C- or ^{14}C-labeled fatty acids are given in meals, the isotopically labeled carbon atoms from the oxidation of triglyceride fatty acids are converted to $^{13}CO_2$ or $^{14}CO_2$. The majority of the labeled CO_2 produced is excreted in the expired air, so that breath samples can be analyzed to measure meal fatty acid oxidation. Yet, some difficulties exist when one chooses to use carbon-labeled fatty acids. A controlled environment is needed for frequent collection of breath samples in order to determine the production rates of the labeled CO_2 per unit time and to calculate cumulative recovery over the study period. Additionally, with the use of carbon tracers, respiratory gas exchange measurements are needed because the CO_2 flux is needed to calculate production rates. This is time consuming and restrictive of daily activity (1). Finally, the potential exists for isotopic exchange of the carbon tracer at several steps along the tricarboxylic acid cycle (87, 88), resulting in an incomplete label ($^{14}CO_2$ or $^{13}CO_2$) excretion and, therefore, an underestimation of fatty acid oxidation. The label fixation also appears to differ depending upon whether the fatty acid is labeled on an even or an odd carbon; as a result, many studies use fatty acids labeled on the first carbon, e.g., [1-^{14}C]oleate. A solution to these problems has been to adjust fatty acid oxidation from CO_2 recovery using a correction factor, which requires an additional study day (84, 85, 87, 88). The advantage of this approach, however, is the ability to measure rates of meal fatty acid oxidation over time and to assess how interventions affect rates of oxidation.

Given some of the difficulties in using carbon tracers of meal fat, the use of deuterium- or tritium-labeled fatty acids provides a good alternative. The loss of deuterium/tritium label in the tricarboxylic acid cycle is minimal and therefore should not require a correction for exchange reactions (68, 77, 97). The use of hydrogen labeling eliminates the need for frequent sampling as well as the measurement of respiratory gas exchange. Hydrogen labels, when oxidized, appear as ^2H_2O or ^3H_2O and mix with the body water pool. Other than minimal losses as urine and insensible water (82, 83), the remaining tracer provides a cumulative record of fat oxidation that is easily collected by obtaining urine samples. The disadvantage of using hydrogen-labeled fatty acids is that measuring oxidation rates still requires frequent sampling of body water (blood, saliva, or urine). In general, however, carbon or hydrogen tracers may be used to measure meal fat oxidation and uptake, as long as the limitations of each method are acknowledged.

A meal triglyceride or fatty acid may take several potential pathways upon ingestion. One of these is oxidation, which is the easiest pathway to measure in human study participants. By using these methods (44, 77, 83, 93, 97) it is possible to trace the fate of the fat from a single meal toward oxidation and, therefore, how a variety of interventions or conditions may affect meal (exogenous) fat oxidation (4, 6, 7, 93, 95). Furthermore, exogenous fat oxidation may be combined with indirect calorimetry to assess the contribution of endogenous fats as well.

It is also possible to measure the appearance of the labeled triglycerides into the plasma chylomicron pool. Meal fatty acids first appear in chylomicrons (77, 99), but also in the free fatty acid (FFA) fraction (78) and then in VLDL-triglycerides (31, 32). Thus, the metabolic fate of ingested fat can be quite complex. In general, meal fat is largely cleared from the plasma compartment within 24 hours (40), presumably partitioned between oxidation and storage elsewhere in the body.

Tracer methodology can also be used to assess triglyceride storage by adipose tissue. Adipose tissue lipoprotein lipase (LPL) activity (20) and arteriovenous balance (14–16, 63) measurements are used as measures of the ability to take up and store triglyceride. Unfortunately, LPL activity measures only one component of the processes that regulate the storage of fatty acids in adipose tissue, and measuring the rate of uptake using arterial-venous balance techniques is usually done over more limited periods of time, which may miss some of the integrated uptake of dietary fat. An approach developed by Björntorp et al. (9) involved administering meals containing a radiolabeled fatty acid tracer and performing adipose tissue biopsies following meal

VLDL: very-low-density lipoproteins

LPL: lipoprotein lipase

absorption. This allowed investigators to have an integrated measure of meal fatty acid storage in adipose tissue. This technique has been applied by several groups (40, 54–56, 77, 93, 99) to directly measure the uptake of dietary fat by adipose tissue in humans in vivo under a variety of conditions. Uptake of dietary fatty acids into visceral fat depots can be assessed, but this requires combining the meal tracer study with planned surgical interventions (40, 55) and is therefore more difficult. Meal fat uptake into skeletal muscle can also be assessed through biopsies (5). Meal fat uptake into an organ such as liver, adipose tissue, or muscle can also be ascertained by measuring the arterio-venous differences across the regions of interest (15, 63). This, however, requires many assumptions and calculations, whereas biopsies provide a direct measure of meal fat uptake.

Update on Research Findings

When assessing regional disposal of meal fat, the measurement of tracer oxidation is imperative to gaining a more complete understanding of the processes that occur. Some of the earlier studies of meal fat uptake into adipose tissue did not measure meal fat oxidation (9, 55, 56) and thus provided an incomplete picture of meal fat trafficking. The oxidation of meal fats is influenced by a myriad of factors. For example, physical activity or inactivity can alter the portion of meal fat that is targeted to oxidation versus nonoxidative pathways, at least over the short term (**Figure 1**). Another consistent finding that must be taken into account when designing studies to address meal fat utilization is that the level of oxidation is specific to fatty acid type. In general, oxidation decreases with fatty acid chain length and degree of saturation (17, 43, 44, 53, 80, 98). **Figure 2** illustrates some of the variability in the percent of the individual fatty acid doses recovered from a single meal after 9–13 hours using ^{13}C tracers that were not corrected for sequestration (4, 43, 62, 95–98). Some of these differences may be attributable to variations in gastro-intestinal handling (41, 62), but there may also be differences in the handling of fatty acids on a cellular level (11). Additionally, the amount of fat given in a test meal may affect the partitioning of fat toward oxidation. Sonko et al. (89) reported an inverse relationship in the size of the fat load and postprandial oxidation when the meal fat

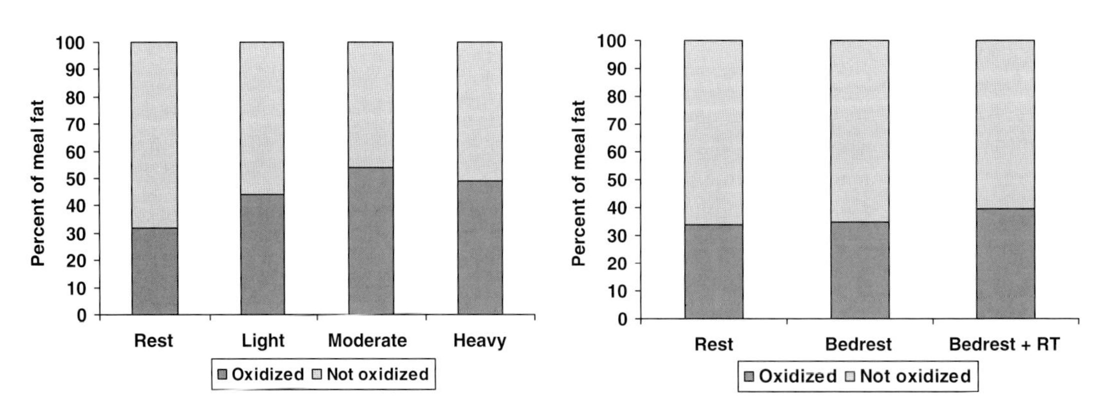

Figure 1

The partitioning of meal fat tracers between oxidation and temporary storage. The 11.5-hour cumulative oxidation of oleate given in a meal 30 minutes after the completion of isocaloric cycling exercise at light, moderate, or heavy intensity compared with rest is shown in the left panel (adapted from Reference 98). The right panel is a depiction of the seven-hour postdose meal oleate oxidation at ambulatory rest and after three months of head-down tilt bed rest, without and with added resistance training (RT) (adapted from Reference 4).

amount was greater than 50 grams (**Figure 3**). We have also recently reported that ingestion of a 70% of energy from fat, hypercaloric meal resulted in a decrease of ~13% in the fraction of the meal fat being oxidized over 24 hours compared with an isocaloric meal containing 30% of energy from fat (99).

Meal fat that is not oxidized is largely stored in adipose tissue. When ingested, meal fat is processed into chylomicrons in the gut and delivered to the circulation. Muscle and adipose tissue LPL has been postulated to be the major regulator of uptake of meal triglycerides (22). LPL activity in human adipose tissue is modulated by physiological conditions such as feeding and fasting, with decreases in LPL activity taking place following weight loss (35, 91) and increases in adipose tissue LPL activity occurring during the postprandial period (23, 99, 104). Until recently, there was little evidence that regional differences in adipose tissue LPL activity are actually linked to the storage of dietary fat. We found that excess energy intake, achieved by a high-fat meal, results in preferential storage of dietary fat in lower-body subcutaneous (LBSQ) fat in lean women compared with lean men and that this is linked to greater postprandial LPL activation in leg fat (99). What we found most impressive is the great interindividual variability in fed state regional LPL activity (99). The source of this huge (10-fold in women) interindividual variability is unknown but likely plays a major role in determining interindividual differences in meal fat storage and potentially body fat distribution.

Meal-derived triglycerides that do not enter tissues due to incomplete chylomicron hydrolysis (chylomicron remnants) can be taken up by the liver, where they can be incorporated into VLDL particles. Heath et al. (32) provided direct evidence with a tracer study that up to 20% of meal fatty acids provided at breakfast have entered the VLDL triglyceride (VLDL-TG) pool after six hours. More recently, the same group showed that tracers of breakfast meal fat begin appearing in VLDL-TG one hour after the meal and in-

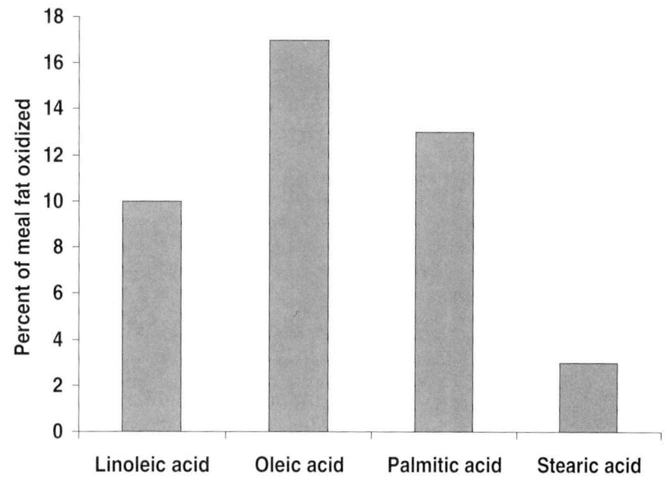

Figure 2

The mean percent oxidation of separate meal fatty acid tracers given in a single test meal. All cumulative recoveries were calculated between 9 and 13 hours postdose. A ^{13}C tracer at the C1 position was used for all tracers, and a correction factor for sequestration was not applied (4, 43, 62, 95–98).

crease to 40% of tracer incorporation at nine hours (31). Moreover, a lunch meal fat tracer given on the same day also rapidly appears in the VLDL-TG fraction. Whether this truly represents chylomicron remnant metabolism or the hepatic uptake of meal fatty acids that have entered the FFA pool during chylomicron hydrolysis (78) is unknown.

Meal fat uptake into adipose tissue can be directly assessed through needle biopsies. Björntorp et al. (9) reported that in three men undergoing gallbladder surgery, the uptake of ^{14}C-palmitate from a meal increased in relation to fat cell size. Subsequently, Mårin et al. (56) recruited premenopausal women with a wide range of adiposity to determine meal fat uptake into the abdominal and thigh subcutaneous fat after either an overnight fast or a prior high-carbohydrate breakfast. The experimental meal provided ~73% of energy from fat using heavy cream, and meal fat uptake into adipose tissue was assessed with U-^{14}C-oleate 4 hours, 24 hours, 1 week, and 1 month after the test meal. At four hours after the test meal, uptake was greater in the abdomen than the thigh and greater in the previously fed versus fasted volunteers.

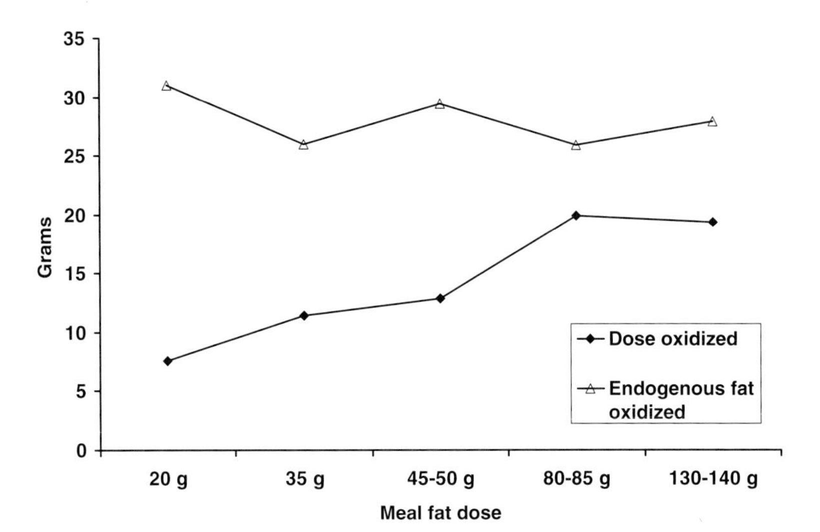

Figure 3

Evidence of meal fat oxidation with increasing meal fat content. Data adapted from Reference 89.

The specific activity in both adipose depots continued to increase until one month, suggesting a redistribution of meal fat from temporary storage in other tissues. The same group later reported that in men given a high-fat test meal, meal fat uptake into omental fat was greater than into subcutaneous abdominal fat. Although this may suggest that meal fat uptake into visceral fat is the cause of greater visceral adiposity in males compared with females (54), direct comparisons with females are largely lacking. We recently found that women also have greater omental than abdominal subcutaneous meal uptake of fatty acids (40).

Studies from our lab have looked at meal fat uptake and how it relates to regional differences in body fat distribution between males and females. Romanski et al. (77) found that meal fatty acid uptake was greater in abdominal subcutaneous fat than in thigh adipose tissue in both men and women, implying that differential meal fat storage does not entirely explain the sex differences in body fat distribution. The main sex difference was a greater percentage of dietary fat stored in subcutaneous adipose tissue in females compared with males. We have subsequently confirmed this pattern of meal fatty acid uptake (93), but also noted substantial intraindividual variability in femoral adipose tissue meal fat uptake in women that could not be explained by menstrual cycle effects.

Based upon studies using a high-fat meal (55, 56), we hypothesized that sex differences in regional fat uptake after a meal would become more apparent in conditions of energy imbalance (99) (**Figure 4**). We've recently reported that, when compared with a normal fat meal, a high fat meal results in more efficient uptake of meal triglyceride in leg adipose tissue in females than in males, whereas the uptake efficiency in abdominal fat does not differ between sexes. This suggests that when meal fat consumption results in net fat storage, females preferentially increase uptake in leg adipose tissue.

FFA KINETICS AND BODY FAT DISTRIBUTION

The relationship between obesity (as measured by body mass index) and components of the metabolic syndrome is even stronger if an upper-body fat distribution phenotype (as measured by waist circumference, waist-to-hip circumference ratio) (13, 18, 19, 25, 27, 28, 30, 67, 72, 92) is taken into account. Intra-abdominal fat (primarily omental and mesenteric—collectively referred to as visceral fat) is usually associated more strongly with these metabolic abnormalities (12, 45,

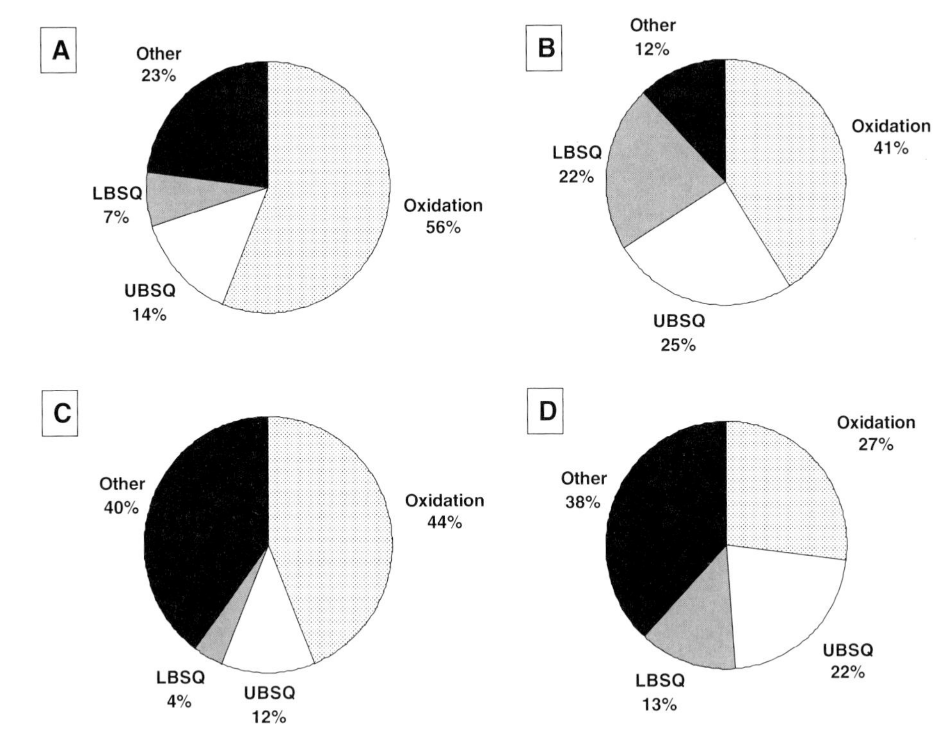

Figure 4

Fate, after 24 hours, of a ^{14}C-triolein meal fat tracer in men given a normal-fat meal (*A*) or a high-fat meal (*C*) and women given a normal-fat meal (*B*) or a high-fat meal (*D*). Meal fat disposal as oxidation or storage into lower-body subcutaneous (LBSQ) and upper-body subcutaneous (UBSQ) was measured. Tracer that was unaccounted for at 24 hours is depicted as "other." Data from Reference 99.

66, 75, 86) than is subcutaneous or total body fat, with some notable exceptions (26). The documented adverse effects of excess FFA on metabolic function and the finding that in vitro omental adipocyte lipolysis is increased compared with subcutaneous lipolysis prompted the hypothesis that excess visceral adipose tissue FFA release is the source of higher FFA concentrations in upper-body/visceral obesity.

Early studies of the relationship between adipocyte characteristics and obesity indicated that large fat cells are characteristic of upper-body obesity and the complications of obesity (10, 49, 51). Large fat cells are reported to have greater rates of basal lipolysis in vitro (49, 74), perhaps especially when they are from visceral depots (33) and men (70). Other studies have shown that visceral fat cells have the same lipolytic activity as abdominal subcutaneous adipocytes when adjusted for size (73) and are less active if visceral fat cells are smaller (70, 73). Despite the sometimes contradictory findings of in vitro studies, it was widely believed that large visceral fat depots flooded the liver and the systemic circulation with FFA (8, 48).

The effect of abnormally high FFA concentrations on glucose metabolism has been thoroughly documented. Elevation of FFA concentrations can induce peripheral (skeletal muscle) and hepatic insulin resistance (24, 46), increased VLDL triglyceride production (52), altered vascular reactivity (90), and dysfunctional pancreatic beta cell function (105). Lowering FFA concentrations in type 2 diabetes can improve insulin action with respect to glucose metabolism (79). The metabolic effects of high FFA concentrations at the level of the muscle appear to involve early steps in the insulin-signaling pathway (21, 76).

If elevation of FFA concentrations can impair insulin action and have other untoward metabolic effects, an understanding of the factors that regulate FFA concentrations is vital. Suppression of lipolysis, whether by insulin (38) or by pharmacological agents (59), results in reduced FFA concentrations, whereas stimulation of lipolysis (epinephrine, growth hormone) increases FFA concentrations. An

FFAs: free fatty acids

exception is what occurs during the onset of exercise, when FFA concentrations fall because the uptake of FFA from the circulation increases to a greater extent than the increase in adipose tissue lipolysis (100). Another exception to the general rule that concentrations reflect lipolysis is the discrepancy between FFA concentrations and flux between women and men; women have 40% greater rates of lipolysis than men at the same plasma FFA concentrations (64) even when adjusted for resting energy expenditure (the best correlate of FFA flux). If one takes into account sex-specific biologic relationships, plasma FFA concentrations are largely determined by the integrated rate of adipose tissue lipolysis (except with exercise). FFA concentrations in turn can affect the ability of insulin to modulate glucose production and uptake. The in vitro differences in regional adipocyte lipolysis suggest, but do not prove, that regional variations in FFA release in vivo could have a major influence on plasma FFA concentrations, with visceral fat playing a disproportionate role.

To the extent that abnormally high FFAs create the metabolic abnormalities associated with obesity, understanding the regional differences in adipose tissue lipolysis in vivo should help resolve the issue as to whether visceral fat is the source of excess FFA in upper-body obesity. A series of studies conducted in our laboratory have documented heterogeneity of adipose tissue lipolysis in vivo, assessed the contribution of upper body subcutaneous, leg, and visceral fat to systemic FFA availability, and evaluated the contribution of visceral adipose tissue lipolysis to hepatic FFA delivery. We used isotope dilution techniques to measure systemic and regional FFA uptake/release in volunteers with hepatic vein, femoral vein, and femoral artery catheters in place. Body composition was measured using the combination of DEXA and CT imaging of the abdomen to quantify regional fat mass (39), and plasma flow was determined using indocyanine green. Systemic FFA (as reflected by arterial FFA concentrations) will affect muscle, pancreatic beta cells, and vascular function, whereas portal FFA concentrations will affect hepatic glucose (69) and VLDL triglyceride (52, 94) production. One can imagine that while portal FFA concentrations may be largely driven by visceral adipose tissue lipolysis (2, 37), systemic FFA concentrations may be less affected by visceral fat because the liver takes up a significant proportion (~50%) of the FFA delivered to it. Sorting out these issues is quite difficult because it is not feasible to measure portal FFA concentrations in humans, except under unique circumstances (94). We did find, however, that it is possible to estimate the proportion of hepatic FFA delivery that originates from visceral adipose tissue lipolysis (37).

We have found that lipolytic activity is greater in upper-body subcutaneous than in leg adipose tissue (per kg of fat) in lean and obese women (36, 60) and in lean and obese men (36, 65). Leg fat contributes ~15%–20% of basal, systemic FFA release in nonobese adults and an average was 28% of FFA release in obese men and women. Leg adipose tissue is exquisitely sensitive to insulin (58) and meal (29, 36) suppression. Upper-body subcutaneous fat accounts for the majority (~70%) of systemic FFA under basal (36, 57, 65) and insulin-suppressed conditions (3, 29, 36, 58). In fact, the greater postprandial FFA concentrations in upper-body obesity compared with lower-body obesity are completely accounted for by excess FFA release from upper-body subcutaneous, not visceral fat (29).

Although the net release of new FFA into the systemic circulation from the splanchnic bed accounts for only ~15% of systemic FFA, this does not fully reflect visceral adipose tissue lipolysis. As noted, the liver takes up a considerable fraction of FFA in the portal vein. Because some of the FFAs entering the splanchnic bed via the arterial supply are taken up by nonhepatic tissues before reaching the portal vein, FFA concentrations in the portal vein are not substantially greater than those typically seen in the arterial circulation (94). That said, the appearance of new FFA in the hepatic vein is a direct measure of the contribution of visceral adipose tissue lipolysis to systemic FFA availability and thus of plasma FFA concentrations. Only 6%–17% of systemic FFAs come from the splanchnic bed under overnight postabsorptive conditions (65), although this can exceed 40% under hyperinsulinemic conditions (58). The latter observation suggests that visceral fat is more resistant to the antilipolytic effects of insulin than is subcutaneous fat, which is consistent with results from dog studies (61).

The issue of whether visceral obesity increases hepatic FFA delivery in humans appeared to be unanswerable without access to the portal vein. Through the use of mathematical modeling (that was able to be validated using animal models), we were able to test whether the proportion of hepatic FFA delivery that originates from visceral lipolysis could be predicted using data collected from hepatic vein catheterization (37). We compared the measured proportion of hepatic FFA delivery from visceral adipose lipolysis as measured by a portal vein catheter to that predicted using a modeling approach (37). The good agreement between measured and predicted values allowed us to apply this model to data collected in lean and obese men and women (65). From these experiments, we found that the percent of hepatic FFA delivery that comes from visceral adipose tissue lipolysis increases with the amount of visceral fat. In most nonobese adults, only 5%–10% of hepatic FFA delivery is predicted to come from visceral lipolysis, whereas this increases to an average of 20%–25% in visceral obesity (maximum values near 50% in some individuals). Of note, the contribution of visceral lipolysis to hepatic FFA delivery increased to a greater extent in women than in men as a function of visceral fat (65).

Although increasing visceral fat is associated with a greater potential delivery of FFA to the liver, systemic FFA still accounts for an average of >75% of hepatic FFA delivery even in persons with visceral obesity. In summary, visceral fat probably plays a role in the hepatic manifestations of visceral obesity, but to the extent that systemic FFA concentrations affect muscle, pancreatic beta cells, and vascular function, it is the abnormal function of upper-body nonsplanchnic fat that should draw our attention.

FUTURE DIRECTIONS

The factors that determine body fat distribution are still not known. How do environmental, hormonal, and genetic factors combine to promote greater fat gain in some depots relative to other depots in humans? What is the contribution of VLDL-triglyceride uptake by different depots to body fat distribution? Are there pathways of fatty acid accumulation in fat cells, such as de novo lipogenesis or direct FFA reuptake, that help to determine regional fatty acid balance? Finally, accumulation of fat up to a certain degree can be accomplished solely by adipocyte hypertrophy, but eventually new fat cells must be recruited. Some investigators believe that preadipocytes from various depots are differentially capable of proliferation and differentiation. How might these differences help determine body fat distribution? New methods and new experimental approaches are required to address these issues. If scientists successfully develop an understanding of the factors that regulate fat distribution, however, new opportunities may be created for novel therapies that create "healthy" fat distributions, if we cannot find the cure for obesity first.

SUMMARY POINTS

1. Adipose tissue uptake of meal-derived fatty acids is associated with postprandial lipoprotein lipase activity.

2. Upper-body subcutaneous fat is the major source of systemic free fatty acid (FFA).
3. Visceral fat contributes substantially to hepatic FFA delivery in those with excess visceral fat.
4. Physical activity increases the oxidation of dietary fatty acids.
5. Regional differences in meal fatty acid uptake into adipose tissue do not seem to account for sex-based differences in body fat distribution under energy balance conditions.
6. Regional differences in adipose tissue FFA release do not seem to account for sex-based differences in body fat distribution under fasted, fed, or exercise conditions.

ACKNOWLEDGMENTS

The efforts of our collaborators, the laboratory staff, the Mayo GCRC staff, and the volunteers for the studies are greatly appreciated. The authors are supported by grants DK40484, DK45343, DK50456, and RR-0585 from the U.S. Public Health Service and by the Mayo Foundation.

LITERATURE CITED

1. Amarri S. 1998. Importance of measuring CO2 production rate when using 13C-breath tests to measure fat digestion. *Br. J. Nutr.* 79:541–45
2. Basso LV, Havel RJ. 1970. Hepatic metabolism of free fatty acids in normal and diabetic dogs. *J. Clin. Invest.* 49:537–47
3. Basu A, Basu R, Shah P, Vella A, Rizza RA, Jensen MD. 2001. Systemic and regional free fatty acid metabolism in type 2 diabetes. *Am. J. Physiol. Endocrinol. Metab.* 280:E1000–6
4. Bergouignan A, Schoeller D, Normand S, Gauquelin-Koch G, Laville M, et al. 2006. Effect of physical inactivity on the oxidation of saturated and monounsaturated dietary fatty acids: results of a randomized trial. *PLOS Clin. Trials* 1:e27. DOI: 10.1371/journal.pctr.0010027
5. Bessesen DH, Vensor SH, Jackman MR. 2000. Trafficking of dietary oleic, linolenic, and stearic acids in fasted or fed lean rats. *Am. J. Physiol. Endocrinol. Metab.* 278:E1124–32
6. Binnert C, Pachiaudi C, Beylot M, Croset M, Cohen R, et al. 1996. Metabolic fate of an oral long-chain triglyceride load in humans. *Am. J. Physiol.* 270:E445–50
7. Binnert C, Pachiaudi C, Beylot M, Hans D, Vandermander J, et al. 1998. Influence of human obesity on the metabolic fate of dietary long- and medium-chain triacylglycerols. *Am. J. Clin. Nutr.* 67:595–601
8. Björntorp P. 1990. "Portal" adipose tissue as a generator of risk factors for cardiovascular disease and diabetes. *Arteriosclerosis* 10:493–96
9. Björntorp P, Enzi G, Ohlson R, Persson B, Sponbergs P, Smith U. 1975. Lipoprotein lipase activity and uptake of exogenous triglycerides in fat cells of different size. *Horm. Metab. Res.* 7:230–37
10. Björntorp P, Sjostrom L. 1971. Number and size of adipose tissue fat cells in relation to metabolism in human obesity. *Metabolism* 20:703–13
11. Bonen A, Luiken J, Liu S, Dyck D, Kiens B, et al. 1998. Palmitate transport and fatty acid transporters in red and white muscles. *Am. J. Physiol.* 275:E471–78

12. Boyko EJ, Leonetti DL, Bergstrom RW, Newell-Morris L, Fujimoto WY. 1995. Visceral adiposity, fasting plasma insulin, and blood pressure in Japanese-Americans. *Diab. Care* 18:174–81
13. Carey VJ, Walters EE, Colditz GA, Solomon CG, Willett WC, et al. 1997. Body fat distribution and risk of non-insulin dependent diabetes mellitus in women. *Am. J. Epidemiol.* 145:614–19
14. Christie W. 1985. Rapid separation and quantification of lipid classes by high pressure liquid chromatography and mass detection. *J. Lipid Res.* 26:507–12
15. Coppack SW, Evans RD, Fisher RM, Frayn KN, Gibbons GF, et al. 1992. Adipose tissue metabolism in obesity: lipase action in vivo before and after a mixed meal. *Metabolism* 41:264–72
16. Coppack SW, Fisher RM, Gibbons GF, Humphreys SM, McDonough MJ, et al. 1990. Postprandial substrate deposition in human forearm and adipose tissues in vivo. *Clin. Sci.* 79:339–48
17. DeLany J, Windhauser M, Champagne C, Bray G. 2000. Differential oxidation of individual dietary fatty acids in humans. *Am. J. Clin. Nutr.* 72:905–11
18. Despres JP, Allard C, Tremblay A, Talbot J, Bouchard C. 1985. Evidence for a regional component of body fatness in the association with serum lipids in men and women. *Metabolism* 34:967–73
19. Despres JP, Moorjani S, Tremblay A, Ferland M, Lupien PJ, et al. 1989. Relation of high plasma triglyceride levels associated with obesity and regional adipose tissue distribution to plasma lipoprotein-lipid composition in premenopausal women. *Clin. Invest. Med.* 12:374–80
20. Dole V. 1955. A relation between non-esterified fatty acids in plasma and the metabolism of glucose. *J. Clin. Invest.* 35:150–54
21. Dresner A, Laurent D, Marcucci M, Griffin ME, Dufour S, et al. 1999. Effects of free fatty acids on glucose transport and IRS-1-associated phosphatidylinositol 3-kinase activity. *J. Clin. Invest.* 103:253–59
22. Eckel RH. 1989. Lipoprotein lipase. A multifunctional enzyme relevant to common metabolic diseases. *N. Engl. J. Med.* 320:1060–68
23. Eriksson J, Buren J, Svensson M, Olivecrona T, Olivecrona G. 2003. Postprandial regulation of blood lipids and adipose tissue lipoprotein lipase in type 2 diabetes patients and healthy control subjects. *Atherosclerosis* 166:359–67
24. Ferrannini E, Barrett EJ, Bevilacqva S, DeFronzo RA. 1983. Effect of fatty acids on glucose production and utilization in man. *J. Clin. Invest.* 72:1737–47
25. Folsom AR, Burke GL, Ballew C, Jacobs DRJ, Haskell WL, et al. 1989. Relation of body fatness and its distribution to cardiovascular risk factors in young blacks and whites. The role of insulin. *Am. J. Epidemiol.* 130:911–24
26. Garg A. 2004. Regional adiposity and insulin resistance. *J. Clin. Endocrinol. Metab.* 89:4206–10
27. Garvey WT, Maianu L, Hancock JA, Golichowski AM, Baron AD. 1992. Gene expression of GLUT4 in skeletal muscle from insulin-resistant patients with obesity, IGT, GDM, and NIDDM. *Diabetes* 41:465–75
28. Gillum RF. 1987. The association of body fat distribution with hypertension, hypertensive heart disease, coronary heart disease, diabetes and cardiovascular risk factors in men and women aged 18–79 years. *J. Chron. Dis.* 40:421–28
29. Guo ZK, Hensrud DD, Johnson CM, Jensen MD. 1999. Regional postprandial fatty acid metabolism in different obesity phenotypes. *Diabetes* 48:1586–92

30. Hartz AJ, Rupley DC, Rimm AA. 1984. The association of girth measurements with disease in 32,856 women. *Am. J. Epidemiol.* 119:71–80
31. Heath RB, Karpe F, Milne RW, Burdge GC, Wootton S, Frayn KN. 2006. Dietary fatty acids make a rapid and substantial contribution to VLDL-triacylglycerol in the fed state. *Am. J. Physiol. Endocrinol. Metab.* DOI: 10.1152/ajpendo.00409.2006
32. Heath RB, Karpe F, Milne RW, Burdge GC, Wootton SA, Frayn KN. 2003. Selective partitioning of dietary fatty acids into the VLDL TG pool in the early postprandial period. *J. Lipid Res.* 44:2065–72
33. Hellmer J, Marcus C, Sonnenfeld T, Arner P. 1992. Mechanisms for differences in lipolysis between human subcutaneous and omental fat cells. *J. Clin. Endocrinol. Metab.* 75:15–20
34. Hu H, Yamamoto H, Sohmiya M, Abe T, Murakami Y, Kato Y. 1994. Body composition assessed by bioelectrical impedance analysis (BIA) and the correlation with plasma insulin-like growth factor 1 (IGF-1) in normal Japanese subjects and patients with acromegaly and GH deficiency. *Endocr. J.* 41:63–69
35. Imbeault P, Almeras N, Richard D, Despres J, Tremblay A, Mauriege P. 1999. Effect of moderate weight loss on adipose tissue lipoprotein lipase activity and expression: existence of sexual variation and regional differences. *Int. J. Obes.* 23:957–65
36. Jensen MD. 1995. Gender differences in regional fatty acid metabolism before and after meal ingestion. *J. Clin. Invest.* 96:2297–303
37. Jensen MD, Cardin S, Edgerton D, Cherrington A. 2003. Splanchnic free fatty acid kinetics. *Am. J. Physiol. Endocrinol. Metab.* 284:E1140–48
38. Jensen MD, Caruso M, Heiling V, Miles JM. 1989. Insulin regulation of lipolysis in nondiabetic and IDDM subjects. *Diabetes* 38:1595–601
39. Jensen MD, Kanaley JA, Reed JE, Sheedy PF. 1995. Measurement of abdominal and visceral fat with computed tomography and dual-energy x-ray absorptiometry. *Am. J. Clin. Nutr.* 61:274–78
40. Jensen MD, Sarr MG, Dumesic DA, Southorn PA, Levine JA. 2003. Regional uptake of meal fatty acids in humans. *Am. J. Physiol. Endocrinol. Metab.* 285:E1282–88
41. Jones A, Stolinski M, Smith R, Murphy J, Wootton S. 1999. Effect of fatty acid chain length and saturation on the gastrointestinal handling and metabolic disposal of dietary fatty acids in women. *Br. J. Nutr.* 81:37–43
42. Jones P. 1985. Model for determination of 13C substrate oxidation rates in humans in the fed state. *Am. J. Clin. Nutr.* 41:1277–82
43. Jones P, Pencharz P, Clandinin M. 1985. Absorption of 13C-labeled stearic, oleic, and linoleic acids in humans: application to breath tests. *J. Lab. Clin. Med.* 105:647–52
44. Jones P, Pencharz P, Clandinin M. 1985. Whole body oxidation of dietary fatty acids: implications for energy utilization. *Am. J. Clin. Nutr.* 42:769–77
45. Kanai H, Matsuzawa Y, Kotani K, Keno Y, Kobatake T, et al. 1990. Close correlation of intra-abdominal fat accumulation to hypertension in obese women. *Hypertension* 16:484–90
46. Kelley DE, Mokan M, Simoneau JA, Mandarino LJ. 1993. Interaction between glucose and free fatty acid metabolism in human skeletal muscle. *J. Clin. Invest.* 92:91–98
47. Kissebah AH, Krakower GR. 1994. Regional adiposity and morbidity. *Physiol. Rev.* 74:761–811
48. Kissebah AH, Peiris AN. 1989. Biology of regional body fat distribution: relationship to non-insulin-dependent diabetes mellitus. *Diab. Metab. Rev.* 5:83–109
49. Kissebah AH, Vydelingum N, Murray R, Evans DJ, Hartz AJ, et al. 1982. Relation of body fat distribution to metabolic complications of obesity. *J. Clin. Endocrinol. Metab.* 54:254–60

50. Klein S, Wolfe R. 1987. The use of isotopic tracers in studying lipid metabolism in human subjects. *Bailliere's Clin. Endocrinol. Metab.* 1:797–816
51. Krotkiewski M, Björntorp P, Sjostrom L, Smith U. 1983. Impact of obesity on metabolism in men and women: importance of regional adipose tissue distribution. *J. Clin. Invest.* 72:1150–62
52. Lewis GF, Uffelman KD, Szeto LW, Weller B, Steiner G. 1995. Interaction between free fatty acids and insulin in the acute control of very low density lipoprotein production in humans. *J. Clin. Invest.* 95:158–66
53. MacDougall D, Jones P, Vogt J, Phang P, Kitts D. 1996. Utilization of myristic and palmitic acid in humans fed different dietary fats. *Eur. J. Clin. Invest.* 26:755–62
54. Mårin P, Andersson B, Ottosson M, Olbe L, Chowdhury B, et al. 1992. The morphology and metabolism of intraabdominal adipose tissue in men. *Metabolism* 41:1242–48
55. Mårin P, Oden B, Olbe L, Bengtsson B, Björntorp P. 1996. Assimilation of triglycerides in subcutaneous and intraabdominal adipose tissues in vivo in men: effects of testosterone. *J. Clin. Endocrinol. Metab.* 81:1018–22
56. Mårin P, Rebuffe-Scrive M, Björntorp P. 1990. Uptake of triglyceride fatty acids in adipose tissue in vivo in man. *Eur. J. Clin. Invest.* 20:158–65
57. Martin ML, Jensen MD. 1991. Effects of body fat distribution on regional lipolysis in obesity. *J. Clin. Invest.* 88:609–13
58. Meek S, Nair KS, Jensen MD. 1999. Insulin regulation of regional free fatty acid metabolism. *Diabetes* 48:10–14
59. Miles JM, Ellman MG, McClean KL, Jensen MD. 1987. Validation of a new method for determination of free fatty acid turnover. *Am. J. Physiol. Endocrinol. Metab.* 252:E431–38
60. Miles JM, Jensen MD. 1991. Determination of plasma-free fatty acid kinetics with tracers: methodologic considerations. *JPEN* 15:90–93S
61. Mittelman SD, Van Citters GW, Kirkman EL, Bergman RN. 2002. Extreme insulin resistance of the central adipose depot in vivo. *Diabetes* 51:755–61
62. Murphy J, Jones A, Brookes S, Wootton S. 1995. The gastrointestinal handling and metabolism of [1-13C] palmitic acid in healthy women. *Lipids* 30:291–98
63. Nguyen TT, Mijares AH, Johnson CM, Jensen MD. 1996. Postprandial leg and splanchnic fatty acid metabolism in nonobese men and women. *Am. J. Physiol. Endocrinol. Metab.* 271:E965–72
64. Nielsen S, Guo Z, Albu JB, Klein S, O'Brien PC, Jensen MD. 2003. Energy expenditure, sex, and endogenous fuel availability in humans. *J. Clin. Invest.* 111:981–88
65. Nielsen S, Guo ZK, Johnson CM, Hensrud DD, Jensen MD. 2004. Splanchnic lipolysis in human obesity. *J. Clin. Invest.* 113:1582–88
66. Pouliot M, Despres JP, Nadeau A, Moorjani S, Prud'Homme D, et al. 1992. Visceral obesity in men. Associations with glucose tolerance, plasma insulin, and lipoprotein levels. *Diabetes* 41:826–34
67. Prineas RJ, Folsom AR, Kaye SA. 1993. Central adiposity and increased risk of coronary artery disease mortality in older women. *Ann. Epidemiol.* 3:35–41
68. Raman A, Blanc S, Adams A, Schoeller DA. 2004. Validation of deuterium-labeled fatty acids for the measurement of dietary fat oxidation during physical activity. *J. Lipid Res.* 45:2339–44
69. Rebrin K, Steil GM, Mittelman SD, Bergman RN. 1996. Casual linkage between insulin suppression of lipolysis and suppression of liver glucose output in dogs. *J. Clin. Invest.* 98:741–49
70. Rebuffe-Scrive M, Andersson B, Olbe L, Björntorp P. 1989. Metabolism of adipose tissue in intraabdominal depots of nonobese men and women. *Metabolism* 38:453–58

71. Rebuffe-Scrive M, Enk L, Crona N, Lonnroth P, Abrahamsson L, et al. 1985. Fat cell metabolism in different regions in women: effect of menstrual cycle, pregnancy, and lactation. *J. Clin. Invest.* 75:1973–76
72. Rexrode KM, Carey VJ, Hennekens CH, Walters EE, Colditz GA, et al. 1998. Abdominal adiposity and coronary heart disease in women. *JAMA* 280:1843–48
73. Reynisdottir S, Dauzats M, Thorne A, Langin D. 1997. Comparison of hormone-sensitive lipase activity in visceral and subcutaneous human adipose tissue. *J. Clin. Endocrinol. Metab.* 82:4162–66
74. Rice T, Despres JP, Daw EW, Gagnon J, Borecki IB, et al. 1997. Familial resemblance for abdominal visceral fat: the HERITAGE family study. *Int. J. Obes. Relat. Metab. Disord.* 21:1024–31
75. Rissanen J, Hudson R, Ross R. 1994. Visceral adiposity, androgens, and plasma lipids in obese men. *Metabolism* 43:1318–23
76. Roden M, Price TB, Perseghin G, Petersen KF, Rothman DL, et al. 1996. Mechanism of free fatty acid-induced insulin resistance in humans. *J. Clin. Invest.* 97:2859–65
77. Romanski SA, Nelson R, Jensen MD. 2000. Meal fatty acid uptake in adipose tissue: gender effects in non-obese humans. *Am. J. Physiol. Endocrinol. Metab.* 279:E455–62
78. Roust LR, Jensen MD. 1993. Postprandial free fatty acid kinetics are abnormal in upper body obesity. *Diabetes* 42:1567–73
79. Saloranta C, Franssila-Kallunki A, Ekstrand A, Taskinen MR, Groop L. 1991. Modulation of hepatic glucose production by non-esterified fatty acids in type 2 (non-insulin-dependent) diabetes mellitus. *Diabetologia* 34:409–15
80. Schmidt D, Allred J, Kien C. 1999. Fractional oxidation of chylomicron-derived oleate is greater than that of palmitate in healthy adults fed frequent small meals. *J. Lipid Res.* 40:2322–32
81. Schoeller D, Klein P, Watkins J, Heim T, MacLean W. 1980. 13C abundance of nutrients and the effect of variations in 13C isotopic abundances of test meals formulated for 13CO2 breath tests. *Am. J. Clin. Nutr.* 33:2375–85
82. Schoeller D, van-Santen E. 1982. Measurement of energy expenditure in humans by doubly labeled water method. *J. Appl. Physiol.* 53:955–59
83. Schoeller D, van-Santen E, Peterson D, Dietz W, Jaspan J, Klein P. 1980. Total body water measurement in humans with 18O and 2H labeled water. *Am. J. Clin. Nutr.* 33:2686–93
84. Schrauwen P, Aggel-Leijssen D, Lichtenbelt WM, Baak M, Gijsen A, Wagenmakers A. 1998. Validation of the [1,2-13C]acetate recovery factor for correction of [U-13C]palmitate oxidation rate in humans. *J. Physiol.* 513:215–23
85. Schrauwen P, Blaak E, Aggel-Leijssen D, Borghouts L, Wagenmakers A. 2000. Determinants of the acetate recovery factor: implications for estimation of [13C]substrate oxidation. *Clin. Sci.* 98:587–92
86. Seidell JC, Björntorp P, Sjostrom L, Kvist H, Sannerstedt R. 1990. Visceral fat accumulation in men is positively associated with insulin, glucose, and C-peptide levels, but negatively with testosterone levels. *Metabolism* 39:897–901
87. Sidossis L, Coggan A, Gastaldelli A, Wolfe R. 1995. A new correction factor for use in tracer estimations of plasma fatty acid oxidation. *Am. J. Physiol.* 269:E649–56
88. Sidossis L, Coggan A, Gastaldelli A, Wolfe R. 1995. Pathway of free fatty acid oxidation in human subjects: implications for tracer studies. *J. Clin. Investig.* 95:278–84
89. Sonko B, Prentice A, Coward W, Murgatroyd P, Goldberg G. 2001. Dose-response relationship between fat ingestion and oxidation: quantitative estimation using whole-body calorimetry and 13C isotope ratio mass spectrometry. *Eur. J. Clin. Nutr.* 55:10–18

90. Steinberg HO, Tarshoby M, Monestel R, Hook G, Cronin J, et al. 1997. Elevated circulating free fatty acid levels impair endothelium-dependent vasodilation. *J. Clin. Invest.* 100:1230–39
91. Taskinen M, Nikkila E. 1987. Basal and postprandial lipoprotein lipase activity in adipose tissue during caloric restriction and refeeding. *Metabolism* 36:625–30
92. Thompson CJ, Ryu JE, Craven TE, Kahl FR, Crouse JR. 1991. Central adipose distribution is related to coronary atherosclerosis. *Arterioscler. Thromb.* 11:327–33
93. Uranga AP, Levine J, Jensen M. 2005. Isotope tracer measures of meal fatty acid metabolism: reproducibility and effects of the menstrual cycle. *Am. J. Physiol. Endocrinol. Metab.* 288:E547–55
94. Vogelberg KH, Gries FA, Moschinski D. 1980. Hepatic production of VLDL-triglycerides. Dependence of portal substrate and insulin concentration. *Horm. Metab. Res.* 12:688–94
95. Votruba S, Atkinson R, Hirvonen M, Schoeller D. 2002. Prior exercise increases subsequent utilization of dietary fat. *Med. Sci. Sports Exerc.* 34:1757–65
96. Votruba S, Atkinson R, Schoeller D. 2005. Sustained increase in dietary oleic acid oxidation following morning exercise. *Int. J. Obes.* 29:100–7
97. Votruba S, Zeddun S, Schoeller D. 2001. Validation of deuterium labeled fatty acids for the measurement of dietary fat oxidation: a method for measuring fat oxidation in free-living subjects. *Int. J. Obes.* 25:1240–45
98. Votruba SB, Atkinson RL, Schoeller DA. 2003. Prior exercise increases dietary oleate, but not palmitate oxidation. *Obes. Res.* 11:1509–18
99. Votruba SB, Jensen MD. 2006. Sex-specific differences in leg fat uptake are revealed with a high-fat meal. *Am. J. Physiol. Endocrinol. Metab.* 291:E1115–23
100. Wahren J, Sato Y, Ostman J, Hagenfeldt L, Felig P. 1984. Turnover and splanchnic metabolism of free fatty acids and ketones in insulin-dependent diabetics at rest and in response to exercise. *J. Clin. Invest.* 73:1367–76
101. Wahrenberg H, Lonnqvist F, Arner P. 1989. Mechanisms underlying regional differences in lipolysis in human adipose tissue. *J. Clin. Invest.* 84:458–67
102. Wang W, Wang Z, Faith MS, Kotler D, Shih R, Heymsfield SB. 1999. Regional skeletal muscle measurement: evaluation of new dual-energy X-ray absorptiometry model. *J. Appl. Physiol.* 87:1163–71
103. Weinman E. 1952. Conversion of fatty acids to carbohydrate: application of isotope to this problem and role of Krebs cycle as a synthesis pathway. *Physiol. Rev.* 37:252–72
104. Yost T, Jensen D, Haugen B, Eckel R. 1998. Effect of dietary macronutrient composition on tissue-specific lipoprotein lipase activity and insulin action in normal-weight subjects. *Am. J. Clin. Nutr.* 68:296–302
105. Zhou YP, Grill VE. 1994. Long-term exposure of rat pancreatic islets to fatty acids inhibits glucose-induced insulin secretion and biosynthesis through a glucose fatty acid cycle. *J. Clin. Invest.* 93:870–76

Trace Element Transport in the Mammary Gland

Bo Lönnerdal

Department of Nutrition, University of California at Davis, California;
email: bllonnerdal@ucdavis.edu

Annu. Rev. Nutr. 2007. 27:165–77

The *Annual Review of Nutrition* is online at http://nutr.annualreviews.org

This article's doi:
10.1146/annurev.nutr.27.061406.093809

0199-9885/07/0821-0165$20.00

Key Words

iron, copper, zinc, vitamin A, iron transporters, copper transporters, zinc transporters, interactions

Abstract

The mammary gland has a remarkable capacity to adapt to maternal deficiency or excess of iron, copper, and zinc and to homeostatically control milk concentrations of these essential nutrients. Similarly, it can regulate changes in concentrations of iron, copper, and zinc change during lactation. For iron, this regulation is achieved by transferrin receptor, DMT1, and ferroportin, whereas mammary gland copper metabolism is regulated by Ctr1, ATP7A, and ATP7B. Zinc homeostasis is complex, involving both zinc importers (Zip3) and zinc exporters (ZnT-1, ZnT-2, and ZnT-4). Both transcriptional and post-translational regulation can affect protein abundance and cellular localization of these transporters, finely orchestrating uptake, intracellular trafficking, and secretion of iron, copper, and zinc. The control of mammary gland uptake and milk secretion of iron, copper, and zinc protects both the mammary gland and the breast-fed infant against deficiency and excess of these nutrients.

Contents

INTRODUCTION

The newborn infant is dependent on an adequate supply of trace elements for optimal nutrition and health. Iron (Fe) is needed for erythropoiesis and synthesis of Fe-requiring enzymes, and Fe deficiency anemia has been associated with long-term adverse effects on cognitive function and motor development (51). Zinc (Zn) deficiency in infants causes decreased growth, impaired immune function, and increased susceptibility to infection (7, 25). Copper (Cu) deficiency can cause anemia, bone and connective tissue abnormalities, and impaired immune function (48, 61). Deficiencies of these elements are very rare in breast-fed infants, at least for the first six months of life, indicating that breast milk provides adequate amounts of trace elements for the exclusively breast-fed infant. Numerous studies have shown that concentrations of trace elements (Fe, Zn, Cu) in breast milk are remarkably similar among women at a given stage of lactation, even if they consume diets low in trace elements or with low bioavailability (50, 47). Similarly, trace element concentrations in breast milk remain the same even if the mother is receiving trace element supplements at generous levels. Thus, it is evident that the mammary gland has a remarkable capacity to tightly regulate concentrations of trace elements secreted in milk (33). Concentrations of trace elements in milk do vary considerably during the lactation period, starting with high concentrations in early lactation (**Figure 1**, see color insert), then decreasing as lactation proceeds (15, 28). Obviously, this change in concentrations is also tightly regulated. Recent advances in our knowledge of transporters regulating Fe, Zn, and Cu metabolism at the cellular level have provided a better understanding of how the mammary gland can regulate milk trace element concentrations.

Fe: iron

Zn: zinc

Cu: copper

MAMMARY GLAND IRON METABOLISM

The concentration of Fe in breast milk is often considered as low, both in relation to serum Fe (milk Fe concentration is ~20%–30% of serum Fe) and to estimated Fe requirements of infants. An argument is frequently made that the healthy, term infant is born with ample stores and that these are mobilized and utilized during the first six months of life, making breast milk Fe an "irrelevant" source of Fe. However, infants fed formula that has not been fortified with Fe frequently have poor Fe status, in spite of the fact that formula usually contains up to three times more Fe than does breast milk (65). Thus, the amount of Fe provided by breast milk certainly contributes to meeting the Fe needs of breast-fed infants. It is possible that the relatively low concentration of Fe in breast milk also helps to protect the infant against Fe toxicity. In a recent study on exclusively breast-fed infants given Fe supplements at 1 mg/kg/day (the currently recommended level), a significant adverse effect on linear growth was found in infants with adequate Fe status, and a marginally significant effect on diarrheal disease (16). Although the mechanisms behind these adverse effects are not yet known, from an evolutionary perspective, it may have been advantageous to provide ample Fe to infants but protect them from excess Fe.

Iron in serum is virtually exclusively bound to transferrin (Tf), and tissue Fe uptake is usually mediated by cellular transferrin receptors (TfRs). Tissue Fe status tightly regulates cellular TfR expression, and circulating TfR (proteolytic cleavage product from cell TfR) is used as an indicator of Fe status (69). No correlation between milk Fe and mammary gland TfR expression has been found in animal models (67), which strongly suggests that regulation of milk Fe concentrations occurs after uptake of Fe by the mammary gland. Diferric Tf binds to the TfR at the mammary epithelial cell surface and is internalized by clathrin-coated vesicles that fuse with acidic endosomes (**Figure 2**, see color insert). In the endosome, the acidic environment causes release of Fe from the Tf-TfR complex, and Tf is recycled to the plasma membrane with TfR. Iron is most likely exported from the endosome by divalent metal ion transporter 1 (DMT1), as shown for several tissues like liver and placenta (23, 71). DMT1 is also localized to an intracellular compartment in many epithelial cells, but there is not yet any evidence that DMT1 facilitates Fe export from endosomes in mammary epithelial cells. Iron released from the endosome can enter the intracellular chelatable Fe pool and then participate in cellular processes, be sequestered by ferritin for storage, be incorporated into Fe-containing proteins in the endoplasmic reticulum (ER), or be secreted across the luminal membrane into milk. Export of Fe from the mammary gland is most likely achieved by ferroportin (FPN), which is localized to the ER in reticuloendothelial cells, where it is believed to transport Fe into intracellular vesicles prior to secretion (1). We have found that FPN is expressed in the mammary gland of rats (44) and is localized throughout the epithelial cell (32). We therefore believe that FPN in the mammary gland epithelial cell transports Fe into secretory vesicles targeted for export into milk (32).

To date, no genetic defects in the transfer of Fe into milk have been found. The hypotransferrinemic mouse (13), which is lacking Tf in serum, dies at a young age, most likely because it was compromised during fetal life, but there have been no studies on milk Fe in this mutant mouse model. These mice survive if given iron intravenously during early life, which suggests that alternative mechanisms exist for tissue Fe uptake. However, once Fe enters the mammary gland it is likely that the homeostatic mechanisms described above regulate milk Fe export.

The decline in milk Fe concentration that occurs during lactation parallels decreases in TfR and FPN expression (44), which suggests that Fe uptake by the mammary gland and its secretion into milk is functionally decreased and not due to tissue Fe depletion. In contrast, mammary gland Fe concentration and DMT1 expression remained constant during lactation, which suggests that DMT1 plays a role in maintaining cellular Fe (44) and does not directly participate in the secretion of Fe into milk. Maternal Fe deficiency in lactating rats did not significantly affect milk Fe concentration, although mammary gland Fe stores were reduced. The maintained milk Fe levels were associated with a decrease in DMT1 expression, whereas TfR and FPN expression did not change, which suggests that the primary regulators of milk Fe secretion are TfR and FPN. These observations suggest that milk Fe concentration is maintained during Fe deficiency due to an uncoupling of the regulatory mechanisms "normally" responding to tissue Fe status, possibly protecting the newborn from excessive Fe transfer into milk during Fe deficiency (33).

The major Fe-binding protein in human milk is lactoferrin (Lf), which, similar to Tf, can bind two ferric ions per molecule (49). Lf is synthesized by the ER and likely is incorporated early into secretory vesicles. It is not yet known whether Fe is incorporated into Lf during its synthesis or if Fe transported into the secretory vesicles becomes bound to Lf in the vesicle, due to the very high affinity

Tf: transferrin

TfR: transferrin receptor

DMT1: divalent metal ion transporter 1

FPN: ferroportin

of Lf for Fe (K_{ass} ~10^{24}). It should be noted that although Lf binds a significant proportion of Fe in human milk, it is only saturated to 5%–10% (20) and therefore is capable of picking up any "free" Fe transported into the secretory vesicles. Iron in human milk is also bound to xanthine oxidase (22), which is part of the milk fat globule membrane, and as Fe is in the heme form, it is likely incorporated during xanthine oxidase biosynthesis.

Ctr1: copper transporter 1

MAMMARY GLAND COPPER METABOLISM

The concentration of Cu in human milk is about 20%–25% of that in serum. The major part of Cu in serum is tightly bound to ceruloplasmin, whereas a minor fraction is loosely associated to serum albumin, amino acids, and low-molecular-weight chelators (**Figure 3**, see color insert). It is not yet known whether membrane-associated Cu transporters accrue Cu from the low-molecular-weight "accessible" Cu pool or if the ceruloplasmin-bound Cu can be made available, either by an endocytotic pathway or by release of Cu at the plasma membrane. However, during early lactation plasma Cu is high, and Cu is primarily bound to serum albumin and amino acids and has been shown to be directly taken up by the mammary gland (18). In contrast, during late lactation plasma Cu is low, and Cu is primarily bound to ceruloplasmin, which suggests that milk Cu levels may reflect the availability of "loosely bound Cu" for uptake by the mammary gland.

The newborn, term infant has ample stores of Cu, primarily in the liver, and these are mobilized during early life (48, 61), similar to Fe. Thus, a case is often made that the amount of Cu provided by breast milk is insignificant with regard to meeting the Cu requirement of infants. However, infants fed unfortified cow milk or infant formula, which contain only half the concentration of Cu in human milk, develop Cu deficiency if fed such diets for extended periods (12), which strongly suggests that human milk Cu contributes significantly to the Cu needs of breast-fed infants.

The mammary gland has been found to have three Cu-specific transporters; Ctr1, ATP7A, and ATP7B (3, 35, 54). Of these, Ctr1 has been found in all tissues examined (42) and is believed to be essential for cellular Cu import as Ctr1 knockout mice die at an early embryonic stage (43). Studies in cells transfected with CTR1 suggest that this protein imports Cu^{+} with high affinity (41, 73). This high affinity may be needed to acquire Cu from the circulation in amounts adequate to meet cellular needs. Ctr1 forms a multimeric complex containing a barrel structure with a central Cu channel (37). It has been shown that Ctr1 is vesicular and is endocytosed and proteolytically degraded in response to increased Cu levels, thereby providing a means of regulating cellular Cu uptake (63). We have found that Ctr1 in the rat mammary gland is localized to both the cell membrane and intracellular vesicles (30), which is similar to other cell types.

It is likely that Cu uptake by the mammary gland is mediated by Ctr1 (30, 39). Mammary gland Cu uptake was highest during early lactation and increased in response to suckling, but increased Ctr1 abundance does not appear to explain this. In fact, Ctr1 abundance decreased in response to suckling and hyperprolactinemia, possibly due to negative feedback of increased prolactin on prolactin receptor abundance (35). Further, Ctr1 abundance was not affected by prolactin treatment of HC11 cells, a finding that suggests Ctr1 abundance in the mammary gland may be regulated by proteasomal degradation (63) through mechanisms unrelated to prolactin signaling pathways. Our results (35) suggest that minimal Ctr1 is located at the serosal membrane until stimulated by prolactin or suckling. Colocalization of Ctr1 with transferrin receptor suggests that Ctr1 may traffic within recycling endosomes, as proposed by Petris et al. (63).

ATP7B, which belongs to the P-type ATPase family of transmembrane proteins, is involved in mammary gland Cu metabolism

(54). ATP7B was found to be defective in patients with Wilson disease, a genetic disorder of Cu toxicity (14). Wilson's patients have mutations in the ATP7B gene, resulting in an inability of the protein to properly localize to an intracellular compartment in the liver, leading to reduced Cu incorporation into ceruloplasmin, bile secretion, and hepatotoxicity. ATP7B is always localized proximal to the luminal membrane of secretory mammary epithelial cells in the lactating rat, most likely associated with the trans-Golgi network and late endosomes (30, 54), and neither its expression nor localization change during lactation or in cell culture (35, 40). It is possible that Cu transported into late endosomes is recycled back to the trans-Golgi and then incorporated into ceruloplasmin for secretion into milk. Mice with a mutation in ATP7B, which results in this Cu transporter being mislocalized in the mammary gland, have impaired Cu secretion into milk (~50% of normal) (54). In normal mice, ATP7B localization changes from being perinuclear to a cytoplasmic, diffuse location, whereas in mutant mice, ATP7B stays perinuclear, probably impairing the secretion of Cu into milk. This "toxic milk" (*tx*) mutation results in neonatal death due to severe Cu deficiency, which strongly suggests that ATP7B is essential for mammary gland secretion of Cu into milk. However, *tx* mice still have some Cu in their milk and most milk Cu is not ceruloplasmin bound (18), which suggests that Cu can be secreted by other mechanisms also.

Another P-type ATPase, ATP7A, which is homologous to ATP7B, was discovered as the protein being defective in Menkes disease (9, 46), a disorder of Cu accrual resulting in severe tissue Cu depletion (27). Several types of mutations of ATP7A have been found, all associated with impaired cellular Cu export. Thus, newly absorbed Cu becomes "trapped" in the enterocytes of the small intestine and never reaches the circulation. ATP7A is expressed ubiquitously and it is localized to both a vesicular and a perinuclear compartment in the mammary gland of mice and humans in the nonlactating state (3, 24). During lactation, however, expression of ATP7A increases and the protein relocalizes to the cell membrane (3), which suggests that ATP7A actively participates in mammary gland Cu transport during lactation. We have found that both suckling and hyperprolactinemia cause increased secretion of ^{67}Cu into milk and relocalization of ATP7A to the plasma membrane during both early and late lactation (35). However, this response is stronger during early lactation, which suggests that it is due to the higher prolactin concentration during this time. In cultured HC11 cells we found ATP7A associated with both the endoplasmic reticulum and late endosomes. It is therefore likely that what we observed in lactating rats was due to increased ATP7A-containing vesicles at the apical membrane.

The concentration of Cu in milk declines during lactation in humans and rodents (15, 21, 28). We have used the rat as a model to study mechanisms regulating milk Cu levels during lactation (35). It is possible that the decrease in serum Cu that occurs during lactation is partially responsible for decreasing milk Cu levels by reducing the supply of Cu to the mammary gland. However, there is also a modest decline in ATP7B protein levels during this time, possibly reflecting Cu export into milk (35). Our results indicate that mammary gland uptake of Cu and its secretion into milk are higher during early lactation, which is mediated by post-translational relocalization of Ctr1 and ATP7A to the cell membrane in response to suckling. We hypothesize that ATP7B is responsible for constitutive Cu secretion into milk via ceruloplasmin, whereas Ctr1 and ATP7A transiently increase Cu uptake into the gland and secretion into milk to ensure adequate transfer of Cu to the nursing infant.

Prolactin is responsible for regulating milk protein synthesis and maintaining lactation (52). During lactation, circulating prolactin concentrations fall, but they increase in response to suckling episodes (60). We investigated the mechanisms behind the increased

ZIP: zinc import protein

ZnT: zinc transporter

Cu secretion into milk in response to suckling by using a mouse mammary epithelial cell line (HC11) that is unique in that it expresses functional prolactin receptors (8) and therefore differentiates into a secretory phenotype. We found that prolactin treatment of HC11 cells increases Cu secretion from monolayers of differentiated cells (35). This increased Cu secretion is not achieved by changes in Ctr1 (see above) or ATP7A expression, but by transient relocalization of Ctr1 to the plasma membrane and of ATP7A from a perinuclear location to a vesicular compartment, possibly resulting in increased Cu secretion from the cell.

MAMMARY GLAND ZINC METABOLISM

In contrast to Fe and Cu, whose concentrations in human milk are a fraction of those in serum, milk Zn concentrations are considerably higher than in serum, at least for the first several months of lactation. Thus, there must be effective mechanisms ensuring uptake of Zn into the mammary gland and its subsequent secretion into milk. In fact, more than 0.5–1.0 mg of Zn is taken up by the mammary gland and secreted into milk per day. This amount is almost twice that of Zn transferred across the placenta to the fetus during late pregnancy (36), which illustrates the remarkable capacity of the mammary gland to transport Zn. Since milk Zn concentrations are similar in women with low Zn status and those who receive daily supplements (38, 56–58), it is apparent that homeostasis of milk Zn transfer is tightly regulated.

Cellular Zn transporters belong to two families with distinct properties (19). Those belonging to the zinc import protein (ZIP) family (ZIP1–14) are Zn importers and were discovered by gene sequence homology to known Zn transporters in yeast and plants (Zrt1, Irt-like proteins). Zip1 is found in all tissues studied, whereas Zip2–4 are tissue specific (72). Zip3 is found in tissues with high Zn requirements, such as pancreas, thymus, brain, and eye, and we have found it in the mammary gland (34), where it is located on the epithelial cell plasma membrane. By gene silencing, we reduced Zip3 expression in cultured mouse mammary cells (HC11) by ~80% and found significantly decreased Zn uptake, showing that Zip3 facilitates Zn import by mammary epithelial cells (**Figure 4**, see color insert). The decreased cell viability following Zip3 knockdown demonstrated the essentiality of Zip3 for the mammary epithelial cell and possibly reflects the high Zn requirement of this highly specialized cell type (34).

The zinc transporter (ZnT) family (ZnT-1–9) of transporters belongs to the larger cation diffusion facilitator family, and its members are primarily responsible for Zn export (19). They have six transmembrane-spanning domains and a histidine-rich region that is believed to play a key role in Zn binding. ZnT-1 and ZnT-2 are expressed in the mammary gland (29, 31, 45), where they are localized to the luminal membrane of the mammary epithelial cell (31), which suggests that they are responsible for mediating Zn secretion into milk. ZnT-4 is most likely a key transporter in milk Zn secretion, as a mutation in this transporter in mice, the lethal milk (*lm*) mouse, results in early death of their offspring due to severe Zn deficiency (2, 26). Their milk, however, contains ~50% of normal milk Zn concentrations, and as maternal Zn supplementation improves pup survival, it is evident that the mammary gland can utilize other Zn transport mechanisms for Zn secretion into milk.

A disorder similar to that in the *lm* mouse is known to exist in humans. Some women who produce breast milk abnormally low in Zn cause this "transient neonatal Zn deficiency." The condition has been described in numerous case reports (4, 5, 64, 70), and milk Zn concentrations cannot be increased by maternal Zn supplementation. Term breast-fed infants of such women usually experience severe eczema and decreased growth by 2–3 months of age; premature infants experience eczema and decreased growth earlier due to their lower Zn stores at birth (5). Oral Zn supplementation quickly alleviates the symptoms, as does the introduction of infant formula, which is fortified with Zn at generous levels. In contrast to the *lm* mouse, ZnT-4 was not found to be responsible for the condition in humans (55). We found a family with several women having had exclusively breast-fed infants who during early infancy experienced classical signs of Zn deficiency, which was undiagnosed (11). Two of these women were still lactating and had abnormally low breast-milk Zn concentrations. We were able to obtain genetic material and found a point mutation (His→Arg) in the *ZnT-2* gene in the mothers of infants suffering from transient neonatal Zn deficiency. We also showed in HEK293 cells that site-directed mutagenesis of the same residue resulted in ZnT-2 mislocalization to a perinuclear, aggresomal compartment, which strongly suggests that ZnT-2 plays a major role in milk Zn secretion (11). We used gene silencing to reduce *ZnT-2* expression in cultured mouse mammary epithelial cells (HC11) by ~75%, which caused a reduction in Zn secretion by ~59%, demonstrating that ZnT-2 is partially responsible for Zn export into milk. It is not yet known how common this mutation is in various populations, but the abundance of published case reports suggests that it is not rare.

During lactation in both humans and rats, milk Zn concentrations decline (15, 21, 28) whereas plasma Zn increases. We have used the lactating rat as a model to study mechanisms underlying developmental changes in milk Zn secretion. When plasma Zn increases during lactation, mammary gland Zn levels and ZnT-1 and ZnT-2 expression increase, whereas ZnT-4 and Zip3 expression peaks during early lactation and then decreases, but remains higher than during initiation of lactation (31). ZnT-1, ZnT-2, and ZnT-4 were all localized to both the luminal and the serosal membrane, but during early lactation, they were primarily localized to the luminal membrane. As lactation proceeds, their intensity at the luminal membrane decreases and ZnT-4 is relocalized to a homogenous intracellular distribution. Thus, the decreased abundance of these transporters at the luminal membrane and the relocalization observed likely explain the decline in milk Zn concentration that occurs during lactation.

Milk Zn concentration is maintained over a wide range of Zn intake (see above). We have investigated how maternal low Zn intake affects mammary gland Zn transporters and their localization in the rat (30, 31). We found that, similar to observations in humans, plasma Zn is reduced, but milk Zn concentration is maintained. We believe that milk Zn is homeostatically regulated by a combination of decreased Zn efflux across the serosal membrane into the maternal circulation mediated by decreased ZnT-1 expression, and increased milk Zn secretion achieved by increased ZnT-4 expression. It should be noted, though, that there is most likely a threshold for the mammary gland being able to respond to maternal Zn deficiency as milk Zn does decrease with further severity of Zn deficiency, most likely due to decreased expression of Zip3, ZnT-1, ZnT-2, and ZnT-4. However, although such a severe deficiency can be achieved in experimental animals, it is unlikely to occur in lactating women.

Prolactin also affects Zn transport during lactation. In a study on lactating rats, we found that maternal Zn deficiency increases circulating prolactin levels, which suggests that Zn deficiency may have secondary effects on lactogenic hormone-signaling pathways, which are involved in the regulation of mammary gland Zn homeostasis (10). We used cultured mouse mammary epithelial cells (HC11) to investigate mechanisms by which prolactin regulates Zip3 and ZnT-2 and found that prolactin exposure transiently enhanced both serosal Zn uptake and luminal Zn export. This increased Zn transport was associated with increased ZnT-2 but not Zip3 expression, which suggests that increased Zn transporter levels is not the only mechanism used by the mammary gland to regulate Zn transport. Using confocal microscopy we found that Zip3 is localized to the serosal membrane (34) in HC11 cells, which is similar to what we found in lactating rats (31). Prolactin transiently induces the movement of Zip3-associated vesicles to the serosal membrane, thereby likely increasing cellular uptake of Zn. In contrast, ZnT-2, which usually is associated with the Golgi, relocalizes to a dispersed vesicular compartment in response to prolactin. Thus, alterations in hormone signaling play a significant role in the regulation of milk Zn secretion.

INTERACTIONS BETWEEN MICRONUTRIENTS IN THE MAMMARY GLAND

Although it is known that maternal excess intake or deficiency of Fe, Cu, and Zn do not affect concentrations of that particular trace element in milk, there are known examples of how an underlying deficiency of one micronutrient can affect the concentration of another micronutrient in milk.

Effect of Maternal Zinc Deficiency on Milk Copper

Low Zn status is common among pregnant and lactating women because of high Zn requirements during these periods. We have investigated the effects of maternal Zn deficiency in rats on mammary gland Zn metabolism and milk Zn concentration (6, 31). In these studies, we noted significantly increased milk Cu levels; therefore, we also explored the effects of maternal marginal Zn deficiency on mammary gland Cu metabolism (30). We found that the Zn deficiency did not affect maternal tissue Zn or Cu, or milk Zn concentration, but that plasma ceruloplasmin activity was higher in dams fed the Zn-deficient diet. They also had high mammary gland Ctr1, ATP7A, and ATP7B levels, milk ceruloplasmin activity, and Cu concentration. Immunohistochemistry and differential centrifugation showed that Zn deficiency also altered Ctr1 and ATP7A localization in the mammary gland. We found a larger proportion of monomeric Ctr1 proteins, but no increase in the larger dimeric or multimeric complexes believed to be the functional form of Ctr1 (41). This suggests that mature Ctr1 in the mammary gland may undergo endocytosis in response to a low-Zn diet, as has been shown to occur in response to Cu exposure (63). However, our results do not suggest that Ctr1 is degraded as a consequence of internalization in response to low Zn intake, as was observed in response to Cu exposure (63). It has been shown previously that Zn can affect Cu transport in Caco-2 cells as they respond to high Zn levels by increasing Cu uptake and decreasing export, a finding that suggests that Zn may play a role in the regulation of Cu transporters (66).

We also found that ATP7A abundance increased in response to the low-Zn diet, and its localization changed away from smaller vesicles to larger vesicles (30), which may have contributed to the increase in milk Cu. This relocalization of ATP7A is similar to that observed with high Cu exposure (62), which suggests that the mammary gland is responding to the higher serum Cu levels. Abundance of ATP7B also increased in response to the low-Zn diet, but its localization did not change. Since ATP7B is responsible for incorporation of Cu into ceruloplasmin, it is likely that the high abundance of ATP7B was responsible for the higher milk Cu and ceruloplasmin activity.

In summary, our results show that marginal maternal Zn intake during pregnancy and lactation increases the abundance of mammary gland Cu transporters and alters their localization, resulting in high milk Cu concentration, possibly in response to transiently elevated plasma Cu levels. The mechanisms behind these observations are not yet known, but it is possible that the Zn deficiency affects prolactin secretion (described above) and that prolactin affects milk Cu secretion. It is also possible that Zn deficiency directly affects the expression and/or localization of Cu transporters.

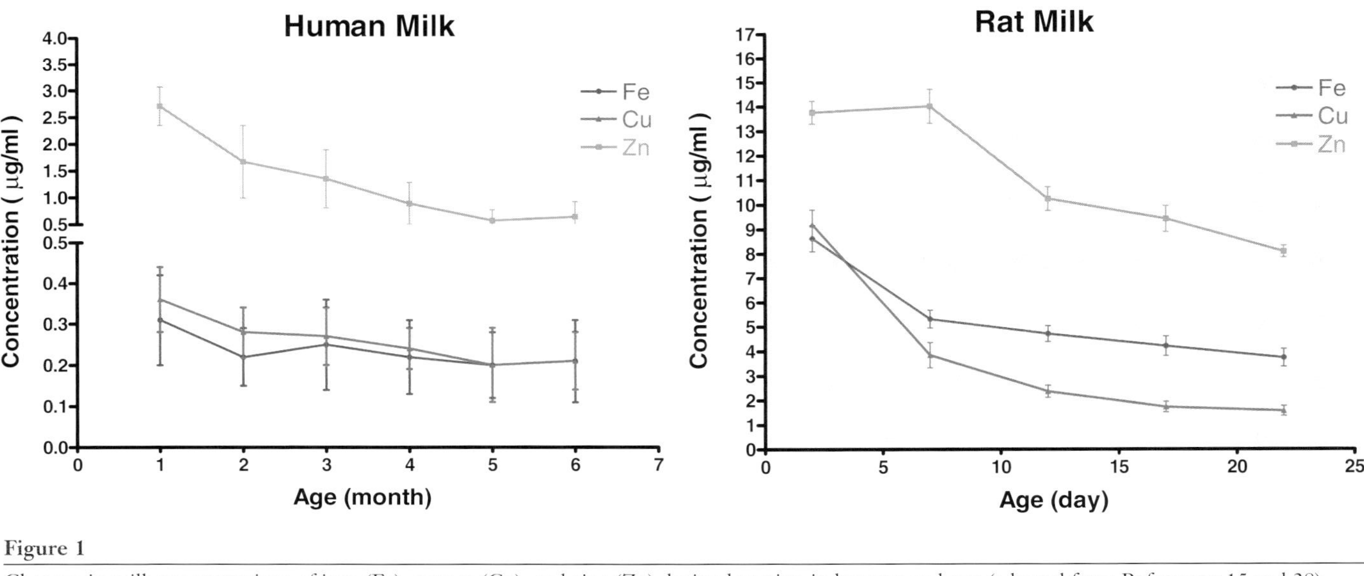

Figure 1

Changes in milk concentrations of iron (Fe), copper (Cu), and zinc (Zn) during lactation in humans and rats (adapted from References 15 and 28).

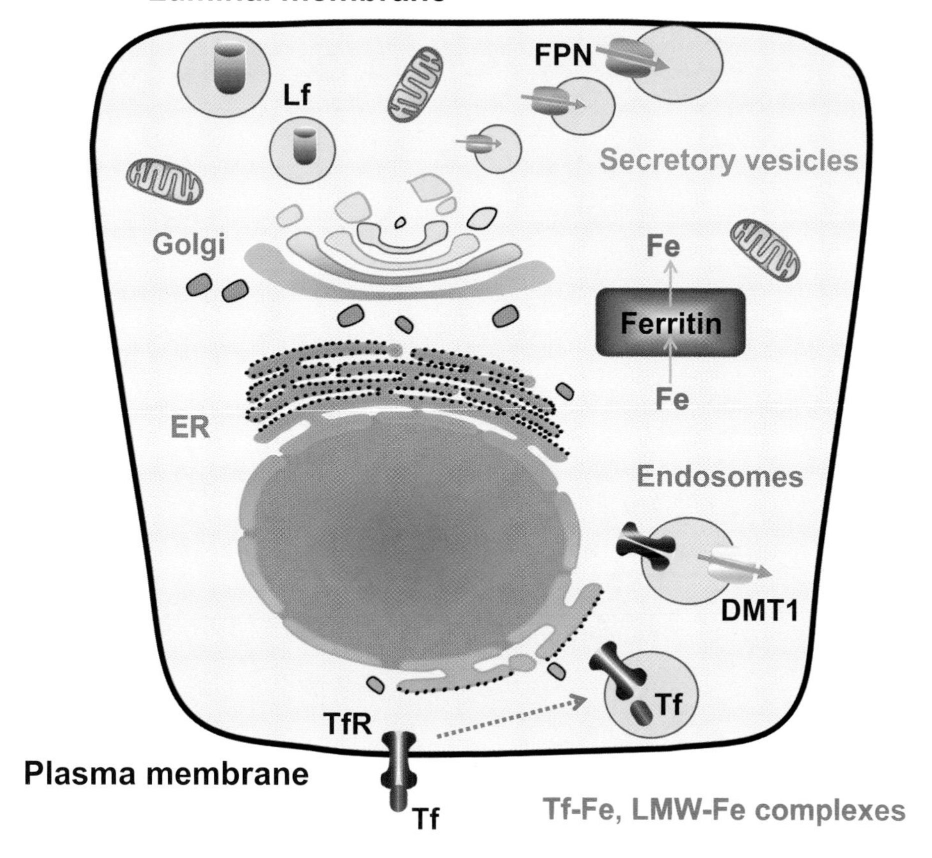

Figure 2

Transport of iron (Fe) in the mammary gland epithelial cell. DMT1, divalent metal transporter 1; ER, endoplasmic reticulum; FPN, ferroportin; LMW, low molecular weight; Tf, transferrin, TfR, transferrin receptor.

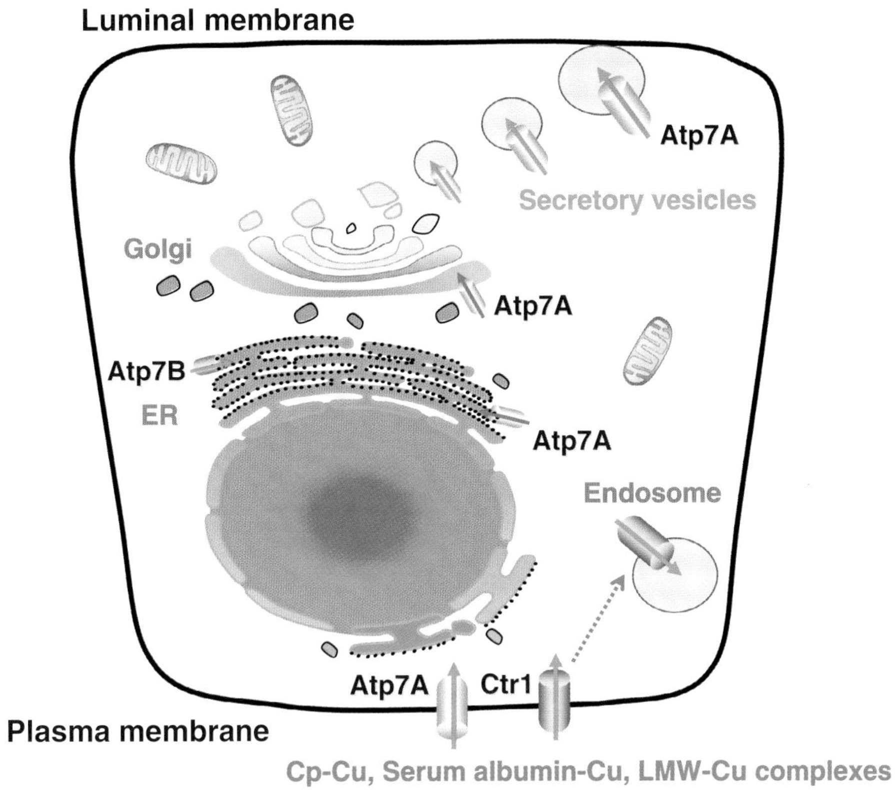

Figure 3

Transport of copper (Cu) in the mammary gland epithelial cell. Atp, adenosine triphosphate; Ctr1, copper transporter 1; ER, endoplasmic reticulum; LMW, low molecular weight.

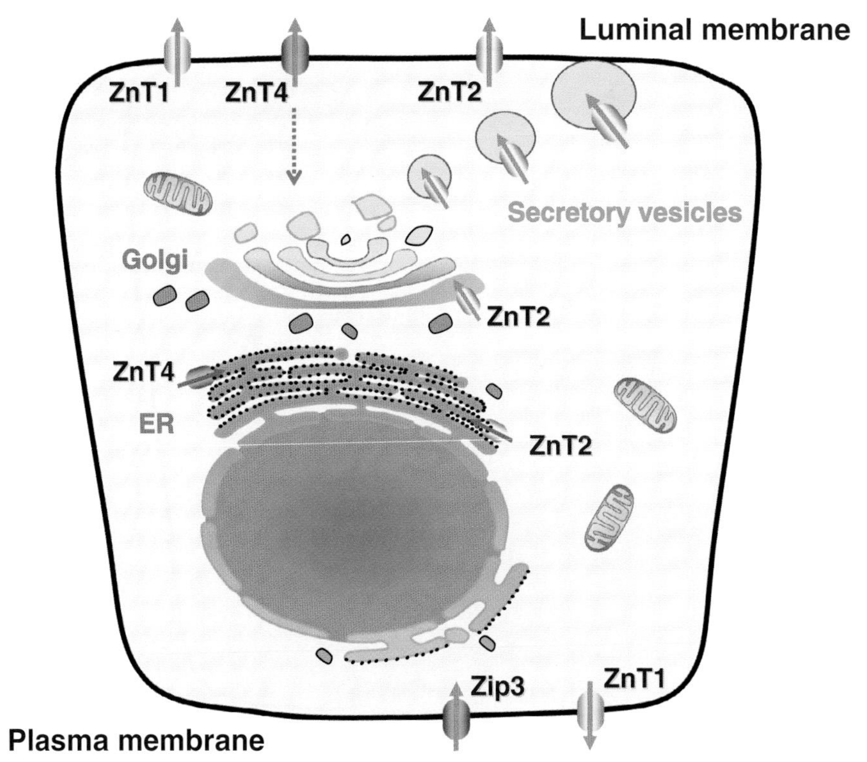

Figure 4

Transport of zinc (Zn) in the mammary gland epithelial cell. ER, endoplasmic reticulum; LMW, low molecular weight; Zip, zinc importer; ZnT, zinc transporter.

It is interesting to note that we found significantly higher milk Cu concentrations in women from Honduras than in Swedish lactating women (17). The Honduran women had lower plasma Zn concentrations than the Swedish women, most likely due to low Zn intake and a corn-based diet with low Zn bioavailability. Thus, marginal Zn deficiency appears to increase milk Cu concentrations in humans also, although the mechanism(s) behind this observation is not yet known.

Effect of Maternal Vitamin A Deficiency on Milk Iron

Vitamin A deficiency is common in developing countries and is known to cause a secondary Fe deficiency and anemia (53, 68). A positive correlation between maternal Fe status and milk Fe has been observed in lactating women supplemented with both vitamin A and Fe but not with Fe alone (59), which suggests there is an effect of vitamin A on mammary gland Fe transport. We investigated the potential mechanisms behind these observations in lactating rats fed a diet marginal in vitamin A (0.4 RE/g) or a control diet (4 RE/g) (32). Milk and liver vitamin A and Fe, and mammary gland Fe concentrations, were lower in rats fed the low–vitamin A diet as compared with control rats. Liver TfR expression was higher, whereas mammary gland TfR expression was lower in rats fed the low–vitamin A diet as compared with controls, which suggests that vitamin A deficiency increased liver Fe acquisition at the expense of the mammary gland. Liver and mammary gland ferritin, DMT1, and FPN protein levels were lower in the low–vitamin A rats, which indicates that there are tissue-specific responses to vitamin A deficiency and that a diet marginally low in vitamin A results in specific effects on Fe transporters. These results suggest that the mammary gland and the liver respond differently to low vitamin A intake during lactation and that milk Fe is significantly decreased due to effects on mammary gland Fe transporters, putting the nursing offspring at risk for Fe deficiency. Whether this occurs in human populations is not yet known, but deficiencies of vitamin A and Fe often coexist in infants, young children, and lactating women.

CONCLUSIONS

It is evident that the mammary gland has a unique capacity to tightly regulate milk secretion of Fe, Cu, and Zn and thereby protect the offspring from maternal deficiency or excess of these trace elements. By up- and down-regulation of transporters and altering their localization within the mammary epithelial cell, homeostasis can be achieved. Lactogenic hormones are involved in this regulation, and their roles, particularly that of prolactin, in this regulation are being unraveled. The consequences of micronutrient interactions on mammary gland trace element homeostasis need to be studied further.

ACKNOWLEDGMENTS

I am grateful to stimulating research collaboration and discussions with Dr. Shannon L. Kelleher and to Ming-yu Jou for her skillful assistance with the illustrations.

LITERATURE CITED

1. Abboud S, Haile DJ. 2000. A novel mammalian iron-regulated protein involved in intracellular metabolism. *J. Biol. Chem.* 275:19906–12
2. Ackland ML, Mercer JF. 1992. The murine mutation, lethal milk, results in production of zinc-deficient milk. *J. Nutr.* 122:1214–18
3. Ackland ML, Anikijenko P, Michalczyk A, Mercer JFB. 1999. Expression of Menkes

copper-transporting ATPase, MNK, in the lactating human breast: possible role in copper transport into milk. *J. Histochem. Cytochem.* 47:1553–61
4. Aggett PJ, Atherton DJ, More J, Davey J, Delves HT, Harries JT. 1980. Symptomatic zinc deficiency in a breast-fed preterm infant. *Arch. Dis. Child.* 55:547–50
5. Atkinson SA, Whelan D, Whyte RK, Lönnerdal B. 1989. Abnormal zinc content in human milk. Risk for development of nutritional zinc deficiency in infants. *Am. J. Dis. Child.* 143:608–11
6. Beshgetoor D, Lönnerdal B. 1997. Effect of marginal maternal zinc deficiency in rats on mammary gland zinc metabolism. *J. Nutr. Biochem.* 8:573–78
7. Black RE. 2003. Zinc deficiency, infectious disease and mortality in the developing world. *J. Nutr.* 133:1485–89S
8. Buck K, Vanek M, Groner B, Ball RK. 1992. Multiple forms of prolactin receptor messenger ribonucleic acid are specifically expressed and regulated in murine tissues and the mammary cell line HC11. *Endocrinology* 130:1108–14
9. Camakaris J, Petris MJ, Bailey L, Shen P, Lockhart P, et al. 1995. Gene amplification of the Menkes (MNK; ATP7A) P-type ATPase gene of CHO cells is associated with copper resistance and enhanced copper efflux. *Hum. Mol. Genet.* 4:2117–23
10. Chowanadisai W, Kelleher SL, Lönnerdal B. 2004. Maternal zinc deficiency raises plasma prolactin levels in lactating rats. *J. Nutr.* 134:1314–19
11. Chowanadisai W, Lönnerdal B, Kelleher SL. 2006. Identification of a mutation in SLC30A2 (ZnT-2) in women with low milk zinc concentration that results in transient neonatal zinc deficiency. *J. Biol. Chem.* 281:39699–707
12. Cordano A. 1998. Clinical manifestations of nutritional copper deficiency in infants and children. *Am. J. Clin. Nutr.* 67(Suppl. 5):1012–16S
13. Craven CM, Alexander J, Eldridge M, Kushner JP, Bernstein S, Kaplan J. 1987. Tissue distribution and clearance kinetics of nontransferrin-bound iron in the hypotransferrinemic mouse: a rodent model for hemochromatosis. *Proc. Natl. Acad. Sci. USA* 84:3457–61
14. Das SK, Ray K. 2006. Wilson's disease: an update. *Nat. Clin. Pract. Neurol.* 2:482–93
15. Dewey KG, Lönnerdal B. 1983. Milk and nutrient intake of breast-fed infants from 1 to 6 months: relation to growth and fatness. *J. Pediatr. Gastroenterol. Nutr.* 2:497–506
16. Dewey KG, Domellöf M, Cohen RJ, Rivera LL, Hernell O, Lönnerdal B. 2002. Iron supplementation affects growth and morbidity of breast-fed infants: results of a randomized trial in Sweden and Honduras. *J. Nutr.* 132:3249–55
17. Domellöf M, Lönnerdal B, Dewey KG, Cohen RJ, Hernell O. 2004. Iron, zinc, and copper concentrations in breast milk are independent of maternal mineral status. *Am. J. Clin. Nutr.* 79:111–15
18. Donley SA, Ilagan BJ, Rim H, Linder MC. 2002. Copper transport to mammary gland and milk during lactation in rats. *Am. J. Physiol. Endocrinol. Metab.* 283:E667–75
19. Eide DJ. 2006. Zinc transporters and the cellular trafficking of zinc. *Biochim. Biophys. Acta* 1763:711–22
20. Fransson GB, Lönnerdal B. 1980. Iron in human milk. *J. Pediatr.* 96:380–84
21. Fransson GB, Lönnerdal B. 1982. Zinc, copper, calcium and magnesium in human milk. *J. Pediatr.* 101:504–8
22. Fransson GB, Lönnerdal B. 1984. Iron, copper, zinc, calcium and magnesium in human milk fat. *Am. J. Clin. Nutr.* 39:185–89
23. Georgieff MK, Wobken JK, Welle J, Burdo JR, Connor JR. 2000. Identification and localization of divalent metal transporter-1 (DMT-1) in term human placenta. *Placenta* 21:799–804

24. Grimes A, Hearn CJ, Lockhart P, Newgreen DF, Mercer JF. 1997. Molecular basis of the brindled mouse mutant (Mo(br)): a murine model of Menkes disease. *Hum. Mol. Genet.* 6:1037–42
25. Hotz C, Brown KH. 2001. Identifying populations at risk of zinc deficiency: the use of supplementation trials. *Nutr. Rev.* 59:80–84
26. Huang L, Gitschier J. 1997. A novel gene involved in zinc transport is deficient in the lethal milk mouse. *Nat. Genet.* 17:292–97
27. Kaler SG. 1998. Metabolic and molecular bases of Menkes disease and occipital horn syndrome. *Pediatr. Dev. Pathol.* 1:85–98
28. Keen CL, Lönnerdal B, Clegg M, Hurley L. 1981. Developmental changes in composition of rat milk: trace elements, minerals, protein, carbohydrate and fat. *J. Nutr.* 111:226–36
29. Kelleher SL, Lönnerdal B. 2002. Zinc transporters in the mammary gland respond to marginal zinc and vitamin A intake during lactation in rats. *J. Nutr.* 132:3280–85
30. Kelleher SL, Lönnerdal B. 2003a. Marginal maternal Zn intake in rats alters mammary gland Cu transporter levels and milk Cu concentration and affects neonatal Cu metabolism. *J. Nutr.* 133:2141–48
31. Kelleher SL, Lönnerdal B. 2003b. Zn transporter levels and localization change throughout lactation in rat mammary gland and are regulated by Zn in mammary cells. *J. Nutr.* 133:3378–85
32. Kelleher SL, Lönnerdal B. 2005a. Low vitamin A intake affects milk iron level and iron transporters in rat mammary gland and liver. *J. Nutr.* 135:27–32
33. Kelleher SL, Lönnerdal B. 2005b. Molecular regulation of milk trace mineral homeostasis. *Mol. Aspects Med.* 26:328–39
34. Kelleher SL, Lönnerdal B. 2005c. Zip3 plays a major role in zinc uptake into mammary epithelial cells and is regulated by prolactin. *Am. J. Physiol. Cell Physiol.* 288:C1042–47
35. Kelleher SL, Lönnerdal B. 2006. Mammary gland copper transport is stimulated by prolactin through alterations in Ctr1 and ATP7A localization. *Am. J. Physiol. Regul. Integr. Comp. Physiol.* 291:R1181–91
36. King JC. 2002. Enhanced zinc utilization during lactation may reduce maternal and infant zinc depletion. *Am. J. Clin. Nutr.* 75:2–3
37. Klomp AEM, Top BBJ, VanDenBerg ET, Berger R, Klomp LWJ. 2002. Biochemical characterization and subcellular localization of human copper transporter 1 (hCTR1). *Biochem. J.* 364:497–505
38. Krebs NF, Reidinger CJ, Hartley S, Robertson AD, Hambidge KM. 1995. Zinc supplementation during lactation: effects on maternal status and milk zinc concentrations. *Am. J. Clin. Nutr.* 61:1030–36
39. Kuo YM, Gybina AA, Pyatskowit JW, Gitschier J, Prohaska JR. 2006. Copper transport protein (CTR1) levels in mice are tissue specific and dependent on copper status. *J. Nutr.* 136:21–26
40. LaFontaine S, Theophilos MB, Firth SD, Gould R, Parton RG, Mercer JFB. 2001. Effect of toxic milk mutation (*tx*) on the function and intracellular localization of Wnd, the murine homologue of the Wilson copper ATPase. *Hum. Mol. Genet.* 10:361–70
41. Lee J, Pena MMO, Nose Y, Thiele DJ. 2002. Biochemical characterization of the human copper transporter Ctr1. *J. Biol. Chem.* 277:4380–87
42. Lee J, Prohaska JR, Dagenais SL, Glover TW, Thiele DJ. 2000. Isolation of a murine copper transporter gene, tissue specific expression and functional complementation of a yeast copper transport mutant. *Gene* 254:87–96
43. Lee J, Prohaska JR, Thiele DJ. 2001. Essential role for mammalian copper transporter Ctr1 in copper homeostasis and embryonic development. *Proc. Natl. Acad. Sci. USA* 98:6842–47

44. Leong WI, Lönnerdal B. 2005. Iron transporters in rat mammary gland: effects of different stages of lactation and maternal iron status. *Am. J. Clin. Nutr.* 81:445–53
45. Liuzzi JP, Bobo JA, Cui L, McMahon RJ, Cousins RJ. 2003. Zinc transporters 1, 2 and 4 are differentially expressed and localized in rats during pregnancy and lactation. *J. Nutr.* 133:342–51
46. Llanos RM, Mercer JFB. 2002. The molecular basis of copper homeostasis and copper-related disorders. *DNA Cell Biol.* 21:259–70
47. Lönnerdal B. 1986. Effects of maternal dietary intake on human milk composition. *J. Nutr.* 116:499–513
48. Lönnerdal B. 1998. Copper nutrition during infancy and childhood. *Am. J. Clin. Nutr.* 67:1046S-53S
49. Lönnerdal B, Iyer S. 1995. Lactoferrin: molecular structure and biological function. *Annu. Rev. Nutr.* 15:93–110
50. Lönnerdal B, Keen CL, Hurley LS. 1981. Iron, copper, zinc and manganese in milk. *Annu. Rev. Nutr.* 1:149–74
51. Lozoff B, Georgieff MK. 2006. Iron deficiency and brain development. *Semin. Pediatr. Neurol.* 13:158–65
52. McManaman JL, Hanson L, Neville MC, Wright RM. 2000. Lactogenic hormones regulate xanthine oxidoreductase and beta-casein levels in mammary epithelial cells by distinct mechanisms. *Arch. Biochem. Biophys.* 373:318–27
53. Mejia LA, Hodges RE, Rucker RB. 1979. Clinical signs of anemia in vitamin A deficient rats. *Am. J. Clin. Nutr.* 32:1439–44
54. Michalczyk AA, Reiger J, Allen KJ, Mercer JFB, Ackland ML. 2000. Defective localization of the Wilson disease protein (ATP7B) in the mammary gland of the toxic milk mouse and the effects of copper supplementation. *Biochem. J.* 352:565–71
55. Michalczyk A, Varigos G, Catto-Smith A, Blomeley RC, Ackland ML. 2003. Analysis of zinc transporter, hZnT4 (Slc30A4), gene expression in a mammary gland disorder leading to reduced zinc secretion into milk. *Hum. Gen.* 113:202–10
56. Moore CME, Roberto RDJ, Greene HL. 1984. Zinc supplementation in lactating women: evidence for mammary control of zinc secretion. *J. Pediatr.* 105:600–2
57. Moser PB, Reynolds RD, Acharya S, Howard MP, Andon MB, Lewis SA. 1988. Copper, iron, zinc, and selenium dietary intake and status of Nepalese lactating women and their breast-fed infants. *Am. J. Clin. Nutr.* 47:729–34
58. Moser-Veillon PB, Reynolds RD. 1990. A longitudinal study of pyridoxine and zinc supplementation of lactating women. *Am. J. Clin. Nutr.* 52:135–41
59. Muslimatun S, Schmidt MK, West CE, Schultink W, Hautvast JGAJ, Karyadi D. 2001. Weekly vitamin A and iron supplementation during pregnancy increases vitamin A concentration of breast milk but not iron status in Indonesian lactating women. *J. Nutr.* 131:2664–69
60. Neville MC, McFadden TB, Forsyth I. 2002. Hormonal regulation of mammary differentiation and milk secretion. *J. Mammary Gland Biol. Neoplasia* 7:49–65
61. Olivares M, Araya M, Uauy R. 2000. Copper homeostasis in infant nutrition: deficit and excess. *J. Pediatr. Gastroenterol. Nutr.* 31:102–11
62. Petris MJ, Mercer JFB. 1999. The Menkes protein (ATP7A:MNK) cycles via the plasma membrane both in basal and elevated extracellular copper using a C-terminal di-leucine endocytic signal. *Hum. Mol. Genet.* 8:2107–15
63. Petris MJ, Smith K, Lee J, Thiele DJ. 2002. Copper-stimulated endocytosis and degradation of the human copper transporter, hCtr1. *J. Biol. Chem.* 278:9639–46

64. Piela Z, Szuber M, Mach B, Janniger CK. 1998. Zinc deficiency in exclusively breast-fed infants. *Cutis* 61:197–200
65. Pizzaro F, Yip R, Dallman PR, Olivares M, Hertrampf E, Walter T. 1991. Iron status with different infant feeding regimens: relevance to screening and prevention of iron deficiency. *J. Pediatr.* 118:687–92
66. Reeves PG, Briske-Anderson M, Johnson L. 1998. Physiologic concentrations of zinc affect the kinetics of copper uptake and transport in the human intestinal cell model, Caco-2. *J. Nutr.* 128:1794–801
67. Sigman M, Lönnerdal B. 1990. Response of rat mammary gland transferrin receptors to maternal dietary iron during pregnancy and lactation. *Am. J. Clin. Nutr.* 52:446–50
68. Sijtsma KW, Berg GJVD, Lemmens AG, West CE, Beynen AC. 1993. Iron status in rats fed on diets containing marginal amounts of vitamin A. *Br. J. Nutr.* 70:777–85
69. Skikne BS, Flowers CH, Cook JD. 1990. Serum transferrin receptor: a quantitative measure of tissue iron deficiency. *Blood* 75:1870–76
70. Stevens J, Lubitz L. 1998. Symptomatic zinc deficiency in breast-fed term and premature infants. *J. Pediatr. Child. Health* 34:97–100
71. Tabuchi M, Yoshimori T, Yamaguchi K, Yoshida T, Kishi F. 2000. Human NRAMP2/DMT1, which mediates iron transport across endosomal membranes, is localized to late endosomes and lysosomes in HEp-2 cells. *J. Biol. Chem.* 275:22220–28
72. Wang F, Dufner-Beattie J, Kim BE, Petris MJ, Andrews GK, Eide DJ. 2004. Zinc-stimulated endocytosis controls activity of the mouse ZIP1 and ZIP3 zinc uptake transporters. *J. Biol. Chem.* 279:24631–39
73. Zhou B, Gitschier J. 1997. hCTR1: a human gene for copper uptake identified by complementation in yeast. *Proc. Natl. Acad. Sci USA* 94:7481–86

ChREBP, a Transcriptional Regulator of Glucose and Lipid Metabolism

Catherine Postic,[1,2] Renaud Dentin,[1,2] Pierre-Damien Denechaud,[1,2] and Jean Girard[1,2]

[1] Institut Cochin, Département d'Endocrinologie, Métabolisme et Cancer, Université Paris Descartes, CNRS (UMR 8104), Paris, France

[2] Inserm, U567, Paris, France; email: postic@cochin.inserm.fr

Annu. Rev. Nutr. 2007. 27:179–92

First published online as a Review in Advance on April 11, 2007

The *Annual Review of Nutrition* is online at http://nutr.annualreviews.org

This article's doi: 10.1146/annurev.nutr.27.061406.093618

0199-9885/07/0821-0179$20.00

Key Words

transcriptional regulation by glucose, insulin resistance, hepatic steatosis, type 2 diabetes

Abstract

Dysregulations in hepatic lipid synthesis are often associated with obesity and type 2 diabetes, and therefore a perfect understanding of the regulation of this metabolic pathway appears essential to identify potential therapeutic targets. Recently, the transcription factor ChREBP (carbohydrate-responsive element-binding protein) has emerged as a major mediator of glucose action on lipogenic gene expression and as a key determinant of lipid synthesis in vivo. Indeed, liver-specific inhibition of ChREBP improves hepatic steatosis and insulin resistance in obese *ob/ob* mice. Since ChREBP cellular localization is a determinant of its functional activity, a better knowledge of the mechanisms involved in regulating its nucleo-cytoplasmic shuttling and/or its post-translational activation is crucial in both physiology and physiopathology. Here, we review some of the studies that have begun to elucidate the regulation and function of this key transcription factor in liver.

Contents

INTRODUCTION

In mammals, the liver is crucial for maintaining overall energy homeostasis and for the conversion of carbohydrate into fat (**Figure 1**, see color insert). The absorption of a high-carbohydrate diet induces several metabolic events aimed at decreasing endogenous glucose production by the liver and increasing glucose uptake and storage in the form of glycogen. When glucose is delivered into the portal vein in large quantities and hepatic glycogen concentrations are restored, glucose is converted in the liver into lipids (through de novo lipogenesis), which are exported as very-low-density lipoprotein (VLDL) and ultimately stored as triglycerides (TGs) in adipose tissue. The activity of the metabolic pathways leading to the synthesis of lipids in liver is strongly dependent upon the nutritional conditions. Indeed, a diet rich in carbohydrates stimulates the glycolytic and lipogenic pathways (**Figure 1**), whereas starvation or a diet rich in lipids decreases their activity. The genes encoding enzymes involved in these pathways include glucokinase (GK) (24), L-pyruvate kinase (L-PK) (55) for glycolysis, ATP citrate lyase (11), stearoyl-CoA desaturase (SCD-1) (43), acetyl CoA carboxylase (ACC) (29), and fatty acid synthase (FAS) (30) for lipogenesis (**Figure 1**). Most of these enzymes are acutely regulated by post-translational and allosteric mechanisms but are also controlled on a long-term basis by a modulation of their transcription rate. Indeed, it is now clear that glycolytic and lipogenic gene transcription requires both insulin and a high glucose concentration to be fully induced (14).

The absorption of carbohydrate in the diet leads to changes in glucose concentrations but is also concomitant with changes in the concentrations of pancreatic hormones, insulin, and glucagon. The transcriptional effect of insulin, long thought to be the main inductor of glycolytic and lipogenic gene transcription, is mediated by sterol regulatory element binding protein-1c (SREBP-1c), a transcription factor of the basic-helix-loop-helix-leucine zipper (bHLH/LZ) transcription factor family. SREBP-1c induces lipogenic genes by its capacity to bind to a sterol regulatory element (SRE) present in the promoter sequence of its target genes (2, 32, 38). SREBP-1c itself is regulated by changes in the nutritional status in liver of rodents (20), and in vitro studies in isolated hepatocytes have demonstrated that the transcription of SREBP-1c is induced by insulin and inhibited by glucagon (13). Transgenic mice that overexpress

VLDL: very-low-density lipoprotein

TG: triglyceride

GK: glucokinase

L-PK: liver-pyruvate kinase

SCD-1: stearoyl-CoA desaturase-1

ACC: acetyl-CoA carboxylase

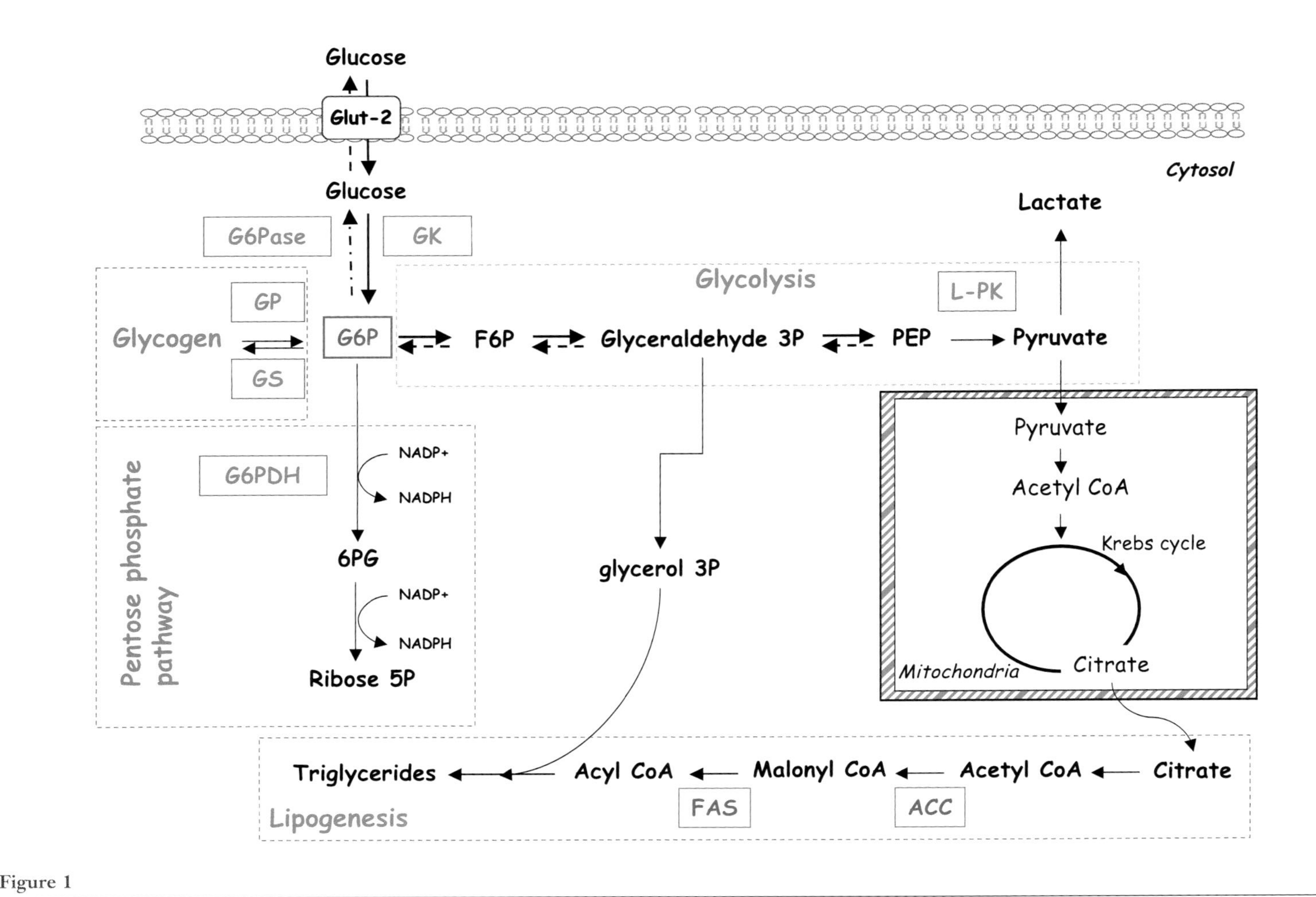

Figure 1

Metabolic pathways leading to the synthesis of triglycerides in liver. Abbreviations: ACC, acetyl-CoA carboxylase; FAS, fatty acid synthase; F6P, fructose 6-phosphate; GK, glucokinase; G6P, glucose 6-phosphate; G6Pase, glucose 6-phosphatase; G6PDH, glucose 6-phosphate dehydrogenase; GP, glycogen phosphorylase; GS, glycogen synthase, L-PK, liver-pyruvate kinase; PEP, phosphoenol pyruvate; TG, triglycerides; X5P, xylulose 5-phosphate.

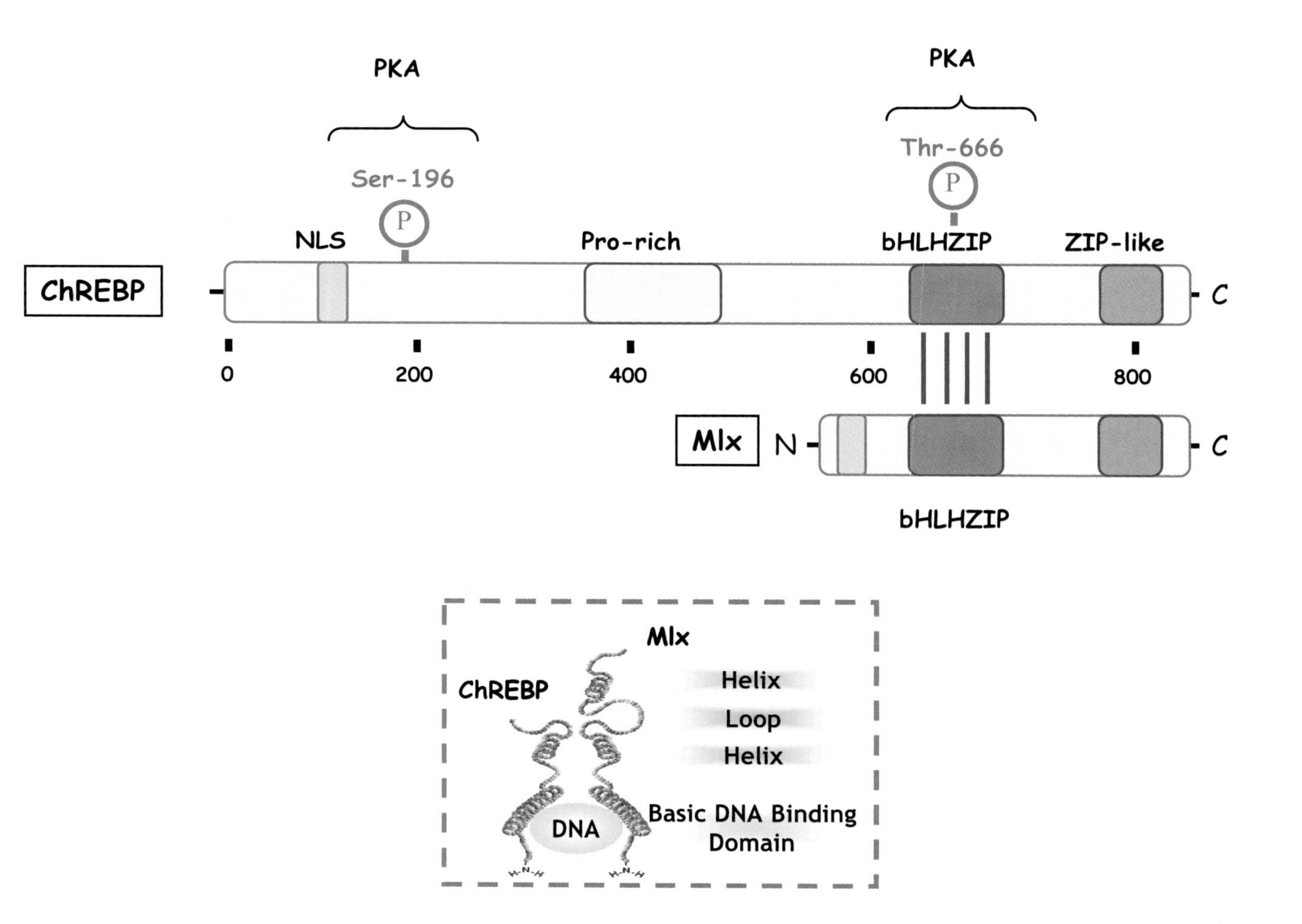

Figure 2
ChREBP and Mlx protein structures. Abbreviations: bHLH/LZ, basic loop-helix-leucine-zipper; ChREBP, carbohydrate-responsive element-binding protein; Mlx, Max-like protein X; NLS, nuclear localization signal; PKA, cAMP-dependent protein kinase.

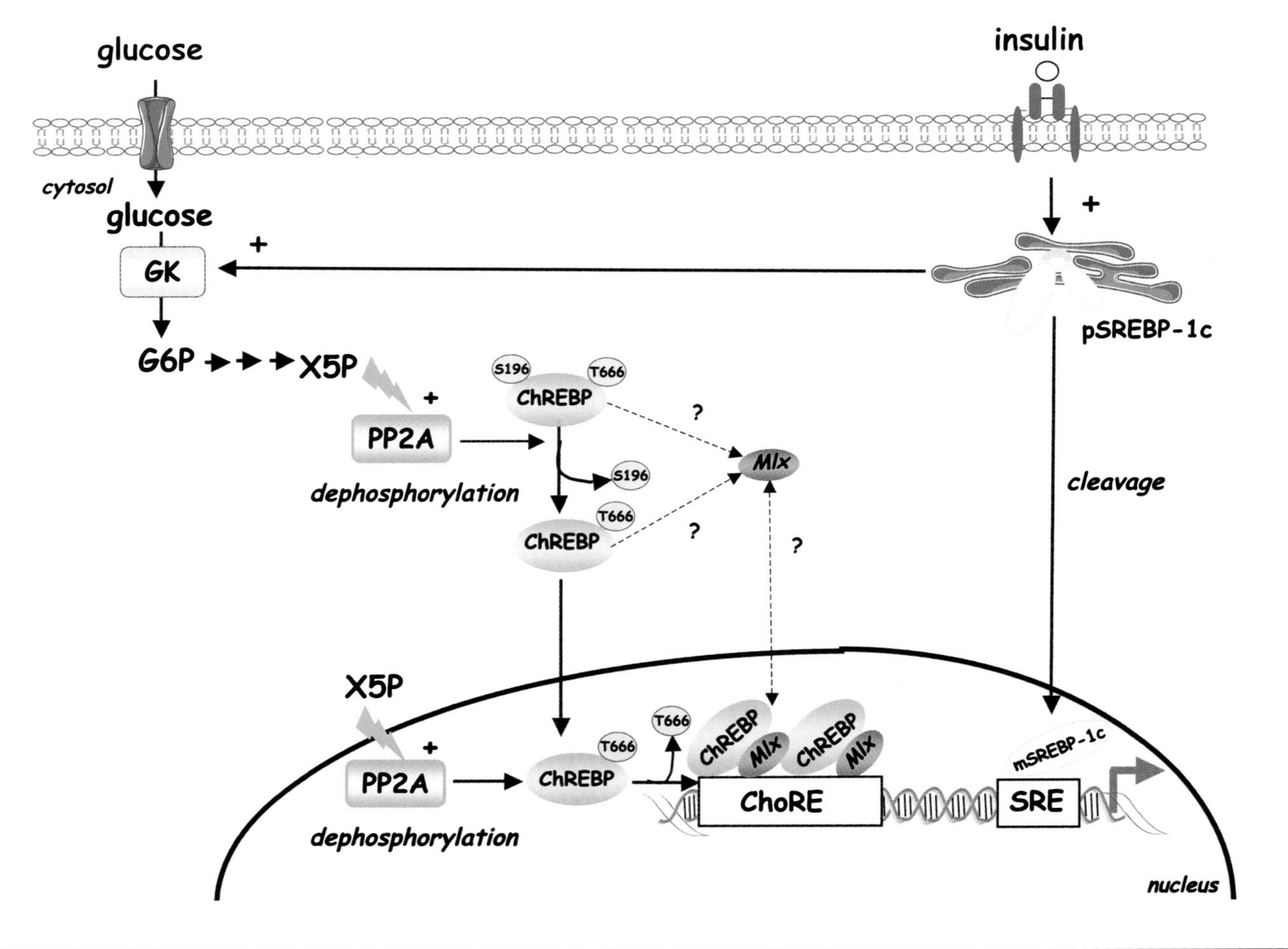

Figure 3

Transcriptional activation of glycolytic and lipogenic genes by ChREBP/Mlx and SREBP-1c in liver. Abbreviations: ChoRE, carbohydrate-responsive element; ChREBP, carbohydrate-responsive element-binding protein; GK, glucokinase; G6P, glucose 6-phosphate; Mlx, Max-like protein X; PP2A, protein phosphatase 2A; SRE, sterol regulatory element; SREBP-1c, sterol regulatory element-binding protein-1c; X5P, xylulose 5-phosphate.

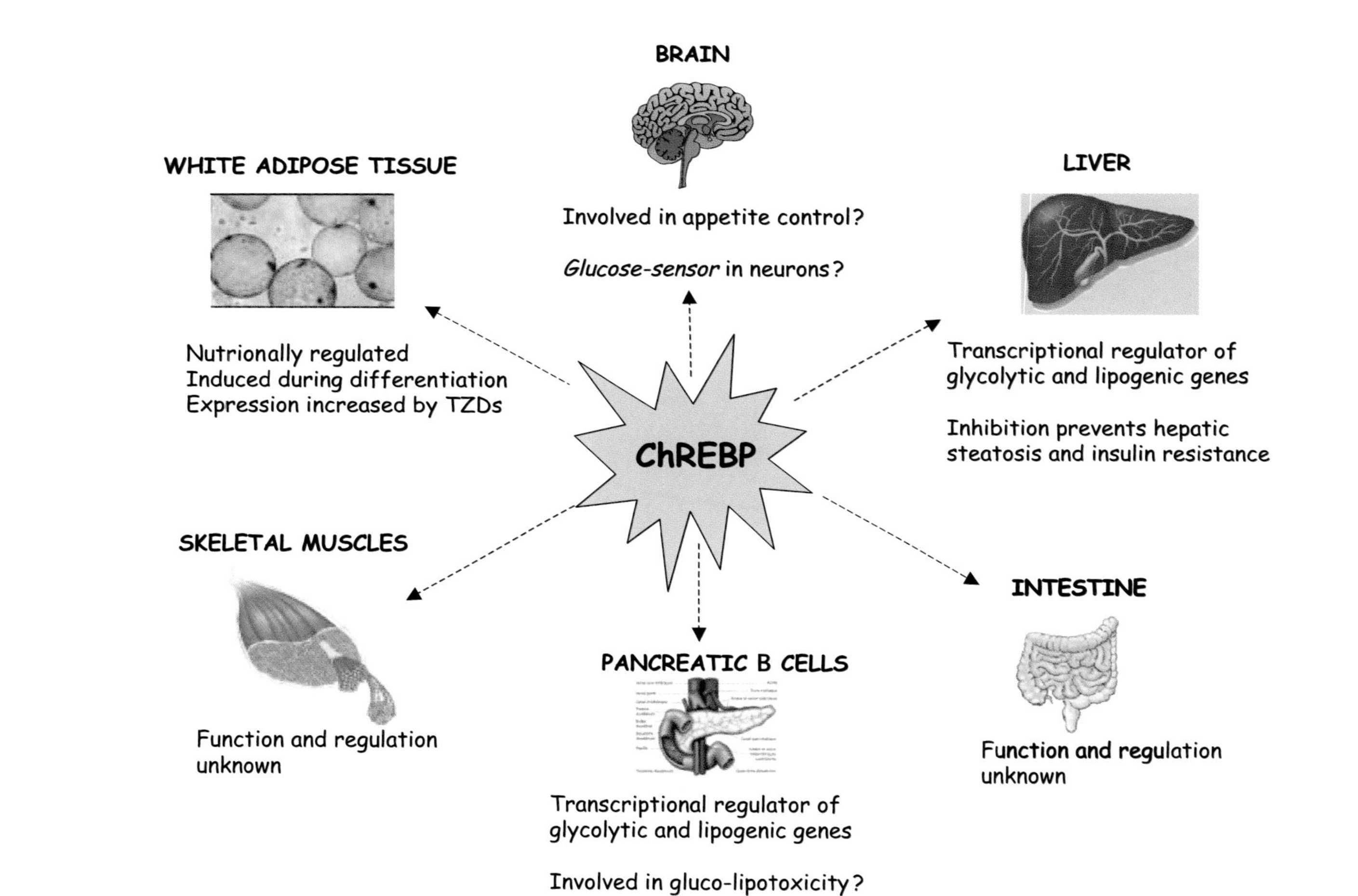

Figure 4

The multiple functions of carbohydrate-responsive element-binding protein (ChREBP). The metabolic and physiological roles of ChREBP may not be limited to the liver. In fact, the function of this transcription may be broader and of particular interest in other sites of expression, including white adipose tissue, brain, and pancreatic β cells (6).

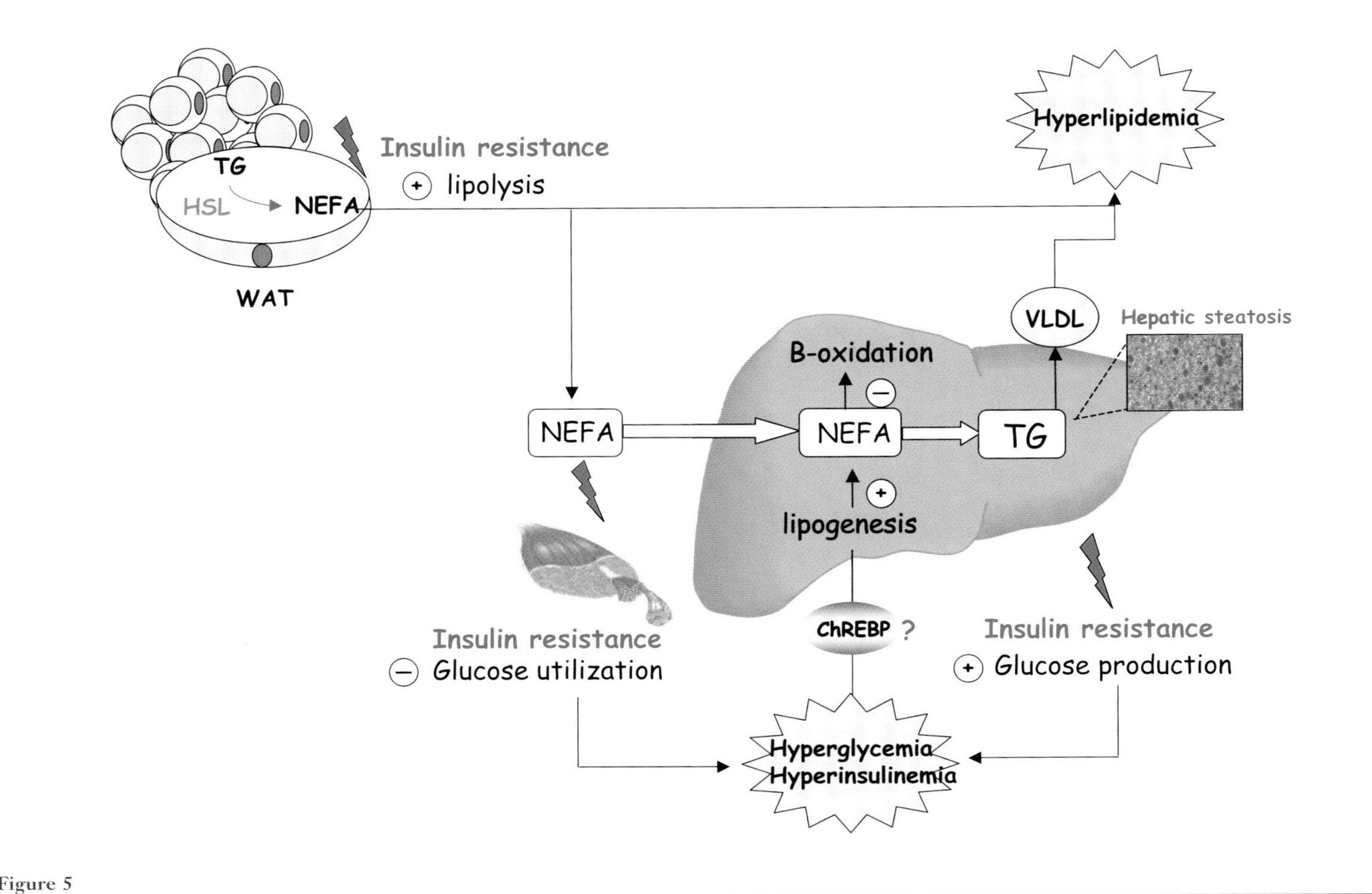

Figure 5

Metabolic defects leading to the development of hepatic steatosis and insulin resistance. Different sources of fatty acids contribute to the development of fatty liver. Under conditions of insulin resistance, insulin does not efficiently suppress lipolysis in the adipose tissue; therefore, peripheral fats stored in adipose tissue flow to the liver by way of plasma nonesterified fatty acids (NEFAs). Because of the circulating NEFAs, skeletal muscles become insulin resistant, and glucose utilization is reduced in this tissue. In addition, the combination of elevated plasma concentrations of glucose and insulin promotes de novo lipid synthesis and impairs β oxidation, thereby participating in the development of hepatic steatosis. The intrahepatic accumulation also has deleterious effects on insulin signaling in liver. Hepatic glucose production is exacerbated, leading to the development of the hyperglycemic phenotype. Recent studies have shown that hepatic lipogenesis contributes significantly to triglyceride (TG) synthesis in humans and that this metabolic pathway is increased in individuals with obesity and insulin resistance (10). Although the molecular mechanisms leading to excess fatty acid accumulation in insulin-resistant states have not been clearly resolved, recent studies have established that alterations in carbohydrate-responsive element-binding protein (ChREBP) expression can be correlated to the physiopathology of hepatic steatosis in genetically obese *ob/ob* mice (7, 22).

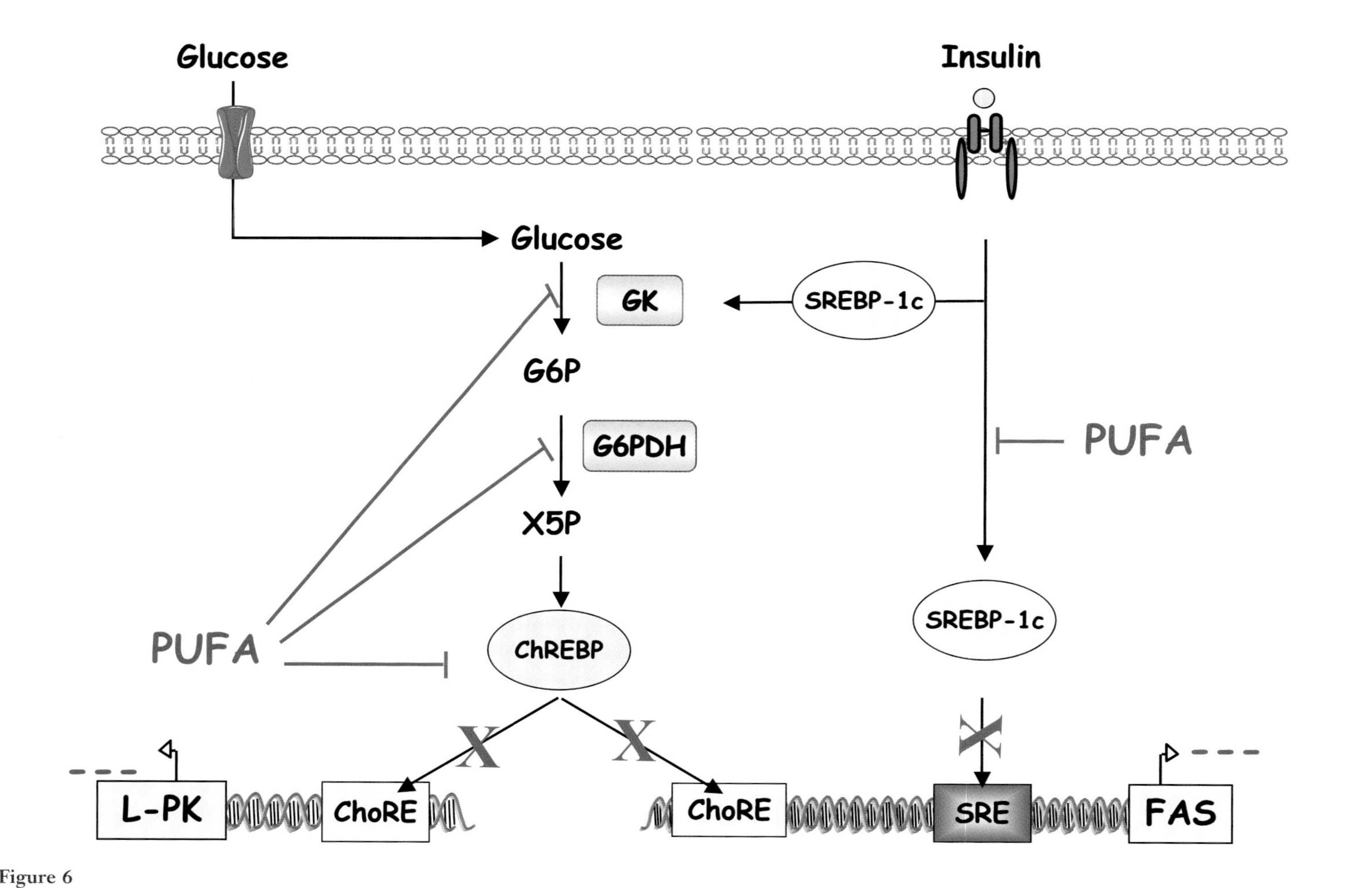

Figure 6

Inhibitory effect of PUFA on ChREBP and SREBP-1c expression and activation. Polyunsaturated fatty acids (PUFA) are potent inhibitors of hepatic glycolysis and de novo lipogenesis, through the inhibition of genes involved in glucose utilization and lipid synthesis, including L-PK, FAS, and ACC. With the identification of the transcription factor SREBP-1c, the molecular mechanism responsible for the PUFA inhibition of lipogenic genes has made important progress. Indeed, PUFA inhibit SREBP-1 gene transcription, enhance SREBP-1c mRNA turnover and interfere with the proteolytic processing of SREBP-1c protein (27). However, the PUFA-mediated suppression of L-PK gene expression cannot be directly attributed to SREBP-1c since L-PK expression is not subjected to SREBP-1c regulation (53) and its promoter does not contain a sterol regulatory element-binding site (SRE) (42). We have recently demonstrated that PUFA suppress ChREBP activity by increasing ChREBP mRNA decay and by altering ChREBP protein translocation from the cytosol to the nucleus, independently of an activation of the AMP-activated protein kinase (AMPK), previously shown to regulate ChREBP activity (8). In the presence of PUFA, ChREBP is retained in the cytosol through the specific inhibition of GK and G6PDH activities, two key enzymes of glycolysis and of the pentose phosphate pathway, respectively.

SREBP-1c in the liver have increased mRNA of most lipogenic genes (50) and develop liver steatosis. Although it is clear that SREBP-1c plays a major role in the long-term control of glucose and lipid homeostasis by insulin, SREBP-1c activity alone does not appear to fully account for the stimulation of glycolytic and lipogenic gene expression in response to carbohydrate diet. In fact, SREBP-1c gene deletion in mice only results in a 50% reduction in fatty acid synthesis (34). In addition, overexpression of a constitutive active form of SREBP-1c in hepatocytes lacking GK (i.e., the enzyme that catalyzes the first step of glucose metabolism in liver) does not allow for a full induction of glycolytic and lipogenic gene expression by glucose and insulin (9).

Although it is clear that increased metabolism through GK is required to initiate glucose signaling, the intracellular mechanism and/or the transcription factor of the glucose-signaling pathway until recently was not fully understood (15, 56). Glucose- or carbohydrate-response elements (ChoREs) that mediate the transcriptional response of glucose have been identified in the promoters of most lipogenic genes through promoter-mapping analysis (48, 49). This element is composed of two E-box (CACGTG) or E-box-like sequences separated by 5 bp. The presence of E-box motifs in these response elements suggests that a bHLH protein family member recognizes the ChoRE and mediates the response to glucose. The recent discovery of a glucose-responsive bHLH/LZ transcription factor, named carbohydrate responsive element-binding protein (ChREBP) (60), has helped explain the mechanism whereby glucose affects gene transcription. This review examines the studies that have helped elucidate the function and regulation of this fascinating transcription factor in liver. We also discuss the recent implication of ChREBP in the physiopathology of hepatic steatosis and insulin resistance.

ChREBP PLAYS A CENTRAL ROLE IN GLUCOSE SIGNALING

Indentification and Function of ChREBP in Liver

In 2001, using affinity chromatography and mass spectrometry, K. Uyeda's group (60) purified a large protein (864 amino acids and $Mr = 94{,}600$) that contains several domains, including a nuclear localization signal (NLS) near the N-terminus, polyproline domains, a basic loop-helix-leucine-zipper (b/HLH/Zip), and a leucine-zipper-like (Zip-like) domain (**Figure 2**, see color insert). This protein, ChREBP, was soon identified as the long-sought glucose-responsive transcription factor. Indeed, when overexpressed in primary culture of hepatocytes, ChREBP induces the activation of an L-PK reporter construct (31). Studies from our laboratory later determined, and for the first time in a physiological context, that ChREBP mediates the transcriptional effect of glucose on both glycolytic (L-PK) and lipogenic (ACC, FAS) gene expression (9). We used small interfering RNA (siRNA) to selectively inhibit ChREBP expression in mouse hepatocytes. When cells were transfected with the ChREBP siRNA, the effect of high glucose concentrations (25 mM) on L-PK, ACC, and FAS gene expression was no longer observed (9). Chromatin immunoprecipitation analysis was later used to confirm that ChREBP directly binds to the promoter sequences of these genes (23).

ChREBP does not homodimerize or bind to the ChoRE as a homodimer (37, 52). Using the yeast two-hybrid system, Towle and coworkers (52) identified a bHLH/LZ protein, Mlx (Max-like protein X) that interacts with the bHLH/LZ domain of ChREBP (**Figure 2**). Mlx is a member of the Myc/Max/Mad family of transcription factors that can serve as a common interaction partner of a transcription factor network (41). The evidence that Mlx is the functional partner of ChREBP was demonstrated using an

FAS: fatty acid synthase

SREBP-1c: sterol regulatory element-binding protein-1c

bHLH/LZ: basic/helix-loop-helix/leucine zipper

SRE: sterol regulatory element

ChoRE: carbohydrate-responsive element

ChREBP: carbohydrate-responsive element-binding protein

Mlx: Max-like protein X

PKA: cAMP-dependant protein kinase

adenovirus expressing a dominant negative form of Mlx (37). The inhibition of Mlx directly interferes with the endogenous ChREBP/Mlx complex and abrogates the glucose response of the ACC reporter gene in primary cultures of hepatocytes (37). This glucose response, however, can be partially restored when ChREBP is overexpressed. The fact that this rescue only occurs at high glucose concentrations of recombinant ChREBP adenovirus suggests that sufficient ChREBP needs to be provided in the cell in order to titrate out the dominant negative effect of Mlx. Over the past three years, Towle's laboratory (35–37, 52) has explored in detail the regulatory domains of the ChREBP and/or Mlx proteins. According to a recent model proposed by Ma et al. (36), two ChREBP-Mlx heterodimers would bind to the two E boxes of the ChoRE to provide a transcriptional complex necessary for glucose regulation. The authors used a ChREBP/Mlx structural model followed by specific mutation experiments to identify three critical residues (F164, I166, and K170) within the Mlx loop that play a crucial role in the binding of the ChREBP/Mlx complex to the ChoRE (35). Therefore, it appears that the Mlx loop region, but not the loop region of ChREBP, is determinant for mediating the response of glucose. Mlx has a significantly longer loop domain than that of most other bHLH/LZ proteins, potentially allowing it to interact across the interface between heterodimer pairs. Therefore, it is possible that other proteins, via interactions involving the Mlx loop, could assist the binding of the ChREBP/Mlx complex to the ChoRE.

Regulation of ChREBP by Translocation and Phosphorylation-Dephosphorylation

ChREBP gene expression is induced by glucose in liver both in vitro (primary cultures of hepatocytes) and in vivo (9), but there are post-translational modifications that allow for a rapid activation of ChREBP. By transfecting a ChREBP-GFP fusion protein in primary cultures of hepatocytes, Uyeda and coworkers (31) first demonstrated that this transcription factor is rapidly translocated from the cytosol into the nucleus in response to high glucose concentrations (27.5 mM). We later confirmed these findings and showed that the endogenous ChREBP protein is indeed addressed into the nucleus in response to high glucose concentrations in primary cultures of mouse hepatocytes and in response to a high-carbohydrate diet in liver of mice (8). Although never demonstrated on the endogenous protein, the mechanism responsible for ChREBP nuclear translocation is thought to involve the dephosphorylation of serine residue 196 (Ser-196), target of cAMP-dependent protein kinase (PKA) and located near the NLS (**Figure 2**). According to the current model, under basal conditions (i.e., low glucose concentrations) ChREBP is phosphorylated on Ser-196 and localized in the cytosol. Under high glucose concentrations, protein phosphatase 2A (PP2A) is selectively activated by xylulose 5-phosphate (X5P), an intermediate of the nonoxidative branch of the pentose phosphate pathway, dephosphorylates ChREBP on this particular residue, and allows for its translocation in the nucleus (28) (**Figure 3**, see color insert). However, because the importance of the PP2A-mediated dephosphorylation of Ser-196 in controlling the translocation process of ChREBP remains to be demonstrated in a physiological context, our laboratory has recently developed a phospho-specific antibody directed against ChREBP residue Ser-196.

Once in the nucleus, ChREBP undergoes a second PP2A-mediated dephosphorylation on residue Threonine 666 (Thr-666) that permits its binding to its ChoRE binding site and hence the transcriptional activation of its target genes (**Figure 3**). Lange and coworkers (58) have observed that the phosphorylation status of the endogenous ChREBP protein (using an in-gel phosphoprotein assay) is decreased under conditions of increased glucose flux through hepatic GK. The fact that the overexpression of GK and the lower phosphorylation state of ChREBP were correlated to a 1.5-fold increase in X5P concentrations seems in agreement with the model initially proposed by Uyeda and colleagues (58). Although there is no doubt that ChREBP is a phosphoprotein, the fact that its activity is activated by dephosphorylation has brought some controversy. Studies from the laboratories of Towle and Chan have strongly challenged these concepts and have suggested that dephosphorylation is not responsible for the activation of ChREBP. The first insight came from the observation that although global phosphorylation of the endogenous ChREBP protein was increased under cAMP conditions, it did not change when hepatocytes were switched from low to high glucose concentrations (54). In addition, mutants of ChREBP, in which one or several of the proposed PKA phosphorylation sites are lacking (including Ser-196 and Thr666), retain the ability to respond to high glucose concentrations (54). More importantly, preventing PKA-mediated phosphorylation at these residues did not create a constitutive active form of ChREBP under low glucose concentrations (54). Taken together, these studies suggest that the post-translational regulation of ChREBP is complex and that mechanisms other than PKA phosphorylation may be required to mediate the glucose activation of ChREBP.

An alternative mechanism to the regulation of ChREBP by phosphorylation/dephosphorylation was also recently proposed (33). Using a structure-function analysis, Li et al. (33) identified within the ChREBP protein sequence a glucose-sensing module composed of a low-glucose inhibitory domain as well as a glucose-response activation conserved element. The specific inhibition of the transactivation activity of the glucose-response activation conserved element by the low-glucose inhibitory domain would confer the inactivity to ChREBP, this inhibition being modulated under high glucose concentrations. Therefore, according to this model, the glucose responsiveness of ChREBP would occur by an intramolecular mechanism independent of a regulation by phosphorylation or dephosphorylation. An interesting finding of this study is that a mutant of ChREBP deleted of its first 197 amino acids behaves as a constitutive active isoform of ChREBP, being transcriptionally active even at low glucose concentrations (33). This region does not contain the Ser-196, thereby excluding a regulatory role for this residue in ChREBP activation. It should be noted, however, that these studies were performed in INS-1-derived 832/13 cells and not in hepatocytes (33). Therefore, the possibility that the activation of ChREBP differs depending on its site of expression should not be excluded.

Finally, as mentioned above, ChREBP interacts with a functional partner, Mlx, to mediate the transcriptional glucose response of its target genes. Although the functional relevance of Mlx is now well established, several questions concerning its regulation remain unaddressed. To our knowledge, nothing is known about the regulation of Mlx by glucose (either transcriptional or post-translational). For example, it would be interesting to determine whether Mlx, like ChREBP, undergoes a nuclear translocation in response to glucose and in which cell compartment (cytosol or nucleus) the association between these two transcription factors occurs (**Figure 3**).

ROLE OF ChREBP IN THE PHYSIOPATHOLOGY OF HEPATIC STEATOSIS AND INSULIN RESISTANCE

Global Inactivation of ChREBP in Vivo

Only a few studies have addressed the role of ChREBP under either physiological or physiopathological conditions in vivo. Global ChREBP gene knockout mice (ChREBP$^{-/-}$) were generated in 2004 by Uyeda's laboratory, and the analysis of these mice has revealed the role of ChREBP in the control of glucose and lipid homeostasis (21). ChREBP$^{-/-}$ mice

NAFLD: nonalcoholic fatty liver disease

have impaired glycolytic and lipogenic pathways in liver and exhibit glucose and insulin intolerance (21). Although this study demonstrates the tight control exerted by ChREBP on hepatic lipogenesis in vivo, the tissue distribution of ChREBP makes the analysis of the phenotype complex. Indeed, the effect on glucose tolerance and insulin sensitivity cannot exclusively be attributed to the inactivation of ChREBP in liver, since this transcription factor is also expressed in other tissues that greatly contribute to the control of glucose homeostasis (i.e., skeletal muscles, white adipose tissue, brain, and pancreatic β cells) (**Figure 4**, see color insert). In addition, the fact that $ChREBP^{-/-}$ mice also show reduced fat pads suggests that ChREBP may play a role in the development and/or function of this tissue. This hypothesis is confirmed by the fact that ChREBP expression is induced during 3T3-L1 preadipocyte differentiation (18). More research clearly is needed to determine the tissue-specific contribution of ChREBP in controlling the phenotypes observed in $ChREBP^{-/-}$ mice (**Figure 4**).

Finally, an unpredicted phenotype of the $ChREBP^{-/-}$ mice is their marked intolerance to fructose. In fact, the exclusive consumption of a diet enriched in fructose leads to premature death in these mice (21). The increase in fructose consumption in Western countries over the past 10–20 years has been linked with a rise in obesity and metabolic disorders. In rodents, fructose stimulates lipogenesis, leading to hepatic and extrahepatic insulin resistance as well as dyslipidemia (57). The cellular and/or molecular mechanisms leading to these deleterious metabolic effects remain largely unknown, but are associated with production of reactive oxygen species and activation of cellular stress pathways, engaging in particular the c-jun N-terminal kinase (57). An interesting finding is that administration of a high-sucrose diet (in which 68% of energy comes from sucrose) leads to higher hepatic concentrations of X5P than do standard diets (in which 68% of energy comes from cornstarch). This indicates that high-sucrose diets are highly lipogenic and stimulate the lipogenic pathway, at least in part, through the specific activation of ChREBP in liver. Nevertheless, further studies are required to delineate the deleterious effects of fructose in $ChREBP^{-/-}$ mice.

Molecular Mechanisms Leading to Hepatic Steatosis

The emergence of ChREBP in the control of lipogenic gene expression in liver prompted us to address its role in the physiopathology of hepatic steatosis. Indeed, fatty acids utilized for the synthesis of TG in liver are available from the plasma nonesterified fatty acid pool as well as from fatty acids newly synthesized through hepatic de novo lipogenesis. TGs can then be stored as lipid droplets within the hepatocytes or secreted into the blood as VLDLs; they can also be hydrolyzed and the fatty acids channeled toward β oxidation. Excessive accumulation of TG is one the main characteristics of hepatic steatosis, a pathological pattern that is now considered as a component of the metabolic syndrome (39) (**Figure 5**, see color insert). Nonalcoholic fatty liver disease (NAFLD) is emerging as the most common chronic liver disease in the Western countries. NAFLD, which describes a large spectrum of liver histopathological features including simple steatosis, nonalcoholic steatohepatitis, cirrhosis, and hepatocellular carcinoma (5), is associated, in the vast majority of the cases, with obesity, insulin resistance, and type 2 diabetes. Therefore, with the epidemics of obesity and type 2 diabetes, NAFLD has become an important public health issue.

Although the molecular mechanism leading to the development of hepatic steatosis is complex, animal models have brought important information for the understanding of hepatic steatosis. For example, mice invalidated for the nuclear receptor PPARα develop steatosis during fasting, which illustrates the crucial role of β oxidation for the removal of fatty acids in the liver (17). Furthermore, a deficiency in choline (which is essential for the export of triglycerides as VLDL) results in the development of a "fatty liver." Hepatic steatosis is also particularly developed in rodent models of obesity, such as *ob/ob* mice, *db/db* mice, and Zucker obese rats, in which an exaggerated lipogenesis has been observed in liver (3). Previously, transcription factors SREBP-1c (51, 59) and PPARγ (the PPARγ2 isoform) have been shown to contribute to the high rates of lipogenesis in livers of these mice (47). When *ob/ob* mice are crossed with either SREBP-1c knockout mice (51) or liver-specific knockout mice of PPARγ2 (40), they show a significant improvement in their hepatic steatosis but not of their overall insulin resistance. We thought that ChREBP, given its importance in the control of lipogenesis, could represent a good candidate to explain the development of the fatty liver phenotype of *ob/ob* mice (**Figure 5**).

Liver-Specific Inhibition of ChREBP in *ob/ob* Mice

We first established a possible molecular link between ChREBP and hepatic steatosis in *ob/ob* mice by determining that ChREBP gene expression and nuclear protein content were markedly increased in livers of these mice (7). We next took the approach of shRNA in vivo (through an adenoviral expression) to specifically inhibit the expression of ChREBP in liver. Our study demonstrated that ChREBP knockdown, both under short-term (two days) and long-term (seven days) conditions, significantly improves the fatty liver phenotype of *ob/ob* mice by decreasing rates of lipogenesis, thereby decreasing hepatic fat accumulation. As expected, the liver-specific inhibition of ChREBP not only markedly affected the expression of ACC and FAS, but also that of SCD-1, the rate-limiting enzyme catalyzing the conversion of saturated long-chain fatty acids into monounsaturated fatty acids, which are the major components of TG (12). Several recent studies have addressed the role of SCD-1 in the development of obesity and insulin resistance (16, 25). The inhibition of SCD-1 using antisense oligonucleotide inhibition (targeting both liver and adipose tissues) has been shown to prevent many of the high-fat-diet metabolic complications, including hepatic steatosis and postprandial hyperglycemia (16, 25). In these studies, the protective effect of SCD-1 on hepatic steatosis was attributed to a combined decrease in SREBP-1c gene expression (i.e., reduced lipogenic rates) and to the up-regulation of L-carnitine palmitoyl transferase I (L-CPT-I) gene expression (i.e., activation of the β-oxidation pathway). Since we did not observe any alteration in SREBP-1c mature protein content in livers of shChREBP RNA-treated *ob/ob* mice, we attributed the improvement of the fatty liver phenotype exclusively to ChREBP knockdown (7). Clearly, more studies are needed to determine the exact contribution of SREBP-1c and ChREBP in controlling fatty acid synthesis.

Interestingly, ChREBP knockdown not only affected the rate of de novo lipogenesis but also had consequences on β oxidation. Lipogenesis and β oxidation are directly correlated because malonyl-CoA, the allosteric inhibitor of CPT-1 (the rate-limiting enzyme of β oxidation) is synthesized by the lipogenic enzyme ACC. The fact that both ACC1 and ACC2 protein content was significantly lower in liver of fasted ChREBP-deficient mice probably led to a constitutive activation of L-CPT1 activity in liver. The significant decrease in malonyl-CoA concentrations and the increase in plasma β hydroxybutyrate levels measured in fasted mice support this hypothesis. Therefore, the coordinate modulation in fatty acid synthesis and oxidation in liver led to overall improvement of lipid homeostasis in ChREBP-deficient mice. Our study is in agreement with the fact that ACC2 gene knockout is also associated with increased rates of β oxidation in liver, leading to the improvement of overall lipid homeostasis in these mice (1).

Interestingly, our study also shows that ChREBP is not only required for the

G6P: glucose 6-phosphate

carbohydrate-induced transcriptional activation of enzymes involved in de novo fatty synthesis but also in TG synthesis, since gene expression was significantly decreased after shChREBP RNA treatment in *ob/ob* mice. Therefore, ChREBP appears to act as a central modulator of fatty acid concentrations in liver by transcriptionally controlling most of the lipogenic program (ACC, FAS, SCD-1), TG synthesis (at the level of glyceraldehyde 3-phosphate acyltransferase), and potentially VLDL export (R. Dentin & C. Postic, unpublished observations).

Improvement in Overall Glucose Tolerance and Insulin Sensitivity After ChREBP Knockdown

Excessive accumulation of hepatic fatty acids in liver is known to lead to deleterious effects on insulin signaling. In agreement with this concept, by markedly preventing fat accumulation in liver, ChREBP knockdown also significantly restored insulin sensitivity in liver. Although the phosphorylation by insulin of Akt, ERK1, ERK2, and Foxo1 was markedly decreased in liver of control *ob/ob* mice, ChREBP knockdown resulted in a significant improvement of insulin signaling in liver of treated *ob/ob* mice as evidenced by the restoration of Akt, ERK1, ERK2, and Foxo1 phosphorylation by insulin (7). Since the phosphorylation of Foxo1 by Akt inhibits its ability to activate gluconeogenesis (46), we hypothesized that restored Foxo1 phosphorylation may lead to an efficient inhibition of gluconeogenic genes in liver of Ad-shChREBP treated *ob/ob* mice. Indeed, after Ad-shChREBP treatment, glucose 6-phosphatase and phosphoenol pyruvate carboxykinase mRNA levels were significantly decreased in livers of *ob/ob* mice, demonstrating that the liver-specific inhibition of ChREBP was associated with a normalization of hepatic insulin signaling in treated *ob/ob* mice.

Interestingly, insulin sensitivity was restored not only in liver but also in skeletal muscles and adipose tissue, in which we also observed a significant improvement in Akt phosphorylation in response to the insulin bolus (7). As a result, glycogen content was restored to control levels in skeletal muscles from shChREBP RNA-treated *ob/ob* mice. Skeletal muscle is known to play a determinant role in the physiopathology of insulin-resistance, and defects in glycogen synthesis have been particularly implicated in the development of the pathogenesis (45). The beneficial effect of ChREBP knockdown was apparent on overall glucose tolerance and insulin sensitivity, with a significant improvement in hyperlipidemia, hyperglycemia, and hyperinsulinemia.

Our findings were also corroborated with the study of Uyeda and coworkers (22) in which the importance of ChREBP in the development of obesity and type 2 diabetes was addressed by intercrossing ChREBP-deficient mice with *ob/ob* mice (*ob/ob*-ChREBP$^{-/-}$ mice). Similar to what we observed, fat accumulation was prevented in liver of these mice, and their hyperlipidemic phenotype was significantly improved (22). An interesting role for ChREBP in the control of appetite was also uncovered by this study. ChREBP gene expression was reported in the brain, a tissue in which this transcription factor could play a role in the sensing of glucose (21) (**Figure 4**). Because of leptin deficiency, *ob/ob* mice are hyperphagic. Interestingly, food consumption was significantly reduced in *ob/ob*-ChREBP$^{-/-}$ mice and was associated with a 30% decrease in the expression of the appetite-stimulating neuropeptide AgRP. Whether ChREBP directly controls food intake or indirectly controls it through AgRP expression needs to be further addressed.

It should be noted that our study (7) and the study of Uyeda and coworkers (22) only addressed the role of ChREBP in the physiopathology of obesity and insulin resistance in the *ob/ob* mouse model. The limitation of this model, as mentioned above, is the fact that *ob/ob* mice are obese and insulin resistant because of genetic deficiency of leptin. A model of diet-induced obesity in C57BL/6J mice would better address the role of ChREBP in a leptin-deficiency independent context. Nevertheless, these studies (7, 22) provide strong support for an important role of ChREBP in insulin resistance and diabetes associated with genetic obesity, and they suggest that ChREBP may represent a potential therapeutic target for the treatment of fatty liver disease and insulin resistance in the future.

PROTECTIVE EFFECT OF POLYUNSATURATED FATTY ACIDS: A ROLE FOR ChREBP

From a therapeutic point of view, dietary polyunsaturated fatty acids (PUFAs), which are potent negative regulators of lipogenesis, were previously shown to ameliorate not only hepatic steatosis of *ob/ob* mice but also notably to attenuate their insulin resistance. PUFAs are potent inhibitors of hepatic glycolysis and de novo lipogenesis, through the inhibition of genes involved in glucose utilization and lipid synthesis, including L-PK, FAS, and ACC. By regulating this pathway, PUFAs promote a shift from fatty acid synthesis and storage to oxidation (26). The positive effects of PUFA on hepatic steatosis are at least partially mediated by SREBP-1c because PUFAs markedly decrease the mature form of SREBP-1c in liver of *ob/ob* mice (**Figure 6**, see color insert). However, since it has been previously reported that disruption of SREBP-1c in *ob/ob* mice does not influence their state of insulin resistance, we can speculate that ChREBP may be responsible for insulin sensitization by PUFA. Indeed, we have recently shown that ChREBP is central for the coordinated inhibition of glycolytic and lipogenic genes by PUFA (8). PUFA [linoleate (C18:2), eicosapentaenoic acid (C20:5), and docosahexaenoic acid (C22:6)] suppresses ChREBP activity by increasing its mRNA decay and by altering ChREBP protein translocation from the cytosol to the nucleus both in primary cultures of hepatocytes and in liver in vivo. The PUFA-mediated alteration in ChREBP translocation is the result of a decrease in glucose metabolism (i.e., an inhibition of the activities of GK and G6PDH, the rate-limiting enzyme of the pentose phosphate pathway) (8) (**Figures 1** and **6**). It remains to be determined whether PUFAs also exert a transcriptional effect on ChREBP gene expression. In the case of SREBP-1c, one of the mechanisms by which PUFAs suppress its gene transcription is through liver X receptor (LXR). PUFAs, by displacing oxysterol from LXR, antagonize the transactivation of LXR, at least in HEK293 cells (44). The recent observation that LXR transcriptionally regulates ChREBP gene expression (4) in liver may suggest that the inhibitory effect of PUFA on ChREBP occurs in an LXR-dependent manner.

PUFA: polyunsaturated fatty acid

LXR: liver X receptor

CONCLUSIONS AND PERSPECTIVES

Dysregulations in hepatic lipid synthesis are often associated with obesity and type 2 diabetes and, therefore, a perfect understanding of this metabolic pathway is essential in both physiology and physiopathology. With the discovery of ChREBP, our understanding of the long-term regulation of glucose and lipid metabolism in liver has recently made considerable progress. ChREBP deficiency overcomes the fatty liver phenotype and improves glucose tolerance and insulin resistance in *ob/ob* mice, suggesting that a reduction of ChREBP activity may have beneficial effect in the treatment of metabolic diseases associated with hyperglycemia and dyslipidemia. So far, the concept that de novo lipogenesis contributes to hepatic steatosis was only based on studies performed in rodents. Recent studies have shown that lipogenesis contributes significantly to TG synthesis in humans and that this metabolic pathway is increased in individuals with obesity and insulin resistance (10). Therefore, the implication of ChREBP in the development of hepatic steatosis in human disease remains to be clearly addressed.

Since ChREBP cellular localization is a key determinant of its functional activity, a better knowledge of the mechanisms involved in regulating its nucleo-cytoplasmic shuttling and/or its post-translation regulation will be crucial in the future to develop novel therapeutic approaches for the study of diseases characterized by dysregulations of glucose and/or lipid metabolism. Indeed, although ChREBP is translocated in the nucleus under high glucose and insulin concentrations in cultured hepatocytes, it is in contrast retained in the cytosol in the presence of PUFAs, well-known inhibitors of lipogenesis. However, the exact mechanisms and/or potentially novel proteic partners involved in the sequestration of ChREBP under nutritional and hormonal conditions remain largely unknown.

In addition, the recent observations on ChREBP function suggest that the physiological roles of ChREBP may be broader and may not be limited to liver (**Figure 4**). The function of ChREBP in white adipose tissue may be of particular interest from a therapeutic point of view. The fact that troglitazone induces ChREBP gene expression during 3T3-L1 preadipocyte differentiation is an interesting observation that suggests that ChREBP may be directly regulated by thiazolidinediones or indirectly regulated through PPARγ (18). Nevertheless, the thiazolidinedione-mediated induction of ChREBP in adipose tissue may represent a way to decrease the hyperglycemic phenotype in diabetic patients.

ACKNOWLEDGMENTS

The work from the authors' laboratory was supported by grants from Alfediam/Sanofi-Synthelabo from the Agence Nationale pour la Recherche (ANR-05-PCOD-035-02) and from the Program National de Recherche sur le Diabète (PNRD-2005).

LITERATURE CITED

1. Abu-Elheiga L, Oh W, Kordari P, Wakil SJ. 2003. Acetyl-CoA carboxylase 2 mutant mice are protected against obesity and diabetes induced by high-fat/high-carbohydrate diets. *Proc. Natl. Acad. Sci. USA* 100:10207–12
2. Bennett MK, Lopez JM, Sanchez HB, Osborne TF. 1995. Sterol regulation of fatty acid synthase promoter. Coordinate feedback regulation of two major lipid pathways. *J. Biol. Chem.* 270:25578–83
3. Bray GA. 1977. Experimental models for the study of obesity: introductory remarks. *Fed. Proc.* 36:137–38
4. Cha JY, Repa JJ. 2006. The liver X receptor and hepatic lipogenesis: the carbohydrate-response element binding protein is a target gene of LXR. *J. Biol. Chem.* 1:743–51
5. Charlton M. 2004. Nonalcoholic fatty liver disease: a review of current understanding and future impact. *Clin. Gastroenterol. Hepatol.* 2:1048–58
6. da Silva Xavier G, Rutter GA, Diraison F, Andreolas C, Leclerc I. 2006. Carbohydrate responsive-element binding protein (chREBP) binding to fatty acid synthase and L-type pyruvate kinase genes is stimulated by glucose in pancreatic MIN6 beta-cells. *J. Lipid Res.* 47:2482–91
7. Dentin R, Benhamed F, Hainault I, Fauveau V, Foufelle F, et al. 2006. Liver-specific inhibition of ChREBP improves hepatic steatosis and insulin resistance in ob/ob mice. *Diabetes* 55:2159–70

8. Dentin R, Benhamed F, Pegorier JP, Foufelle F, Viollet B, et al. 2005. Polyunsaturated fatty acids suppress glycolytic and lipogenic genes through the inhibition of ChREBP nuclear protein translocation. *J. Clin. Invest.* 115:2843–54
9. Dentin R, Pegorier JP, Benhamed F, Foufelle F, Ferre P, et al. 2004. Hepatic glucokinase is required for the synergistic action of ChREBP and SREBP-1c on glycolytic and lipogenic gene expression. *J. Biol. Chem.* 279:20314–26
10. Donnelly KL, Smith CI, Schwarzenberg SJ, Jessurun J, Boldt MD, Parks EJ. 2005. Sources of fatty acids stored in liver and secreted via lipoproteins in patients with nonalcoholic fatty liver disease. *J. Clin. Invest.* 115:1343–51
11. Elshourbagy NA, Near JC, Kmetz PJ, Sathe GM, Southan C, et al. 1990. Rat ATP citrate-lyase. Molecular cloning and sequence analysis of a full-length cDNA and mRNA abundance as a function of diet, organ, and age. *J. Biol. Chem.* 265:1430–35
12. Flowers MT, Miyazaki M, Liu X, Ntambi JM. 2006. Probing the role of stearoyl-CoA desaturase-1 in hepatic insulin resistance. *J. Clin. Invest.* 116:1478–81
13. Foretz M, Guichard C, Ferré P, Foufelle F. 1999. Sterol regulatory element binding protein-1c is a major mediator of insulin action on the hepatic expression of glucokinase and lipogenesis-related genes. *Proc. Natl. Acad. Sci. USA* 96:12737–42
14. Foufelle F, Ferré P. 2002. New perspectives in the regulation of hepatic glycolytic and lipogenic genes by insulin and glucose: a role for the transcription factor sterol regulatory element binding protein-1c. *Biochem. J.* 366:377–91
15. Girard J, Ferré P, Foufelle F. 1997. Mechanisms by which carbohydrates regulate expression of genes for glycolytic and lipogenic enzymes. *Annu. Rev. Nutr.* 17:325–52
16. Gutierrez-Juarez R, Pocai A, Mulas C, Ono H, Bhanot S, et al. 2006. Critical role of stearoyl-CoA desaturase-1 (SCD1) in the onset of diet-induced hepatic insulin resistance. *J. Clin. Invest.* 116:1686–95
17. Hashimoto T, Cook WS, Qi C, Yeldandi AV, Reddy JK, Rao MS. 2000. Defect in peroxisome proliferator-activated receptor alpha-inducible fatty acid oxidation determines the severity of hepatic steatosis in response to fasting. *J. Biol. Chem.* 275:28918–28
18. He Z, Jiang T, Wang Z, Levi M, Li J. 2004. Modulation of carbohydrate response element-binding protein gene expression in 3T3-L1 adipocytes and rat adipose tissue. *Am. J. Physiol. Endocrinol. Metab.* 287:E424–30
19. Hegarty BD, Bobard A, Hainault I, Ferre P, Bossard P, Foufelle F. 2005. Distinct roles of insulin and liver X receptor in the induction and cleavage of sterol regulatory element-binding protein-1c. *Proc. Natl. Acad. Sci. USA* 102:791–96
20. Horton JD, Bashmakov Y, Shimomura I, Shimano H. 1998. Regulation of sterol regulatory element binding proteins in livers of fasted and refed mice. *Proc. Natl. Acad. Sci. USA* 95:5987–92
21. Iizuka K, Bruick RK, Liang G, Horton JD, Uyeda K. 2004. Deficiency of carbohydrate response element-binding protein (ChREBP) reduces lipogenesis as well as glycolysis. *Proc. Natl. Acad. Sci. USA* 101:7281–86
22. Iizuka K, Miller B, Uyeda K. 2006. Deficiency of carbohydrate-activated transcription factor ChREBP prevents obesity and improves plasma glucose control in leptin-deficient (ob/ob) mice. *Am. J. Physiol. Endocrinol. Metab.* 291:E358–64
23. Ishii S, Iizuka K, Miller BC, Uyeda K. 2004. Carbohydrate response element binding protein directly promotes lipogenic enzyme gene transcription. *Proc. Natl. Acad. Sci. USA* 101(44):15597–602
24. Iynedjian PB, Ucla C, Mach B. 1987. Molecular cloning of glucokinase cDNA. Developmental and dietary regulation of glucokinase mRNA in rat liver. *J. Biol. Chem.* 62:6032–38

25. Jiang G, Li Z, Liu F, Ellsworth K, Dallas-Yang Q, et al. 2005. Prevention of obesity in mice by antisense oligonucleotide inhibitors of stearoyl-CoA desaturase-1. *J. Clin. Invest.* 115:1030–38
26. Jump DB. 2004. Fatty acid regulation of gene transcription. *Crit. Rev. Clin. Lab. Sci.* 41:41–78
27. Jump DB, Botolin D, Wang Y, Xu J, Christian B, Demeure O. 2005. Fatty acid regulation of hepatic gene transcription. *J. Nutr.* 135:2503–6
28. Kabashima T, Kawaguchi T, Wadzinski BE, Uyeda K. 2003. Xylulose 5-phosphate mediates glucose-induced lipogenesis by xylulose 5-phosphate-activated protein phosphatase in rat liver. *Proc. Natl. Acad. Sci. USA* 100:5107–12
29. Katsurada A, Iritani N, Fukuda H, Matsumura Y, Nishimoto N, et al. 1990. Effects of nutrients and hormones on transcriptional and post-transcriptional regulation of acetyl-CoA carboxylase in rat liver. *Eur. J. Biochem.* 190:435–41
30. Katsurada A, Iritani N, Fukuda H, Matsumura Y, Noguchi T, Tanaka T. 1989. Effects of nutrients and insulin on transcriptional and post-transcriptional regulation of glucose-6-phosphate dehydrogenase synthesis in rat liver. *Biochim. Biophys. Acta* 1006:104–10
31. Kawaguchi T, Takenoshita M, Kabashima T, Uyeda K. 2001. Glucose and cAMP regulate the L-type pyruvate kinase gene by phosphorylation/dephosphorylation of the carbohydrate response element binding protein. *Proc. Natl. Acad. Sci. USA* 98:13710–15
32. Koo SH, Dutcher AK, Towle HC. 2001. Glucose and insulin function through two distinct transcription factors to stimulate expression of lipogenic enzyme genes in liver. *J. Biol. Chem.* 276:9437–45
33. Li MV, Chang B, Imamura M, Poungvarin N, Chan L. 2006. Glucose-dependent transcriptional regulation by an evolutionarily conserved glucose-sensing module. *Diabetes* 55:1179–89
34. Liang G, Yang J, Horton JD, Hammer RE, Goldstein JL, Brown MS. 2002. Diminished hepatic response to fasting/refeeding and liver X receptor agonists in mice with selective deficiency of sterol regulatory element-binding protein-1c. *J. Biol. Chem.* 277:9520–28
35. Ma L, Robinson LN, Towle HC. 2006. ChREBP/Mlx is the principal mediator of glucose-induced gene expression in the liver. *J. Biol. Chem.* 281:28721–30
36. Ma L, Sham YY, Walters KJ, Towle HC. 2007. A critical role for the loop region of the basic helix-loop-helix/leucine zipper protein Mlx in DNA binding and glucose-regulated transcription. *Nucleic Acids Res.* 35(1):35–44
37. Ma L, Tsatsos NG, Towle HC. 2005. Direct role of ChREBP/Mlx in regulating hepatic glucose-responsive genes. *J. Biol. Chem.* 280:12019–27
38. Magana MM, Osborne TF. 1996. Two tandem binding sites for sterol regulatory element binding proteins are required for sterol regulation of fatty-acid synthase promoter. *J. Biol. Chem.* 271:32689–94
39. Marchesini G, Brizi M, Bianchi G, Tomassetti S, Bugianesi E, et al. 2001. Nonalcoholic fatty liver disease: a feature of the metabolic syndrome. *Diabetes* 50:1844–50
40. Matsusue K, Haluzik M, Lambert G, Yim SH, Gavrilova O, et al. 2003. Liver-specific disruption of PPARgamma in leptin-deficient mice improves fatty liver but aggravates diabetic phenotypes. *J. Clin. Invest.* 111:737–47
41. Meroni G, Cairo S, Merla G, Messali S, Brent R, et al. 2000. Mlx, a new Max-like bHLHZip family member: the center stage of a novel transcription factors regulatory pathway? *Oncogene* 19:3266–77

42. Moriizumi S, Gourdon L, Lefrancois-Martinez AM, Kahn A, Raymondjean M. 1998. Effect of different basic helix-loop-helix leucine zipper factors on the glucose response unit of the L-type pyruvate kinase gene. *Gene Expr.* 7:103–13
43. Ntambi JM. 1992. Dietary regulation of stearoyl-CoA desaturase 1 gene expression in mouse liver. *J. Biol. Chem.* 267:10925–30
44. Pawar A, Xu J, Jerks E, Mangelsdorf DJ, Jump DB. 2002. Fatty acid regulation of liver X receptors (LXR) and peroxisome proliferator-activated receptor alpha (PPARalpha) in HEK293 cells. *J. Biol. Chem.* 277:39243–50
45. Petersen KF, Shulman GI. 2002. Pathogenesis of skeletal muscle insulin resistance in type 2 diabetes mellitus. *Am. J. Cardiol.* 90:11–18G
46. Puigserver P, Spiegelman BM. 2003. Peroxisome proliferator-activated receptor-gamma coactivator 1 alpha (PGC-1 alpha): transcriptional coactivator and metabolic regulator. *Endocr. Rev.* 24:78–90
47. Rahimian R, Masih-Khan E, Lo M, van Breemen C, McManus BM, Dube GP. 2001. Hepatic over-expression of peroxisome proliferator activated receptor gamma2 in the ob/ob mouse model of non-insulin dependent diabetes mellitus. *Mol. Cell Biochem.* 224:29–37
48. Rufo C, Teran-Garcia M, Nakamura MT, Koo SH, Towle HC, Clarke SD. 2001. Involvement of a unique carbohydrate-responsive factor in the glucose regulation of rat liver fatty-acid synthase gene transcription. *J. Biol. Chem.* 276:21969–75
49. Shih HM, Liu Z, Towle HC. 1995. Two CACGTG motifs with proper spacing dictate the carbohydrate regulation of hepatic gene transcription. *J. Biol. Chem.* 270:21991–97
50. Shimano H, Horton JD, Shimomura I, Hammer RE, Brown MS, Goldstein JL. 1997. Isoform 1c of sterol regulatory element binding protein is less active than isoform 1a in livers of transgenic mice and in cultured cells. *J. Clin. Invest.* 99:846–54
51. Shimomura I, Bashmakov Y, Horton JD. 1999. Increased levels of nuclear SREBP-1c associated with fatty livers in two mouse models of diabetes mellitus. *J. Biol. Chem.* 274:30028–32
52. Stoeckman AK, Ma L, Towle HC. 2004. Mlx is the functional heteromeric partner of the carbohydrate response element-binding protein in glucose regulation of lipogenic enzyme genes. *J. Biol. Chem.* 279:15662–69
53. Stoeckman AK, Towle HC. 2002. The role of SREBP-1c in nutritional regulation of lipogenic enzyme gene expression. *J. Biol. Chem.* 277:27029–35
54. Tsatsos NG, Towle HC. 2006. Glucose activation of ChREBP in hepatocytes occurs via a two-step mechanism. *Biochem. Biophys. Res. Commun.* 340:449–56
55. Vaulont S, Munnich A, Decaux JF, Kahn A. 1986. Transcriptional and post-transcriptional regulation of L-type pyruvate kinase gene expression in rat liver. *J. Biol. Chem.* 261:7621–25
56. Vaulont S, Vasseur-Cognet M, Kahn A. 2000. Glucose regulation of gene transcription. *J. Biol. Chem.* 275:31555–58
57. Wei Y, Wang D, Topczewski F, Pagliassotti MJ. 2007. Fructose-mediated stress signaling in the liver: implications for hepatic insulin resistance. *J. Nutr. Biochem.* 18:1–9
58. Wu C, Kang JE, Peng LJ, Li H, Khan SA, et al. 2005. Enhancing hepatic glycolysis reduces obesity: differential effects on lipogenesis depend on site of glycolytic modulation. *Cell Metab.* 2:131–40

59. Yahagi N, Shimano H, Hasty AH, Matsuzaka T, Ide T, et al. 2002. Absence of sterol regulatory element-binding protein-1 (SREBP-1) ameliorates fatty livers but not obesity or insulin resistance in Lep(ob)/Lep(ob) mice. *J. Biol. Chem.* 277:19353–57
60. Yamashita H, Takenoshita M, Sakurai M, Bruick RK, Henzel WJ, et al. 2001. A glucose-responsive transcription factor that regulates carbohydrate metabolism in the liver. *Proc. Natl. Acad. Sci. USA* 98:9116–21

Conserved and Tissue-Specific Genic and Physiologic Responses to Caloric Restriction and Altered IGFI Signaling in Mitotic and Postmitotic Tissues

Stephen R. Spindler[1] and Joseph M. Dhahbi[2]

[1]Department of Biochemistry, University of California, Riverside, California 92521; email: spindler@ucr.edu

[2]Children's Hospital Oakland Research Institute, Oakland, California 94609; email: jdhahbi@chori.org

Annu. Rev. Nutr. 2007. 27:193–217

First published online as a Review in Advance on April 11, 2007

The *Annual Review of Nutrition* is online at http://nutr.annualreviews.org

This article's doi: 10.1146/annurev.nutr.27.061406.093743

0199-9885/07/0821-0193$20.00

Key Words

lifespan, microarray, liver, heart, gene expression, apoptosis

Abstract

Caloric restriction (CR), the consumption of fewer calories without malnutrition, and reduced insulin and/or IGFI receptor signaling delay many age-related physiological changes and extend the lifespan of many model organisms. Here, we present and review microarray and biochemical studies indicating that the potent anticancer effects of CR and disrupted insulin/IGFI receptor signaling evolved as a byproduct of the role of many mitotic tissues as reservoirs of metabolic energy. We argue that the longevity effects of CR are derived from repeated cycles of apoptosis and autophagic cell death in mitotically competent tissues and protein turnover and cellular repair in postmitotic tissues. We review studies showing that CR initiated late in life can rapidly induce many of the benefits of lifelong CR, including its anticancer effects. We also discuss evidence from liver and heart indicating that many benefits of lifelong CR are recapitulated in mitotic and postmitotic tissues when CR is initiated late in life.

Contents

INTRODUCTION

Caloric restriction (CR), the consumption of fewer calories while avoiding malnutrition, has long been known to delay many age-related physiological changes and extend maximum lifespan (the average age of the longest-lived 10% of a cohort) and average lifespan in a phylogenetically diverse group of model organisms, including some species of nematodes, flies, and rodents (82). Long-term CR (LTCR), usually begun shortly after weaning, is a highly effective means of reducing cancer incidence and increasing the mean age of onset of many age-related changes and diseases, including immunosenescence, diabetes, renal disease, and some neurodegenerative diseases (82). LTCR, short-term CR (STCR), and a family of longevity-enhancing mutations in mice can dramatically delay tumor-associated mortality and increase apoptosis in at least some mitotic tissues, including the liver and lung (25, 62). Many of the physiological effects of CR were described 65 years ago (85, 86), and the anticancer benefits were described almost a century ago (96). A combination of genetic and other approaches in lower eukaryotes and mammals have identified genetic, metabolic, and hormonal changes that may underlie some of the health and longevity effects of CR (63).

CR: caloric restriction

LTCR: long-term caloric restriction

STCR: short-term caloric restriction

Evolutionary theory holds that responses to CR evolved early in metazoans as an adaptation to boom and bust cycles in the food supply (48, 104). Because selection acts on reproductively active members of a population, it is difficult to rationalize the potent anticancer effects of CR with this theory. Cancer rates are low during the reproductive period of most mammals, and few individuals live long enough in the wild to die of cancer (104). Thus, the anticancer effects of CR may have evolved as a secondary consequence of another trait that was subject to selection. We argue below that this trait is the metabolic role of some mitotic tissues as reservoirs of metabolic energy.

Potent mechanisms of tumor suppression have evolved to suppress the development of cancer until after the reproductive lifespan has ended (see, e.g., 115). Unfortunately, these mechanisms also appear to reduce the potential for tissue regeneration later in life (8, 58, 71, 94). In long-lived rodents, which die primarily of neoplasms, the anticancer effects of CR underlie its lifespan benefits (121). Gerontologists often conjecture that CR slows the "underlying rate of aging" because it increases maximum lifespan. However, in mice, CR can rapidly extend maximum and average lifespan by decreasing the rate of tumor growth (22 and S.R. Spindler, unpublished results). Whether this is rightly viewed as decreasing the rate of aging is open to debate. Thus, it is an open question whether the concept of "underlying rate of aging," which has never been well defined, has any real meaning.

CONSERVED ADAPTATIONS TO CR IN MITOTIC AND POSTMITOTIC TISSUES

Holliday (48) first proposed that CR is an evolutionary adaptation that diverts limited energy resources from breeding to maintenance. In this part of the review, we present a reanalysis of our published Affymetrix microarray data. It suggests that CR produces a common genic response in heart and liver that is related to a redistribution of metabolic energy. In these tissues, CR appears to decrease protein flux through the endoplasmic reticulum (ER) and Golgi, protein import into the mitochondria, glycoprotein degradation, protein and RNA trafficking between the nucleus and cytoplasm, nucleotide and nucleic acid metabolism, and inflammation. These results are consistent with the general reduction in the rates of protein, RNA, lipid, and DNA synthesis that are found in CR animals (e.g., 14, 15, 75, 89). We argue here that it is the role of tissue protein and lipid as reversible sources of metabolic energy that leads to many of the anticancer and longevity-related effects of CR.

Microarray Data Analysis

The data obtained in large-scale microarray studies is often misinterpreted. Gene lists produced using different analytical platforms and statistical tools are sometimes compared to identify similarly changed genes. One such comparison of microarray results obtained with tissues from mice, rats, pigs, monkeys, yeast, and flies found no common genes that were responsive to CR (43). But, this result would be expected, even if similarly changed genes exist. All large-scale microarray studies require sophisticated analytical and statistical tools to remove false positives and maximize the number of real positives identified. As the statistical stringency of the analysis increases to cull false positives from the set of found genes, fewer real positives remain. Further, even when identical data sets are analyzed with different statistical tools, only partially overlapping gene sets are identified (110). For example, we used two different statistical methods on a single data set and only found ~50% overlap between the sets of genes that were identified (28).

A better way to make such comparisons is to use data from a single array platform, globally normalize all probe set results, and apply identical analytical and statistical tests to all the normalized data. We used this approach to reanalyze our Affymetrix data from heart and liver (14, 22, 23, 28, 126). This new analysis identified 32 genes that were similarly responsive to CR in heart and liver (**Table 1**). All but two of these genes were downregulated. The genes fall into a number of functional groups (**Tables 1** and **2**).

ER: endoplasmic reticulum

Conserved Responses

CR decreases the rate of DNA and protein synthesis and decreases the RNA content of the liver, kidney, heart, and small intestine in rats (32, 38, 75, 88–92). Despite decreased synthetic rates, LTCR animals appear to maintain their organ mass by decreasing the rate of protein degradation (see below). In LTCR animals, the sum of these effects appears to produce higher rates of protein turnover and smaller visceral organ sizes (132). CR begun in older control mice reduces organ sizes and increases the rate of protein turnover (see below).

Chaperones. LTCR downregulated five major cytoplasmic and ER chaperones in heart and liver (**Table 1**). This was found even though LTCR protects cardiomyocytes from apoptotic and necrotic cell death throughout life (28). The three ER chaperone genes downregulated in liver and heart, *Hspa5* (also known as GRP78 or BiP), *Calr* (calreticulin), and *Pdia3* (Grp58), have major roles

Table 1 Genes changed by long-term caloric restriction in both liver and heart[a]

Symbol	Name	Heart CR/Con FC[b]	Liver CR/Con FC	Function
Glycoprotein catabolism				
Aga	Aspartylglucose-aminidase	−1.6	−1.4	One of the final steps in lysosomal breakdown of glycoproteins. It cleaves the amide bond between asparagine and the oligosaccharide.
Aspa	Aspartoacylase (aminoacylase) 2	−1.4	−1.3	Nuclear and cytoplasmic membrane enzyme that catabolizes the terminal N-acylpeptides or N-acylated amino acids. It is a scavenger of N-acetylaspartic acid.
Asrgl1	Asparaginase-like 1	−1.3	−1.3	Mainly a mitochondrial enzyme that catalyzes the conversion of L-asparagine to aspartic acid and ammonia.
Dpp3	Dipeptidylpeptidase 3	−1.4	−1.3	Releases an N-terminal dipeptide from a peptide composed of four or more amino acids, including angiotensin and enkephalin. Has a broad specificity.
Fbxo6b	F box–only protein 6b (Frap)	−1.5	−1.4	ER-associated enzyme that targets sugar chains in N-linked glycoproteins for ubiquitination and degradation. Involved in ER quality control and the calnexin-calreticulin cycle. Plays a role in the differentiation and hepatocyte proliferation.
Hexa	Hexosaminidase A (alpha polypeptide)	−1.7	−1.5	α subunit of the lysosomal β-hexosaminidase that catalyzes the degradation of molecules containing terminal N-acetyl hexosamines.
Manba	Mannosidase, beta A, lysosomal	−1.4	−1.3	Catalyzes the penultimate step in lysosomal N-linked oligosaccharide catabolism. Cleaves the single β-linked mannose residue from the nonreducing end of all N-linked glycoprotein oligosaccharides.
Nagk	N-acetyl-glucosamine kinase	−1.5	−1.4	Converts endogenous GlcNAc produced by lysosomal degradation or from nutritional sources into GlcNAc 6-phosphate, which can enter further catabolic or anabolic pathways.
Protein processing/repair				
Mipep	Mitochondrial intermediate peptidase	−1.6	−1.4	Releases an N-terminal octapeptide as the second stage in processing some proteins imported into the mitochondria.
Msrb2	Methionine sulfoxide reductase B2	−1.3	−1.4	Mainly a mitochondrial enzyme that repairs oxidative damage to methionine residues. Implicated as one of the primary defenses against oxidative stress.
Psen2	Presenilin 2	−1.8	−1.4	ER and *cis*-Golgi localized, catalytic subunit of the endoprotease γ-secretase complex that catalyzes the intramembrane cleavage of integral membrane proteins such as the Notch receptors and the β-amyloid precursor protein.
Chaperones				
Calr	Calreticulin	−1.3	−1.4	Major lumenal ER chaperone. Major Ca^{2+}-binding and storage protein. It has a key role in the calreticulin/calnexin quality control cycle. In the nucleus it inhibits retinoic acid, glucocorticoid, and androgen receptor action.

(*Continued*)

Table 1 (*Continued*)

Symbol	Name	Heart CR/Con FC[b]	Liver CR/Con FC	Function
Fkbp3	FK506-binding protein 3; peptidylprolyl isomerase; cyclophilin; (rotamases)	−1.3	−1.3	Nuclear immunophilin involved in protein folding and trafficking. Its inhibition in cancer cells suppresses proliferation, the transformed phenotype, and tumorigenicity.
Fkbp5	FK506-binding protein 5; peptidylprolyl *cis*-trans isomerases (rotamases)	2.0	2.1	Immunophilin involved in protein folding and trafficking. It is part of a heteromultimeric cytoplasmic complex with HSP90, HSP70, and some steroid hormone receptors. Dissociates when glucocorticoid receptor binds its ligand. Induced by progestins and androgens.
Hspa5	GRP78; BiP; heat shock 70kD protein 5	−1.8 to −1.5	−1.6	Major lumenal ER chaperone. When induced can be antiapoptotic by binding some caspases.
Pdia3	GRP58; protein disulfide isomerase family A, member 3	−1.9	−1.4	Major luminal ER protein disulfide isomerase that binds calreticulin and calnexin to modulate folding of newly synthesized glycoproteins. Involved in quality control. Interacts with the DNA-binding domain of the glucocorticoid receptor to mediate its nuclear export.
Triap1	TP53-regulated inhibitor of apoptosis 1	−1.6	−1.3	p53-inducible gene involved in the p53-dependent cell-survival pathway. In response to low levels of DNA damage, it inhibits apoptosis by inhibiting activation of caspase-9.
Transporters				
Slc44a1	Solute carrier family 44, member 1	−1.4	−1.3	Probable choline transporter in the plasma membrane. Choline is a major source of methyl groups that participates in S-adenosylmethionine biosynthesis.
Inflammation				
Comt	Catechol-O-methyltransferase	−1.6	−1.3	Involved in catecholamine degradation and in detoxification. Likely low because serum catecholamine levels are low.
Hpgd	Hydroxyprostaglandin dehydrogenase 15 (NAD)	−1.4	−1.5	Rate-limiting enzyme for PGE2 and PGF2α catabolism. Likely low because PGE2, which is produced by macrophages, is low.
Il13ra1	Interleukin-13 receptor alpha-1 chain precursor	−2.7	−1.4	Plasma membrane receptor capable of transducing a proliferative signal in response to IL13. In eosinophils, IFNG, TNFA, and particularly TGFB enhance its expression. Overexpressed in tumor cells.
Lyzs	Lysozyme (renal amyloidosis)	−2.2	−1.6	A myeloid cell-specific marker induced by macrophage activation.
Protein and nucleic acid nuclear export/import				
Cblb	Casitas B-lineage lymphoma b; Cas-Br-M (murine) ecotropic retroviral transforming sequence b	1.6	1.3	Key role in protein import into the nucleus. E3 ubiquitin-protein ligase accepts ubiquitin from specific E2 ubiquitin-conjugating enzymes and transfers it to substrates, generally promoting their degradation by the proteosome.

(*Continued*)

Table 1 (*Continued*)

Symbol	Name	Heart CR/Con FC[b]	Liver CR/Con FC	Function
Ddx39	DEAD (Asp-Glu-Ala-Asp)-box polypeptide 39	−1.3	−1.4	Involved in pre-mRNA splicing and the export of mature mRNA from the nucleus. Upregulated in proliferating cells. Lower levels in quiescent cells.
G3BP2	Ras-GTPase activating protein SH3 domain-binding protein 2	−1.4	−1.3	Implicated in Ras, NFκB signaling, the ubiquitin proteasome pathway, and RNA processing. Retains IκBα and IκBα/NFκB complexes in the cytoplasm.
Ipo11	Importin 11	−1.4	−1.3	Functions in nuclear protein import as a receptor for nuclear localization signals in cargo substrates. Thought to mediate docking of the importin/substrate complex to the nuclear pore complex.
Ncbp1; Refbp2	Nuclear cap–binding protein subunit 1, 80 kDa	−1.6	−1.3	Present in a U snRNA export complex with m7G-capped RNA. Subunit of the exon junction complex.
Pttg1ip	Pituitary tumor–transforming 1 interacting protein precursor	−1.3	−1.5	A multifunctional human securin oncogene, with roles in mitosis, cell transformation, DNA repair, gene regulation, and fetal development. Overexpression has been reported in multiple tumor types. Interacts with p53 and blocks its activity by blocking its binding to DNA.
Nucleotide/nucleic acid metabolism				
Dtymk	Thymidylate kinase; dTMP kinase	−1.7	−1.4	Thymidylate kinase activity parallel rates of cell cycle progression and growth.
Nudt1	Nudix (nucleoside diphosphate-linked moiety X)-type motif 1	−1.5	−1.7	Hydrolyzes 8-oxo-dGTP to 8-oxo-dGMP, preventing its misincorporation into DNA, which would lead to A:T to C:G transversions.
Nudt2	Nudix (nucleoside diphosphate-linked moiety X)-type motif 2	−1.4	−1.5	Asymmetrically hydrolyzes Ap4A to yield AMP and ATP. Plays a major role in maintaining nucleotide homeostasis. Ap4A and other dinucleotides participate in blood pressure regulation.
Pnkp	Polynucleotide kinase 3′-phosphatase (ATP-dependent poly-deoxyribonucleotide 5′-hydroxyl-kinase) Ap4a (murine)	−1.6	−1.4	Catalyzes the phosphorylation of nuclear DNA at 5′-hydroxyl termini and can dephosphorylate the 3′-phosphate termini. Has an important function in DNA repair following oxidative damage.

[a]Probe set data from our published studies were reanalyzed to identify genes that were similarly responsive to LTCR in both liver and heart (14, 22, 28, 122, 126). The Entrez, GeneCard, Bioinformatic Harvester, NCBI OMIM, and PubMed databases were used to identify functions.
[b]Abbreviations: AMP, adenosine monophosphate; ATP, adenosine triphosphate; Con, control; CR, caloric restriction; ER, endoplasmic reticulum; FC, fold change; LTCR, long-term caloric restriction.

in the ER stress response, protein folding, glycosylation, the calreticulin/calnexin cycle, and quality control. We previously reported that STCR and/or LTCR downregulate many ER and several cytoplasmic chaperones in the liver, skeletal muscle, kidney, and heart of mice (14, 20–22, 24, 28, 123, 126). A number of ER and cytoplasmic chaperones

Table 2 Comparison of the categories of the genes altered by long-term caloric restriction and short-term caloric restriction in the liver and heart of mice

Liver specific[a]	Conserved in liver and heart	Heart specific
Down[b]	**Down**	**Down**
Glycolysis	Chaperones and stress response	Fibrosis- and tissue-remodeling related
Intracellular signaling	Glycoprotein catabolism	Extracellular matrix, cytoskeletal structure and dynamics
Up	Protein and RNA nuclear import and export	Cell motility
Fatty acid oxidation and lipid catabolism	Inflammation and immune activation	Blood pressure and hemodynamic stress
Gluconeogenesis	**Mixed**	Signal transduction, differentiation, cell division
Proapoptotic	Xenobiotic, oxidant and toxicant metabolism	Protein degradation
Ureagenesis		**Up**
		PPARα signaling (enhanced energy homeostasis)
		cAMP (enhanced cardiac contractility)
		Mixed (but mostly downregulated)
		Proapoptotic

[a]The genes were assigned to functional groups by reference to our previous publications (14, 22, 28, 122, 126) and using the Entrez, GeneCard, Bioinformatic Harvester, NCBI OMIM, and PubMed databases.
[b]Down, decreased by CR; up, increased by CR relative to control; mixed, genes were both up- and downregulated.

are additively downregulated by the combination of LTCR and the Ames dwarf mutation (126). Ames dwarf mice are homozygous for a loss-of-function mutation in the Prop1 gene, leading to reduced serum levels of insulin like growth factor I (IGFI) and other hormones produced by or released in response to signaling from the anterior pituitary (119). Fasting also downregulates and refeeding upregulates cytoplasmic and ER chaperones, possibly in response to changes in blood insulin and glucagon levels (20, 21). Two chaperone genes recently were reported to be downregulated by CR in mouse heart, liver, and hypothalamus (37). These results are consistent with a reduced level of protein synthesis and trafficking in the mitotic and postmitotic tissues of fasted, CR, and Ames dwarf mice.

It is often posited that chaperone overexpression should extend lifespan (e.g., 44, 45). Transient induction of heat shock proteins does extend the lifespan of nematodes (101). However, it is highly unlikely that heat shock proteins [which are undetectable at all times in control and CR mice (unpublished results)] are ever induced in animals that are conventionally maintained in a vivarium. Many of the chaperones that normally are expressed in vivo are downregulated by LTCR, STCR, and starvation, as described above. There is no reason to expect that constitutive overexpression of chaperones should extend mammalian lifespan. Chaperones are pleiotropic in their actions. Some initiate protein degradation as well as protein folding and maturation (113). A number of chaperones bind caspases, negatively regulate apoptosis, and promote carcinogenesis (109, 113, 137). For example, calreticulin has roles in secretory pathway quality control, intracellular Ca^{2+} homeostasis, ER Ca^{2+} storage, early cardiac development, autoimmunity, and cancer (134). In mice, most chaperones are downregulated by LTCR at all times, especially before feeding (20, 21, 24, 97). Feeding induces the expression of some chaperones, matching their abundance to that of their substrates, which are postprandially synthesized proteins (20, 21).

IGFI: insulin-like growth factor I

Intracellular protein and RNA trafficking. Seven glycoprotein-catabolism–related genes were downregulated in heart and liver (**Table 1**). Downregulation of the *Psen2* (presenilin 2) gene is consistent with the general downregulation of protein trafficking in the ER. Presenilin 2 is the catalytic subunit of the γ-secretase complex, the maturase that processes membrane proteins like β-amyloid precursor protein and the Notch receptors. Together, these results suggest that CR reduces the rates of glycoprotein synthesis and catabolism in heart and liver. These changes must be viewed in the context of a general decrease in macromolecular synthesis and turnover, which nonetheless results in enhanced rates of protein turnover for energy production (see below). Pulse-chase studies in hepatocytes isolated from LTCR mice demonstrated that downregulation of ER chaperones paradoxically increases the efficiency of trans-ER-Golgi transport and protein secretion, probably by decreasing protein degradation in the ER (21). Thus, the liver appears to adapt to reduced dietary energy by increasing the efficiency of protein secretion.

Further evidence for reduced synthesis and trafficking of macromolecules in the liver and heart of CR mice comes from the downregulation of six genes involved in protein and RNA import and export from the nucleus, and four genes involved in DNA and RNA synthesis and repair (**Table 1**). For example, the product of the downregulated Ddx39 gene, an RNA helicase, is required for pre-mRNA splicing and nuclear export. It is downregulated in quiescent cells, consistent with other data suggesting there is a decrease in the rate of cell growth and division in CR animals (46, 61). However, despite decreased rates of cell division in CR animals, the liver cells of CR rats appear to respond more promptly to toxic challenge and promitogenic signaling than those of controls (4).

Inflammation. The downregulation of four inflammation-related genes in LTCR liver and heart is consistent with the reduced inflammation often reported for LTCR mice (15; **Table 1**). For example, Lyzs (lysozyme) is an inducible marker of macrophage activation and inflammatory disease (16, 64). IL13R (interleukin 13 receptor) is overexpressed in human tumor cells (116), and IL-13 is a major inducer of fibrosis through induction of transforming growth factor β1 in macrophages (34). Thus, downregulation of these genes is consistent with reduced inflammation and macrophage activation in the heart and liver of CR mice. Other conserved changes reported above may represent changes in macrophage and/or white blood cell–related gene expression.

CR, CANCER, AND MITOTIC TISSUES

We do not know how CR extends the lifespan of any organism, not even that of the intensively studied model organisms such as *C. elegans* and mouse. Genetic studies in *C. elegans* have elegantly defined genes and genetic pathways capable of extending lifespan (63). However, we do not know why nematodes die of old age; therefore, we do not know how these longevity pathways extend lifespan. There is a similar problem with mice. Most laboratory strains of mice die of a few, strain-specific types of tumors, often hepatomas and/or lymphomas (22, 121, 127). However, since the discovery of the potent anticancer effects of LTCR nearly a century ago, there have been almost no mechanistic studies of how CR prevents death from the spontaneous tumors that actually kill the mice. Essentially all CR-related studies of cancer use transplanted or induced tumors (53). Although this work has been illuminating, there is no clear evidence that these models recapitulate the mechanisms at work in the spontaneous tumors that actually limit, and thereby determine, the lifespan of mice.

As discussed above, a decrease in the rate of tumor growth increases the maximum lifespan of mice. The extension of maximum lifespan is normally thought to be indicative of decelerated aging. However, for the reasons discussed above, screening for longevity therapeutics in mice will likely identify mostly compounds that intervene in tumorigenesis (23, 122). Paradoxically, this may also identify therapeutics with other longevity-enhancing effects. Many of the molecular pathways controlling lifespan in nematodes, which do not normally die of tumors, also reduce the growth rate of a mutationally induced tumor in this organism (106). Thus, the ancient pathways controlling longevity in metazoans are highly pleiotropic in their effects. Most of the interventions known to extend lifespan also alter key signaling systems controlling the expression of relatively large batteries of "effector" genes (7, 76, 126). Thus, the pathways capable of extending lifespan in metazoans appear to have been selected for their ability to directly target the wide array of disease processes that lead to death.

CANCER, CR, AND REDUCED ANTERIOR PITUITARY SIGNALING

Relatively few cancers arise from postmitotic cells (135). Cell division is required to genetically fix oncogenic mutations. As discussed above, selection acts on reproductively active members of a population, and few mice live long enough to die of cancer in the wild (104). Highly effective molecular mechanisms have evolved to suppress the development of cancer until after reproduction ceases. These include mechanisms for high fidelity DNA replication and repair, and tumor suppressor genes such as $p16^{INK4a}$ and ARF. The expression of $p16^{INK4a}$ and ARF increases with age in stem and possibly other cell types, upregulating the retinoblastoma and p53 pathways, respectively (58, 71, 94). In mice, this upregulation may suppress the development of cancer until after the end of the reproductive lifespan (115). Thus, the anticancer effects of CR may have coevolved with another phenotype, which was subject to natural selection. Below we discuss published studies suggesting that CR drives higher rates of protein and lipid turnover in postmitotic and mitotic tissues, and the apoptotic and/or autophagic turnover of cells in mitotically competent tissues. We postulate that this turnover drives many of the beneficial effects of CR on health and lifespan.

A widely accepted model proposes that carcinogenesis involves three steps: initiation, an initial mutation in a tumor suppressor gene; promotion, the accumulation of mutations in cell growth or proliferation-related genes; and progression, a gain in tumor mass through increased rates of cell proliferation and/or reduced rates of apoptosis (53). The relative rates of proliferation and apoptosis during promotion and progression are major determinants of the rates of tumor onset and growth. LTCR reduces carcinogenesis at every stage of this model (53). LTCR increases the age of onset and decreases the rate of growth and number of metastases produced by model tumors, including hepatomas, mammary carcinomas, and prostatic tumors (53, 133). LTCR suppresses the carcinogenic action of several classes of chemicals, inhibits several forms of radiation-induced cancer, and inhibits neoplasia in early-tumor-onset knockout and transgenic mouse models (53). There is compelling evidence that in mitotic tissues, LTCR enhances the rate of apoptosis in preneoplastic, tumor, and normal cells. Preneoplastic and tumor cells appear to be more susceptible to apoptosis than normal cells. For example, the rate of apoptosis, as measured using terminal dUTP nick end labeling (TUNEL) of apoptotic bodies, is three times higher in hepatocytes of CR mice at all ages (55, 56, 98). Increased hepatocyte apoptosis is associated with a significantly lower incidence of spontaneous hepatomas throughout the life of LTCR mice, although the mechanism remains unknown. Even brief periods of CR enhance apoptosis and reduce tumor incidence. For example, one to three months of food restriction can significantly increase the latency and reduce the incidence of spontaneous cancer over the entire lifespan of a mouse (65). Just one week of CR induces apoptosis of the glutathione S-transferase-II-positive (an immunohistochemical marker of preneoplastic liver cells) hepatocytes of old mice (99). Forty-percent food restriction for three months eliminates 20% to 30% of liver cells through apoptosis and reduces the number and volume of chemically induced preneoplastic foci by 85% (40). CR also enhances apoptosis in mitotically competent cells of other organs, including jejunum, colon, bladder, and dexamethasone-treated lymph node and spleen lymphocytes of MRL/lpr mice (49, 78). We found that CR begun at 19 months of age in C3B6F1 mice (at the beginning of the accelerated mortality phase of their lifespan) decreases tumor-associated mortality by 3.1-fold within eight weeks and extends both mean and maximum lifespan (22, 121). These effects appear to be due to a reduction in the rate of tumor growth (22, 121). Because CR does not appear to reduce the rate of tumor-cell division, it probably increases their rate of apoptosis or autophagic cell death (S.R. Spindler, Y. Higami, & I. Shimokawa, unpublished results).

Tumorigenesis can involve inactivation of tumor suppressor genes, activation of oncogenes, overexpression of growth factors, and inappropriate growth factor signaling. LTCR, STCR, methionine restriction, and a family of mutations in mice dramatically extend lifespan and reduce insulin and IGFI serum levels and postreceptor signaling (6, 7, 25, 62, 68, 80). They also delay tumor-associated mortality and increase apoptosis in mitotic tissues, including the liver (25, 29, 62, 67). The IGFI receptor plays the major role in mitogenesis, transformation, tumorigenicity, and protection from apoptosis in vivo (1, 2, 12, 50–52, 103). For example, neoplastic lesions and the incidence of adenocarcinoma are reduced in lung, and the growth of spontaneous and transplanted tumors is reduced in Ames dwarf mice (54). Serum IGFI levels are reduced by many of the interventions that extend mammalian lifespan in rodents (6, 7, 76, 111). In tumor cells, IGFI acts as an autocrine/paracrine growth factor as well as an inhibitor of apoptosis (111). IGFI receptor is emerging as a critical factor in hepatocarcinogenesis (112). Defects in IGFI receptor expression and/or activation inhibit tumorigenicity, reverse the transformed phenotype, and cause massive apoptosis in vitro and in vivo (13, 111). CR has a well-described anticarcinogenic effect on spontaneous and chemically induced tumors (53). Reduced proliferation and increased apoptosis are thought to be responsible (53). Downregulation of fatty acid synthase and fatty acid biosynthesis by CR and the dwarf mutations also may be a source of its antioncogenic effects (14, 72, 108, 126). Both are required for the survival of many human cancer cell lines. The inhibition of fatty acid synthase rapidly leads to apoptosis in tumor cells (72, 108).

In one genomewide microarray study of liver gene expression, we found that 21% of the genes that changed expression in response to LTCR are associated with apoptosis, cell growth, or cell survival (14). For example, LTCR induced the expression of the BAK1 and VDAC1 genes. The products of these genes interact to release cytochrome c from mitochondria, initiating apoptosis (117). The rapid induction of Vdac1 after four weeks of CR is consistent with the increase in apoptosis and reduction in chemical carcinogenesis also found in fasting rodents (14, 47, 65, 107).

PROTEIN TURNOVER AND GLUCONEOGENESIS

Cellular turnover in metazoans involves degradation of cytoplasmic and nuclear proteins by cellular calpains (118) and the proteosome (100); degradation of mitochondria by mitochondrial proteases (5); autophagic degradation of membranes, mitochondria, ribosomes, ER, and peroxisomes (10, 30, 60); and cellular turnover initiated by apoptotic, necrotic, and autophagic cell death (59). Nutritional stress increases the rate of these processes (35). LTCR (30%) reduces the weight of the heart, liver, kidney, spleen, prostate, and skeletal muscle of rats by 25% to 50% (132).

This reduction appears to be due to both decreased rates of macromolecular synthesis and cell division (32, 38, 75, 88–92) and increased rates of cell death and macromolecular degradation. Mitotically competent tissues such as liver and lung undergo a profound, rapid, and reversible loss of cell number (via necrosis, apoptosis, and/or autophagic cell death), protein, and lipid after the initiation of either CR or fasting (69, 83). For example, fasting for 48 hours reduces liver weight by half and liver proliferative index by 85% while increasing its apoptotic index by 2.5-fold (70). The number of lung alveoli in mice is reduced by 35% after 72 hours of 33% CR (83). Fifteen days of CR reduces alveolar number by 45% (83). Refeeding for 72 hours fully restores alveolar number (83). Thus, CR appears to tip the regulatory balance in some mitotic tissues toward apoptosis and the degradation of cellular carbohydrate, protein, and lipid.

AGING AND ENERGY METABOLISM

Aging produces a decline in the autophagic and apoptotic turnover of cells, organelles, membranes, carbohydrates, and proteins (10, 30). It also decreases the enzymatic capacity for utilizing protein for the production of metabolic energy (120). During the postabsorptive state, when blood insulin and glucose levels begin to wane and glucagon, glucocorticoids, and catecholamines increase, most tissues begin to utilize glycogen and amino acids derived from protein turnover to generate energy via the tricarboxylic acid cycle. This drives the autophagic degradation of proteins, organelles, and membranes. Amino acid catabolism is initiated by two enzymatic steps, collectively called transdeamination (**Figure 1**). The enzymatic capacities for many of these transdeamination reactions are enhanced in the liver of LTCR mice (41). Transdeamination leads to the liberation of the amino nitrogen as ammonia, which is transferred to glutamate by glutamine synthetase (GS) to produce glutamine. Glutamine is the major shuttle for nitrogen and carbon between tissues in most mammals. In the liver, it is used for both gluconeogenesis and ureagenesis. Aging decreases the expression of muscle GS in mice (26), suggesting that the enzymatic capacity for the metabolism of the products of protein turnover decreases with age. In rats, muscle GS levels increase with age, except for 55% of the oldest animals, where levels are reduced (105). These results suggest that the enzymatic adjustments to muscle protein turnover with age may be more complex in rats than in mice.

CPSI: carbamylphosphate synthase-1

Glutamine produced in muscle is metabolized by glutaminase in the liver to glutamate and ammonia (**Figure 1**). Because of its extreme toxicity, the ammonia is channeled into the urea cycle for detoxification and disposal. The decrease in muscle GS found in aged mice is consistent with the decrease in hepatic carbamylphosphate synthase-1 (CPSI), GS, and tyrosine amino transferase with age (14, 25, 26, 120, 125; **Figure 1**).

Glutamate (and other amino acids) undergoes transdeamination in the liver and enters the tricarboxylic acid cycle as oxaloacetate (or pyruvate; **Figure 2**). Once oxaloacetate is converted to phosphoenolpyruvate by phosphoenolpyruvate carboxykinase (PEPCK), it will be converted to glucose by hepatocytes. PEPCK is the key gating enzyme of gluconeogenesis. Glucose-6-phosphatase (G6Pase) hydrolyzes glucose 6-phosphate to glucose, thereby releasing it from hepatocytes into the circulation (**Figure 2**). This glucose is utilized for energy by the brain and other organs. Aging decreases the expression of liver and kidney PEPCK and G6Pase and decreases PEPCK levels in the skeletal muscle of mice (20, 26, 120; **Figure 2**). Others have confirmed many of these results (41, 42). These changes are consistent with the decrease in whole-body protein turnover that occurs with age (39, 75).

At the level of enzymatic capacity, the changes in metabolic enzyme expression described above are most likely the result of

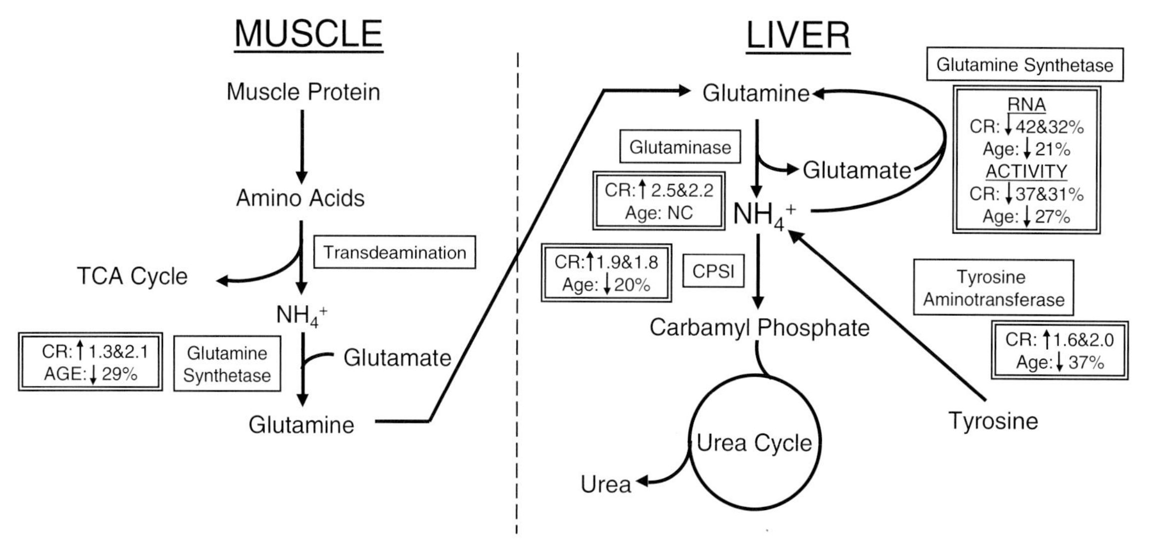

Figure 1

Summary of the effects of age and diet on muscle and liver nitrogen metabolism. In muscle and many other tissues, the degradation of proteins to amino acids is utilized for generating metabolic energy. Transdeamination of amino acids produces tricarboxylic acid cycle intermediates and ammonia. Glutamine synthetase synthesizes glutamine from glutamate and ammonia. Glutamine is transported to the liver in the blood, where glutaminase releases the ammonia, regenerating glutamate. Carbamylphosphate synthase-1 (CPSI) converts this ammonia to carbamylphosphate, which is converted to urea by the urea cycle. The amino group of excess tyrosine is released by tyrosine aminotransferase as ammonia, which is also detoxified beginning with the action of CPSI. In the figure, substrates are not boxed, enzyme names are in shaded boxes, and summaries of experimental results are in double-bordered boxes. When two values are given following "CR," they represent the fold change in young and old mice, respectively. The value after "Age" is the main effect of age. A down arrow indicates the percent decrease; an up arrow indicates the fold increase. The value given for age is a combination of both dietary groups. NC is no change.

CR-related adjustments of insulin, glucocorticoid, thyroid hormone, and IGFI levels, and not of changes in substrate availability (27, 124). Thus, the adjustments in enzymatic capacity are a cause rather than an effect of decreased protein turnover during aging (129, 130). Although the studies reviewed focused on the liver and muscle, protein turnover in all or most tissues of the body appears to decline with age (32, 38, 75, 88, 91, 92). Decreased macromolecular turnover may underlie the age-related accumulation of oxidatively damaged protein. This decrease may exacerbate the effects of the oft-reported age-related increase in oxidant production by isolated muscle mitochondria (e.g., 9, 81).

LTCR, STCR, AND AMES DWARFISM: GLUCONEOGENESIS, GLYCOLYSIS, AND LIPOGENESIS

In 1989, Feuers et al. (33) published the first study suggesting that the enzymatic capacity of the liver for gluconeogenesis increases, and the enzymatic capacity for glycolysis decreases, in LTCR mice. Using a variety of biochemical and genic approaches, we were able to confirm and extend these studies (25–27, 124–126). We found that LTCR, STCR, and the Ames dwarf mutation induce the fasting and fed levels of PEPCK and G6Pase activity and/or mRNA in liver (14, 25, 120, 124, 126; **Figures 1** and **2**). G6Pase mRNA is more abundant in LTCR mice, at all times, even 1.5 hours after feeding (25, 26). STCR and LTCR elevated PEPCK mRNA in both young and old mice (25, 26). PEPCK mRNA and activity decrease within 1.5 hours of feeding, but by 5 hours after feeding, CR mice accumulated twice as much PEPCK mRNA and activity as did control mice (25). LTCR and dwarfism together additively enhanced PEPCK, glucose-6-phosphate isomerase, and glycerol-6-phosphate transporter mRNA (126). The latter two enzymes also have important roles in gluconeogenesis. Thus, LTCR, STCR, and reduced anterior pituitary signaling oppose the age-related decrease in protein turnover by reversing many age-related effects on the activity and/or mRNA of key gluconeogenic enzymes (25–27, 124–126).

Evidence that LTCR enhances protein turnover and utilization for energy production is also found in the expression of nitrogen metabolizing genes. LTCR increases GS expression in muscle and decreases GS activity and mRNA in the liver (**Figure 1**), even 1.5 hours after feeding (25, 26). Dwarfism also reduces hepatic glutamine synthetase expression (126). These effects spare glutamate reutilization for glutamine production, thereby fueling hepatic gluconeogenesis and ureagenesis. LTCR leads to a 2.5-fold increase in hepatic glutaminase mRNA (26; **Figure 1**). The level of this mRNA closely reflects hepatic glutaminase activity (136). CPSI mRNA in young and old CR mice is two to five times its level in control mice (25, 26, 125). CPSI gene transcription responds rapidly to reduced caloric intake, leading to a rapid increase in CPSI mRNA, protein, and activity (125). The initiation of CR also rapidly induces three other urea cycle enzymes, argininosuccinate synthetase 1, argininosuccinate lyase, and arginase 1 (22). Together, these results indicate that CR animals have a significantly enhanced capacity for protein turnover, gluconeogenesis, and nitrogen disposal for energy generation, even soon after feeding. A number of these results have been confirmed by others (33, 41, 66, 77).

The changes in gene expression discussed above are most likely the result of CR- or dwarfism-related alterations in insulin, glucocorticoid, thyroid hormone, and/or IGFI levels (reviewed in 27, 124). This suggests that CR mice catabolize protein derived from proteolysis, autophagy, and the autophagic and apoptotic death of mitotically competent cells to generate substrates for energy production. CR mice are approximately four times more insulin sensitive than control mice, leading to greatly reduced serum insulin levels (25). Insulin also can be a strongly antiapoptotic comitogen in the liver and other tissues (11). After feeding, increased blood insulin levels drive a compensatory wave of macromolecular biosynthesis and cell division (25). Thereafter, as glucoregulatory hormone levels respond to fasting, carbon and nitrogen from liver and other tissues begin to flow back to the liver for gluconeogenesis and disposal, respectively. In this way, CR appears to drive balanced waves of catabolism and compensatory resynthesis, resulting in both decreased tumor initiation and growth and reduced accumulation of damaged macromolecules. In both LTCR and dwarf mice, these cycles appear to produce smaller mice with smaller organs.

LTCR and Ames dwarf mice also underexpress the key gating enzymes of glycolysis (glucokinase, pyruvate kinase, and acetyl-CoA carboxykinase), which suggests that both decrease substrate availability for de novo liver lipogenesis (25, 126). Both of these longevity enhancers decreased the hepatic expression of 16 lipid- and cholesterol-related genes, including genes involved in lipid, fatty acid, and cholesterol biosynthesis, lipid transport, and HDL metabolism (126). Further, they induce eight genes for key fatty acid β-oxidation enzymes, several of which are additively induced by the combined treatments. LTCR also decreases the mRNA and activity of the key gating enzyme of fatty acid biosynthesis, pyruvate dehydrogenase, even in the hours following feeding (25, 26, 120). Together, these results suggest that two means of lifespan extension produce a sustained decrease in lipogenesis and enhancement of lipolysis in the liver. Others have confirmed a number of these results (42). As mentioned above, fatty acid biosynthesis appears to be required for the survival of many cancer cells (72, 108).

STRESS RESISTANCE IN POSTMITOTIC CELLS

Although there are similarities in the genic responses of heart and liver to LTCR, the differences may be most apposite to its differential effects on mitotic and postmitotic tissues (**Table 2**). For example, although CR shifted liver toward a genic profile consistent with increased apoptotic cell death, no such shift was found in heart (28). CR is known to suppress apoptotic cell death and increase the stress resistance of the cardiovascular and cerebrovascular systems in vivo (84). Apoptotic or autophagic loss of postmitotic cells in these tissues would be highly disadvantageous, and the oncogenic transformation of

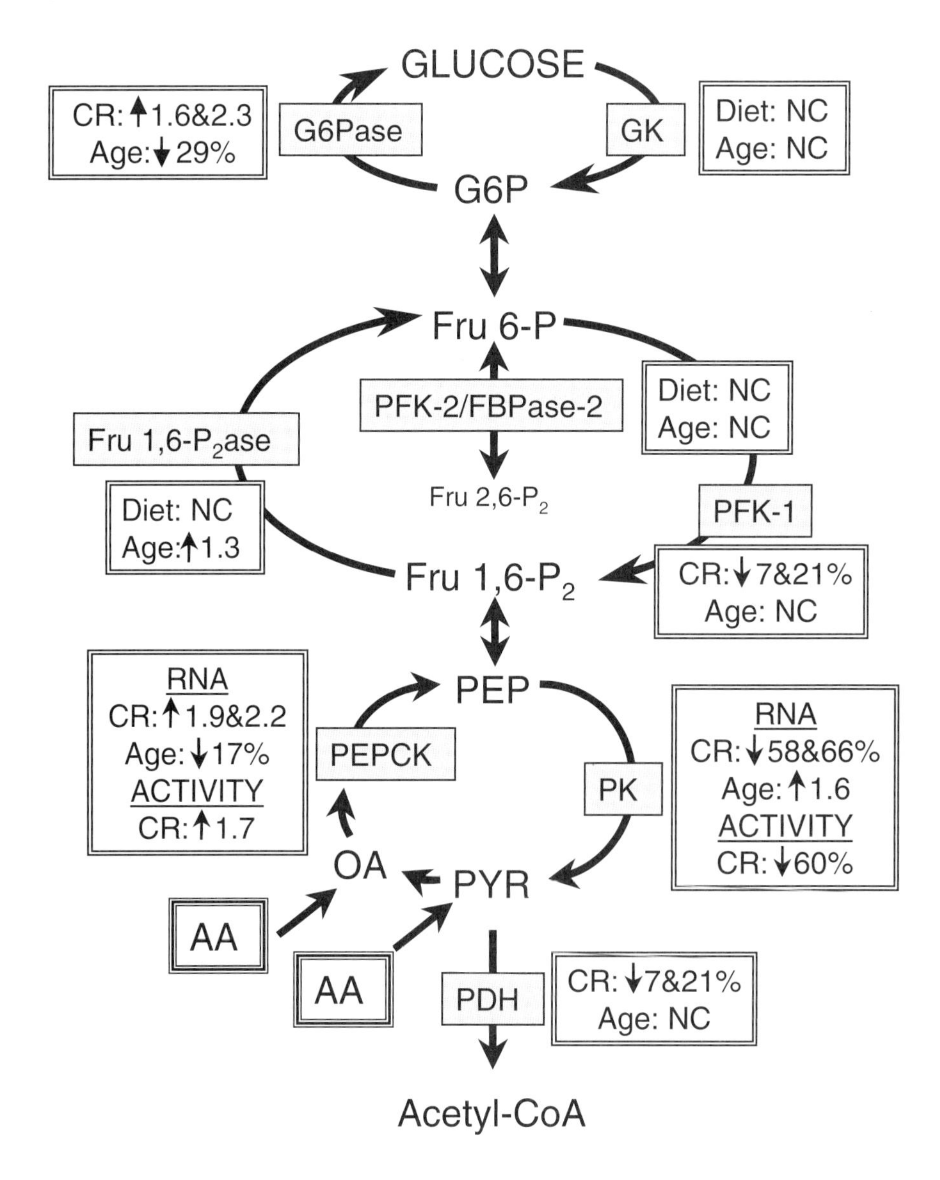

postmitotic cells is rare. Thus, reduced stress and increased stress resistance is closely associated with reduced functional impairment in these organs. An illustration of this can be found in the heart. Aging impairs cardiac capacity, contractility, and diastolic and systolic function (87). Approximately 40% of male C57BL/6 mice develop cardiomyopathy by 1000 days of age (127). In rodents and humans, three major age-associated changes markedly affect myocardial performance. First, myocardial fibrosis, a hallmark of cardiac aging in humans and rats, is initiated by cellular necrosis and apoptosis, which induce reparative interstitial and perivascular collagen deposition (3, 19, 31). Fibrosis decreases cardiac distensibility and increases diastolic pressure, impairing coronary hemodynamics, and lowering coronary reserve (57, 131). Second, there is an age-related decline in the number of cardiomyocytes, which leads to compensatory myocyte hypertrophy (17, 28, 79). Left ventricular hypertrophy is the most common cardiac manifestation of aging (73). Third, aging produces impairment in mitochondrial bioenergetics, which appears to contribute to myocardial stiffness, apoptosis, atrophy, and compensatory hypertrophy (95, 128). These changes may underlie age-related cardiac arrhythmias, dysfunction, and failure. LTCR enhances cardiovascular function and reduces these manifestations of aging (84). LTCR reduces risk factors for coronary artery disease and stroke in humans and other animals (36, 84, 93). Moderate CR improves cardiac remodeling and diastolic dysfunction in the Dahl-SS rat, which develops age-related hypertension-associated diastolic dysfunction (114).

We and others investigated the effects of LTCR on global gene expression in mouse heart (28, 37, 74). We conducted high-density microarray, biochemical, and histochemical studies of STCR and LTCR. Although there are changes in gene expression common to heart and liver (37; **Table 2**), most responses to CR are tissue-specific and tailored to the age-related dysfunctions of each organ. In heart, many downregulated genes are associated with reduced fibrosis, tissue remodeling, and blood pressure. Many of the changes in signal transduction–related gene expression

Figure 2

Summary of the effects of age and caloric restriction (CR) on the glycolytic and gluconeogenic pathways of the liver. Glycolytic metabolism in the liver involves three irreversible, regulated steps. Glucokinase (GK) initiates glucose metabolism by phosphorylation of C6, yielding glucose 6-phosphate (G6P). The committed step in glycolysis, and the second irreversible and regulated step, is the phosphorylation of fructose 6-phosphate (Fru 6-P) by phosphofructokinase (PFK-1) to produce fructose 1,6-bisphosphate (Fru 1,6-P_2). The third irreversible step controls the outflow of the pathway. Phosphoenolpyruvate (PEP) and adenosine diphosphate (ADP) are utilized by pyruvate kinase (PK) to produce pyruvate (PYR) and adenosine triphosphate (ATP). Pyruvate dehydrogenase (PDH) oxidatively decarboxylates pyruvate to form acetyl-CoA, which is a bridge between glycolysis and the tricarboxylic acid cycle or fatty acid biosynthesis. Phosphoenolpyruvate carboxykinase (PEPCK) catalyzes the first committed step in gluconeogenesis. The main noncarbohydrate precursors for gluconeogenesis are amino acids from the diet and from protein breakdown in muscle and other organs. Most of these amino acids are converted to oxaloacetate (OA), which is metabolized to PEP by PEPCK. In the second regulated and essentially irreversible step in gluconeogenesis, fructose 1,6-bisphosphatase (Fru 1,6-P_2ase) catalyzes the formation of Fru 6-P from Fru 1,6-P_2. Finally, in the third essentially irreversible reaction of gluconeogenesis, glucose is formed by the hydrolysis of G6P in a reaction catalyzed by glucose 6-phosphatase (G6Pase). In the figure, substrates are not boxed, enzyme names are in shaded boxes, summaries of experimental results are in double-bordered boxes, and amino acids are indicated by "AA" in triple-bordered boxes. When two values are given following "CR," they represent the fold change in young and old mice, respectively. The value after "Age" is the main effect of age. A down arrow indicates the percent decrease; an up arrow indicates the fold increase. The value given for age is a combination of both dietary groups. NC is no change.

appear to be focused around the differentiated functions of heart, including enhanced lipid catabolism for energy production and enhanced contractility (28). We found no evidence for enhanced apoptosis-related gene expression in heart, in sharp contrast to the changes found in liver.

In heart, STCR induces a relatively small subset of the LTCR-responsive genes (28). However, these changes appear to be important and consistent with the rapid effects of CR on cardiac physiology. Just four months of CR reduces oxidative, glycoxidative, and lipoxidative damage to rat heart mitochondrial proteins (102). Just eight weeks of CR produces many LTCR-like changes in the expression of most extracellular matrix genes and in many genes related to the cytoskeleton, cell motility, signal transduction, differentiation, cell division, immune function, inflammation, chaperones, and stress (28). When LTCR mice were fed a control diet for just eight weeks, 97% of the LTCR-responsive genes returned to control expression levels (28). Thus, even in heart, gene expression can be rapidly responsive to shifts to and from a CR-associated genic profile.

SHIFTING FROM THE CONTROL TO THE CR STATE

The results reviewed above raise an important question. How rapid and complete is the shift from the control to the CR state when CR is initiated later in life? Another way of asking this question is, Can STCR induce all of the benefits of LTCR? The studies reviewed here suggest at least three categories of changes are induced later in life. First are changes that respond rapidly and completely. These include the rapid genic responses to CR in liver and heart that are reviewed above. Second are the changes that take longer than eight weeks. These include processes like the depletion of perivascular collagen in cardiac vessels (28). Eight weeks of CR in old mice downregulated the expression of many extracellular matrix genes but did not significantly reduce the level of perivascular collagen deposited around cardiac vessels. The turnover of extracellular matrix is relatively slow and probably requires longer than eight weeks to decrease significantly. A third type of LTCR-related change probably cannot be reproduced by late-onset CR. Such changes include the loss of cardiomyocytes in the left ventricle of the heart during aging. This change is unlikely to be altered by late-life CR.

CONCLUSIONS

Metazoan evolution has selected a complex web of physiological changes in response to shortages in nutritional energy. Genomewide microarray and conventional molecular and biochemical studies indicate that aging is accompanied by a genic drift toward gene-expression patterns associated with the characteristic age-related pathologies of specific tissues and toward increased inflammation, cellular stress, and fibrosis. LTCR, STCR, and other means of extending lifespan appear to shift intracellular and extracellular signaling toward a physiologic and genic state that reverses or resists these changes. Although many of the genic changes induced by CR are conserved between functionally different tissues such as liver and heart, most appear to be tailored to organ-specific functions. Broadly, mitotically competent tissues shift toward susceptibility to apoptotic and autophagic cell death, whereas postmitotic tissues enhance stress resistance and cellular repair. Many of the genic responses to CR shared by tissues appear to involve accommodation to reduced macromolecular biosynthesis. Despite these reductions, CR increases the overall rate of macromolecular turnover to mobilize metabolic energy. Evidence for this can be found in the liver, where alterations in the enzymatic capacity for glycolysis, gluconeogenesis, and ureagenesis result in reduced lipid biosynthesis and increased glucose biosynthesis and nitrogen disposal. Together these changes show that lifespan extension is a multifaceted process derived in part from repeated cycles of cell and tissue turnover in mitotically competent tissues and tissue turnover and repair in postmitotic tissues.

SUMMARY POINTS

1. LTCR produces a subset of genic and physiologic effects common to the mitotic liver and postmitotic heart. These responses suggest that CR produces a widespread reduction in protein, RNA, DNA, and lipid biosynthesis and adjusts the rates of protein degradation, particularly glycoprotein degradation, to compensate.
2. Most of the genic responses to CR are tissue specific and tailored to the age-related physiologic changes and age-related diseases of each tissue.
3. In heart, CR rapidly produces changes in gene expression consistent with reduced fibrosis, remodeling, cytoskeletal dynamics, cell motility, inflammation, immune activation, blood pressure, and protein degradation.
4. In liver, CR produces changes in gene expression consistent with reduced glycolysis and increased gluconeogenesis, ureagenesis, and susceptibility to apoptosis. Many of these changes are enhanced or recapitulated by the Ames longevity mutation.
5. LTCR and STCR initiated late in life suppress the growth rate of tumors, apparently by increasing the rate of apoptosis of tumor cells.
6. The whole-body protein turnover driven by CR can be detected by the enhanced expression of gluconeogenic and ureagenic enzymes in the liver.
7. CR initiated late in life can recapitulate many, but probably not all, of the beneficial effects of LTCR in heart. It can induce gene expression changes consistent with reduced blood pressure and extracellular matrix overexpression and enhanced lipid β-oxidation for energy generation.
8. CR initiated late in life can recapitulate the anticancer and most of the other effects of LTCR.

FUTURE ISSUES

1. Studies need to define how CR enhances the apoptotic potential of tumors and some mitotic tissues while reducing the apoptotic potential of many postmitotic tissues.
2. Studies need to determine how CR induces higher rates of apoptosis in tumors, especially in spontaneous hepatomas. Untreated patients with hepatoma usually die in 3–4 months, whereas treated patients live 6–18 months, if they respond to therapy. Clearly, novel targets are needed.
3. Studies of the gluconeogenic, glycolytic, and nitrogen disposal pathways need to investigate how the changes in the enzymatic capacity of specific steps in these pathways actually change carbon and nitrogen flux through the pathways.
4. Studies need to continue the identification of the signal-transmission pathways altered by CR that lead to its anticancer and cardiovascular benefits.

5. Continuing research is needed to identify pharmacologic agents that target the pathways used by CR to produce its anticancer and other health benefits.
6. The effects on lifespan of mutational or pharmacological manipulation of the pathways of intermediary metabolism need to be conducted to define the scope of their probable effects on lifespan and health span.
7. When studies have progressed sufficiently, potential longevity therapeutics identified in animals should be studied for their effects in humans.

LITERATURE CITED

1. Alexia C, Fourmatgeat P, Delautier D, Groyer A. 2006. Insulin-like growth factor-I stimulates H(4)II rat hepatoma cell proliferation: dominant role of PI-3′K/Akt signaling. *Exp. Cell. Res.* 312:1142–52
2. Alexia C, Lasfer M, Groyer A. 2004. Role of constitutively activated and insulin-like growth factor–stimulated ERK1/2 signaling in human hepatoma cell proliferation and apoptosis: evidence for heterogeneity of tumor cell lines. *Ann. N. Y. Acad. Sci.* 1030:219–29
3. Anversa P, Palackal T, Sonnenblick EH, Olivetti G, Meggs LG, Capasso JM. 1990. Myocyte cell loss and myocyte cellular hyperplasia in the hypertrophied aging rat heart. *Circ. Res.* 67:871–85
4. Apte UM, Limaye PB, Ramaiah SK, Vaidya VS, Bucci TJ, et al. 2002. Upregulated promitogenic signaling via cytokines and growth factors: potential mechanism of robust liver tissue repair in calorie-restricted rats upon toxic challenge. *Toxicol. Sci.* 69:448–59
5. Bakala H, Delaval E, Hamelin M, Bismuth J, Borot-Laloi C, et al. 2003. Changes in rat liver mitochondria with aging. Lon protease-like reactivity and N^{ϵ}-carboxymethyllysine accumulation in the matrix. *Eur. J. Biochem.* 270:2295–302
6. Bartke A. 2005. Minireview: role of the growth hormone/insulin-like growth factor system in mammalian aging. *Endocrinology* 146:3718–23
7. Bartke A. 2006. Long-lived Klotho mice: new insights into the roles of IGF-1 and insulin in aging. *Trends Endocrinol. Metab.* 17:33–35
8. Beausejour CM, Campisi J. 2006. Ageing: balancing regeneration and cancer. *Nature* 443:404–5
9. Bejma J, Ji LL. 1999. Aging and acute exercise enhance free radical generation in rat skeletal muscle. *J. Appl. Physiol.* 87:465–70
10. Bergamini E. 2006. Autophagy: a cell repair mechanism that retards ageing and age-associated diseases and can be intensified pharmacologically. *Mol. Aspects Med.* 27:403–10
11. Bilodeau M, Tousignant J, Ethier C, Rocheleau B, Raymond VA, Lapointe R. 2004. Anti-apoptotic effect of insulin on normal hepatocytes in vitro and in vivo. *Apoptosis* 9:609–17
12. Boissan M, Beurel E, Wendum D, Rey C, Lecluse Y, et al. 2005. Overexpression of insulin receptor substrate-2 in human and murine hepatocellular carcinoma. *Am. J. Pathol.* 167:869–77
13. Burfeind P, Chernicky CL, Rininsland F, Ilan J, Ilan J. 1996. Antisense RNA to the type I insulin-like growth factor receptor suppresses tumor growth and prevents invasion by rat prostate cancer cells in vivo. *Proc. Natl. Acad. Sci. USA* 93:7263–68
14. Cao SX, Dhahbi JM, Mote PL, Spindler SR. 2001. Genomic profiling of short- and long-term caloric restriction effects in the liver of aging mice. *Proc. Natl. Acad. Sci. USA* 98:10630–35

15. Chung HY, Sung B, Jung KJ, Zou Y, Yu BP. 2006. The molecular inflammatory process in aging. *Antioxid. Redox. Signal.* 8:572–81
16. Clarke S, Greaves DR, Chung LP, Tree P, Gordon S. 1996. The human lysozyme promoter directs reporter gene expression to activated myelomonocytic cells in transgenic mice. *Proc. Natl. Acad. Sci. USA* 93:1434–38
17. Colucci WS. 1997. Molecular and cellular mechanisms of myocardial failure. *Am. J. Cardiol.* 80:15–25L
18. Deleted in proof
19. De Souza RR. 2002. Aging of myocardial collagen. *Biogerontology* 3:325–35
20. Dhahbi JM, Cao SX, Mote PL, Rowley BC, Wingo JE, Spindler SR. 2002. Postprandial induction of chaperone gene expression is rapid in mice. *J. Nutr.* 132:31–37
21. Dhahbi JM, Cao SX, Tillman JB, Mote PL, Madore M, et al. 2001. Chaperone-mediated regulation of hepatic protein secretion by caloric restriction. *Biochem. Biophys. Res. Commun.* 284:335–39
22. Dhahbi JM, Kim HJ, Mote PL, Beaver RJ, Spindler SR. 2004. Temporal linkage between the phenotypic and genomic responses to caloric restriction. *Proc. Natl. Acad. Sci. USA* 101:5524–29
23. Dhahbi JM, Mote PL, Fahy GM, Spindler SR. 2005. Identification of potential caloric restriction mimetics by microarray profiling. *Physiol. Genomics* 23:343–50
24. Dhahbi JM, Mote PL, Tillman JB, Walford RL, Spindler SR. 1997. Dietary energy tissue specifically regulates endoplasmic reticulum chaperone gene expression in the liver of mice. *J. Nutr.* 127:1758–64
25. Dhahbi JM, Mote PL, Wingo J, Rowley BC, Cao SX, et al. 2001. Caloric restriction alters the feeding response of key metabolic enzyme genes. *Mech. Ageing Dev.* 122:35–50
26. Dhahbi JM, Mote PL, Wingo J, Tillman JB, Walford RL, Spindler SR. 1999. Calories and aging alter gene expression for gluconeogenic, glycolytic, and nitrogen-metabolizing enzymes. *Am. J. Physiol.* 277:E352–60
27. Dhahbi JM, Spindler SR. 2003. Aging of the liver. In *Aging of the Organs and Systems*, ed. R Aspinall, 12:271–91. Dordrecht, Netherlands: Kluwer Acad.
28. Dhahbi JM, Tsuchiya T, Kim HJ, Mote PL, Spindler SR. 2006. Gene expression and physiologic responses of the heart to the initiation and withdrawal of caloric restriction. *J. Gerontol. A Biol. Sci. Med. Sci.* 61:218–31
29. Dominici FP, Hauck S, Argentino DP, Bartke A, Turyn D. 2002. Increased insulin sensitivity and upregulation of insulin receptor, insulin receptor substrate (IRS)-1 and IRS-2 in liver of Ames dwarf mice. *J. Endocrinol.* 173:81–94
30. Donati A. 2006. The involvement of macroautophagy in aging and antiaging interventions. *Mol. Aspects Med.* 27:455–70
31. Eghbali M, Eghbali M, Robinson TF, Seifter S, Blumenfeld OO. 1989. Collagen accumulation in heart ventricles as a function of growth and aging. *Cardiovasc. Res.* 23:723–29
32. el Haj AJ, Lewis SE, Goldspink DF, Merry BJ, Holehan AM. 1986. The effect of chronic and acute dietary restriction on the growth and protein turnover of fast and slow types of rat skeletal muscle. *Comp. Biochem. Physiol. A* 85:281–87
33. Feuers RJ, Duffy PH, Leakey JA, Turturro A, Mittelstaedt RA, Hart RW. 1989. Effect of chronic caloric restriction on hepatic enzymes of intermediary metabolism in the male Fischer 344 rat. *Mech. Ageing Dev.* 48:179–89
34. Fichtner-Feigl S, Strober W, Kawakami K, Puri RK, Kitani A. 2006. IL-13 signaling through the IL-13α2 receptor is involved in induction of TGF-β1 production and fibrosis. *Nat. Med.* 12:99–106

35. Finn PF, Dice JF. 2006. Proteolytic and lipolytic responses to starvation. *Nutrition* 22:830–44
36. Fontana L, Meyer TE, Klein S, Holloszy JO. 2004. Long-term calorie restriction is highly effective in reducing the risk for atherosclerosis in humans. *Proc. Natl. Acad. Sci. USA* 101:6659–63
37. Fu C, Hickey M, Morrison M, McCarter R, Han ES. 2006. Tissue specific and nonspecific changes in gene expression by aging and by early stage CR. *Mech. Ageing Dev.* 127:905–16
38. Goldspink DF, el Haj AJ, Lewis SE, Merry BJ, Holehan AM. 1987. The influence of chronic dietary intervention on protein turnover and growth of the diaphragm and extensor *digitorum longus* muscles of the rat. *Exp. Gerontol.* 22:67–78
39. Goodman MN, Larsen PR, Kaplan MM, Aoki TT, Young VR, Ruderman NB. 1980. Starvation in the rat. II. Effect of age and obesity on protein sparing and fuel metabolism. *Am. J. Physiol.* 239:E277–86
40. Grasl-Kraupp B, Bursch W, Ruttkay-Nedecky B, Wagner A, Lauer B, Schulte-Hermann R. 1994. Food restriction eliminates preneoplastic cells through apoptosis and antagonizes carcinogenesis in rat liver. *Proc. Natl. Acad. Sci. USA* 91:9995–99
41. Hagopian K, Ramsey JJ, Weindruch R. 2003. Caloric restriction increases gluconeogenic and transaminase enzyme activities in mouse liver. *Exp. Gerontol.* 38:267–78
42. Hagopian K, Ramsey JJ, Weindruch R. 2003. Influence of age and caloric restriction on liver glycolytic enzyme activities and metabolite concentrations in mice. *Exp. Gerontol.* 38:253–66
43. Han ES, Hickey M. 2005. Microarray evaluation of dietary restriction. *J. Nutr.* 135:1343–46
44. Harper JM, Salmon AB, Chang Y, Bonkowski M, Bartke A, Miller RA. 2006. Stress resistance and aging: influence of genes and nutrition. *Mech. Ageing Dev.* 127:687–94
45. Heydari AR, Conrad CC, Richardson A. 1995. Expression of heat shock genes in hepatocytes is affected by age and food restriction in rats. *J. Nutr.* 125:410–18
46. Higami Y, Shimokawa I, Ando K, Tanaka K, Tsuchiya T. 2000. Dietary restriction reduces hepatocyte proliferation and enhances p53 expression but does not increase apoptosis in normal rats during development. *Cell Tissue Res.* 299:363–69
47. Hikita H, Vaughan J, Babcock K, Pitot HC. 1999. Short-term fasting and the reversal of the stage of promotion in rat hepatocarcinogenesis: role of cell replication, apoptosis, and gene expression. *Toxicol. Sci.* 52:17–23
48. Holliday R. 1989. Food, reproduction and longevity: Is the extended lifespan of calorie-restricted animals an evolutionary adaptation? *Bioessays* 10:125–27
49. Holt PR, Moss SF, Heydari AR, Richardson A. 1998. Diet restriction increases apoptosis in the gut of aging rats. *J. Gerontol. Biol. Sci.* 53A:B168–72
50. Hopfner M, Huether A, Sutter AP, Baradari V, Schuppan D, Scherubl H. 2006. Blockade of IGF-1 receptor tyrosine kinase has antineoplastic effects in hepatocellular carcinoma cells. *Biochem. Pharmacol.* 71:1435–48
51. Huether A, Hopfner M, Baradari V, Schuppan D, Scherubl H. 2005. EGFR blockade by cetuximab alone or as combination therapy for growth control of hepatocellular cancer. *Biochem. Pharmacol.* 70:1568–78
52. Huether A, Hopfner M, Sutter AP, Schuppan D, Scherubl H. 2005. Erlotinib induces cell cycle arrest and apoptosis in hepatocellular cancer cells and enhances chemosensitivity towards cytostatics. *J. Hepatol.* 43:661–69

53. Hursting SD, Lavigne JA, Berrigan D, Perkins SN, Barrett JC. 2003. Calorie restriction, aging, and cancer prevention: mechanisms of action and applicability to humans. *Annu. Rev. Med.* 54:131–52
54. Ikeno Y, Bronson RT, Hubbard GB, Lee S, Bartke A. 2003. Delayed occurrence of fatal neoplastic diseases in Ames dwarf mice: correlation to extended longevity. *J. Gerontol. A Biol. Sci. Med. Sci.* 58:291–96
55. James SJ, Muskhelishvili L. 1994. Rates of apoptosis and proliferation vary with caloric intake and may influence incidence of spontaneous hepatoma in C57BL/6 × C3H F1 mice. *Cancer Res.* 54:5508–10
56. James SJ, Muskhelishvili L, Gaylor DW, Turturro A, Hart R. 1998. Upregulation of apoptosis with dietary restriction: implications for carcinogenesis and aging. *Environ. Health Persp.* 106:307–12
57. Janicki JS. 1992. Myocardial collagen remodeling and left ventricular diastolic function. *Braz. J. Med. Biol. Res.* 25:975–82
58. Janzen V, Forkert R, Fleming HE, Saito Y, Waring MT, et al. 2006. Stem-cell ageing modified by the cyclin-dependent kinase inhibitor p16INK4a. *Nature* 443:421–26
59. Jin Z, El Deiry WS. 2005. Overview of cell death signaling pathways. *Cancer Biol. Ther.* 4:139–63
60. Kadowaki M, Karim MR, Carpi A, Miotto G. 2006. Nutrient control of macroautophagy in mammalian cells. *Mol. Aspects Med.* 27:426–43
61. Kapadia F, Pryor A, Chang TH, Johnson LF. 2006. Nuclear localization of poly(A)+ mRNA following siRNA reduction of expression of the mammalian RNA helicases UAP56 and URH49. *Gene* 384:37–44
62. Kennedy MA, Rakoczy SG, Brown-Borg HM. 2003. Long-living Ames dwarf mouse hepatocytes readily undergo apoptosis. *Exp. Gerontol.* 38:997–1008
63. Kenyon C. 2005. The plasticity of aging: insights from long-lived mutants. *Cell* 120:449–60
64. Keshav S, Chung P, Milon G, Gordon S. 1991. Lysozyme is an inducible marker of macrophage activation in murine tissues as demonstrated by in situ hybridization. *J. Exp. Med.* 174:1049–58
65. Klebanov S. 2007. Can short-term dietary restriction and fasting have a long-term anti-carcinogenic effect? *Interdiscip. Top. Gerontol.* 35:176–92
66. Klionsky DJ, Emr SD. 2000. Autophagy as a regulated pathway of cellular degradation. *Science* 290:1717–21
67. Komninou D, Leutzinger Y, Reddy BS, Richie JP Jr. 2006. Methionine restriction inhibits colon carcinogenesis. *Nutr. Cancer* 54:202–8
68. Koubova J, Guarente L. 2003. How does calorie restriction work? *Genes Dev.* 17:313–21
69. Kouda K, Nakamura H, Kohno H, Ha-Kawa SK, Tokunaga R, Sawada S. 2004. Dietary restriction: effects of short-term fasting on protein uptake and cell death/proliferation in the rat liver. *Mech. Ageing Dev.* 125:375–80
70. Deleted in proof
71. Krishnamurthy J, Ramsey MR, Ligon KL, Torrice C, Koh A, et al. 2006. p16INK4a induces an age-dependent decline in islet regenerative potential. *Nature* 443:453–57
72. Kuhajda FP, Pizer ES, Li JN, Mani NS, Frehywot GL, Townsend CA. 2000. Synthesis and antitumor activity of an inhibitor of fatty acid synthase. *Proc. Natl. Acad. Sci. USA* 97:3450–54
73. Lakatta EG. 2000. Cardiovascular aging in health. *Clin. Geriatr. Med.* 16:419–44

74. Lee CK, Allison DB, Brand J, Weindruch R, Prolla TA. 2002. Transcriptional profiles associated with aging and middle age–onset caloric restriction in mouse hearts. *Proc. Natl. Acad. Sci. USA* 99:14988–93
75. Lewis SE, Goldspink DF, Phillips JG, Merry BJ, Holehan AM. 1985. The effects of aging and chronic dietary restriction on whole body growth and protein turnover in the rat. *Exp. Gerontol.* 20:253–63
76. Liang H, Masoro EJ, Nelson JF, Strong R, McMahan CA, Richardson A. 2003. Genetic mouse models of extended lifespan. *Exp. Gerontol.* 38:1353–64
77. Liu Z, Barrett EJ, Dalkin AC, Zwart AD, Chou JY. 1994. Effect of acute diabetes on rat hepatic glucose-6-phosphatase activity and its messenger RNA level. *Biochem. Biophys. Res. Commun.* 205:680–86
78. Luan X, Zhao W, Chandrasekar B, Fernandes G. 1995. Calorie restriction modulates lymphocyte subset phenotype and increases apoptosis in MRL/lpr mice. *Immunol. Lett.* 47:181–86
79. Lushnikova EL, Nepomnyashchikh LM, Klinnikova MG. 2001. Morphological characteristics of myocardial remodeling during compensatory hypertrophy in aging Wistar rats. *Bull. Exp. Biol. Med.* 132:1201–6
80. Malloy VL, Krajcik RA, Bailey SJ, Hristopoulos G, Plummer JD, Orentreich N. 2006. Methionine restriction decreases visceral fat mass and preserves insulin action in aging male Fischer 344 rats independent of energy restriction. *Aging Cell* 5:305–14
81. Mansouri A, Muller FL, Liu Y, Ng R, Faulkner J, et al. 2006. Alterations in mitochondrial function, hydrogen peroxide release and oxidative damage in mouse hind-limb skeletal muscle during aging. *Mech. Ageing Dev.* 127:298–306
82. Masoro EJ. 2005. Overview of caloric restriction and ageing. *Mech. Ageing Dev.* 126:913–22
83. Massaro D, DeCarlo MG, Baras A, Hoffman EP, Clerch LB. 2004. Calorie-related rapid onset of alveolar loss, regeneration, and changes in mouse lung gene expression. *Am. J. Physiol. Lung Cell Mol. Physiol.* 286:L896–906
84. Mattson MP, Wan R. 2005. Beneficial effects of intermittent fasting and caloric restriction on the cardiovascular and cerebrovascular systems. *J. Nutr. Biochem.* 16:129–37
85. McCay CM, Crowell MF, Maynard LA. 1935. The effect of retarded growth upon the length of the life span and upon the ultimate body size. *J. Nutr.* 10:63–79
86. McCay CM, Crowell MF, Maynard LA. 1989. The effect of retarded growth upon the length of life span and upon the ultimate body size. 1935. *Nutrition* 5:155–71
87. McGuire DK, Levine BD, Williamson JW, Snell PG, Blomqvist CG, et al. 2001. A 30-year follow-up of the Dallas Bedrest and Training Study: I. Effect of age on the cardiovascular response to exercise. *Circulation* 104:1350–57
88. Merry BJ, Goldspink DF, Lewis SE. 1991. The effects of age and chronic restricted feeding on protein synthesis and growth of the large intestine of the rat. *Comp. Biochem. Physiol. A* 98:559–62
89. Merry BJ, Holehan AM. 1985. In vivo DNA synthesis in the dietary restricted long-lived rat. *Exp. Gerontol.* 20:15–28
90. Merry BJ, Holehan AM. 1991. Effect of age and restricted feeding on polypeptide chain assembly kinetics in liver protein synthesis in vivo. *Mech. Ageing Dev.* 58:139–50
91. Merry BJ, Holehan AM, Lewis SE, Goldspink DF. 1987. The effects of ageing and chronic dietary restriction on in vivo hepatic protein synthesis in the rat. *Mech. Ageing Dev.* 39:189–99

92. Merry BJ, Lewis SE, Goldspink DF. 1992. The influence of age and chronic restricted feeding on protein synthesis in the small intestine of the rat. *Exp. Gerontol.* 27:191–200
93. Meyer TE, Kovacs SJ, Ehsani AA, Klein S, Holloszy JO, Fontana L. 2006. Long-term caloric restriction ameliorates the decline in diastolic function in humans. *J. Am. Coll. Cardiol.* 47:398–402
94. Molofsky AV, Slutsky SG, Joseph NM, He S, Pardal R, et al. 2006. Increasing p16INK4a expression decreases forebrain progenitors and neurogenesis during ageing. *Nature* 443:448–52
95. Moreau R, Heath SH, Doneanu CE, Harris RA, Hagen TM. 2004. Age-related compensatory activation of pyruvate dehydrogenase complex in rat heart. *Biochem. Biophys. Res. Commun.* 325:48–58
96. Moreschi C. 1909. Beziehungen zwischen ernahrung und tumorwachstum [Relationship between nutrition and tumor growth]. *Z. Immunitatsforsch.* 2:651
97. Mote PL, Tillman JB, Spindler SR. 1998. Glucose regulation of GRP78 gene expression. *Mech. Ageing Dev.* 104:149–58
98. Muskhelishvili L, Hart RW, Turturro A, James SJ. 1995. Age-related changes in the intrinsic rate of apoptosis in livers of diet-restricted and ad libitum–fed B6C3F1 mice. *Am. J. Pathol.* 147:20–24
99. Muskhelishvili L, Turturro A, Hart RW, James SJ. 1996. Pi-class glutathione-S-transferase-positive hepatocytes in aging B6C3F1 mice undergo apoptosis induced by dietary restriction. *Am. J. Pathol.* 149:1585–91
100. Myung J, Kim KB, Crews CM. 2001. The ubiquitin-proteasome pathway and proteasome inhibitors. *Med. Res. Rev.* 21:245–73
101. Olsen A, Vantipalli MC, Lithgow GJ. 2006. Lifespan extension of *Caenorhabditis elegans* following repeated mild hormetic heat treatments. *Biogerontology* 7:221–30
102. Pamplona R, Portero-Otin M, Requena J, Gredilla R, Barja G. 2002. Oxidative, glycoxidative and lipoxidative damage to rat heart mitochondrial proteins is lower after 4 months of caloric restriction than in age-matched controls. *Mech. Ageing Dev.* 123:1437–46
103. Pandini G, Conte E, Medico E, Sciacca L, Vigneri R, Belfiore A. 2004. IGF-II binding to insulin receptor isoform A induces a partially different gene expression profile from insulin binding. *Ann. N. Y. Acad. Sci.* 1028:450–56
104. Phelan JP, Austad SN. 1989. Natural selection, dietary restriction, and extended longevity. *Growth Dev. Aging* 53:4–6
105. Pinel C, Coxam V, Mignon M, Taillandier D, Cubizolles C, et al. 2006. Alterations in glutamine synthetase activity in rat skeletal muscle are associated with advanced age. *Nutrition* 22:778–85
106. Pinkston JM, Garigan D, Hansen M, Kenyon C. 2006. Mutations that increase the life span of *C. elegans* inhibit tumor growth. *Science* 313:971–75
107. Pitot HC, Hikita H, Dragan Y, Sargent L, Haas M. 2000. Review article: the stages of gastrointestinal carcinogenesis—application of rodent models to human disease. *Aliment Pharmacol. Ther.* 14(Suppl. 1):153–60
108. Pizer ES, Chrest FJ, DiGiuseppe JA, Han WF. 1998. Pharmacological inhibitors of mammalian fatty acid synthase suppress DNA replication and induce apoptosis in tumor cell lines. *Cancer Res.* 58:4611–15
109. Rao RV, Peel A, Logvinova A, del Rio G, Hermel E, et al. 2002. Coupling endoplasmic reticulum stress to the cell death program: role of the ER chaperone GRP78. *FEBS Lett.* 514:122–28

110. Rosati B, Grau F, Kuehler A, Rodriguez S, McKinnon D. 2004. Comparison of different probe-level analysis techniques for oligonucleotide microarrays. *Biotechniques* 36:316–22
111. Rubini M, D'Ambrosio C, Carturan S, Yumet G, Catalano E, et al. 1999. Characterization of an antibody that can detect an activated IGF-I receptor in human cancers. *Exp. Cell Res.* 251:22–32
112. Scharf JG, Braulke T. 2003. The role of the IGF axis in hepatocarcinogenesis. *Horm. Metab. Res.* 35:685–93
113. Schroder M, Kaufman RJ. 2005. The mammalian unfolded protein response. *Annu. Rev. Biochem.* 74:739–89
114. Seymour EM, Parikh RV, Singer AA, Bolling SF. 2006. Moderate calorie restriction improves cardiac remodeling and diastolic dysfunction in the Dahl-SS rat. *J. Mol. Cell. Cardiol.* 41:661–68
115. Sharpless NE. 2005. INK4a/ARF: a multifunctional tumor suppressor locus. *Mutat. Res.* 576:22–38
116. Shimamura T, Husain SR, Puri RK. 2006. The IL-4 and IL-13 pseudomonas exotoxins: new hope for brain tumor therapy. *Neurosurg. Focus* 20:E11
117. Shimizu S, Tsujimoto Y. 2000. Proapoptotic BH3-only Bcl-2 family members induce cytochrome c release, but not mitochondrial membrane potential loss, and do not directly modulate voltage-dependent anion channel activity. *Proc. Natl. Acad. Sci. USA* 97:577–82
118. Sorimachi H, Ishiura S, Suzuki K. 1997. Structure and physiological function of calpains. *Biochem. J.* 328:721–32
119. Sornson MW, Wu W, Dasen JS, Flynn SE, Norman DJ, et al. 1996. Pituitary lineage determination by the Prophet of Pit-1 homeodomain factor defective in Ames dwarfism. *Nature* 384:327–33
120. Spindler SR. 2001. Caloric restriction enhances the expression of key metabolic enzymes associated with protein renewal during aging. *Ann. N. Y. Acad. Sci.* 928:296–304
121. Spindler SR. 2005. Rapid and reversible induction of the longevity, anticancer and genomic effects of caloric restriction. *Mech. Ageing Dev.* 126:960–66
122. Spindler SR. 2006. Use of microarray biomarkers to identify longevity therapeutics. *Aging Cell* 5:39–50
123. Spindler SR, Crew MD, Mote PL, Grizzle JM, Walford RL. 1990. Dietary energy restriction in mice reduces hepatic expression of glucose-regulated protein 78 (BiP) and 94 mRNA. *J. Nutr.* 120:1412–17
124. Spindler SR, Dhahbi JM, Mote PL. 2003. Protein turnover, energy metabolism and aging. In *Energy Metabolism and Lifespan Determination: Advances in Cell Aging and Gerontology, Volume 14*, ed. MP Mattson, 4:69–86. Amsterdam, Netherlands: Elsevier
125. Tillman JB, Dhahbi JM, Mote PL, Walford RL, Spindler SR. 1996. Dietary calorie restriction in mice induces carbamyl phosphate synthetase I gene transcription tissue specifically. *J. Biol. Chem.* 271:3500–6
126. Tsuchiya T, Dhahbi JM, Cui X, Mote PL, Bartke A, Spindler SR. 2004. Additive regulation of hepatic gene expression by dwarfism and caloric restriction. *Physiol. Genomics* 17:307–15
127. Turturro A, Duffy P, Hass B, Kodell R, Hart R. 2002. Survival characteristics and age-adjusted disease incidences in C57BL/6 mice fed a commonly used cereal-based diet modulated by dietary restriction. *J. Gerontol. A Biol. Sci. Med. Sci.* 57:B379–89
128. van Raalte DH, Li M, Pritchard PH, Wasan KM. 2004. Peroxisome proliferator-activated receptor (PPAR)-alpha: a pharmacological target with a promising future. *Pharm. Res.* 21:1531–38

129. Van Remmen H, Ward WF. 1998. Effect of dietary restriction on hepatic and renal phosphoenolpyruvate carboxykinase induction in young and old Fischer 344 rats. *Mech. Ageing Dev.* 104:263–75
130. Van Remmen H, Ward WF, Sabia RV, Richardson A. 1995. Gene expression and protein degradation. In *Handbook of Physiology. Section 11: Aging*, ed. EJ Masoro, 9:171–234. New York: Oxford Univ. Press
131. Varagic J, Susic D, Frohlich E. 2001. Heart, aging, and hypertension. *Curr. Opin. Cardiol.* 16:336–41
132. Weindruch R, Sohal RS. 1997. Seminars in medicine of the Beth Israel Deaconess Medical Center. Caloric intake and aging. *N. Engl. J. Med.* 337:986–94
133. Weindruch R, Walford RL. 1988. *The Retardation of Aging and Disease by Dietary Restriction*. Springfield, IL: Thomas. 436 pp.
134. Williams DB. 2006. Beyond lectins: the calnexin/calreticulin chaperone system of the endoplasmic reticulum. *J. Cell. Sci.* 119:615–23
135. Wright KM, Deshmukh M. 2006. Restricting apoptosis for postmitotic cell survival and its relevance to cancer. *Cell. Cycle* 5:1616–20
136. Zhan Z, Vincent NC, Watford M. 1994. Transcriptional regulation of the hepatic glutaminase gene in the streptozotocin-diabetic rat. *Int. J. Biochem.* 26:263–68
137. Zhang K, Kaufman RJ. 2006. The unfolded protein response: a stress signaling pathway critical for health and disease. *Neurology* 66:S102–9

The Clockwork of Metabolism

Kathryn Moynihan Ramsey,[1,2,3] Biliana Marcheva,[1,3] Akira Kohsaka,[2,3] and Joseph Bass[1,2,3]

[1] Department of Medicine, Feinberg School of Medicine, Northwestern University, Evanston, Illinois 60208

[2] Department of Neurobiology and Physiology, Northwestern University, Evanston, Illinois 60208

[3] Evanston Northwestern Healthcare (ENH) Research Institute and Department of Medicine, Evanston Hospital, Evanston, Illinois 60208;
email: j-bass@northwestern.edu

Annu. Rev. Nutr. 2007. 27:219–40

First published online as a Review in Advance on April 12, 2007

The *Annual Review of Nutrition* is online at http://nutr.annualreviews.org

This article's doi:
10.1146/annurev.nutr.27.061406.093546

0199-9885/07/0821-0219$20.00

Key Words

circadian, clock, suprachiasmatic nucleus, diabetes, obesity, sleep

Abstract

The observation that cycles of sleep and wakefulness occur with a periodicity fixed in time to match the rotation of the Earth on its axis provided a key to unlock the first genetic code for a neurobehavioral pathway in flies and ultimately in mice. As a remarkable outcome of this discovery, we have gained an unprecedented view of the conserved genetic program that encodes a sense of time across all kingdoms of life. The tools are now in hand to begin to understand how important processes such as energy homeostasis and fuel utilization are coordinated to anticipate daily changes in environment caused by the rising and setting of the sun. A better understanding of the impact of circadian gene networks on nutrient balance at the molecular, cellular, and system levels promises to shed light on the emerging association between disorders of diabetes, obesity, sleep, and circadian timing.

Contents

OPENING QUOTE

> We have unlocked time, as in the seventeenth century we unlocked space, and now have at our disposal what are, in effect, temporal microscopes and temporal telescopes of prodigious power.... In this way, stuck though we are in our own speed and time, we can, in imagination, enter all speeds, all time.—Oliver Sacks (127)

INTRODUCTION: THE TEMPORAL BIOLOGY OF METABOLISM

Circadian rhythm: a biological rhythm that persists under constant conditions with a period length of ~24 hours

Clock: a central mechanism controlling circadian rhythms

Zeitgeber: an entraining agent such as light or food; German for "time giver"

Although humans have been acutely aware of the cyclical nature of their external environment since ancient times, the idea of the existence of an internal timekeeping system was not considered until the early 1700s when French astronomer Jean Jacques d'Ortous de Marian observed that daily leaf movement of the *Mimosa* plant persisted for several days in constant darkness. Nearly a century later, Alphonse de Candolle demonstrated not only that endogenous rhythmicity was sustained in the absence of external environmental cues, but also that in constant darkness, this rhythmicity advanced to an earlier start each day. However, despite these early observations, it was not until the mid-1900s that it became accepted that circadian rhythms were not merely passive reflections of the environmental light/dark cycle, but were rather dependent upon an underlying internal endogenous clock.

Circadian rhythms are such an innate part of our behavior that we rarely pause to speculate why they even exist. Many physiological processes, such as sleep-wake cycles, locomotor activity, body temperature, hormone secretion, and metabolism, are under the control of circadian clocks. The approximately 24-hour nature of the endogenous clock maintains a periodicity fixed in time to match the Earth's rotation around its axis, hence the term circadian (derived from the Latin phrase *circa diem*, or about a day). To remain in sync with their environment, circadian clocks are reset or entrained on a daily basis by zeitgebers, environmental cues such as light that provide information about the external time. A presumed advantage of the circadian system is that it enables organisms to anticipate, rather than simply react to, daily changes in the external light/dark environment, and it also allows synchronization of behavioral and physiological processes to the environment in order to optimize energy utilization, reproduction, and survival. The ubiquity of the circadian clock in organisms as diverse as cyanobacteria, fungi, fruit flies, birds, and mammals implies that it confers an adaptive advantage to the organism. In plants, for example, transcripts encoding proteins involved in flowering, nitrogen fixation, and photosynthesis are synthesized and degraded according to a 24-hour cycle that matches the availability of sunlight and conserves protein biogenesis during darkness (62). Direct demonstration for a distinct survival and competitive advantage to having properly tuned circadian clocks and "circadian resonance" came from clever experiments performed in *Arabidopsis thaliana* (49). When plants harboring mutations that result in altered period lengths were placed in an environment with light/dark cycles that were shorter, equal to, or longer than the endogenous period length, those plants whose endogenous clock matched that of the external light/dark cycle had increased photosynthesis, growth, and survival (49).

In vertebrates, reproductive function has been shown to be under circadian control (24, 171). Furthermore, mice with genetically disrupted circadian rhythms have reduced gonadotropin production, irregular estrous cycles, and high pregnancy failure rates (106). A more general example suggesting a link between clock function and fitness in vertebrates is offered by the observation that chronic reversal of the light/dark cycle results in decreased survival time in cardiomyopathic hamsters (117). These observations suggest that the ability to sustain an internal timekeeping mechanism may have important implications for maintenance of fitness, health, and longevity of the organism.

LINKS BETWEEN CIRCADIAN RHYTHMS, SLEEP, AND HUMAN HEALTH

There is now reason to speculate that disruption of circadian rhythms of physiology and behavior may have broader implications for human health. A long history of clinical epidemiology in humans indicates that myocardial infarction, pulmonary edema, and hypertensive crises all peak at certain times during the day (98, 149). With advances in automation, communication, and travel, the pressure to extend wakefulness or repeatedly invert the normal sleep-wake cycle has become widespread. Interestingly, association studies have demonstrated an increased incidence of obesity and cardiovascular disease among shift workers, who are routinely subjected to extended and/or fragmented working hours (47, 77, 78). Furthermore, the average nighttime sleep duration has decreased dramatically in the past few decades, in parallel with a rampant increase in obesity (147). Indeed, a number of epidemiological investigations have reported that voluntary short sleep duration is associated with increased body mass index and elevated incidence of type 2 diabetes (65, 68, 102, 108, 155). Clinical studies have also identified changes in many aspects of energy metabolism following even just a few days of partial sleep restriction. For example, healthy subjects restricted to four hours of sleep for six consecutive nights exhibited impaired glucose tolerance and reduced insulin responsiveness following a glucose challenge, a pattern indicative of aging and early diabetes (169). Furthermore, self-reported short sleepers had significantly reduced circulating levels of the anorectic hormone leptin and increased levels of the orexigenic hormone ghrelin (155). These neuroendocrine changes could explain, in part, reports of increased appetite following sleep loss (148). Other changes related to metabolic function in the short sleepers included increased sympathoadrenal tone, hypercortisolemia, and altered thyroid hormone turnover (148). Although these

Period: duration of one complete cycle in a rhythmic variation

Dawn phenomenon: an increase in blood glucose levels that occurs prior to the onset of the activity period

Suprachiasmatic nucleus (SCN): hypothalamic region containing the "master circadian pacemaker"

epidemiological and clinical studies have provided clues to possible links between sleep and metabolic regulatory processes, specific mechanisms underlying the effects of sleep loss on energy metabolism need to be further elucidated.

Circadian control of glucose metabolism was recognized from early studies demonstrating variation in glucose tolerance and insulin action across the day (61, 163). In humans, it has been repeatedly demonstrated that oral glucose tolerance is impaired in the afternoon and evening compared to the morning hours (10, 22, 29, 74, 123). A similar decrease in glucose tolerance toward the evening hours was observed in subjects exposed to a constant rate of intravenous glucose infusion for 24 hours (137, 162). The cyclical nature of glucose tolerance has been ascribed to a circadian effect on insulin sensitivity of the peripheral tissues (13, 85, 88, 166) as well as to a relative decrease in insulin secretion during the evening hours (19, 29, 88, 103). Although circadian fluctuations in plasma levels of corticosterone have also been hypothesized to account for the circadian rhythms of glucose metabolism, this hypothesis remains controversial because corticosterone, which is known to decrease insulin sensitivity, peaks at a time of day when insulin sensitivity is greatest (10, 48, 163). Another example of circadian regulation of glucose metabolism is demonstrated by the so-called dawn phenomenon, whereby glucose levels peak before the onset of the activity period (11, 20). Together, these data suggest that humans are most tolerant to glucose when the plasma glucose concentrations are highest prior to the onset of activity. Finally, circadian regulation of glucose metabolism is further indicated by recent studies showing that destruction of the hypothalamic suprachiasmatic nucleus (SCN), believed to contain the "master circadian pacemaker," abolishes diurnal variation in glucose metabolism in rats (85), and that degeneration of the autonomic tracts linking the SCN to liver similarly diminishes the 24-hour rhythms in glucose levels (27). However, despite the well-documented diurnal variation in glucose tolerance and insulin sensitivity, the molecular mechanisms underlying these phenomena are not yet well understood.

Finally, evidence suggests that loss of circadian rhythmicity of glucose metabolism may contribute to the development of metabolic disorders, such as type 2 diabetes, in both rodents (115, 142, 165) and humans (146, 163). For example, daily cycles of insulin secretion and glucose tolerance are lost in patients with type 2 diabetes (18, 163), as are daily variations in plasma corticosterone levels and locomotor activity in streptozotocin-induced diabetic rats (115, 165). These findings indicate that a critical relationship exists between endogenous circadian rhythms and diabetes. The findings also suggest that time of day may be an important consideration for the diagnosis and treatment of metabolic disorders such as type 2 diabetes (134, 159). As discussed below, clues from studies on the molecular genetics of circadian clock genes may offer insight into the molecular mechanisms underlying the diurnal variation in glucose metabolism.

MOLECULAR CLOCK COMPONENTS

Amid much skepticism that single gene mutations could affect such complex behavioral processes as circadian rhythms, the first clock mutant, *period*, was identified in *Drosophila melanogaster* in 1971 (82). However, it was not until more than two decades later that the first mammalian circadian gene, *circadian locomotor output cycles kaput* (*Clock*), was identified in a large-scale chemical mutagenesis screen for circadian variants in mice (167). *Clock* is a semidominant mutation, and homozygous *Clock* mutant animals have an initial free-running period of approximately 27–28 hours and become arrhythmic in constant darkness. Positional cloning and genetic rescue experiments identified *Clock* as a member of the basic helix-loop-helix period-ARNT-single-minded (bHLH-PAS) transcription factor family (80, 167). Since this initial discovery more than a decade ago, the identification of additional genes that are expressed with pronounced circadian rhythmicity has progressed rapidly and has revealed that circadian gene expression in mammals is controlled by autoregulatory transcription-translation feedback loops, similar to those found in other prokaryotes and eukaryotes (17).

CLOCK heterodimerizes with another bHLH-PAS family protein, BMAL1 (brain and muscle ARNT-like; also known as MOP3), and this heterodimer constitutes the positive limb of the circadian feedback loop mechanism (**Figure 1**, see color insert). The CLOCK/BMAL1 complex activates transcription of target genes containing E-box *cis*-regulatory enhancer elements (5′-CACGTG-3′), including the *period* (*Per1*, *2*, and *3*) and *cryptochrome* (*Cry 1* and *2*) genes (26, 64, 79, 84, 180). The PER and CRY proteins comprise the negative limb of the feedback loop; upon translation, PER and CRY proteins multimerize and subsequently translocate to the nucleus and directly inhibit the transcriptional activity of the CLOCK/BMAL1 complex (64, 89, 113, 133, 138). PER and CRY are phosphorylated and degraded, in part through the action of the casein kinases I epsilon and delta (CKIε/δ) (6, 51, 89, 94), and as a result, the CLOCK/BMAL1 heterodimer is released from inhibition and is free to reinitiate transcription. In addition to the *Per* and *Cry* targets, CLOCK/BMAL also activates transcription of the orphan nuclear receptors *Rev-erbα* and *Rorα* (5, 118, 132, 158). REV-ERBα and retinoic acid–related orphan receptor RORα subsequently compete for binding to the retinoic acid–related orphan receptor response elements (ROREs) in order to repress or activate, respectively, transcription of *Bmal1* (5, 66, 118, 132). This entire autoregulatory cycle takes approximately 24 hours to complete before cycling anew.

Targeted gene knockout strategies have revealed functional roles for each of the core clock components in the generation of circadian rhythms. Mice lacking *Bmal1* exhibit a complete loss of circadian rhythmicity in constant darkness (25), and as described above, mice with a dominant-negative *Clock* mutation have a four-hour increase in period length and become arrhythmic in constant darkness (80, 167). However, a recent report has questioned the absolute requirement for CLOCK in the generation of circadian rhythms because of the finding that *Clock* knockout mice retain rhythmic activity (50). A possible explanation for the lack of an observable effect on circadian rhythms in these animals is that the *Clock* homolog neuronal PAS domain protein 2 (*Npas2*) could functionally compensate for the lack of *Clock* (50). Knockout studies targeting components in the negative limb of the circadian clock have revealed additional examples of functional redundancy within the clock machinery. Although mice lacking any one of the *Per* or *Cry* genes individually have subtle circadian phenotypes that alter period length by ~1 hour or less (with the exception of *Per2*, which shortens the period by 1.5 hours and leads to eventual arrhythmicity in constant darkness), the double mutants *Per1/Per2* and *Cry1/Cry2* experience a complete loss of circadian rhythmicity (12, 30, 164, 168, 180, 181). While our knowledge of the clock machinery has attained a level of detail perhaps exceeding that of any other neurobehavioral gene pathway, it is likely that additional genes and components of the core clock machinery have yet to be identified.

LOCALIZATION OF THE CIRCADIAN CLOCK

Studies of the molecular components of the clock have provided a powerful new framework to better understand the temporal control of physiology and behavior at the cell and whole animal levels. The concept that distinct circadian centers, or pacemakers, direct organismal timekeeping was validated by studies performed in the 1960s and 1970s that identified circadian pacemaker centers in insects (in the optic lobe), mollusks (in the eye), and birds (in the pineal gland) (56, 63,

Oscillator: a system of components that produces a circadian rhythm

Clock-controlled gene: a gene whose expression is rhythmically regulated by a clock

109). In mammals, lesioning studies in rats revealed that rhythmic locomotor and feeding activity required the central circadian pacemaker in the SCN within the anterior ventral hypothalamus. Evidence for a definitive role for the SCN as a "master pacemaker" came from studies wherein the circadian locomotor activity rhythm of SCN-lesioned hamsters with a short period was restored by transplantation of the SCN from a wild-type animal (121). Interestingly, such transplantation studies also revealed that the restored rhythms of the host always matched the rhythms of the donor, implying that circadian period length is determined by the SCN (121). Furthermore, despite lack of neuronal connections between the grafted SCN and the host brain, transplantation of donor SCN tissue into hosts with lesioned SCN partially restored their circadian rhythms, suggesting that a diffusible secreted molecule, such as transforming growth factor-α or prokineticin-2, might be responsible for generation of circadian rhythms from the SCN (2, 34, 83, 143). However, while circadian locomotor activity is restored by SCN transplants, circadian endocrine rhythms of corticosteroid or melatonin secretion are not (104), suggesting that in addition to secreted factors, neural efferents must also be critical for generation of certain circadian rhythms.

Intriguingly, a major transformation in our understanding of circadian biology came from the discovery that circadian rhythms and the core clock machinery are also present in most, if not all, peripheral tissues, as well as in extra-SCN regions of the brain (**Figure 2**, see color insert). Maintenance of sustained rhythms in cultured fibroblasts following a serum shock was the first demonstration that non-neuronal mammalian cells have the autonomous capacity for generating circadian rhythms (14). It was subsequently demonstrated that self-sustaining oscillations could be observed in explants in a variety of tissues including muscle and liver by using luciferase as a reporter of *Per1* or *Per2* expression (173, 174, 177, 178). The SCN, which is directly entrained by photic input from the retinohypothalamic tract, synchronizes the timing of the clocks in the peripheral tissues; destruction of the SCN in rats abolishes synchronization of peripheral oscillators (128). Furthermore, the phase of peripheral clocks is delayed approximately four hours compared to that of the SCN (14). Interestingly, the phase of the peripheral clocks can be uncoupled from that of the SCN in response to hormonal signals (such as glucocorticoids) and restricted feeding (15, 41, 151). Restricting the availability of food to a limited period during the light cycle rapidly entrains the peripheral tissues of mice; within two days of the start of a restricted feeding regimen, circadian rhythms in the periphery are essentially inverted while rhythms in the SCN remained unchanged (41, 151). Thus, feeding time, rather than light, appears to be the dominant zeitgeber for peripheral clocks.

Although the mammalian core circadian components are well defined, the molecular effectors acting downstream of the core circadian clock machinery that link the circadian regulation to metabolism and physiological processes are much less clear. One example of a well-studied *Clock-controlled gene* is the *D-element binding protein* (*Dbp*), encoding a helix-loop-helix winged transcription factor that regulates the transcription of genes containing an insulin-response element. Oscillations in the *Clock* gene in liver induce 100-fold changes in the expression of *Dbp*, which, in turn, regulates the rhythmic transcription of key genes involved in gluconeogenesis and lipogenesis (87).

The development of DNA microarray technology has greatly expanded our ability to examine the downstream effectors of the core clock machinery, particularly in peripheral tissues. Gene expression profiling has revealed that a surprisingly large number of transcripts (approximately 5%–10% of the transcriptome) display a 24-hour variation in mRNA expression levels within the SCN, liver, heart, vasculature, and fat (116, 119, 152, 161). Furthermore, very few of these genes show coordinate circadian regulation between tissues, suggesting a high degree of tissue specificity in the output of the *Clock-controlled genes*. Profiling of the circadian proteome has further revealed that up to 20% of proteins are subject to circadian control in the liver (122). Surprisingly, however, almost half of these cycling proteins did not have correspondingly cycling transcripts, suggesting that circadian regulation also exists at a post-transcriptional level (122). Importantly, both the transcriptome and proteome studies have highlighted a key role for the circadian regulation of a number of genes and/or proteins involved in intermediary metabolic processes, including oxidative phosphorylation, carbohydrate metabolism and transport, lipid biogenesis, cholesterol biosynthesis, and proprotein processing (116, 119, 152, 161). These studies suggest that circadian regulation may provide a temporal mechanism to coordinate and/or separate a diverse range of interdependent chemical reactions in the cell.

COMMUNICATION BETWEEN SCN AND CNS CENTERS CONTROLLING ENERGY BALANCE AND METABOLISM

Map of Circadian Centers

There are several levels at which circadian and metabolic systems may affect metabolism within the whole animal. In taking a top-down approach, it is useful to consider first how circadian signaling centers within the brain are connected to regions involved in appetite control, energy expenditure, and metabolism (**Figure 3**, see color insert). For example, neural tracing studies have revealed numerous projections from the SCN to hypothalamic cell clusters that express orexigenic and anorexigenic neuropeptides (154, 170). The largest output of SCN projections is directed toward the subparaventricular zone (SPZ) and the dorsomedial nucleus of the hypothalamus (DMH) (131). The role of each of these hypothalamic regions in the regulation of circadian rhythms was determined by elegant studies using neurotrophic toxins (35, 95). Destruction of the ventral SPZ (vSPZ) reduced circadian rhythms of sleep-wakefulness and locomotor activity but had little effect on circadian regulation of body temperature (95). Conversely, degeneration of the dorsal SPZ (dSPZ) disrupted circadian regulation of body temperature with minimal effect on sleep-wakefulness and locomotor activity (95), thus demonstrating a dissociation of circadian regulation of sleep-wakefulness and body temperature (131). Electrode ablation of the DMH cell bodies, which receive inputs from both the SCN and the SPZ, resulted in severe impairment of circadian-regulated sleep-wakefulness, locomotor activity, corticosteroid secretion, and feeding (35). Furthermore, the DMH has many outputs to other regions of the brain, including the ventrolateral preoptic nucleus, the paraventricular nucleus, and the lateral hypothalamus, which regulate sleep, corticosteroid release, and wakefulness/feeding, respectively. Thus, the DMH constitutes a gateway between the master pacemaker neurons of the SCN and cell bodies located within brain centers important in energy homeostasis (**Figure 3**). Interestingly, the DMH has also been implicated in the ability of organisms to be entrained by restricted feeding; a subset of DMH neurons show robust *Per2* oscillations following restricted feeding, and ablation of the DMH eliminates the altered sleep-wake, activity, and feeding rhythms characteristic of food-restricted animals (64a, 105). However, controversy remains concerning the precise anatomic localization of the food-entrainable oscillator because Landry et al. (85a) have reported that DMH ablation fails to disrupt this phenomena.

SPZ: subparaventricular zone

DMH: dorsomedial hypothalamus

Map of Energy Centers

While studies of SCN architecture have advanced our understanding of CNS timekeeping, a distinct line of investigation has focused on the localization of neuronal centers

ARC: arcuate nucleus

CART: cocaine- and amphetamine-regulated transcript

α-MSH: α-melanocyte-stimulating hormone

NPY: neuropeptide Y

AgRP: agouti-related protein

involved in energy balance and feeding behavior (71). Classical lesioning studies performed more than 50 years ago demonstrated that distinct regions of the hypothalamus control hunger and satiety. Destruction of the ventromedial hypothalamic (VMH), PVH, and DMH regions resulted in obesity (7, 23, 69, 70), whereas ablation of the lateral hypothalamus (LH) resulted in anorexia (7). Although these relatively nonselective approaches did not provide a molecular entrée into understanding the hypothalamic regulation of appetite and food intake, they did provide an anatomical framework for future studies examining the integration of hormonal and nutrient signals at the level of specific hypothalamic regions. The suggestion that humoral factors might be responsible for the control of appetite and energy expenditure was first made by Coleman and colleagues (37, 38) in the late 1960s and early 1970s, following parabiosis experiments between two genetic mouse models of obesity, the *obese* (*ob/ob*) and *diabetic* (*db/db*) mice, that suggested that the *ob/ob* gene encoded a secreted factor, whereas the *db/db* gene encoded its cognate receptor. Ultimately, a major breakthrough in our molecular understanding of hypothalamic regulation of energy balance came with the positional cloning of leptin, a secreted adipocyte-derived factor, as the product of the *ob/ob* gene (179). Subsequently, expression and positional cloning identified the protein product deficient in *db/db* mice as the leptin receptor (33, 36, 90, 156). Administration of leptin to *ob/ob* mice decreased food intake and body weight and corrected neuroendocrine abnormalities (28, 67, 117). Importantly, Ahima et al. (3) showed that low levels of leptin during fasting suppress reproductive function and energy expenditure. The fact that leptin is secreted from adipocytes in proportion to total body adipose mass (59, 96), that leptin is expressed in a circadian fashion in addition to fluctuating in response to fasting and feeding (4, 76, 91, 92, 135, 145), and that the leptin receptor is highly expressed in various regions within the hypothalamus, including the arcuate nucleus (ARC), DMH, and VMH nuclei (54), suggests that humoral signals derived from peripheral tissues may communicate the nutritional status of the organism to the hypothalamic centers controlling hunger and satiety in a circadian-dependent manner.

Additional insight into the neural control of energy homeostasis came with the discovery of the melanocortin system as downstream of leptin (57, 72). Leptin, a satiety signal, stimulates pro-opiomelanocortin (POMC) and cocaine- and amphetamine-regulated transcript (CART)-expressing neurons within the ARC to produce α-melanocyte-stimulating hormone (α-MSH), which subsequently activates the melanocortin receptor subtype 4 (MC4) and results in decreased food intake and increased energy expenditure (1, 39). Leptin also suppresses a distinct set of neuropeptide Y (NPY) and agouti-related protein (AgRP)-expressing ARC neurons that, when active, antagonize the effect of α-MSH on the MC4 receptor through release of AgRP (114, 120, 124) and inhibit the POMC/CART-expressing neurons through release of the small inhibitory amino acid neurotransmitter γ-aminobutyric acid (40). In the absence of leptin, such as during the fasted state, the orexigenic NPY/AgRP neuropeptides cause decreased energy expenditure and increased appetite (16, 52, 53, 99, 150). The integration of signaling by agonists (α-MSH) and antagonists (AgRP) of the melanocortin receptor is pivotal in the weight-regulating effects of leptin in the central nervous system.

Both POMC/CART and NPY/AgRP ARC neurons project to multiple nuclei involved in feeding behavior, some of which also receive input from the SCN and display pronounced circadian rhythms of gene expression (40, 52, 54, 55). These include neurons in the lateral hypothalamic area that produce the hunger-stimulating neuropeptides melanin-concentrating hormone (MCH) and orexins A and B (58, 60, 136). Targeted deletion studies of MCH resulted in hypophagic lean mice with a high metabolic rate and demonstrated that MCH acts downstream of leptin and the melanocortin system (140). Orexins A and B are two neuropeptides generated from a single transcript that display a circadian rhythm of expression and are strongly induced by fasting (153, 172). Intracerebroventricular injection of orexin A stimulates food intake acutely in rats, in part through excitation of NPY in the ARC (130, 153); however, the long-term effects of orexins on energy balance are not yet fully established.

Genetic studies have also uncovered a role for the orexins in the regulation of sleep-wake rhythms. Mutations in the orexin B receptor were found to cause narcolepsy in two independent canine populations (93, 172), and deletion of the orexin gene results in narcolepsy in mice (31). Narcoleptic humans also have decreased orexin levels (111) and, interestingly, increased body mass index levels (110). Furthermore, the finding that orexin-producing neurons project to extensive regions within both the cortex and brainstem is consistent with a role for these neuropeptides in modulating arousal and autonomic function (45, 46). It is also important to note that additional neuromodulators involved in both feeding and alertness, including the histaminergic and serotinergic transmitters, may have combined effects on alertness, circadian rhythmicity, and metabolism (100, 101, 157). The complete identity of both chemical and anatomic pathways through which organisms balance the homeostatic needs of sleep and fuel metabolism remains an active area of investigation.

INTERCONNECTIONS BETWEEN CIRCADIAN GENE PATHWAYS AND METABOLISM

A unifying principle to have emerged from studies of circadian timekeeping and energy balance is that both of these dynamic processes exhibit a hierarchical organization in which the brain drives the function of peripheral tissues. Furthermore, as reviewed above, the circadian and energetic centers are intimately connected at both a neuroanatomical and neuroendocrine level. More recent studies suggest that such interconnections also extend to coregulation of metabolic and circadian transcription networks within individual peripheral tissues and cells. A major advance in our awareness of the temporal organization of metabolic processes stemmed from the landmark discovery by Schibler and colleagues (14) that peripheral tissues express self-sustained periodic oscillators. The following sections focus on recent evidence that suggests that a reciprocal relationship exists between the circadian and metabolic gene pathways.

Circadian Transcriptional Networks Promote Metabolic Homeostasis

Mounting evidence suggests that many essential metabolic pathways are subject to circadian control. For example, a vast number of nuclear receptor (NR) proteins exhibit circadian patterns of gene expression in a variety of metabolic tissues (175). NR proteins are transcription factors activated by the binding of endocrine hormones, such as steroid and thyroid hormones, vitamins, and dietary lipids, and these proteins regulate a diverse range of metabolic processes, including lipid and carbohydrate metabolism (32). Thus, it is possible that the circadian rhythmicity of NRs will contribute in part to the well-documented diurnal variations in lipid and glucose metabolism.

As described above, CLOCK/BMAL heterodimers positively regulate the transcription of the orphan nuclear receptor *Rev-erbα*, which subsequently inhibits transcription of *Bmal1* as part of a cell-autonomous feedback loop (66, 118). In addition to its regulation by the core clock complex, *Rev-erbα* is also regulated by a host of metabolic processes, including adipogenesis and carbohydrate metabolism, which in turn may affect the circadian clock through their actions on *Rev-erbα*. For example, *Rev-erbα* mRNA levels increase dramatically during adipocyte differentiation (31), and REV-ERBα is phosphorylated and stabilized by glycogen synthase kinase 3 (176). Furthermore, *Rev-erbα* transcription is inhibited by retinoic acid (31), levels of which are increased in the metabolic syndrome (175), and the retinoic acid–related orphan receptor RORα has been shown to regulate lipogenesis and lipid storage in muscle in addition to its role as a positive transcriptional regulator of *Bmal1* (95).

The circadian rhythmicity of another NR family member, peroxisome proliferator-activated receptor α (PPARα), provides a further example of a reciprocal link between circadian and metabolic processes. As with RORα, the CLOCK/BMAL heterodimer activates transcription of PPARα, which subsequently binds to the peroxisome-proliferator response element and activates transcription of *Bmal1*. PPARα regulates the transcription of genes involved in lipid and glucose metabolism upon binding of endogenous free fatty acids to its receptor. These data are concordant with the finding that BMAL1-deficient embryonic fibroblasts fail to differentiate into adipocytes (141) and demonstrate that PPARα may also play a unique role at the intersection of circadian and metabolic pathways.

Emerging studies from experimental genetic models support a central role for clock genes in the regulation of energy balance and metabolism. Both *Clock* mutant and $Bmal1^{-/-}$ mice develop not only circadian defects, but also metabolic deficits in glucose and lipid homeostasis (125, 160). An analysis performed on C57BL/6J *Clock/Clock* mutant and coisogenic wild-type mice revealed that *Clock* mutant mice have an attenuated diurnal feeding pattern, are hyperphagic and obese, and develop metabolic abnormalities, including hyperleptinemia, hyperlipidemia, hepatic steatosis, hyperglycemia, and hypoinsulinemia. Furthermore, *Clock* mutant mice had reduced levels of the orexigenic neuropeptides orexin and ghrelin (160). On mixed genetic backgrounds, Rudic et al. (125) reported decreased gluconeogenesis in both *Clock* mutant and $Bmal1^{-/-}$ mice, in addition to suppression of the normal diurnal variation in glucose and triglycerides. Additional studies, recently reviewed by Kohsaka & Bass (81), have also pointed to a role for the clock genes in adipocyte hypertrophy and the response to diet-induced obesity in vivo, in addition to the importance of considering strain background. A fascinating question remains as to whether the metabolic phenotypes of the *Clock* and *Bmal1* mutant animals are dependent or independent on the circadian function of these conserved genes. A deeper understanding of the cell-autonomous function of each gene will lead to better insight into their phenotypes and open new windows on manipulations to enhance metabolic function under circumstances of circadian disruption. Finally, it is interesting to speculate that clock genes represent an example of convergent evolution because the pressure to preserve energy and to adhere to a light/dark cycle may have coexisted during the origins of life.

Nutrient and Metabolic Signaling in Circadian Rhythms and Sleep

Feeding and sleep/circadian rhythmicity. Although the aforementioned studies clearly demonstrate that many central metabolic pathways are subject to circadian control, several studies have revealed that the reciprocal relationship also holds true: i.e., alterations in metabolism disrupt sleep-wake patterns and/or circadian rhythmicity. For example, mice fed a high-fat diet have increased sleep time, particularly in the nonrapid eye movement (NREM) stage, but decreased sleep consolidation (75). On the other hand, food deprivation results in decreased sleep time (43, 107) and a more fragmented sleep pattern in rats (21). The refeeding period following food deprivation in these animals is accompanied by lengthened sleep time (139) and varies as a function of the nutritional content of the food (107). In addition to diet-induced alterations in sleep architecture, genetic mouse models of obesity have similarly demonstrated disrupted sleep-wake patterns. The

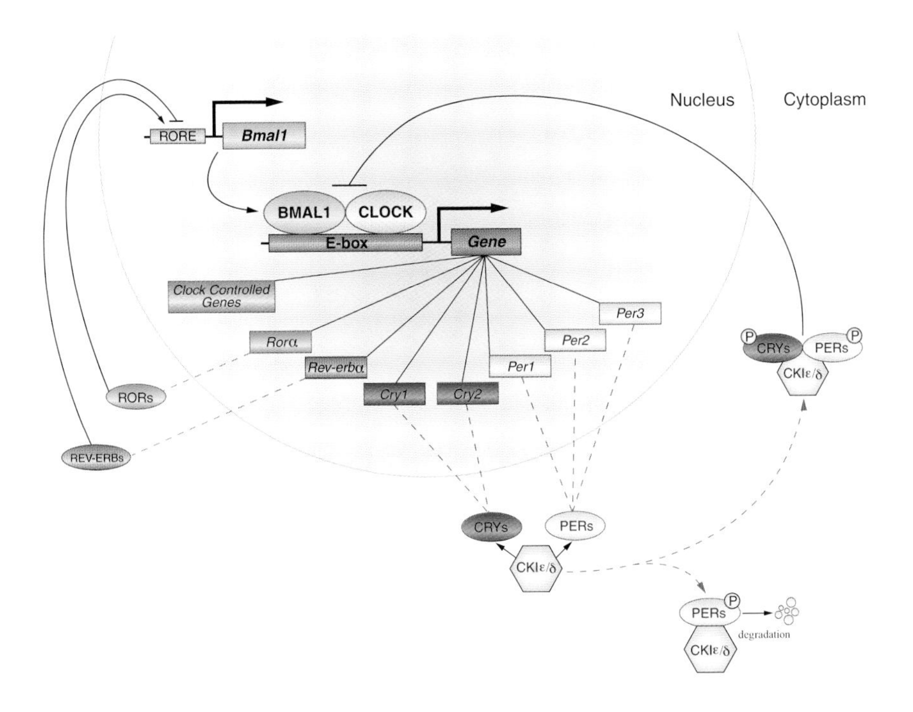

Figure 1

Central mechanism of the clock in all cells. The mammalian circadian clock consists of a network of transcription-translation feedback loops. The transcription factors circadian locomotor output cycles kaput (CLOCK) and brain and muscle ARNT-like (BMAL)1 heterodimerize and activate transcription of downstream targets, including the *period*, *cryptochrome*, *Ror*, and *Rev-Erb* genes, which contain E-box enhancer elements within their promoters. Upon translation, the period (PER) and cryptochrome (CRY) proteins multimerize and inhibit the action of the CLOCK/BMAL1 complex. Phosphorylation of PERs and CRYs by casein kinases I epsilon and delta (CKIε/δ), and the subsequent degradation of the PERs, is an important modulator of circadian rhythmicity. The retinoic acid–related orphan receptors (RORs) and REV-ERBs constitute another regulatory feedback loop through regulation of *Bmal1* transcription.

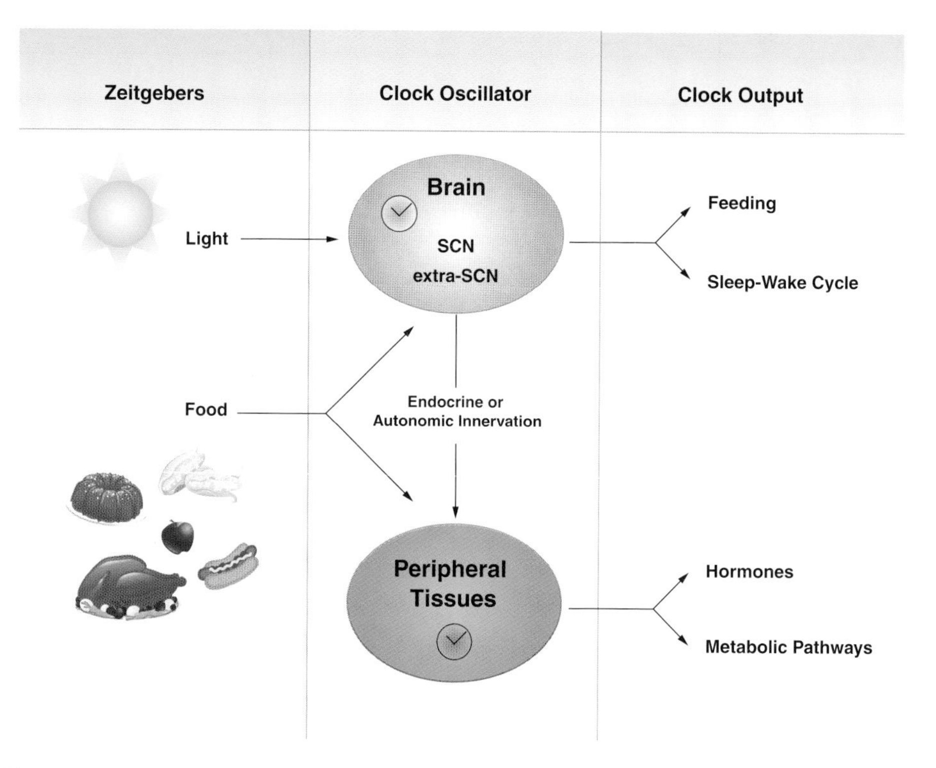

Figure 2

Clocks coordinate feeding and metabolism with environmental cues. Although the mammalian master pacemaker is located in the suprachiasmatic nucleus (SCN), the core clock machinery has been identified in most peripheral tissues, as well as in extra-SCN regions of the brain. These oscillators are entrainable, responding to extrinsic stimuli such as light and food, and the master pacemaker coordinates peripheral clocks through both endocrine signals and autonomic innervation. The clock output includes behavioral and metabolic responses, such as feeding, sleep-wakefulness, hormone secretion, and metabolic homeostasis. Not drawn are extensive reciprocal loops that connect clock output in both brain and peripheral tissues with the clock oscillators.

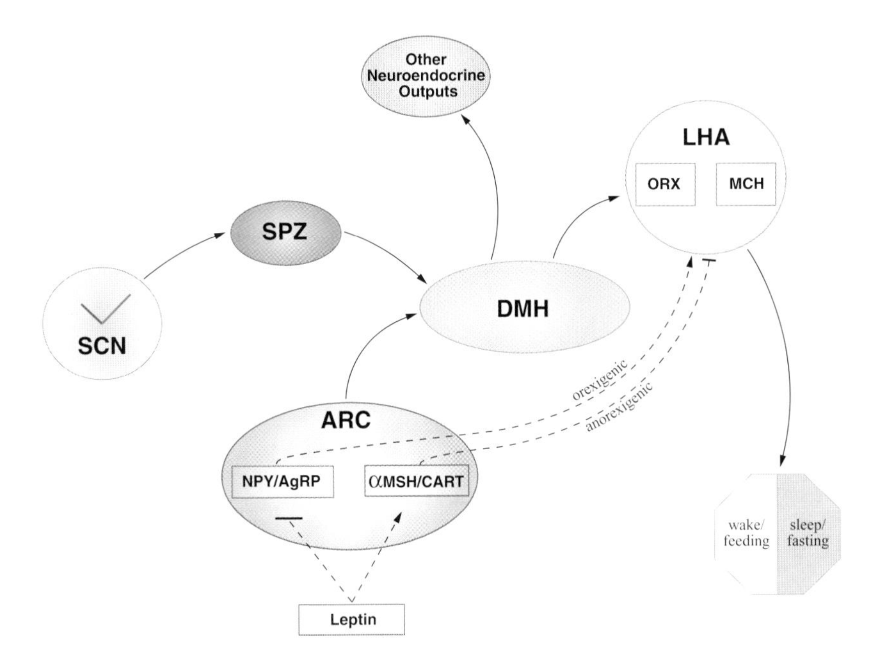

Figure 3

Neuroanatomic and neuroendocrine connections within the hypothalamus. The largest output of neural projections from the suprachiasmatic nucleus (SCN) extends toward the subparaventricular zone (SPZ) and continues from the SPZ to the dorsomedial hypothalamus (DMH). The DMH has many outputs to other regions of the brain, including the lateral hypothalamus (LHA), which controls circadian regulation of coordination of the alternans of sleep/wakefulness and fasting/feeding. The LHA also receives neuroendocrine input from the arcuate nucleus (ARC). Leptin activates neuronal cells within the ARC that express the anorexigenic neuropeptides α-MSH/CART, which in turn results in inhibition of production of orexigenic peptides orexin (ORX) and melanin concentrating hormone (MCH) in the LHA. In the absence of leptin, orexigenic neurons in the ARC produce neuropeptide Y (NPY)/agouti-related protein (AgRP) and stimulate hunger and decreased energy expenditure via signaling to the LHA.

leptin-deficient *ob/ob* mouse exhibits hyperphagia, obesity, and stigmata of the metabolic syndrome, including hyperglycemia, insulin resistance, and dyslipidemia (73, 179). These mice have recently been shown to have increased NREM sleep time, decreased sleep consolidation, decreased locomotor activity, and a smaller compensatory rebound response to acute sleep deprivation (86). Similarly, rats harboring mutations in the leptin receptor display increased sleep time and decreased sleep consolidation (42, 102). Evidence has begun to emerge suggesting that metabolic disorders may also affect circadian rhythmicity. For example, the circadian expression of a number of genes is attenuated in the fat and liver of obese KK-A(y) mice, a polygenic model for noninsulin-dependent diabetes mellitus (8, 9).

Molecular sensors linking metabolism and circadian rhythmicity. A major question resulting from these studies concerns the nature of the molecular link between the regulation of metabolism and circadian rhythmicity, particularly in the peripheral tissues. Is there a molecular "sensor" common to the regulation of both of these processes? One possible explanation for the interdependence of metabolic and circadian processes stems from the finding that changes in the cellular redox status of cells, represented by the nicotinamide adenine dinucleotide cofactors NAD(H) and NADP(H), regulate the transcriptional activity of the bHLH proteins CLOCK and its homolog NPAS2. The reduced forms of these redox cofactors enhance DNA binding of the CLOCK/BMAL1 and NPAS2/BMAL1 heterodimers, whereas the oxidized forms inhibit binding (126). Thus, it is possible that direct modulation of the redox state in response to feeding, for example, may provide an additional level of regulation of the circadian clock and may serve as a molecular link between metabolic and circadian processes. However, how metabolic sensors affect circadian processes in vivo remains an area of active investigation.

Hormones and sleep. Within the whole animal, numerous studies have revealed that various hormones and neuromodulators have overlapping roles in regulating metabolism and sleep, and by extension, may be involved in synchronizing these processes. For example, acute administration of leptin, an adipocyte-derived circulating hormone that acts at specific receptors in the hypothalamus to suppress appetite and increase metabolism, decreases REM and increases NREM sleep time in rats (144). Furthermore, leptin-deficient mice have significantly disrupted sleep architecture with impaired sleep consolidation and diurnal rhythmicity, as described above (86). Increased levels of other anorectic hormones, including gastrointestinal tract–derived cholecystokinin and pancreatic β cell–derived insulin also increase sleep time in rodents (44, 97). Ghrelin, an orexigenic stomach-derived hormone, has been shown to increase NREM sleep in both rodents and humans (112, 171), whereas orexin/hypocretin neuropeptides, produced by a small subset of neurons within the lateral, posterior, and perifornical hypothalamus in response to fasting, stimulate food intake, locomotor activity, and wakefulness (46, 129). Interestingly, the receptor for orexin/hypocretin has been shown to be the causative genetic defect in the most common form of canine narcolepsy (93). The regulation of both metabolism and wakefulness by these neuroendocrine factors suggests that coordination of periods of fasting with sleep and feeding with wakefulness is important. These observations also have potential implications for the pharmacological development of therapies for both sleep and metabolic disease. Lack of sleep or altered metabolism may disrupt these homeostatic conditions, resulting in activation of metabolic pathways that lead to increased food intake or altered sleep architecture, respectively.

CONCLUSIONS/PERSPECTIVES

Remarkable advances in mammalian experimental genetics heralded by the discoveries of leptin in 1994 and the *Clock* gene in 1997 have transformed our understanding of both metabolism and circadian rhythmicity. A major theme to have emerged has been the finding that perturbation of either CNS pathways or those within peripheral metabolic tissues contribute to diabetes and obesity and are important in basal homeostasis. Compelling new evidence reviewed above has uncovered an interconnection between temporal regulation and metabolic processes that may have implications for understanding human diseases such as sleep disorders and diabetes. With the molecular road map now in hand to unlock the key to internal timekeeping, new opportunities are available to integrate studies of behavior and metabolism. One conclusion that can already be drawn is that metabolic processes are highly dynamic and subject to strong variation across the 24-hour light/dark cycle at both the molecular and physiologic levels. One implication is that introducing temporal analyses in studies of metabolism may lead to the discovery of previously unrecognized phenotypes. At the cellular level, the challenge will be to define the impact of the clock gene network on specific metabolic processes. At the organismal level, the integration of circadian and metabolic analyses may lead us closer to a unified understanding of how internal systems have evolved to optimize survival across the daily light/dark changes in environment.

DISCLOSURE STATEMENT

Joseph Bass is a consultant for Abbot Laboratories, Amylin Pharmaceuticals, Astells, Astra Zeneca, Aventis, Bristol-Myers Squibb, Clinical Advisors, Gerson Lehrman Group, Hinshaw, Merck, Novartis (Genomics Institute of the Novartis Foundation), Novo Nordisk, Regeneron, Schering-Plough, and Takeda.

ACKNOWLEDGMENTS

This work was supported by National Institutes of Health grants to JB. KMR is supported in part by NIH/NIDDK Training Grant DK007169. This work was also supported by the National Center for Research Resources grant number 1CO6RR015497-0141. We thank Drs. R. Allada, A. Laposky, J. Takahashi, F. Turek, and M. Vitaterna, as well as other members of the Bass lab, for their ongoing and helpful discussions.

LITERATURE CITED

1. Adan RA, Cone RD, Burbach JP, Gispen WH. 1994. Differential effects of melanocortin peptides on neural melanocortin receptors. *Mol. Pharmacol.* 46:1182–90
2. Aguilar-Roblero R, Morin LP, Moore RY. 1994. Morphological correlates of circadian rhythm restoration induced by transplantation of the suprachiasmatic nucleus in hamsters. *Exp. Neurol.* 130:250–60
3. Ahima RS, Prabakaran D, Mantzoros C, Qu D, Lowell B, et al. 1996. Role of leptin in the neuroendocrine response to fasting. *Nature* 382:250–52
4. Ahren B. 2000. Diurnal variation in circulating leptin is dependent on gender, food intake and circulating insulin in mice. *Acta Physiol. Scand.* 169:325–31
5. Akashi M, Takumi T. 2005. The orphan nuclear receptor RORα regulates circadian transcription of the mammalian core-clock Bmal1. *Nat. Struct. Mol. Biol.* 12:441–48
6. Akashi M, Tsuchiya Y, Yoshino T, Nishida E. 2002. Control of intracellular dynamics of mammalian period proteins by casein kinase I epsilon (CKIε) and CKIδ in cultured cells. *Mol. Cell. Biol.* 22:1693–703

7. Anand BK, Brobeck JR. 1951. Localization of a "feeding center" in the hypothalamus of the rat. *Proc. Soc. Exp. Biol. Med.* 77:323–24
8. Ando H, Oshima Y, Yanagihara H, Hayashi Y, Takamura T, et al. 2006. Profile of rhythmic gene expression in the livers of obese diabetic KK-A(y) mice. *Biochem. Biophys. Res. Commun.* 346:1297–302
9. Ando H, Yanagihara H, Hayashi Y, Obi Y, Tsuruoka S, et al. 2005. Rhythmic messenger ribonucleic acid expression of clock genes and adipocytokines in mouse visceral adipose tissue. *Endocrinology* 146:5631–36
10. Aparicio NJ, Puchulu FE, Gagliardino JJ, Ruiz M, Llorens JM, et al. 1974. Circadian variation of the blood glucose, plasma insulin and human growth hormone levels in response to an oral glucose load in normal subjects. *Diabetes* 23:132–37
11. Arslanian S, Ohki Y, Becker DJ, Drash AL. 1990. Demonstration of a dawn phenomenon in normal adolescents. *Horm. Res.* 34:27–32
12. Bae K, Jin X, Maywood ES, Hastings MH, Reppert SM, Weaver DR. 2001. Differential functions of mPer1, mPer2, and mPer3 in the SCN circadian clock. *Neuron* 30:525–36
13. Baker IA, Jarrett RJ. 1972. Diurnal variation in the blood-sugar and plasma-insulin response to tolbutamide. *Lancet* 2:945–47
14. Balsalobre A, Damiola F, Schibler U. 1998. A serum shock induces circadian gene expression in mammalian tissue culture cells. *Cell* 93:929–37
15. Balsalobre A, Marcacci L, Schibler U. 2000. Multiple signaling pathways elicit circadian gene expression in cultured Rat-1 fibroblasts. *Curr. Biol.* 10:1291–94
16. Baskin DG, Breininger JF, Schwartz MW. 1999. Leptin receptor mRNA identifies a subpopulation of neuropeptide Y neurons activated by fasting in rat hypothalamus. *Diabetes* 48:828–33
17. Bell-Pedersen D, Cassone VM, Earnest DJ, Golden SS, Hardin PE, et al. 2005. Circadian rhythms from multiple oscillators: lessons from diverse organisms. *Nat. Rev. Genet.* 6:544–56
18. Boden G, Chen X, Polansky M. 1999. Disruption of circadian insulin secretion is associated with reduced glucose uptake in first-degree relatives of patients with type 2 diabetes. *Diabetes* 48:2182–88
19. Boden G, Ruiz J, Urbain JL, Chen X. 1996. Evidence for a circadian rhythm of insulin secretion. *Am. J. Physiol.* 271:E246–52
20. Bolli GB, De Feo P, De Cosmo S, Perriello G, Ventura MM, et al. 1984. Demonstration of a dawn phenomenon in normal human volunteers. *Diabetes* 33:1150–53
21. Borbely AA. 1977. Sleep in the rat during food deprivation and subsequent restitution of food. *Brain Res.* 124:457–71
22. Bowen AJ, Reeves RL. 1967. Diurnal variation in glucose tolerance. *Arch. Intern. Med.* 119:261–64
23. Brobeck JR. 1946. Mechanisms of the development of obesity in animals with hypothalamic lesions. *Physiol. Rev.* 26:541–49
24. Brown SA, Fleury-Olela F, Nagoshi E, Hauser C, Juge C, et al. 2005. The period length of fibroblast circadian gene expression varies widely among human individuals. *PLOS Biol.* 3:e338
25. Bunger MK, Walisser JA, Sullivan R, Manley PA, Moran SM, et al. 2005. Progressive arthropathy in mice with a targeted disruption of the Mop3/Bmal-1 locus. *Genesis* 41:122–32
26. Bunger MK, Wilsbacher LD, Moran SM, Clendenin C, Radcliffe LA, et al. 2000. Mop3 is an essential component of the master circadian pacemaker in mammals. *Cell* 103:1009–17

27. Cailotto C, La Fleur SE, Van Heijningen C, Wortel J, Kalsbeek A, et al. 2005. The suprachiasmatic nucleus controls the daily variation of plasma glucose via the autonomic output to the liver: Are the clock genes involved? *Eur. J. Neurosci.* 22:2531–40
28. Campfield LA, Smith FJ, Guisez Y, Devos R, Burn P. 1995. Recombinant mouse OB protein: evidence for a peripheral signal linking adiposity and central neural networks. *Science* 269:546–49
29. Carroll KF, Nestel PJ. 1973. Diurnal variation in glucose tolerance and in insulin secretion in man. *Diabetes* 22:333–48
30. Cermakian N, Monaco L, Pando MP, Dierich A, Sassone-Corsi P. 2001. Altered behavioral rhythms and clock gene expression in mice with a targeted mutation in the Period1 gene. *EMBO J.* 20:3967–74
31. Chawla A, Lazar MA. 1993. Induction of Rev-ErbA alpha, an orphan receptor encoded on the opposite strand of the alpha-thyroid hormone receptor gene, during adipocyte differentiation. *J. Biol. Chem.* 268:16265–69
32. Chawla A, Repa JJ, Evans RM, Mangelsdorf DJ. 2001. Nuclear receptors and lipid physiology: opening the X-files. *Science* 294:1866–70
33. Chen H, Charlat O, Tartaglia LA, Woolf EA, Weng X, et al. 1996. Evidence that the diabetes gene encodes the leptin receptor: identification of a mutation in the leptin receptor gene in db/db mice. *Cell* 84:491–95
34. Cheng MY, Bullock CM, Li C, Lee AG, Bermak JC, et al. 2002. Prokineticin 2 transmits the behavioural circadian rhythm of the suprachiasmatic nucleus. *Nature* 417:405–10
35. Chou TC, Scammell TE, Gooley JJ, Gaus SE, Saper CB, Lu J. 2003. Critical role of dorsomedial hypothalamic nucleus in a wide range of behavioral circadian rhythms. *J. Neurosci.* 23:10691–702
36. Chua SCJ, Chung WK, Wu-Peng XS, Zhang Y, Liu SM, et al. 1996. Phenotypes of mouse diabetes and rat fatty due to mutations in the OB (leptin) receptor. *Science* 271:994–96
37. Coleman DL. 1973. Effects of parabiosis of obese with diabetes and normal mice. *Diabetologia* 9:294–98
38. Coleman DL, Hummel KP. 1969. Effects of parabiosis of normal with genetically diabetic mice. *Am. J. Physiol.* 217:1298–304
39. Cone RD. 2005. Anatomy and regulation of the central melanocortin system. *Nat. Neurosci.* 8:571–78
40. Cowley MA, Smart JL, Rubinstein M, Cerdan MG, Diano S, et al. 2001. Leptin activates anorexigenic POMC neurons through a neural network in the arcuate nucleus. *Nature* 411:480–84
41. Damiola F, Le Minh N, Preitner N, Kornmann B, Fleury-Olela F, Schibler U. 2000. Restricted feeding uncouples circadian oscillators in peripheral tissues from the central pacemaker in the suprachiasmatic nucleus. *Genes Dev.* 14:2950–61
42. Danguir J. 1989. Sleep patterns in the genetically obese Zucker rat: effect of acarbose treatment. *Am. J. Physiol.* 256:R281–83
43. Danguir J, Nicolaidis S. 1979. Dependence of sleep on nutrients' availability. *Physiol. Behav.* 22:735–40
44. Danguir J, Nicolaidis S. 1984. Chronic intracerebroventricular infusion of insulin causes selective increase of slow wave sleep in rats. *Brain Res.* 306:97–103
45. Date Y, Ueta Y, Yamashita H, Yamaguchi H, Matsukura S, et al. 1999. Orexins, orexigenic hypothalamic peptides, interact with autonomic, neuroendocrine and neuroregulatory systems. *Proc. Natl. Acad. Sci. USA* 96:748–53

46. de Lecea L, Kilduff TS, Peyron C, Gao X, Foye PE, et al. 1998. The hypocretins: hypothalamus-specific peptides with neuroexcitatory activity. *Proc. Natl. Acad. Sci. USA* 95:322–27
47. Di Lorenzo L, De Pergola G, Zocchetti C, L'Abbate N, Basso A, et al. 2003. Effect of shift work on body mass index: results of a study performed in 319 glucose-tolerant men working in a Southern Italian industry. *Int. J. Obes. Relat. Metab. Disord.* 27:1353–58
48. Dinneen S, Alzaid A, Miles J, Rizza R. 1995. Effects of the normal nocturnal rise in cortisol on carbohydrate and fat metabolism in IDDM. *Am. J. Physiol.* 268:E595–603
49. Dodd AN, Salathia N, Hall A, Kevei E, Toth R, et al. 2005. Plant circadian clocks increase photosynthesis, growth, survival, and competitive advantage. *Science* 309:630–33
50. Easton A, Meerlo P, Bergmann B, Turek FW. 2004. The suprachiasmatic nucleus regulates sleep timing and amount in mice. *Sleep* 27:1307–18
51. Eide EJ, Vielhaber EL, Hinz WA, Virshup DM. 2002. The circadian regulatory proteins BMAL1 and cryptochromes are substrates of casein kinase I-epsilon. *J. Biol. Chem.* 277:17248–54
52. Elias CF, Aschkenasi C, Lee C, Kelly J, Ahima RS, et al. 1999. Leptin differentially regulates NPY and POMC neurons projecting to the lateral hypothalamic area. *Neuron* 23:775–86
53. Elias CF, Kelly JF, Lee CE, Ahima RS, Drucker DJ, et al. 2000. Chemical characterization of leptin-activated neurons in the rat brain. *J. Comp. Neurol.* 423:261–81
54. Elmquist JK, Ahima RS, Elias CF, Flier JS, Saper CB. 1998. Leptin activates distinct projections from the dorsomedial and ventromedial hypothalamic nuclei. *Proc. Natl. Acad. Sci. USA* 95:741–46
55. Elmquist JK, Elias CF, Saper CB. 1999. From lesions to leptin: hypothalamic control of food intake and body weight. *Neuron* 22:221–32
56. Eskin A. 1979. Identification and physiology of circadian pacemakers. Introduction. *Fed. Proc.* 38:2570–72
57. Fan W, Boston BA, Kesterson RA, Hruby VJ, Cone RD. 1997. Role of melanocortinergic neurons in feeding and the agouti obesity syndrome. *Nature* 385:165–68
58. Flier JS, Maratos-Flier E. 1998. Obesity and the hypothalamus: novel peptides for new pathways. *Cell* 92:437–40
59. Frederich RC, Hamann A, Anderson S, Lollmann B, Lowell BB, Flier JS. 1995. Leptin levels reflect body lipid content in mice: evidence for diet-induced resistance to leptin action. *Nat. Med.* 1:1311–14
60. Friedman JM, Halaas JL. 1998. Leptin and the regulation of body weight in mammals. *Nature* 395:763–70
61. Gagliardino JJ, Hernandez RE, Rebolledo OR. 1984. Chronobiological aspects of blood glucose regulation: a new scope for the study of diabetes mellitus. *Chronobiologia* 11:357–79
62. Gardner MJ, Hubbard KE, Hotta CT, Dodd AN, Webb AA. 2006. How plants tell the time. *Biochem. J.* 397:15–24
63. Gaston S, Menaker M. 1968. Pineal function: the biological clock in the sparrow? *Science* 160:1125–27
64. Gekakis N, Staknis D, Nguyen HB, Davis FC, Wilsbacher LD, et al. 1998. Role of the CLOCK protein in the mammalian circadian mechanism. *Science* 280:1564–69
64a. Gooley JJ, Schomer A, Saper CB. 2006. The dorsomedial hypothalamic nucleus is critical for the expression of food-entrainable circadian rhythms. *Nat. Neurosci.* 9:398–407

65. Gottlieb DJ, Punjabi NM, Newman AB, Resnick HE, Redline S, et al. 2005. Association of sleep time with diabetes mellitus and impaired glucose tolerance. *Arch. Intern. Med.* 165:863–67
66. Guillaumond F, Dardente H, Giguere V, Cermakian N. 2005. Differential control of Bmal1 circadian transcription by REV-ERB and ROR nuclear receptors. *J. Biol. Rhythms* 20:391–403
67. Halaas JL, Gajiwala KS, Maffei M, Cohen SL, Chait BT, et al. 1995. Weight-reducing effects of the plasma protein encoded by the obese gene. *Science* 269:543–46
68. Hasler G, Buysse DJ, Klaghofer R, Gamma A, Ajdacic V, et al. 2004. The association between short sleep duration and obesity in young adults: a 13-year prospective study. *Sleep* 27:661–66
69. Hetherington AW, Ranson SW. 1940. Hypothalamic lesion and adiposity in the rat. *Anat. Rec.* 78:149–72
70. Hetherington AW, Ranson SW. 1942. The relation of various hypothalamic lesions to adiposity in the rat. *J. Comp. Neurol.* 76:475–99
71. Horvath TL. 2005. The hardship of obesity: a soft-wired hypothalamus. *Nat. Neurosci.* 8:561–65
72. Huszar D, Lynch CA, Fairchild-Huntress V, Dunmore JH, Fang Q, et al. 1997. Targeted disruption of the melanocortin-4 receptor results in obesity in mice. *Cell* 88:131–41
73. Ingalls AM, Dickie MM, Snell GD. 1950. Obese, a new mutation in the house mouse. *J. Hered.* 41:317–18
74. Jarrett RJ, Keen H. 1969. Diurnal variation of oral glucose tolerance: a possible pointer to the evolution of diabetes mellitus. *Br. Med. J.* 2:341–44
75. Jenkins JB, Omori T, Guan Z, Vgontzas AN, Bixler EO, Fang J. 2005. Sleep is increased in mice with obesity induced by high-fat food. *Physiol. Behav.* 87(2):255–62
76. Kalsbeek A, Fliers E, Romijn JA, La Fleur SE, Wortel J, et al. 2001. The suprachiasmatic nucleus generates the diurnal changes in plasma leptin levels. *Endocrinology* 142:2677–85
77. Karlsson B, Knutsson A, Lindahl B. 2001. Is there an association between shift work and having a metabolic syndrome? Results from a population based study of 27485 people. *Occup. Environ. Med.* 58:747–52
78. Karlsson BH, Knutsson AK, Lindahl BO, Alfredsson LS. 2003. Metabolic disturbances in male workers with rotating three-shift work. Results of the WOLF study. *Int. Arch. Occup. Environ. Health* 76:424–30
79. King DP, Vitaterna MH, Chang AM, Dove WF, Pinto LH, et al. 1997. The mouse Clock mutation behaves as an antimorph and maps within the W19H deletion, distal of Kit. *Genetics* 146:1049–60
80. King DP, Zhao Y, Sangoram AM, Wilsbacher LD, Tanaka M, et al. 1997. Positional cloning of the mouse circadian Clock gene. *Cell* 89:641–53
81. Kohsaka A, Bass J. 2007. A sense of time: how molecular clocks organize metabolism. *Trends Endocrinol. Metab.* 18(1):4–11
82. Kondratov RV, Chernov MV, Kondratova AA, Gorbacheva VY, Gudkov AV, Antoch MP. 2003. BMAL1-dependent circadian oscillation of nuclear CLOCK: posttranslational events induced by dimerization of transcriptional activators of the mammalian clock system. *Genes Dev.* 17:1921–32
83. Kramer A, Yang FC, Snodgrass P, Li X, Scammell TE, et al. 2001. Regulation of daily locomotor activity and sleep by hypothalamic EGF receptor signaling. *Science* 294:2511–15

84. Kume K, Zylka MJ, Sriram S, Shearman LP, Weaver DR, et al. 1999. mCRY1 and mCRY2 are essential components of the negative limb of the circadian clock feedback loop. *Cell* 98:193–205
85. la Fleur SE, Kalsbeek A, Wortel J, Fekkes ML, Buijs RM. 2001. A daily rhythm in glucose tolerance: a role for the suprachiasmatic nucleus. *Diabetes* 50:1237–43
85a. Landry GJ, Simon MM, Webb IC, Mistlberger RE. 2006. Persistence of a behavioral food-anticipatory circadian rhythm following dorsomedial hypothalamic ablation in rats. *Am. J. Physiol. Regul. Integr. Comp. Physiol.* 290:R1527–34
86. Laposky AD, Shelton J, Bass J, Dugovic C, Perrino N, Turek FW. 2006. Altered sleep regulation in leptin-deficient mice. *Am. J. Physiol. Regul. Integr. Comp. Physiol.* 290:R894–903
87. Lavery DJ, Lopez-Molina L, Margueron R, Fleury-Olela F, Conquet F, et al. 1999. Circadian expression of the steroid 15 alpha-hydroxylase (Cyp2a4) and coumarin 7-hydroxylase (Cyp2a5) genes in mouse liver is regulated by the PAR leucine zipper transcription factor DBP. *Mol. Cell Biol.* 19:6488–99
88. Lee A, Ader M, Bray GA, Bergman RN. 1992. Diurnal variation in glucose tolerance. Cyclic suppression of insulin action and insulin secretion in normal-weight, but not obese, subjects. *Diabetes* 41:742–49
89. Lee C, Etchegaray JP, Cagampang FR, Loudon AS, Reppert SM. 2001. Posttranslational mechanisms regulate the mammalian circadian clock. *Cell* 107:855–67
90. Lee GH, Proenca R, Montez JM, Carroll KM, Darvishzadeh JG, et al. 1996. Abnormal splicing of the leptin receptor in diabetic mice. *Nature* 379:632–35
91. Licinio J, Mantzoros C, Negrao AB, Cizza G, Wong ML, et al. 1997. Human leptin levels are pulsatile and inversely related to pituitary-adrenal function. *Nat. Med.* 3:575–79
92. Licinio J, Negrao AB, Mantzoros C, Kaklamani V, Wong ML, et al. 1998. Synchronicity of frequently sampled, 24-h concentrations of circulating leptin, luteinizing hormone, and estradiol in healthy women. *Proc. Natl. Acad. Sci. USA* 95:2541–46
93. Lin L, Faraco J, Li R, Kadotani H, Rogers W, et al. 1999. The sleep disorder canine narcolepsy is caused by a mutation in *Hypocretin* (orexin) receptor 2 gene. *Cell* 98:365–76
94. Lowrey PL, Shimomura K, Antoch MP, Yamazaki S, Zemenides PD, et al. 2000. Positional syntenic cloning and functional characterization of the mammalian circadian mutation tau. *Science* 288:483–92
95. Lu J, Zhang YH, Chou TC, Gaus SE, Elmquist JK, et al. 2001. Contrasting effects of ibotenate lesions of the paraventricular nucleus and subparaventricular zone on sleep-wake cycle and temperature regulation. *J. Neurosci.* 21:4864–74
96. Maffei M, Fei H, Lee GH, Dani C, Leroy P, et al. 1995. Increased expression in adipocytes of ob RNA in mice with lesions of the hypothalamus and with mutations at the db locus. *Proc. Natl. Acad. Sci. USA* 92:6957–60
97. Mansbach RS, Lorenz DN. 1983. Cholecystokinin (CCK-8) elicits prandial sleep in rats. *Physiol. Behav.* 30:179–83
98. Maron BJ, Kogan J, Proschan MA, Hecht GM, Roberts WC. 1994. Circadian variability in the occurrence of sudden cardiac death in patients with hypertrophic cardiomyopathy. *J. Am. Coll. Cardiol.* 23:1405–9
99. Marsh DJ, Miura GI, Yagaloff KA, Schwartz MW, Barsh GS, Palmiter RD. 1999. Effects of neuropeptide Y deficiency on hypothalamic agouti-related protein expression and responsiveness to melanocortin analogues. *Brain Res.* 848:66–77

100. Masaki T, Chiba S, Yasuda T, Noguchi H, Kakuma T, et al. 2004. Involvement of hypothalamic histamine H1 receptor in the regulation of feeding rhythm and obesity. *Diabetes* 53:2250–60
101. Masaki T, Yoshimatsu H. 2006. The hypothalamic H1 receptor: a novel therapeutic target for disrupting diurnal feeding rhythm and obesity. *Trends Pharmacol. Sci.* 27:279–84
102. Megirian D, Dmochowski J, Farkas GA. 1998. Mechanism controlling sleep organization of the obese Zucker rats. *J. Appl. Physiol.* 84:253–56
103. Melani F, Verrillo A, Marasco M, Rivellese A, Osorio J, Bertolini MG. 1976. Diurnal variation in blood sugar and serum insulin in response to glucose and/or glucagon in healthy subjects. *Horm. Metab. Res.* 8:85–88
104. Meyer-Bernstein EL, Jetton AE, Matsumoto SI, Markuns JF, Lehman MN, Bittman EL. 1999. Effects of suprachiasmatic transplants on circadian rhythms of neuroendocrine function in golden hamsters. *Endocrinology* 140:207–18
105. Mieda M, Williams SC, Richardson JA, Tanaka K, Yanagisawa M. 2006. The dorsomedial hypothalamic nucleus as a putative food-entrainable circadian pacemaker. *Proc. Natl. Acad. Sci. USA* 103:12150–55
106. Miller BH, Olson SL, Turek FW, Levine JE, Horton TH, Takahashi JS. 2004. Circadian clock mutation disrupts estrous cyclicity and maintenance of pregnancy. *Curr. Biol.* 14:1367–73
107. Minet-Ringuet J, Le Ruyet PM, Tome D, Even PC. 2004. A tryptophan-rich protein diet efficiently restores sleep after food deprivation in the rat. *Behav. Brain Res.* 152:335–40
108. Nilsson PM, Roost M, Engstrom G, Hedblad B, Berglund G. 2004. Incidence of diabetes in middle-aged men is related to sleep disturbances. *Diab. Care* 27:2464–69
109. Nishiisutsuji-Uwo J, Pittendrigh CS. 1968. Central nervous system control of circadian rhythmicity in the cockroach. *Z. Vergl. Physiol.* 58:14–46
110. Nishino S, Mignot E. 2002. Article reviewed: plasma orexin-A is lower in patients with narcolepsy. *Sleep Med.* 3:377–78
111. Nishino S, Ripley B, Overeem S, Lammers GJ, Mignot E. 2000. Hypocretin (orexin) deficiency in human narcolepsy. *Lancet* 355:39–40
112. Obal FJ, Alt J, Taishi P, Gardi J, Krueger JM. 2003. Sleep in mice with nonfunctional growth hormone-releasing hormone receptors. *Am. J. Physiol. Regul. Integr. Comp. Physiol.* 284:R131–39
113. Okamura H, Miyake S, Sumi Y, Yamaguchi S, Yasui A, et al. 1999. Photic induction of *mPer1* and *mPer2* in *Cry*-deficient mice lacking a biological clock. *Science* 286:2531–34
114. Ollmann MM, Wilson BD, Yang YK, Kerns JA, Chen Y, et al. 1997. Antagonism of central melanocortin receptors in vitro and in vivo by agouti-related protein. *Science* 278:135–38
115. Oster MH, Castonguay TW, Keen CL, Stern JS. 1988. Circadian rhythm of corticosterone in diabetic rats. *Life Sci.* 43:1643–45
116. Panda S, Antoch MP, Miller BH, Su AI, Schook AB, et al. 2002. Coordinated transcription of key pathways in the mouse by the circadian clock. *Cell* 109:307–20
117. Pelleymounter MA, Cullen MJ, Baker MB, Hecht R, Winters D, et al. 1995. Effects of the obese gene product on body weight regulation in ob/ob mice. *Science* 269:540–43
118. Preitner N, Damiola F, Lopez-Molina L, Zakany J, Duboule D, et al. 2002. The orphan nuclear receptor REV-ERBα controls circadian transcription within the positive limb of the mammalian circadian oscillator. *Cell* 110:251–60
119. Ptitsyn AA, Zvonic S, Conrad SA, Scott LK, Mynatt RL, Gimble JM. 2006. Circadian clocks are resounding in peripheral tissues. *PLOS Comput. Biol.* 2:e16

120. Quillan JM, Sadee W, Wei ET, Jimenez C, Ji L, Chang JK. 1998. A synthetic human Agouti-related protein-(83-132)-NH2 fragment is a potent inhibitor of melanocortin receptor function. *FEBS Lett.* 428:59–62
121. Ralph MR, Foster RG, Davis FC, Menaker M. 1990. Transplanted suprachiasmatic nucleus determines circadian period. *Science* 247:975–78
122. Reddy AB, Karp NA, Maywood ES, Sage EA, Deery M, et al. 2006. Circadian orchestration of the hepatic proteome. *Curr. Biol.* 16:1107–15
123. Roberts HJ. 1964. Afternoon glucose tolerance testing: a key to the pathogenesis, early diagnosis and prognosis of diabetogenic hyperinsulinism. *J. Am. Geriatr. Soc.* 12:423–72
124. Rossi M, Kim MS, Morgan DG, Small CJ, Edwards CM, et al. 1998. A C-terminal fragment of Agouti-related protein increases feeding and antagonizes the effect of alpha-melanocyte stimulating hormone in vivo. *Endocrinology* 139:4428–31
125. Rudic RD, McNamara P, Curtis AM, Boston RC, Panda S, et al. 2004. BMAL1 and CLOCK, two essential components of the circadian clock, are involved in glucose homeostasis. *PLOS Biol.* 2:e377
126. Rutter J, Reick M, Wu LC, McKnight SL. 2001. Regulation of clock and NPAS2 DNA binding by the redox state of NAD cofactors. *Science* 293:510–14
127. Sacks O. 2004 (Aug. 23). A neurologist's notebook: speed—aberrations of time and movement. *The New Yorker*, pp. 60–69
128. Sakamoto K, Nagase T, Fukui H, Horikawa K, Okada T, et al. 1998. Multitissue circadian expression of rat period homolog (rPer2) mRNA is governed by the mammalian circadian clock, the suprachiasmatic nucleus in the brain. *J. Biol. Chem.* 273:27039–42
129. Sakurai T, Amemiya A, Ishii M, Matsuzaki I, Chemelli RM, et al. 1998. Orexins and orexin receptors: a family of hypothalamic neuropeptides and G protein-coupled receptors that regulate feeding behavior. *Cell* 92:573–85
130. Samson WK, Resch ZT. 2000. The hypocretin/orexin story. *Trends Endocrinol. Metab.* 11:257–62
131. Saper CB, Scammell TE, Lu J. 2005. Hypothalamic regulation of sleep and circadian rhythms. *Nature* 437:1257–63
132. Sato TK, Panda S, Miraglia LJ, Reyes TM, Rudic RD, et al. 2004. A functional genomics strategy reveals RORa as a component of the mammalian circadian clock. *Neuron* 43:527–37
133. Sato TK, Yamada RG, Ukai H, Baggs JE, Miraglia LJ, et al. 2006. Feedback repression is required for mammalian circadian clock function. *Nat. Genet.* 38:312–19
134. Schmidt MI, Hadji-Georgopoulos A, Rendell M, Margolis S, Kowarski A. 1981. The dawn phenomenon, an early morning glucose rise: implications for diabetic intraday blood glucose variation. *Diab. Care* 4:579–85
135. Schoeller DA, Cella LK, Sinha MK, Caro JF. 1997. Entrainment of the diurnal rhythm of plasma leptin to meal timing. *J. Clin. Invest.* 100:1882–87
136. Schwartz MW, Woods SC, Porte DJ, Seeley RJ, Baskin DG. 2000. Central nervous system control of food intake. *Nature* 404:661–71
137. Shapiro ET, Tillil H, Polonsky KS, Fang VS, Rubenstein AH, Van Cauter E. 1988. Oscillations in insulin secretion during constant glucose infusion in normal man: relationship to changes in plasma glucose. *J. Clin. Endocrinol. Metab.* 67:307–14
138. Shearman LP, Sriram S, Weaver DR, Maywood ES, Chaves I, et al. 2000. Interacting molecular loops in the mammalian circadian clock. *Science* 288:1013–19

139. Shemyakin A, Kapas L. 2001. L-364718, a cholecystokinin-A receptor antagonist, suppresses feeding-induced sleep in rats. *Am. J. Physiol. Regul. Integr. Comp. Physiol.* 280:R1420–26
140. Shimada M, Tritos NA, Lowell BB, Flier JS, Maratos-Flier E. 1998. Mice lacking melanin-concentrating hormone are hypophagic and lean. *Nature* 396:670–74
141. Shimba S, Ishii N, Ohta Y, Ohno T, Watabe Y, et al. 2005. Brain and muscle Arnt-like protein-1 (BMAL1), a component of the molecular clock, regulates adipogenesis. *Proc. Natl. Acad. Sci. USA* 102:12071–76
142. Shimomura Y, Takahashi M, Shimizu H, Sato N, Uehara Y, et al. 1990. Abnormal feeding behavior and insulin replacement in STZ-induced diabetic rats. *Physiol. Behav.* 47:731–34
143. Silver R, LeSauter J, Tresco PA, Lehman MN. 1996. A diffusible coupling signal from the transplanted suprachiasmatic nucleus controlling circadian locomotor rhythms. *Nature* 382:810–13
144. Sinha MK, Ohannesian JP, Heiman ML, Kriauciunas A, Stephens TW, et al. 1996. Nocturnal rise of leptin in lean, obese, and non-insulin-dependent diabetes mellitus subjects. *J. Clin. Invest.* 97:1344–47
145. Sinha MK, Sturis J, Ohannesian J, Magosin S, Stephens T, et al. 1996. Ultradian oscillations of leptin secretion in humans. *Biochem. Biophys. Res. Commun.* 228:733–38
146. Spallone V, Bernardi L, Ricordi L, Solda P, Maiello MR, et al. 1993. Relationship between the circadian rhythms of blood pressure and sympathovagal balance in diabetic autonomic neuropathy. *Diabetes* 42:1745–52
147. Spiegel K, Knutson K, Leproult R, Tasali E, Van Cauter E. 2005. Sleep loss: a novel risk factor for insulin resistance and type 2 diabetes. *J. Appl. Physiol.* 99:2008–19
148. Spiegel K, Leproult R, Van Cauter E. 1999. Impact of sleep debt on metabolic and endocrine function. *Lancet* 354:1435–39
149. Staels B. 2006. When the Clock stops ticking, metabolic syndrome explodes. *Nat. Med.* 12:54–55
150. Stephens TW, Basinski M, Bristow PK, Bue-Valleskey JM, Burgett SG, et al. 1995. The role of neuropeptide Y in the antiobesity action of the obese gene product. *Nature* 377:530–32
151. Stokkan KA, Yamazaki S, Tei H, Sakaki Y, Menaker M. 2001. Entrainment of the circadian clock in the liver by feeding. *Science* 291:490–93
152. Storch KF, Lipan O, Leykin I, Viswanathan N, Davis FC, et al. 2002. Extensive and divergent circadian gene expression in liver and heart. *Nature* 417:78–83
153. Sutcliffe JG, de Lecea L. 2000. The hypocretins: excitatory neuromodulatory peptides for multiple homeostatic systems, including sleep and feeding. *J. Neurosci. Res.* 62:161–68
154. Swanson LW, Cowan WM. 1975. The efferent connections of the suprachiasmatic nucleus of the hypothalamus. *J. Comp. Neurol.* 160:1–12
155. Taheri S, Lin L, Austin D, Young T, Mignot E. 2004. Short sleep duration is associated with reduced leptin, elevated ghrelin, and increased body mass index. *PLOS Med.* 1:e62
156. Tartaglia LA, Dembski M, Weng X, Deng N, Culpepper J, et al. 1995. Identification and expression cloning of a leptin receptor, OB-R. *Cell* 83:1263–71
157. Tecott LH, Abdallah L. 2003. Mouse genetic approaches to feeding regulation: serotonin 5-HT2C receptor mutant mice. *CNS Spectr.* 8:584–88
158. Triqueneaux G, Thenot S, Kakizawa T, Antoch MP, Safi R, et al. 2004. The orphan receptor Rev-erbα gene is a target of the circadian clock pacemaker. *J. Mol. Endocrinol.* 33:585–608

159. Troisi RJ, Cowie CC, Harris MI. 2000. Diurnal variation in fasting plasma glucose: implications for diagnosis of diabetes in patients examined in the afternoon. *JAMA* 284:3157–59
160. Turek FW, Joshu C, Kohsaka A, Lin E, Ivanova G, et al. 2005. Obesity and metabolic syndrome in circadian Clock mutant mice. *Science* 308:1043–45
161. Ueda HR, Chen W, Adachi A, Wakamatsu H, Hayashi S, et al. 2002. A transcription factor response element for gene expression during circadian night. *Nature* 418:534–39
162. Van Cauter E. 1989. Physiology and pathology of circadian rhythms. In *Recent Advances in Endocrinology and Metabolism*, ed. CW Edwards, DW Lincoln, pp. 109–34. Edinburgh: Churchill Livingstone
163. Van Cauter E, Polonsky KS, Scheen AJ. 1997. Roles of circadian rhythmicity and sleep in human glucose regulation. *Endocr. Rev.* 18:716–38
164. van der Horst GT, Muijtjens M, Kobayashi K, Takano R, Kanno S, et al. 1999. Mammalian Cry1 and Cry2 are essential for maintenance of circadian rhythms. *Nature* 398:627–30
165. Velasco A, Huerta I, Marin B. 1988. Plasma corticosterone, motor activity and metabolic circadian patterns in streptozotocin-induced diabetic rats. *Chronobiol. Int.* 5:127–35
166. Verrillo A, De Teresa A, Martino C, Di Chiara G, Pinto M, et al. 1989. Differential roles of splanchnic and peripheral tissues in determining diurnal fluctuation of glucose tolerance. *Am. J. Physiol.* 257:E459–65
167. Vitaterna MH, King DP, Chang AM, Kornhauser JM, Lowrey PL, et al. 1994. Mutagenesis and mapping of a mouse gene, Clock, essential for circadian behavior. *Science* 264:719–25
168. Vitaterna MH, Selby CP, Todo T, Niwa H, Thompson C, et al. 1999. Differential regulation of mammalian period genes and circadian rhythmicity by cryptochromes 1 and 2. *Proc. Natl. Acad. Sci. USA* 96:12114–19
169. Wakamatsu H, Yoshinobu Y, Aida R, Moriya T, Akiyama M, Shibata S. 2001. Restricted-feeding-induced anticipatory activity rhythm is associated with a phase-shift of the expression of mPer1 and mPer2 mRNA in the cerebral cortex and hippocampus but not in the suprachiasmatic nucleus of mice. *Eur. J. Neurosci.* 13:1190–96
170. Watts AG, Swanson LW, Sanchez-Watts G. 1987. Efferent projections of the suprachiasmatic nucleus: I. Studies using anterograde transport of *Phaseolus vulgaris leucoagglutinin* in the rat. *J. Comp. Neurol.* 258:204–29
171. Weikel JC, Wichniak A, Ising M, Brunner H, Friess E, et al. 2003. Ghrelin promotes slow-wave sleep in humans. *Am. J. Physiol. Endocrinol. Metab.* 284:E407–15
172. Willie JT, Chemelli RM, Sinton CM, Yanagisawa M. 2001. To eat or to sleep? Orexin in the regulation of feeding and wakefulness. *Annu. Rev. Neurosci.* 24:429–58
173. Wilsbacher LD, Yamazaki S, Herzog ED, Song EJ, Radcliffe LA, et al. 2002. Photic and circadian expression of luciferase in mPeriod1-luc transgenic mice in vivo. *Proc. Natl. Acad. Sci. USA* 99:489–94
174. Yamazaki S, Numano R, Abe M, Hida A, Takahashi R, et al. 2000. Resetting central and peripheral circadian oscillators in transgenic rats. *Science* 288:682–85
175. Yang Q, Graham TE, Mody N, Preitner F, Peroni OD, et al. 2005. Serum retinol binding protein 4 contributes to insulin resistance in obesity and type 2 diabetes. *Nature* 436:356–62
176. Yin L, Wang J, Klein PS, Lazar MA. 2006. Nuclear receptor Rev-erbα is a critical lithium-sensitive component of the circadian clock. *Science* 311:1002–5

177. Yoo SH, Ko CH, Lowrey PL, Buhr ED, Song EJ, et al. 2005. A noncanonical E-box enhancer drives mouse Period2 circadian oscillations in vivo. *Proc. Natl. Acad. Sci. USA* 102:2608–13
178. Yoo SH, Yamazaki S, Lowrey PL, Shimomura K, Ko CH, et al. 2004. PERIOD2::LUCIFERASE real-time reporting of circadian dynamics reveals persistent circadian oscillations in mouse peripheral tissues. *Proc. Natl. Acad. Sci. USA* 101:5339–46
179. Zhang Y, Proenca R, Maffei M, Barone M, Leopold L, Friedman JM. 1994. Positional cloning of the mouse obese gene and its human homologue. *Nature* 372:425–32
180. Zheng B, Albrecht U, Kaasik K, Sage M, Lu W, et al. 2001. Nonredundant roles of the *mPer1* and *mPer2* genes in the mammalian circadian clock. *Cell* 105:683–94
181. Zheng B, Larkin DW, Albrecht U, Sun ZS, Sage M, et al. 1999. The *mPer2* gene encodes a functional component of the mammalian circadian clock. *Nature* 400:169–73

Creatine: Endogenous Metabolite, Dietary, and Therapeutic Supplement

John T. Brosnan and Margaret E. Brosnan

Department of Biochemistry, Memorial University of Newfoundland, St. John's, Newfoundland, A1B 3X9, Canada; email: jbrosnan@mun.ca, mbrosnan@mun.ca

Annu. Rev. Nutr. 2007. 27:241–61

First published online as a Review in Advance on April 12, 2007

The *Annual Review of Nutrition* is online at http://nutr.annualreviews.org

This article's doi: 10.1146/annurev.nutr.27.061406.093621

0199-9885/07/0821-0241$20.00

Key Words

muscle, brain, neurodegenerative diseases, inborn errors, amino acids, ergogenic action

Abstract

Creatine and phosphocreatine serve not only as an intracellular buffer for adenosine triphosphate, but also as an energy shuttle for the movement of high-energy phosphates from mitochondrial sites of production to cytoplasmic sites of utilization. The spontaneous loss of creatine and of phosphocreatine to creatinine requires that creatine be continuously replaced; this occurs by a combination of diet and endogenous synthesis. Vegetarians obtain almost no dietary creatine. Creatine synthesis makes major demands on the metabolism of glycine, arginine, and methionine. Large doses of creatine monohydrate are widely taken, particularly by athletes, as an ergogenic supplement; creatine supplements are also taken by patients suffering from gyrate atrophy, muscular dystrophy, and neurodegenerative diseases. Children with inborn errors of creatine synthesis or transport present with severe neurological symptoms and a profound depletion of brain creatine. It is evident that creatine plays a critical, though underappreciated, role in brain function.

Contents

INTRODUCTION

Interest in creatine has increased markedly in recent years. Much of this interest has been due to the use of creatine as a supplement by athletes and bodybuilders. Recent information indicates that the annual consumption of supplemental creatine (as creatine monohydrate) amounts to some four million kilograms per annum with a value, in the United States alone, close to $400 million. Creatine monohydrate is one of the more widely used dietary supplements. Readers who wish to access the literature on the efficacy of creatine in improving athletic performance will find that the article by Branch (6) provides a convenient entrée. Similarly, issues of the safety of supplemental creatine are dealt with by Schilling et al. (67) and Graham & Hatton (25). This review article is concerned with the function of creatine and phosphocreatine in tissues, the synthesis of creatine (including the metabolic burden of this synthesis), the metabolic and therapeutic effects of supplemental creatine, and the inborn errors of creatine synthesis and transport. We have endeavored, as much as possible, to address recent work. An extensive coverage of the older literature is available in the review by Wyss & Kaddurah-Daouk (96). Readers should apply a cautious attitude to the many commercial and nonscientific Web sites devoted to creatine. However, a Web site maintained by the Office of Dietary Supplements of the National Institutes of Health (**www.ods.od.nih.gov**) is a valuable source of balanced information.

PHYSIOLOGICAL FUNCTION OF THE CREATINE SYSTEM

Creatine is involved in a single enzyme-catalyzed reaction, which is catalyzed by creatine kinase:

$$\begin{aligned} &\mathrm{Mg}\cdot\mathrm{ADP}^{-} + \text{phosphocreatine}^{2-} + \mathrm{H}^{+} \\ &\quad\leftrightarrow \mathrm{Mg}\cdot\mathrm{ATP}^{2-} + \text{creatine} \end{aligned}$$

The conventional textbook description of this system is that it serves as a temporal high-energy phosphate buffer, so that adenosine triphosphate (ATP) may be rapidly replenished from adenosine diphosphate (ADP) and phosphocreatine. This is certainly true. However, we now appreciate that the creatine system plays a more complex role in energy metabolism. It is found in cells with high and fluctuating energy demand, such as skeletal muscle and the heart (96). It is not present in hepatocytes that have a constitutively high metabolic rate. It is also found in the brain. Although the oxygen consumption (and energy demand) of the brain as a whole is relatively constant (compared, for example, with the large excursions in energy demand exhibited by skeletal and cardiac muscle), it should be appreciated that individual, rapidly firing neurons can exhibit quite a large variation in their energy needs (69).

The subcellular distribution of creatine kinase isoforms has stimulated a revision of the function played by the creatine system. Wallimann et al. (93) have provided a cogent account of the different creatine kinase isoenzymes. For the purposes of the present discussion, the key factor is their subcellular location. Mitochondrial creatine kinase is found at contact sites between the inner and outer mitochondrial membranes and, in the presence of creatine, ensures that much of the ATP produced by oxidative phosphorylation is readily converted to phosphocreatine. Cytosolic isoforms are found in the "bulk cytoplasm" and, most critically, at sites of high ATP demand, e.g., in myofibrils, sarcoplasmic reticulum, and plasma membranes (93). These and other observations have given rise to the proposal of a role for creatine and phosphocreatine in an energy shuttle of high-energy phosphates between the mitochondrial sites of ATP production and the cytosolic sites of ATP utilization (93). In this view, phosphocreatine (rather than ATP) diffuses from mitochondria to the major sites of ATP utilization and creatine (rather than ADP) diffuses back. Although the original arguments for such a shuttle were based on the fact that phosphocreatine (MW = 211) would diffuse faster than ATP (MW = 507) and creatine (MW = 131) would diffuse faster than ADP (MW = 427) (20), it is more likely that the key consideration lies in the differences between their free concentrations in the cytosol (ATP, 3–5 mM; ADP, 20–40 μM; phosphocreatine, 20–35 mM; creatine, 5–10 mM) (93).

Temporal high-energy phosphate buffering and spatial high-energy phosphate transport are not mutually exclusive. Indeed, they probably coexist, to different degrees, in different cells, but depending on physiological requirements, one or the other may predominate. Thus, in fast-twitch (primarily glycolytic) muscles, the ATP buffer function predominates, whereas in slow-twitch, oxidative, or cardiac muscle, the energy transport function is more important. Wallimann and coworkers (93) have identified a number of additional functions of the creatine/phosphocreatine system. These include buffering the products of ATP hydrolysis and maintaining cellular ATP/ADP ratios. ATP hydrolysis produces ADP, phosphate, and a hydrogen ion. During very rapid ATP hydrolysis, it is important that both ADP and the hydrogen ion are buffered. The creatine/phosphocreatine system prevents a rise in [ADP] that would both inhibit ATPases and lead to the metabolic loss of adenine nucleotides; elevated [ADP] leads to elevated [AMP], catalyzed by adenylate kinase, and this leads to increased deamination of AMP to IMP. Local or generalized cellular acidification, due to high rates of ATP utilization, is prevented by the requirement for a hydrogen ion when the creatine kinase reaction operates in the direction of ATP synthesis. Finally, it is apparent that by buffering both [ATP] and [ADP], the creatine kinase reaction maintains the constancy of the ATP/ADP ratio, which protects the thermodynamic efficiency of ATP hydrolysis. These different functional aspects of the creatine kinase system are illustrated in **Figure 1** (see color insert).

MtCK: mitochondrial creatine kinase

Our knowledge of the function of individual creatine kinase isoforms has been enhanced by recent studies of knockout mice. These mice are viable and fertile and, indeed, when unstressed, often exhibit a relatively mild phenotype. This is often due to compensatory mechanisms as well as some redundancy. A good example is provided by mice deficient in both the homo-dimeric muscle creatine kinase, which is associated with sites of high ATP utilization, such as myofibrils and sarcoplasmic reticulum and the mitochondrial creatine kinase (MtCK), so that both ends of the phosphocreatine shuttle are ablated. These animals greatly expand their mitochondrial number near the longitudinal sarcoplasmic reticulum and the myosin filaments so that direct energy channeling via ATP and ADP is enhanced (37). Nevertheless, these mice exhibit a markedly reduced

AGAT: L-arginine:glycine amidinotransferase

GAMT: guanidinoacetate methyltransferase

voluntary running capacity (53). Knockout of MtCK results in left ventricular hypertrophy and dilatation (55). Mice in which both mitochondrial creatine kinase and the brain-specific creatine kinase were knocked out showed a number of neurological impairments, including severely diminished spatial learning (79).

CREATINE METABOLISM

Creatine Loss and Replacement

Both creatine and phosphocreatine spontaneously break down to creatinine that is quantitatively lost in the urine. The rate of loss is estimated to be about 1.7% of the total body pool per day (96). As more than 90% of the body's creatine and phosphocreatine is found in skeletal muscle, creatine losses (and creatinine excretion) vary as a function of gender and age. Creatinine excretion is at a maximum in the 18- to 29-year-old age group, with mean rates of 23.6 $mg \cdot kg^{-1} \cdot 24\ h^{-1}$. Mean rates for women are about 80% of rates for men. The rate of creatinine loss decreases almost linearly with age; men aged 70–79 years have mean excretion rates of 12.6 $mg \cdot kg^{-1} \cdot 24\ h^{-1}$ (11).

These data on creatinine excretion define the quantities of creatine that need to be provided by diet or by synthesis. The principal dietary sources of creatine are muscle meats and dairy products. We have employed United States Department of Agriculture data on the consumption of different foods, together with knowledge of the creatine content of different foods, to estimate dietary creatine (75). Our data indicate dietary creatine intakes of 7.9 and 5.0 mmol/day for men and women, respectively, in the 20- to 39-year-old age group. These intakes decrease somewhat with age. Food creatine has the same high bioavailability as does dissolved creatine (29), which has been estimated to be about 80% (49). These data permit us to tease out the quantity of creatine obtained from the diet and, therefore, the amount that must be synthesized. For ease of comparison, our data are normalized to a 70-kg person. Vegans obtain virtually no dietary creatine and vegetarians very little. De novo synthesis must provide essentially all of their creatine. Ingestion of vegetarian diets is associated with decreased serum and muscle creatine levels (14, 47), which may indicate that creatine synthesis is insufficient in these subjects. For individuals ingesting a typical U.S. diet, we estimate rates of creatine synthesis of 7.7, 5.6, and 3.7 $mmol \cdot day^{-1}$ in males in the 20–39, 40–59, and 60+ age brackets, respectively. The rates for women were about 70%–80% of those in men.

Creatine synthesis occurs via a remarkably simple pathway (**Figure 2**, see color insert). However, it involves three different amino acids: glycine, arginine, and methionine. In the first reaction, catalyzed by L-arginine:glycine amidinotransferase (AGAT), an amidino group is transferred from arginine to the amino group of glycine to produce guanidinoacetate and ornithine. The second reaction, catalyzed by guanidinoacetate methyltransferase (GAMT), employs *S*-adenosylmethionine to methylate guanidinoacetate, producing creatine and *S*-adenosylhomocysteine.

These rates of creatine synthesis permit us to estimate the metabolic burden it imparts. Synthesis of 7.7 $mmol \cdot day^{-1}$ (approximately 1.0 g) requires the same molar quantity of glycine, amidino groups, and methyl groups. The mean dietary intakes of these amino acids in U.S. men and women aged 31–50 are 48 mmol glycine, 27 mmol arginine, and 13 mmol methionine (17). Clearly, creatine synthesis makes major demands on amino acid metabolism. However, the nature of the demand varies among the three amino acids. As shown in **Figure 2**, the entire glycine molecule is incorporated into creatine so that creatine synthesis consumes about 16% of dietary glycine. In the case of methionine, only the methyl group is incorporated. Labile methyl groups are available in the diet from methionine, choline, and betaine. In addition, new labile methyl groups may be produced by the process of methylneogenesis (54). Consensus estimates of the total transmethylation flux (i.e., the sum of all of the *S*-adenosylmethionine-requiring methylation reactions) are 17–23 mmol per day in young adults (54). Thus, creatine synthesis accounts for about 40% of all *S*-adenosylmethionine-derived methyl groups in young adults. This percentage decreases somewhat in the elderly. Direct evidence for the role of methylneogenesis in providing methyl groups for creatine synthesis is provided by the impairment of this process in patients with an inborn error of cobalamin metabolism (3).

It is still an open question whether creatine synthesis results in the loss of an entire arginine molecule. The key to this question depends on the fate of the ornithine produced by the AGAT reaction (**Figure 2**). Ornithine could be reconverted to arginine by the enzymes of the urea cycle (7). Since expression of carbamyl phosphate synthase I is restricted to the liver and the small intestine (7), AGAT expression would be required in these tissues. This is an unresolved issue. However, the 1953 study by Sandberg et al. (66) should be noted. After examining their catheterization studies across the human liver, these workers reported that the entire pathway of creatine synthesis occurred in this organ.

Creatine Synthesis and Transport: Tissue Sites and Regulation

The tissue localization of AGAT and GAMT is complex. In mammals, the kidneys express high activities of AGAT but low (or undetectable) activities of GAMT. This has given rise to the view that creatine synthesis is primarily an interorgan process in which guanidinoacetate produced by the kidney is methylated to creatine in the liver. This certainly occurs in the rat (96). However, the relative contribution of other tissues is uncertain. The possible occurrence of AGAT activity in the liver is enigmatic, in large part due to the difficulty of assaying the enzyme in tissues with high arginase activity. For example, immunofluorescence microscopy has identified a protein that reacts to AGAT antiserum in rat liver (51), but unambiguous presence of enzyme activity in this tissue has yet to be demonstrated. It is clear that the pancreas and testes express both AGAT and GAMT and that AGAT is found in tissues such as lung, spleen, and brain. In summary, much of the body's creatine is synthesized via a renal-hepatic axis, but the importance of the synthetic enzymes that are expressed in other tissues remains to be delineated. We address the issue of brain creatine synthesis in Treatment of the Inborn Errors section below.

CRT: creatine transporter

Regulation of creatine synthesis has been best studied in rats. Dietary supplementation of rats with creatine results in a marked decrease in AGAT activity and mRNA levels in the rat kidney (52), indicating regulation at a pretranslational level. The molecular mechanism whereby creatine down-regulates AGAT expression remains to be elucidated. Decreased hepatic creatine production follows from the decreased circulating guanidinoacetate levels.

By and large, the tissues that contain the largest quantities of creatine (e.g., skeletal and cardiac muscle) have essentially no capacity for its synthesis. A creatine transporter (CRT) has been identified that is responsible for the uptake of creatine into tissues such as skeletal muscle, cardiac muscle, kidney, and brain. Uptake occurs against a large concentration gradient; typical creatine concentrations in humans are 50–100 μM in plasma and 5–10 mM in skeletal muscle. The transporter (SLC 6A8) is a member of the Na^+-dependent neurotransmitter transporter family (closely related to γ-aminobutyrate, taurine, and betaine transporters), and this gene is found on the human X chromosome (27). A cDNA clone from human brain with an open reading frame of 1905 base pairs predicts a protein of 635 amino acids (≈70.5 kDa), 12 transmembrane-spanning domains, and putative phosphorylation and glycosylation sites (73). It has about 97% identity with homologous rat, rabbit, and bovine genes (72, 73). The transport properties of CRT have been determined. Creatine (a zwitterion) is cotransported with at least two Na^+ and one Cl^-. This transport therefore is electrogenic and an example of secondary active transport, driven by the sodium gradient established by the Na^+ + K^+-ATPase (12). Creatine transport is enhanced by hormones (e.g., insulin) that activate the Na^+ + K^+-ATPase and presumably increase the driving force for creatine uptake (72).

Studies on the size, tissue expression, and regulation of the CRT gene product have yielded confusing results; for example, estimates of its molecular weight vary from 40 kDa to 150 kDa. Some of this variation may be attributed to glycosylation and to the anomalous behavior of hydrophobic proteins in gels. The meticulous study of Speer et al. (74) clearly demonstrates that much of the difficulty has arisen as a result of the cross-reactivity of different antibodies against other proteins. Until this issue is resolved, data on the abundance, location, and regulation of CRT proteins must be treated with caution. Nevertheless, it is quite likely that different isoforms of CRT do exist as Northern blots have identified two different mRNAs (28).

Creatine transport may be regulated both acutely and chronically. Acute regulation may be brought about either by changes in the creatine concentration or in the sodium gradient or in the insertion of the transporter into the plasma membrane. Chronically, creatine transport may be regulated at the level of gene expression, translation, or post-translational modification. It is clear that creatine uptake is regulated by intracellular creatine concentrations. An inverse relationship exists between the intracellular creatine concentration and creatine uptake (18). It is known that an elevated extracellular creatine concentration leads to an initial increase in transport followed by a down-regulation. The mechanism of down-regulation is not known, but it seems to require protein synthesis (42).

Creatine is also absorbed in the intestine, reabsorbed in the kidney, and released, after synthesis, by the liver. Tosco and coworkers (86) have demonstrated a creatine transporter, electrogenic and Na^+ + Cl^- dependent, in jejunal apical membranes. In view of the small quantities of creatine found in the urine, it can be calculated that human kidneys must reabsorb approximately 13.5 mmol creatine (1.76 g) per day. A Na^+ + Cl^--dependent creatine transporter is known to occur in renal cortical brush-border membranes (24). Creatine synthesized by the liver is released into the blood. However, given the direction of the sodium gradient, this is likely to require a novel transporter that is yet to be identified. Recent work (74) has suggested that creatine transporters occur on mitochondrial membranes. Creatine uptake could be demonstrated by isolated mitochondria. However, the K_m for creatine is quite high (16 mM), the transport may be inhibited competitively by either lysine or arginine, and it is found in mitochondria from tissues (e.g., liver) that do not express creatine kinase (74). The occurrence of a mitochondrial creatine transporter challenges our understanding of creatine physiology. However, definitive demonstration of a physiological role for creatine inside the inner mitochondrial membrane has yet to be provided.

SUPPLEMENTAL AND THERAPEUTIC CREATINE INGESTION

Creatine monohydrate is one of the most common dietary supplements. It is taken by athletes and bodybuilders. A popular intake schedule involves a loading phase of 20 g per day (in four divided doses) for five days, followed by maintenance doses of 2–5 g per day. In addition to its use by athletes, creatine has been used therapeutically in patients suffering from a number of neurological and neuromuscular disorders.

Effects of Creatine Ingestion on Muscle Creatine Levels

Supplemental creatine is appreciably taken up by skeletal muscle over the first 2–3 days

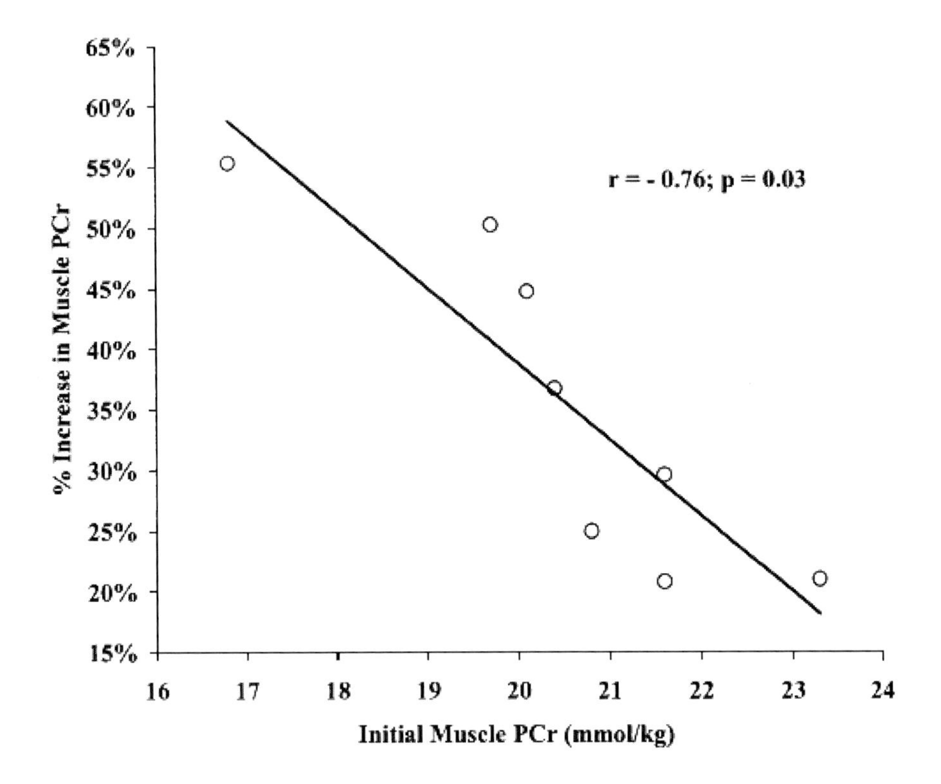

Figure 3

The increase in muscle phosphocreatine (PCr) after creatine supplementation is inversely related to presupplementation PCr levels. Reproduced from Volek & Rawson (90), with permission from Elsevier.

of supplementation. Decreased urine output during this time has been attributed to water retention because of the osmotic effects of creatine uptake (97). Creatine is frequently taken together with carbohydrate as this tends to increase its uptake into muscle, presumably as a consequence of insulin action. However, the amounts of carbohydrate required (~100 g per 5 g of creatine) are impractically large (26). Exercise is a potent stimulus for creatine uptake by skeletal muscle. This was elegantly demonstrated by studies in which a single leg was exercised, resulting in appreciably more creatine uptake than in the unexercised contralateral leg (30). Typical skeletal muscle levels, before supplementation, are about 85 and 41 mmol/kg dry matter, respectively, for phosphocreatine and creatine (30). Therefore, the combined concentration of creatine and phosphocreatine in muscle intracellular water, presupplementation, is of the order of 40–50 mM. Creatine supplementation increased total muscle creatine (creatine plus phosphocreatine) by about 25%, and when accompanied by exercise, by an average of 37%. Clearly, these compounds are major osmotically active intracellular solutes. Creatine supplementation does not affect muscle ATP levels (30).

Considerable variation exists between individuals in the degree of creatine loading into muscles. Although this is not completely understood, it is clear that presupplement muscle creatine levels are an important factor (63). **Figure 3** shows that the increment in muscle phosphocreatine following supplementation in young (age 20–32) men was inversely related to their presupplementation levels. Muscle phosphocreatine levels in older (age 63–83) men were relatively refractory to supplementation, possibly because presupplementation levels were higher than those of the younger subjects (63).

The Ergogenic Effect of Creatine Supplementation

Creatine supplementation enhances our ability to do certain types of work or exercise. This is clearly evident for high-intensity exercise of short duration. Evidence for a beneficial effect in endurance events is not compelling. A meta-analysis of 96 studies that examined the effect of creatine supplementation found marked effects on high-intensity exercise of short duration ($\leq$30 s) but virtually no effect on performance tasks longer than 150 s (6). The effect of creatine supplementation on work performance and lean body mass was more pronounced in vegetarians than in nonvegetarians, presumably because their presupplementation levels of muscle creatine are lower (8). In recent years, the focus of research has shifted from performance evaluation to the elucidation of the mechanism(s) responsible for enhanced performance. Certainly, the elevated phosphocreatine levels are important because, via creatine kinase, they increase the ability to rapidly replete ATP during strenuous exercise. However, other mechanisms involving effects on muscle mass, the metabolism of carbohydrates, as well as metabolic regulation may also play a role. Because training can affect many of these parameters, and increased phosphocreatine levels permit more vigorous training, it is often difficult to determine whether the effects of creatine supplementation are direct or indirect. Studies in vitro avoid some of these problems but are, of course, less physiologically relevant. Comparison of the in vivo studies is often confounded by differences in the subject groups, in the duration or dosage of the creatine supplementation, in the extent to which muscle creatine levels are increased, and in any accompanying exercise protocols.

One of the most striking effects of creatine supplementation is an increase in muscle mass, especially when an exercise program accompanies supplementation. A meta-analysis of 96 studies reports a mean increase in lean body mass of 2.2 kg (6). Twelve weeks of resistance training coupled with creatine supplementation increased muscle fiber diameter by 35%, compared with a 6%–15% increase in a placebo group that also completed the resistance exercises (89). It appears that creatine supplementation in the absence of an exercise program has little effect on muscle mass. An isotopic study of myofibrillar protein synthesis and degradation in subjects who did not exercise found no effects of creatine supplementation (45). The same group was unable to show any additional effect of creatine in subjects who underwent a program of resistance exercise (44). These results are at variance with the studies that found increased muscle mass, although the studies could be reconciled if there were effects of creatine supplementation on proteolysis; however, there are no data on the subject. In rats, creatine ingestion alone did not increase lean body mass; exercise alone increased lean body mass, and this effect was much larger in creatine-supplemented rats who exercised (23). With regard to mechanism, it should be noted that 12 weeks of resistance training of individuals who ingested creatine resulted in enhanced expression of both mRNA levels and protein content of myogenic regulatory factors (myogenin and MRF-4) compared with subjects who ingested a placebo during the exercise program (95).

Effects of creatine ingestion on carbohydrate metabolism have also been reported. In particular, muscle glycogen content increases by about 20% after five days of creatine loading (20 g per day), but this was not maintained during supplementation at 2 g per day. The increases in total muscle creatine and muscle glycogen were closely correlated. The mechanism for the increase in muscle glycogen may involve increased cellular hydration, secondary to total creatine accumulation (87). There is direct evidence that cell swelling can increase glycogen synthesis in rat skeletal muscle (46). The situation with regard to GLUT-4 is more problematic. The van Loon et al. (87) study, which reported elevated muscle glycogen, found that creatine supplementation caused no change in GLUT-4 mRNA or protein content. However, Derave et al. (15) found that creatine supplementation increased GLUT-4 expression during a six-week resistance exercise program that followed a two-week leg immobilization. Creatine supplementation of rats increases GLUT-4 expression as well as transcription factors that regulate GLUT-4 expression in muscle (36). There is uncertainty as to how an increase in GLUT-4 may be achieved. One suggestion is that creatine supplementation proportionately increases muscle creatine levels more than phosphocreatine levels. The AMP-activated protein kinase has been reported to be sensitive to the creatine/phosphocreatine ratio such that an increase in this ratio activates the AMP kinase (58), which in turn could bring about an increase in GLUT-4 (33). However, not every study reports that creatine loading alters the creatine/phosphocreatine ratio (87), and there is controversy as to whether phosphocreatine actually inhibits the AMP kinase (85).

Therapeutic Uses of Creatine

Creatine has been used therapeutically in a variety of human diseases as well as in animal models of human disease. Many, but not all, of these diseases include disorders of energy metabolism. The use of creatine in the treatment of inborn errors of creatine synthesis is addressed below.

Gyrate atrophy is an autosomal recessive disease characterized by chorioretinal degeneration and atrophy of type 2 muscle fibers. The molecular lesion involves mutations in ornithine aminotransferase with consequent hyperornithinemia (62). Plasma ornithine levels can be elevated 10- to 20-fold (0.65–1.35 mM); this elevation causes an inhibition of AGAT (Ki for ornithine is 0.25 mM) and therefore of creatine synthesis. Creatine therapy has been employed with mixed results. Muscle phosphocreatine levels were restored by the creatine therapy (31). However, although the skeletal muscle abnormalities were markedly reduced or even eliminated, the progression of visual impairment continued because the hyperornithinemia was not corrected (88).

Creatine supplementation has been used in a number of neurological and neurodegenerative diseases. Huntington's disease is caused by expanded CAG repeats in the gene that encodes huntingtin. It is one of nine known polyglutamine diseases. In general, fewer than 38 CAG repeats are not associated with pathology. However, beyond this number, a specific degenerative sequence begins in middle age; the longer the number of CAG repeats, the earlier the onset of symptoms. The function of the huntingtin protein is unknown, but it is thought that protein-protein interactions of either the mutant protein or of fragments arising from its proteolysis initiate a pathogenic program that ultimately leads to cell death. Dysfunctional cellular energy metabolism has been identified as one of the prominent early lesions in Huntington's disease and has been suggested to be an important component of the degenerative sequence (64). Positron emission tomography studies have shown reduced glucose metabolism both in presymptomatic and symptomatic patients (50). Striatal lactate is increased in symptomatic patients, and the increase is related to the CAG repeat number (35). Patients with Huntington's disease have reduced skeletal muscle ratios of phosphocreatine to inorganic phosphate (38). There is, therefore, considerable evidence that a defect in energy metabolism is an early event in these patients. There is also direct evidence for a significant reduction in the number of mitochondria and of their size in striatal caudate neurons of presymptomatic patients (64).

Extensive work has been carried out in animal models of Huntington's disease. R6/2 mice are a transgenic line that express *exon 1* of the human *HD* gene, containing 150 CAG repeats (41). These animals develop a sequence of motor and cognitive impairments, many of which recapitulate events in the human disease but in a highly compressed timeframe. Creatine supplementation of these animals prolonged life span, decreased brain atrophy, and delayed atrophy of striatal neurons and the formation of mutant huntingtin protein aggregates (22). Creatine supplementation also reverses the decreased brain levels of creatine and ATP found in these mice; increases of 39% and 65% are found, respectively, upon creatine supplementation of these mice (13).

This preclinical work on creatine supplementation in an animal model has made a strong case for clinical trials. A number of small studies have shown that doses of 3–8 g per day are safe and tolerable (64). A significant (7.2%) increase in brain creatine was found in patients who ingested 5 g/day for four months (64). None of these human studies have as yet shown an effect on the progression or severity of the disease. However, a recent randomized, double-blind placebo-controlled trial of 64 subjects with Huntington's disease showed that serum levels of 8-hydroxy-2′-deoxyguanosine, an indicator of oxidative injury to DNA, which are markedly elevated in Huntington's patients, were reduced by supplementation of 8 g/day of creatine for 16 weeks (32). A strong case has been made for a large-scale trial of creatine supplementation in patients with Huntington's disease with sufficient statistical power to detect meaningful changes in the progression or severity of the disease. Creatine and the creatine kinase system have also been linked to pathological consequences in animal models of amyotrophic lateral sclerosis (94) and Alzheimer's disease (9).

There have also been trials of creatine supplementation in muscle and neuromuscular disorders. Low-dose creatine supplementation improves skeletal muscle function in patients with McArdle's disease (deficiency of muscle glycogen phosphorylase), but high doses do not improve function (91, 92). Tarnopolsky et al. (83) have shown that creatine supplementation of boys with Duchenne muscular dystrophy for four months (0.1 g/kg/day) was well tolerated and led to significant increases in handgrip strength and in fat-free mass. Louis et al. (43) reported increased muscle function (maximal voluntary contraction and resistance to fatigue) but no change in lean body mass in a group of boys suffering from either Duchenne or Becker muscular dystrophy. Bourgeois & Tarnopolsky (4) have reviewed the effects of creatine supplementation in mitochondrial cytopathies. Creatine ingestion has also been shown to reduce the plasma concentration of the atherogenic amino acid, homocysteine, in rats (75) and in humans (39), although one study was unable to confirm the finding (77). The decreased homocysteine is due to the down-regulation of endogenous creatine synthesis that, since it is responsible for 40% of all *S*-adenosylhomocysteine production in humans, is responsible for the production of 40% of the body's homocysteine (76).

INBORN ERRORS OF CREATINE SYNTHESIS AND TRANSPORT

Brain Creatine Depletion and Neurological Symptoms

Inborn errors involving mutations in each of the three proteins required for creatine synthesis and transport (AGAT, GAMT, and CRT) are now known. Although children with these mutations exhibit hypotonia, they present with little in the way of cardiac or skeletal muscular pathology (80). Rather, they present with a cluster of neurological symptoms that include mental retardation, speech delay, and epileptic seizures. Proton nuclear magnetic resonance spectroscopy reveals a massive depletion of brain creatine (80, 81) (**Figure 4**). Muscle creatine levels do not appear to be as severely depleted as do brain creatine levels in patients with deficiencies of either GAMT or CRT (21, 60). This may indicate the occurrence of redundant mechanisms for muscle creatine uptake. The creatine-deficiency diseases may be differentiated on the basis of biochemical findings. All of them are characterized by low urinary creatinine excretion and low plasma creatinine levels. However, these tests are not particularly reliable in very young infants and are not

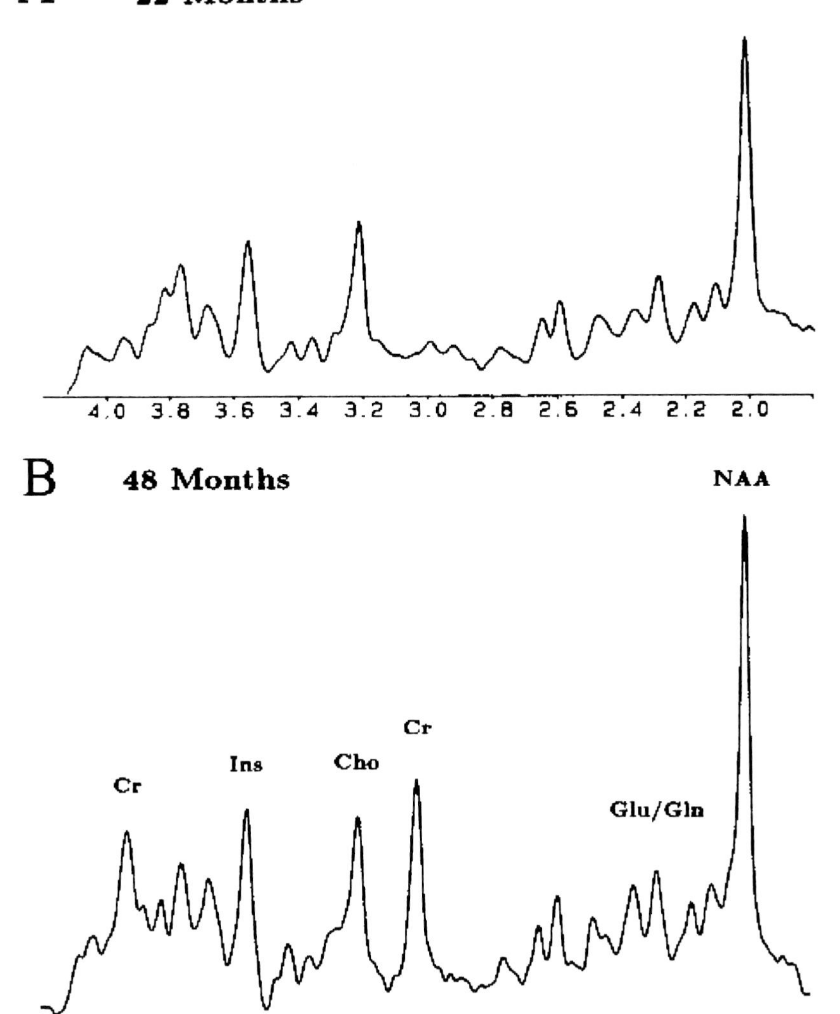

Figure 4

In vivo proton magnetic resonance spectroscopy of the brain of a patient with cerebral creatine deficiency due to guanidinoacetate methyltransferase deficiency. *Panel A* shows an absence of the creatine resonance; *Panel B* shows normalization of the creatine spectrum after six months of supplementation with creatine monohydrate. Cho, choline; Cr, creatine; Gln, glutamine; Glu, glutamate; Ins, myoinositol; NAA, *N*-acetylaspartate. Reproduced from Sykut-Cegielska et al. (81) with permission of the publisher.

absolutely specific for creatine-deficiency diseases; measurement of guanidinoacetate and creatine are more informative. AGAT deficiency is associated with very low plasma guanidinoacetate concentrations as well as low creatine levels. Patients with GAMT deficiency exhibit more severe symptoms, which include intractable epileptic seizures and a movement disorder. It is thought that the elevated guanidinoacetate levels exert an independent pathological action (70). The CRT defect is characterized by elevated creatine and normal guanidinoacetate levels (65). The ultimate diagnosis of these diseases requires functional and genetic confirmation. Functional confirmation of AGAT and GAMT deficiency requires measurements of enzyme activity (80); for the transporter defect, it is necessary to show impaired creatine uptake, usually in cultured fibroblasts

(65). Recent work suggests that the creatine transporter defect may be relatively common, perhaps so common that it may occur in about 1% of males with mental retardation of unknown etiology (10, 56).

Treatment of the Inborn Errors

The fundamental objective in the treatment of children with these inborn errors is the restoration of brain creatine. The experience with AGAT and GAMT deficiency is that brain creatine may be restored, largely or completely, by creatine supplementation. This resulted in marked clinical improvement, but the children never fully recovered; learning and language functions remained impaired (80). Until recently, it has not been clear whether the neurological deficits could have been prevented if creatine supplementation had been instituted sufficiently early. Two recent studies suggest that a measure of guarded optimism may be justified. Battini et al. (2) have reported on a child, homozygous for the W149X mutation in AGAT, in whom an early diagnosis could be made since it was known that two older siblings harbored the same mutation. Treatment with creatine monohydrate was begun upon weaning, at four months of age. As of 18 months of age, the child's growth and development were entirely normal. A second study (71) concerns a child with GAMT deficiency; early diagnosis was also possible because of an older affected sibling. Treatment involved replacement of creatine as well as steps to reduce the synthesis of guanidinoacetate; these included reducing the substrates for AGAT (by feeding an arginine-restricted diet and providing benzoate to reduce glycine levels via the formation of hippuric acid) as well as inhibiting AGAT via provision of ornithine. Fourteen months of this treatment resulted in a normally developed child with none of the symptoms of GAMT deficiency.

Patients with deficiency of the creatine transporter are completely refractory to supplementation with creatine, and at present, no effective therapy exists for this disorder. The severity of the creatine transporter deficiency presents something of a paradox, given that brain does possess a creatine synthetic capacity. Lunardi et al. (48) have suggested that this may be because the brain creatine transporter plays a dual role: the uptake of circulating creatine across the blood-brain barrier and the neuronal uptake of creatine that is synthesized in glia. Certainly, the brain uptake of creatine from the circulation is a slow process. It required six weeks of supplementation with creatine (4–8 g/day) to attain 50% of the normal brain creatine level in a GAMT-deficient infant (78). This contrasts with studies with mice that suggest a major role for the blood pool in providing creatine to the brain (57). The issue of the cell-specificity of brain creatine synthesis has not yet been clarified. Studies in mouse brain suggest very low GAMT activity in neurons but higher activities in oligodendrocytes, glia, and astrocytes; this has provided experimental support for the idea that glia may provide creatine to neurons (82). These results contrast with the studies of Braissant et al. (5), who find little evidence of mRNA for the creatine transporter in astrocytes associated with the blood-brain barrier. However, they find that both AGAT and GAMT are ubiquitously expressed in adult rat brain, and suggest, therefore, that the brain receives the bulk of its creatine via endogenous synthesis and that every cell in the central nervous system is capable of creatine synthesis. We now appreciate that how the brain, particularly the young brain, acquires its creatine is a crucial issue. Further work is needed to resolve these discrepancies.

Recently, Lunardi et al. (48) addressed the issue of providing creatine to the brain in the absence of a functional transporter. Studies with mouse hippocampal slices have shown that their creatine levels may be elevated by incubation with creatine benzyl ester and that this is not affected by an inhibitor of the creatine transporter (48). Presumably, the mechanism involves diffusion of the lipophilic creatine ester into the cell,

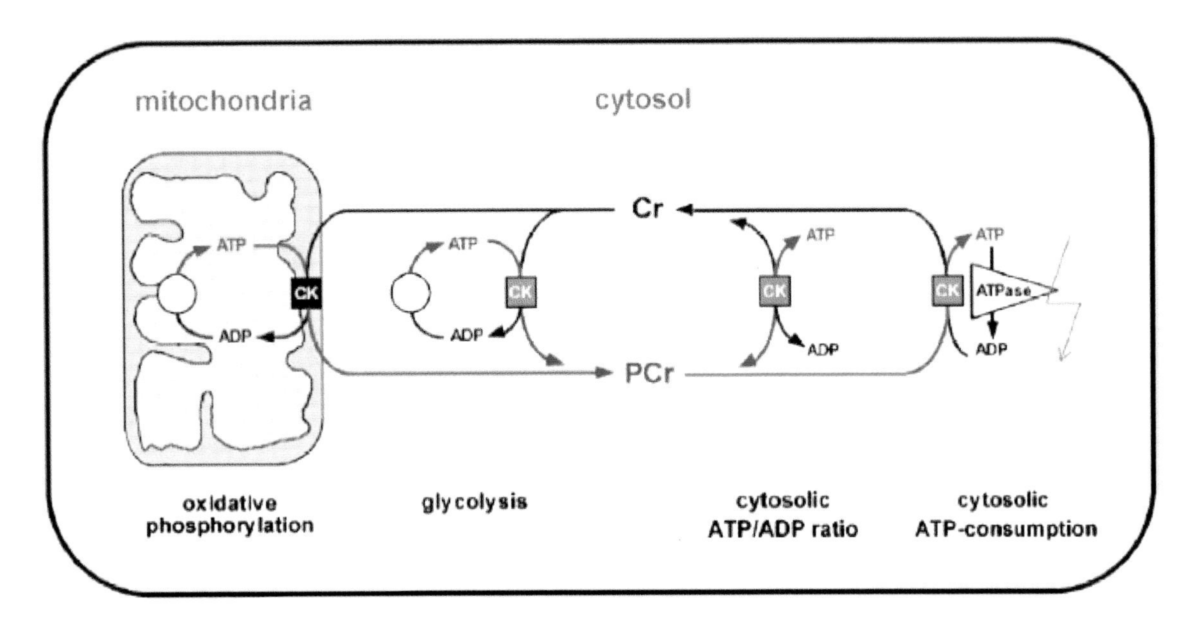

Figure 1

The creatine kinase/phosphocreatine system. ADP, adenosine diphosphate; ATP, adenosine triphosphate; CK, creatine kinase; CR, creatine; PCr, phosphocreatine. Reproduced from Schlattner et al. (68), with permission from Elsevier.

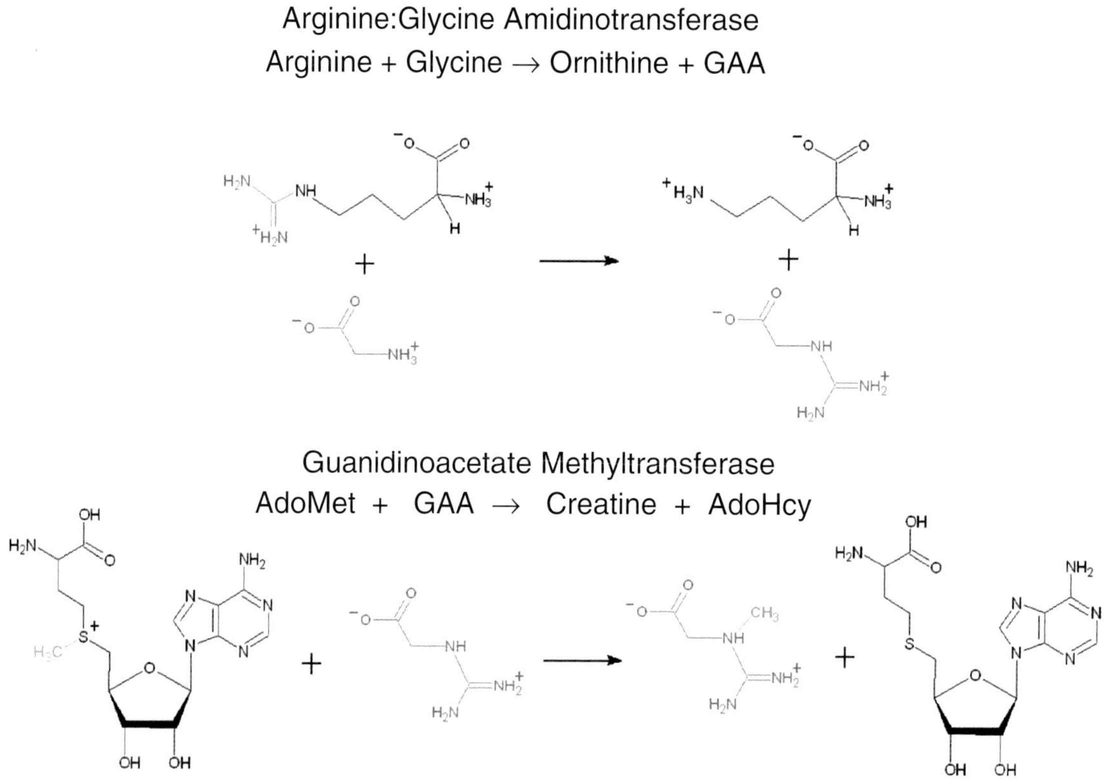

Arginine:Glycine Amidinotransferase

Arginine + Glycine → Ornithine + GAA

Guanidinoacetate Methyltransferase

AdoMet + GAA → Creatine + AdoHcy

Figure 2

Pathway of creatine synthesis. GAA, guanidinoacetate.

followed by hydrolysis by a broad-specificity esterase. Approaches along these lines have the potential of providing creatine to the brains of patients with creatine transporter deficiency (48).

PERSPECTIVE

Creatine and Brain Function

More than 90% of the body's store of creatine is found in skeletal muscle. Nevertheless, recent work has highlighted the crucial role of the creatine system in the brain. The most striking demonstration of the importance of creatine to the brain is provided by the devastating consequences that attend the creatine-deficiency diseases. However, other work also points to the importance of brain creatine. An intriguing study by Rae et al. (61) examined the effects of creatine supplementation on performance in a number of cognitive tests. The subjects, students from the University of Sydney, were either vegetarians or vegans as it was thought that their creatine status may be somewhat compromised because of very low dietary intake of creatine. A double-blind, placebo-controlled, crossover trial was carried out in which the subjects ingested a daily dose of 5 g of creatine monohydrate or placebo for six weeks. Then, after a six-week washout period, the treatments were reversed. A number of cognitive tests that require speed of processing were administered at the beginning of the experiment and after each six-week period. Creatine ingestion resulted in a significantly improved performance on these tests. **Figure 5** illustrates performance on the Auditory Backward Digit Span test. This test requires subjects to listen to a series of numbers and then to recite them backward. It involves short-term storage and active memory, both of which have high energy requirements. The remarkable result, evident in **Figure 5**, is that at the end of the experiment, the subjects who had just completed six weeks of creatine intake could, on average, recite 8.5 digits backward, whereas those who had completed six weeks of placebo intake could, on average, recite 7 digits backward. Studies such as this should stimulate new work on the role of creatine in cognitive processes.

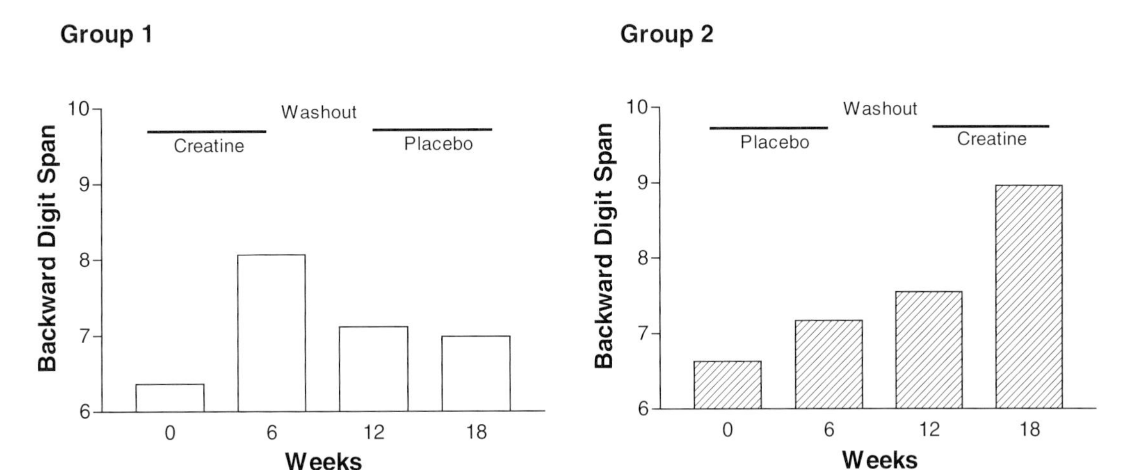

Figure 5

Effect of creatine monohydrate and placebo intake on performance on the Auditory Backward Digit Span test. Group 1 received creatine monohydrate for the first six weeks, followed by a six-week washout period, followed by placebo from weeks 12 to 18. Group 2 received placebo for the first six weeks, followed by a six-week washout period, followed by creatine monohydrate supplementation from weeks 12 to 18. Supplementation with oral creatine monohydrate significantly affected performance compared with the placebo ($P < 0.001$), with no effect of order. Adapted from Rae et al. (61).

MPT: mitochondrial permeability transition

Nonclassical Mechanisms of Creatine Action

Creatine exerts many of its functions by increasing phosphocreatine levels, thereby permitting very rapid regeneration of ATP after a burst of ATP utilization. This is the "classical" function of creatine and is certainly responsible for the ergogenic effect of creatine supplementation in high-intensity, short-duration exercise. However, some of the effects of creatine supplementation may not be so readily explained. The neuroprotection offered by creatine in a mouse model of stroke affords a striking example. In these studies, mice fed a diet supplemented with creatine for three weeks underwent transient focal cerebral ischemia via occlusion of the cerebral middle artery for 45 min. The extraordinary result was that although only minor, nonsignificant changes were found in cerebral creatine, phosphocreatine, or adenine nucleotides, dietary creatine supplementation reduced infarct volume by about 40% (59). Although it is not possible to exclude a substantial increase in phosphocreatine in a small set of key cells, it seems unlikely that the classical mechanism can explain the results. Certainly, Prass et al. (59) suggest that neuroprotection occurred independent of changes in the bioenergetic status of the brain, possibly because of a cerebrovascular effect. It is appropriate, therefore, to review nonclassical actions of creatine.

Creatine and phosphocreatine are major intracellular solutes in muscle cells. Creatine supplementation, by increasing the levels of these metabolites, increases cell hydration. As outlined above, this acts as an anabolic signal that may be responsible for increased glycogen accretion. Creatine can also serve as a compatible osmolyte (similar to betaine, taurine, and myoinositol) in cultured muscle cells exposed to hypertonic stress. Exposure of C2C12 muscle cells to a hypertonic medium increased CRT mRNA about threefold and also increased creatine uptake into these cells (1). Creatine also exerts direct antioxidant effects, in particular toward radical anions such as superoxide and peroxynitrite (40). It is tempting to relate this property to the neuroprotective action of creatine in a number of animal models of neurodegenerative disease (34).

Mitochondrial creatine kinase (either the sarcomeric MtCK found in striated muscle or the ubiquitous MtCK found in other tissues such as brain, kidney, and spermatozoa) plays a remarkable structural role in mitochondria (68). This enzyme occurs as an octamer at contact sites between the inner and outer mitochondrial membranes. These contact sites are formed by proteolipid complexes that contain, in addition to MtCK, the adenine nucleotide translocase (inner membrane protein) and porin (outer membrane protein). Physiologically, it is clear that this physical interaction provides a microcompartment that ensures close functional coupling between the substrates and products of creatine kinase. Porin, also known as the voltage-dependent anion channel, is an outer-membrane component of the system responsible for the mitochondrial permeability transition (MPT), the reversible opening of a large pore in the inner membrane that results in a general loss of small molecules from the matrix. The identity of all of the components of the MPT pore is not known, although the adenine nucleotide translocase has been implicated. Opening of the pore may be triggered by a number of signals, such as an increase in Ca^{2+} or reactive oxygen species; it may lead to cell death either through apoptosis (via the release of proapoptotic proteins such as cytochrome *c*) or necrosis (via energy depletion) (68). It is apparent that mitochondrial creatine kinase restrains the permeability transition. Direct evidence for this idea comes from elegant experiments involving transgenic mice that express the ubiquitous MtCK in their liver, an organ that does not normally express creatine kinase (19). Mitochondria from the transgenic livers were resistant to Ca^{2+}-induced MPT. Moreover, it is clear that MtCK played a functional role, not just a structural one, since the phenomenon required the correctly localized, enzymatically active octameric protein as well as the substrates for creatine kinase (19). When MtCK is enzymatically active, it maintains a high matrix ADP concentration, which inhibits MPT pore opening (68). That creatine and phosphocreatine levels are able to restrain opening of the MPT pore may provide a mechanism for their neuroprotective effects, particularly in conditions associated with excessive production of reactive oxygen and reactive nitrogen species.

Finally, MtCK is involved in another pathological process that is modified by creatine levels. A number of events that affect energy metabolism in skeletal muscle (i.e., ischemia, experimental creatine depletion, and culture of adult rat myocytes in the absence of added creatine) lead to the appearance of enlarged mitochondria with arrays of paracrystalline inclusion bodies (68). These inclusions seem to consist, very largely, of MtCK. Similar inclusion bodies are also found in skeletal muscles of patients suffering from a variety of mitochondrial cytopathies. In some circumstances, the occurrence of these inclusion bodies can be directly linked to creatine status. In the case of animals depleted of creatine by treatment with the CRT inhibitor β-guanidinopropionate, the inclusion bodies disappear upon withdrawal of this agent (16). A particularly intriguing case concerns an athletic patient with a novel cytochrome *b* mutation. Cells from this subject produced high basal rates of reactive oxygen species. A muscle biopsy showed paracrystalline inclusion bodies in mitochondria that disappeared after five weeks of treatment with creatine monohydrate at 10 g/day (84).

It is clear that creatine and creatine supplementation exert potent effects that go beyond the simple buffering of cytoplasmic ATP. Further understanding of these effects may be expected in the next few years. Certainly, the words of Hamlet are apposite: "There are more things in heaven and earth, Horatio, than are dreamt of in your philosophy."

SUMMARY POINTS

1. Creatine and phosphocreatine play important roles in both ATP buffering and high-energy phosphate shuttling in a variety of cells.
2. Because of the spontaneous and irreversible breakdown of both creatine and phosphocreatine to creatinine, creatine needs to be continuously replaced by a combination of diet and synthesis. Vegetarians receive very little creatine in their diet and must obtain almost all of it by synthesis. Creatine synthesis makes major demands on amino acid metabolism.
3. Creatine supplementation is used as an ergogenic agent, particularly by athletes involved in exercise of high intensity and short duration. It is also used therapeutically in the treatment of a number of neuromuscular and neurodegenerative diseases.
4. Though long recognized for its role in muscle, it is now clear that creatine is vital for normal brain function. This is evidenced by the neurological symptoms displayed by children with inborn errors of creatine synthesis or transport.

FUTURE ISSUES

1. How do neonates acquire brain creatine? What is the importance of synthesis within the brain compared with creatine supplied via the circulation?

2. What is the role of the liver in creatine synthesis? Is it capable of the entire synthesis of creatine or does it just methylate guanidinoacetate that it obtains from the circulation? What transporter is responsible for creatine release by the liver?
3. How does creatine exert its neuroprotective effect in animal models of neurodegenerative diseases? Is creatine supplementation as effective in Huntington's disease in humans as it is in animal models of this disease?

ACKNOWLEDGMENTS

This work was supported by grants from the Canadian Institutes of Health Research. We thank Mr. Robin da Silva for his assistance with the figures.

LITERATURE CITED

1. Alfieri RR, Bonelli MA, Cavazzoni A, Brigotti M, Fumarola C, et al. 2006. Creatine as a compatible osmolyte in muscle cells exposed to hypertonic stress. *J. Physiol.* 576:391–401
2. Battini R, Alessandri MG, Leuzzi V, Moro F, Tosetti M, et al. 2006. Arginine:glycine amidinotransferase (AGAT) deficiency in a newborn: early treatment can prevent phenotypic expression of the disease. *J. Pediatr.* 148:828–30
3. Bodamer OA, Sahoo T, Beaudet AL, O'Brien WE, Bottiglieri T, et al. 2005. Creatine metabolism in combined methylmalonic aciduria and homocystinuria. *Ann. Neurol.* 57:557–60
4. Bourgeois JM, Tarnopolsky MA. 2000. Creatine supplementation in mitochondrial cytopathies. In *Creatine: From Basic Science to Clinical Application*, ed. R Paoletti, A Poli, AS Jackson, pp. 91–100. Dordrecht: Kluwer
5. Braissant O, Henry H, Loup M, Eilers B, Bachmann C. 2001. Endogenous synthesis and transport of creatine in the rat brain: an in situ hybridization study. *Brain Res. Mol. Brain Res.* 86:193–201
6. Branch JD. 2003. Effect of creatine supplementation on body composition and performance: a meta-analysis. *Int. J. Sport Nutr. Exerc. Metab.* 13:198–226
7. Brosnan ME, Brosnan JT. 2004. Renal arginine metabolism. *J. Nutr.* 134:2791–95S
8. Burke DG, Chilibeck PD, Parise G, Candow DG, Mahoney D, Tarnopolsky M. 2003. Effect of creatine and weight training on muscle creatine and performance in vegetarians. *Med. Sci. Sports Exerc.* 35:1946–55
9. Bürklen TS, Schlattner U, Homayouni R, Gough K, Rak M, et al. 2006. The creatine kinase/creatine connection to Alzheimer's disease: CK inactivation, APP-CK complexes, and focal creatine deposits. *J. Biomed. Biotechnol.* 2006:1–11
10. Clark AJ, Rosenberg EH, Almeida LS, Wood TC, Jakobs C, et al. 2006. X-linked creatine transporter (SLC6A8) mutations in about 1% of males with mental retardation of unknown etiology. *Hum. Genet.* 119:604–10
11. Cockcroft DW, Gault MH. 1976. Prediction of creatinine clearance from serum creatinine. *Nephron* 16:31–41
12. Dai W, Vinnakota S, Qian X, Kunze DL, Sarkar HK. 1999. Molecular characterization of the human CRT-1 creatine transporter expressed in Xenopus oocytes. *Arch. Biochem. Biophys.* 361:75–84

13. Dedeoglu A, Kubilus JK, Yang L, Ferrante KL, Hersch SM, et al. 2003. Creatine therapy provides neuroprotection after onset of clinical symptoms in Huntington's disease transgenic mice. *J. Neurochem.* 85:1359–67
14. Delanghe J, De Slypere JP, De Buyzere M, Robbrecht J, Wieme R, Vermeulen A. 1989. Normal reference values for creatine, creatinine and carnitine are lower in vegetarians. *Clin. Chem.* 35:1802–3
15. Derave W, Eijnde BO, Verbessem P, Ramaekers M, van Leemputte M, et al. 2003. Combined creatine and protein supplementation in conjunction with resistance training promotes muscle GLUT-4 content and glucose tolerance in humans. *J. Appl. Physiol.* 94:1910–16
16. De Tata V, Cavallini G, Pollera M, Gori Z, Bergamini E. 1993. The induction of mitochondrial myopathy in the rat by feeding beta-guanidinopropionic acid and the reversibility of the induced mitochondrial lesions: a biochemical and ultrastructural investigation. *Int. J. Exp. Pathol.* 74:501–9
17. Dietary Reference Intakes for Energy. 2005. *Carbohydrate, Fiber, Fat, Fatty Acids, Cholesterol, Protein and Amino Acids.* Washington, DC: Natl. Acad. Sci.
18. Dodd JR, Zheng T, Christie DL. 1999. Creatine accumulation and exchange by HEK293 cells stably expressing high levels of a creatine transporter. *Biochim. Biophys. Acta* 1472:128–36
19. Dolder M, Walzel B, Speer O, Schlattner U, Wallimann T. 2003. Inhibition of the mitochondrial permeability transition by creatine kinase substrates. Requirement for microcompartmentation. *J. Biol. Chem.* 278:17760–66
20. Ellington WR. 2001. Evolution and physiological roles of phosphagen systems. *Annu. Rev. Physiol.* 63:289–325
21. Ensenauer R, Thiel T, Schwab KO, Tacke U, Stockler-Ipsiroglu S, et al. 2004. Guanidinoacetate methyltransferase deficiency: differences of creatine uptake in human brain and muscle. *Mol. Genet. Metab.* 82:208–13
22. Ferrante RJ, Andreassen OA, Jenkins BG, Dedeoglu A, Kuemmerle S, et al. 2000. Neuroprotective effects of creatine in a transgenic mouse model of Huntington's disease. *J. Neurosci.* 20:4389–97
23. Ferreira LG, De Toledo Bergamaschi C, Lazaretti-Castro M, Heilberg IP. 2005. Effects of creatine supplementation on body composition and renal function in rats. *Med. Sci. Sports Exerc.* 37:1525–29
24. Garcia-Delgado M, Peral MJ, Cano M, Calonge ML, Ilundain AA. 2001. Creatine transport in brush-border membrane vesicles isolated from rat kidney cortex. *J. Am. Soc. Nephrol.* 12:1819–25
25. Graham AS, Hatton RC. 1999. Creatine: a review of efficacy and safety. *J. Am. Pharm. Assoc.* 39:803–10
26. Green AL, Hultman E, Macdonald IA, Sewell DA, Greenhaff PL. 1996. Carbohydrate ingestion augments skeletal muscle creatine accumulation during creatine supplementation in humans. *Am. J. Physiol.* 271:E821–26
27. Gregor P, Nash SR, Caron MG, Seldin MF, Warren ST. 1995. Assignment of the creatine transporter gene (SLC6A8) to human chromosome Xq28 telomeric to G6PD. *Genomics* 25:332–33
28. Guimbal C, Kilimann MW. 1993. A Na(+)-dependent creatine transporter in rabbit brain, muscle, heart and kidney. cDNA cloning and functional expression. *J. Biol. Chem.* 268:8418–21
29. Harris RC, Nevill M, Harris DB, Fallowfield JL, Bogdanis GC, Wise JA. 2002. Absorption of creatine supplied as a drink, in meat or in solid form. *J. Sports Sci.* 20:147–51

30. Harris RC, Soderlund K, Hultman E. 1992. Elevation of creatine in resting and exercised muscle of normal subjects by creatine supplementation. *Clin. Sci. (Lond.)* 83:367–74
31. Heinanen K, Nanto-Salonen K, Komu M, Erkintalo M, Alanen A, et al. 1999. Creatine corrects muscle 31P spectrum in gyrate atrophy with hyperornithinaemia. *Eur. J. Clin. Invest.* 29:1060–65
32. Hersch SM, Gevorkian S, Marder K, Moskowitz C, Feigin A, et al. 2006. Creatine in Huntington disease is safe, tolerable, bioavailable in brain and reduces serum 8OH2′dG. *Neurology* 66:250–52
33. Holmes BF, Kurth-Kraczek EJ, Winder WW. 1999. Chronic activation of 5′-AMP-activated protein kinase increases GLUT-4, hexokinase and glycogen in muscle. *J. Appl. Physiol.* 87:1990–95
34. Ikeda K, Iwasaki Y, Kinoshita M. 2000. Oral administration of creatine monohydrate retards progression of motor neuron disease in the wobbler mouse. *Amyotroph. Lateral Scler. Other Motor Neuron Disord.* 1:207–12
35. Jenkins BG, Rosas HD, Chen YC, Makabe T, Myers R, et al. 1998. 1H NMR spectroscopy studies of Huntington's disease: correlations with CAG repeat numbers. *Neurology* 50:1357–65
36. Ju JS, Smith JL, Oppelt PJ, Fisher JS. 2005. Creatine feeding increases GLUT4 expression in rat skeletal muscle. *Am. J. Physiol. Endocrinol. Metab.* 288:E347–52
37. Kaasik A, Veksler V, Boehm E, Novotova M, Ventura-Clapier R. 2003. From energy store to energy flux: a study in creatine kinase-deficient fast skeletal muscle. *FASEB J.* 17:708–10
38. Koroshetz WJ, Jenkins BG, Rosen BR, Beal MF. 1997. Energy metabolism defects in Huntington's disease and effects of coenzyme Q10. *Ann. Neurol.* 41:160–65
39. Korzun WJ. 2004. Oral creatine supplements lower plasma homocysteine concentrations in humans. *Clin. Lab. Sci.* 17:102–6
40. Lawler JM, Barnes WS, Wu G, Song W, Demaree S. 2002. Direct antioxidant properties of creatine. *Biochem. Biophys. Res. Commun.* 290:47–52
41. Li JY, Popovic N, Brundin P. 2005. The use of the R6 transgenic mouse models of Huntington's disease in attempts to develop novel therapeutic strategies. *NeuroRx* 2:447–64
42. Loike JD, Zalutsky DL, Kaback E, Miranda AF, Silverstein SC. 1988. Extracellular creatine regulates creatine transport in rat and human muscle cells. *Proc. Nat. Acad. Sci. USA* 85:807–11
43. Louis M, Lebacq J, Poortmans JR, Belpaire-Dethiou MC, Devogelaer JP, et al. 2003. Beneficial effects of creatine supplementation in dystrophic patients. *Muscle Nerve* 27:604–10
44. Louis M, Poortmans JR, Francaux M, Berre J, Boisseau N, et al. 2003. No effect of creatine supplementation on human myofibrillar and sarcoplasmic protein synthesis after resistance exercise. *Am. J. Physiol. Endocrinol. Metab.* 285:E1089–94
45. Louis M, Poortmans JR, Francaux M, Hultman E, Berre J, et al. 2003. Creatine supplementation has no effect on human muscle protein turnover at rest in the postabsorptive or fed states. *Am. J. Physiol. Endocrinol. Metab.* 284:E764–70
46. Low SY, Rennie MJ, Taylor PM. 1996. Modulation of glycogen synthesis in rat skeletal muscle by changes in cell volume. *J. Physiol.* 495:299–303
47. Lukaszuk JM, Robertson RJ, Arch JE, Moore GE, Yaw KM, et al. 2002. Effect of creatine supplementation and a lacto-ovo-vegetarian diet on muscle creatine concentration. *Int. J. Sports Exerc. Metab.* 12:336–48
48. Lunardi G, Parodi A, Perasso L, Pohvozcheva AV, Scarrone S, et al. 2006. The creatine transporter mediates the uptake of creatine by brain tissue, but not the uptake of two creatine-derived compounds. *Neuroscience* 142:991–97

49. MacNeil L, Hill L, MacDonald D, Keefe L, Cormier JF, et al. 2005. Analysis of creatine, creatinine, creatine-d3 and creatinine-d3 in urine, plasma, and red blood cells by HPLC and GC-MS to follow the fate of ingested creatine-d3. *J. Chromatogr. B Analyt. Technol. Biomed. Life Sci.* 827:210–15
50. Mazziotta JC, Phelps ME, Pahl JJ, Huang SC, Baxter LR, et al. 1987. Reduced cerebral glucose metabolism in asymptomatic subjects at risk for Huntington's disease. *N. Engl. J. Med.* 316:357–62
51. McGuire DM, Gross MD, Elde RP, Van Pilsum JF. 1986. Localization of L-arginine-glycine amidinotransferase protein in rat tissues by immunofluorescence microscopy. *J. Histochem. Cytochem.* 34:429–35
52. McGuire DM, Gross MD, Van Pilsum JF, Towle HC. 1984. Repression of rat kidney L-arginine:glycine amidinotransferase synthesis by creatine at a pretranslational level. *J. Biol. Chem.* 259:12034–38
53. Momken I, Lechene P, Koulmann N, Fortin D, Mateo P, et al. 2005. Impaired voluntary running capacity of creatine kinase-deficient mice. *J. Physiol.* 565:951–64
54. Mudd SH, Brosnan JT, Brosnan ME, Jacobs RL, Stabler SP, et al. 2007. Methyl balance and transmethylation fluxes in humans. *Am. J. Clin. Nutr.* 85:19–25
55. Nahrendorf M, Spindler M, Hu K, Bauer L, Ritter O, et al. 2005. Creatine kinase knockout mice show left ventricular hypertrophy and dilatation, but unaltered remodeling post-myocardial infarction. *Cardiovasc. Res.* 65:419–27
56. Newmeyer A, Cecil KM, Schapiro M, Clark JF, Degrauw TJ. 2005. Incidence of brain creatine transporter deficiency in males with developmental delay referred for brain magnetic resonance imaging. *J. Dev. Behav. Pediatr.* 26:276–82
57. Ohtsuki S, Tachikawa M, Takanaga H, Shimizu H, Watanabe M, et al. 2002. The blood-brain barrier creatine transporter is a major pathway for supplying creatine to the brain. *J. Cereb. Blood Flow Metab.* 22:1327–35
58. Ponticos M, Lu QL, Morgan JE, Hardie DG, Partridge TA, Carling D. 1998. Dual regulation of the AMP-activated protein kinase provides a novel mechanism for the control of creatine kinase in skeletal muscle. *EMBO J.* 17:1688–99
59. Prass K, Royl G, Lindauer U, Freyer D, Megow D, et al. 2007. Improved reperfusion and neuroprotection by creatine in a mouse model of stroke. *J. Cereb. Blood Flow Metab.* 27:452–59
60. Pyne-Geithman GJ, de Grauw TJ, Cecil KM, Chuck G, Lyons MA, et al. 2004. Presence of normal creatine in the muscle of a patient with a mutation in the creatine transporter: a case study. *Mol. Cell. Biochem.* 262:35–39
61. Rae C, Digney AL, McEwan SR, Bates TC. 2003. Oral creatine monohydrate supplementation improves brain performance: a double-blind, placebo-controlled, cross-over trial. *Proc. Biol. Sci.* 270:2147–50
62. Ramesh V, Gusella JF, Shih VE. 1991. Molecular pathology of gyrate atrophy of the choroid and retina due to ornithine aminotransferase deficiency. *Mol. Biol. Med.* 8:81–93
63. Rawson ES, Clarkson PM, Price TB, Miles MP. 2002. Differential response of muscle phosphocreatine to creatine supplementation in young and old subjects. *Acta Physiol. Scand.* 174:57–65
64. Ryu H, Rosas HD, Hersch SM, Ferrante RJ. 2005. The therapeutic role of creatine in Huntington's disease. *Pharmacol. Ther.* 108:193–207
65. Salomons GS, van Dooren SJ, Verhoeven NM, Marsden D, Schwartz C, et al. 2003. X-linked creatine transporter defect: an overview. *J. Inherit. Metab. Dis.* 26:309–18
66. Sandberg AA, Hecht HH, Tyler FH. 1953. Studies in disorders of muscle. X. The site of creatine synthesis in the human. *Metabolism* 2:22–29

67. Schilling BK, Stone MH, Utter A, Kearney JT, Johnson M, et al. 2001. Creatine supplementation and health variables: a retrospective study. *Med. Sci. Sports Exerc.* 33:183–88
68. Schlattner U, Tokarska-Schlattner M, Wallimann T. 2006. Mitochondrial creatine kinase in human health and disease. *Biochim. Biophys. Acta* 1762:164–80
69. Scholey AB, Harper S, Kennedy DO. 2001. Cognitive demand and blood glucose. *Physiol. Behav.* 73:585–92
70. Schulze A. 2003. Creatine deficiency syndromes. *Mol. Cell. Biochem.* 244:143–50
71. Schulze A, Hoffmann GF, Bachert P, Kirsch S, Salomons GS, et al. 2006. Presymptomatic treatment of neonatal guanidinoacetate methyltransferase deficiency. *Neurology* 67:719–21
72. Snow RJ, Murphy RM. 2001. Creatine and the creatine transporter: a review. *Mol. Cell. Biochem.* 224:169–81
73. Sora I, Richman J, Santoro G, Wei H, Wang Y, et al. 1994. The cloning and expression of a human creatine transporter. *Biochem. Biophys. Res. Commun.* 204:419–27
74. Speer O, Neukomm LJ, Murphy RM, Zanolla E, Schlattner U, et al. 2004. Creatine transporters: a reappraisal. *Mol. Cell. Biochem.* 256–257:407–24
75. Stead LM, Au KP, Jacobs RL, Brosnan ME, Brosnan JT. 2001. Methylation demand and homocysteine metabolism: effects of dietary provision of creatine and guanidinoacetate. *Am. J. Physiol. Endocrinol. Metab.* 281:E1095–100
76. Stead LM, Brosnan JT, Brosnan ME, Vance DE, Jacobs RL. 2006. Is it time to reevaluate methyl balance in humans? *Am. J. Clin. Nutr.* 83:5–10
77. Steenge GR, Verhoef P, Greenhaff PL. 2001. The effect of creatine and resistance training on plasma homocysteine concentration in healthy volunteers. *Arch. Intern. Med.* 161:1455–56
78. Stockler S, Hanefeld F, Frahm J. 1996. Creatine replacement therapy in guanidinoacetate methyltransferase deficiency, a novel inborn error of metabolism. *Lancet* 348:789–90
79. Streijger F, Oerlemans F, Ellenbroek BA, Jost CR, Wieringa B, van der Zee CE. 2005. Structural and behavioural consequences of double deficiency for creatine kinases BCK and UbCKmit. *Behav. Brain Res.* 157:219–34
80. Stromberger C, Bodamer OA, Stockler-Ipsiroglu S. 2003. Clinical characteristics and diagnostic clues in inborn errors of creatine metabolism. *J. Inherit. Metab. Dis.* 26:299–308
81. Sykut-Cegielska J, Gradowska W, Mercimek-Mahmutoglu S, Stockler-Ipsiroglu S. 2004. Biochemical and clinical characteristics of creatine deficiency syndromes. *Acta Biochim. Pol.* 51:875–82
82. Tachikawa M, Fukaya M, Terasaki T, Ohtsaki S, Watanabe M. 2004. Distinct cellular expressions of creatine synthetic enzyme GAMT and creatine kinases uCK-Mi and CK-B suggest a novel neuron-glial relationship for brain energy homeostasis. *Eur. J. Neurosci.* 20:144–60
83. Tarnopolsky MA, Mahoney DJ, Vajsar J, Rodriguez C, Doherty TJ, et al. 2004. Creatine monohydrate enhances strength and body composition in Duchenne muscular dystrophy. *Neurology* 62:1771–77
84. Tarnopolsky MA, Simon DK, Roy BD, Chorneyko K, Lowther SA, et al. 2004. Attenuation of free radical production and paracrystalline inclusions by creatine supplementation in a patient with a novel cytochrome b mutation. *Muscle Nerve* 29:537–47
85. Taylor EB, Ellingson WJ, Lamb JD, Chesser DG, Compton CL, Winder WW. 2006. Evidence against regulation of AMP-activated protein kinase and LKB1/STRAD/MO25 activity by creatine phosphate. *Am. J. Physiol. Endocrinol. Metab.* 290:E661–69
86. Tosco M, Faelli A, Sironi C, Gastaldi G, Orsenigo MN. 2004. A creatine transporter is operative at the brush border level of the rat jejunal enterocyte. *J. Membr. Biol.* 202:85–95

87. van Loon LJ, Murphy R, Oosterlaar AM, Cameron-Smith D, Hargreaves M, et al. 2004. Creatine supplementation increases glycogen storage but not GLUT-4 expression in human skeletal muscle. *Clin. Sci. (Lond.)* 106:99–106
88. Vannas-Sulonen K, Sipila I, Vannas A, Simell O, Rapola J. 1985. Gyrate atrophy of the choroid and retina. A five-year follow-up of creatine supplementation. *Ophthalmology* 92:1719–27
89. Volek JS, Duncan ND, Mazzetti SA, Staron RS, Putukian M, et al. 1999. Performance and muscle fiber adaptations to creatine supplementation and heavy resistance training. *Med. Sci. Sports Exerc.* 31:1147–56
90. Volek JS, Rawson ES. 2004. Scientific basis and practical aspects of creatine supplementation for athletes. *Nutrition* 20:609–14
91. Vorgerd M, Grehl T, Jager M, Muller K, Freitag G, et al. 2000. Creatine therapy in myophosphorylase deficiency (McArdle disease): a placebo-controlled crossover trial. *Arch. Neurol.* 57:956–63
92. Vorgerd M, Zange J, Kley R, Grehl T, Husing A, et al. 2002. Effect of high-dose creatine therapy on symptoms of exercise intolerance in McArdle disease: double-blind, placebo-controlled crossover study. *Arch. Neurol.* 59:97–101
93. Wallimann T, Wyss M, Brdiczka D, Nicolay K, Eppenberger HM. 1992. Intracellular compartmentation, structure and function of creatine kinase isoenzymes in tissues with high and fluctuating energy demands: the "phosphocreatine circuit" for cellular energy homeostasis. *Biochem. J.* 281:21–40
94. Wendt S, Dedeoglu A, Speer O, Wallimann T, Beal MF, Andreassen OA. 2002. Reduced creatine kinase activity in transgenic amyotrophic lateral sclerosis mice. *Free Radic. Biol. Med.* 32:920–26
95. Willoughby DS, Rosene JM. 2003. Effects of oral creatine and resistance training on myogenic regulatory factor expression. *Med. Sci. Sports Exerc.* 35:923–29
96. Wyss M, Kaddurah-Daouk R. 2000. Creatine and creatinine metabolism. *Physiol. Rev.* 80:1107–213
97. Ziegenfuss TN, Lowery LM, Lemon PWR. 1998. Acute fluid and volume changes in men during three days of creatine supplementation. *J. Exerc. Physiol.* 1: 1–10

The Genetics of Anorexia Nervosa

Cynthia M. Bulik,[1,2]
Margarita C.T. Slof-Op't Landt,[4,5,7]
Eric F. van Furth,[4,6] and Patrick F. Sullivan[1,3]

[1]Department of Psychiatry, [2]Department of Nutrition, and [3]Department of Genetics, University of North Carolina at Chapel Hill, North Carolina 27599; [4]Centrum Eetstoornissen Ursula, National Center for Eating Disorders, Leidschendam, The Netherlands; [5]Molecular Epidemiology Section (Department of Medical Statistics) and [6]Department of Psychiatry, Leiden University Medical Center, The Netherlands; [7]Department of Biological Psychology, Vrije Universiteit, Amsterdam, The Netherlands; email: cbulik@med.unc.edu

Annu. Rev. Nutr. 2007. 27:263–75

First published online as a Review in Advance on April 12, 2007

The *Annual Review of Nutrition* is online at http://nutr.annualreviews.org

This article's doi:
10.1146/annurev.nutr.27.061406.093713

0199-9885/07/0821-0263$20.00

Key Words

twin, linkage, association study

Abstract

Anorexia nervosa is a perplexing illness marked by low body weight and persistent fear of weight gain. Anorexia nervosa has the highest mortality rate of any psychiatric disease. Historically, anorexia nervosa was viewed as a disorder primarily influenced by sociocultural factors; however, over the past decade, this perception has been challenged. Family studies have consistently demonstrated that anorexia nervosa runs in families. Twin studies have underscored the contribution of additive genetic factors to the observed familial aggregation. With these bodies of literature as a starting point, we evaluate critically the current state of research on molecular genetic studies of anorexia nervosa and provide guidance for future research.

Contents

THE GENETICS OF ANOREXIA NERVOSA

For decades, anorexia nervosa (AN) was considered a disorder influenced primarily by family and sociocultural factors; however, recent research has focused on the possibility that genetics also play a critical role in vulnerability to this perplexing and often deadly disorder. In this review, we critically appraise the extant literature focusing on family, twin, and molecular genetic studies of AN.

Presentation of Anorexia Nervosa

AN is a serious psychiatric illness marked by an inability to maintain a normal healthy body weight, with patients often dropping well below 85% of expected. Patients who are still growing fail to make expected increases in height, weight, and bone density. Despite increasing emaciation, individuals with AN continue to obsess about body weight and shape, remain dissatisfied with the perceived size and shape of their bodies, and engage in unhealthy behaviors to perpetuate weight loss (e.g., purging, dieting, excessive exercise, and fasting). A subgroup of individuals with AN develop binge eating and purging. Shape and weight become critical markers of self-worth and self-esteem. Although amenorrhea is a diagnostic criterion, it is of questionable relevance as meaningful differences have not been identified between individuals with AN who do and do not menstruate (12, 43). Typical personality features of individuals with AN include perfectionism, obsessionality, anxiety, harm avoidance, and low self-esteem (61).

The most common comorbid psychiatric conditions include major depression (58) and anxiety disorders (11, 21, 28). Anxiety disorders often predate the onset of the eating disorder (11, 28), and depression often persists postrecovery (55). The average prevalence of AN has been reported to be 0.3% (25). The prevalence of subthreshold AN, defined as one criterion short of threshold, is greater—ranging from 0.37%–1.3% (41, 60). Eating disorders are among the ten leading causes of disability among young women (40), the perceived quality of life of sufferers and former sufferers is poor (18), and anorexia nervosa has the highest mortality rate of all psychiatric disorders, with a standardized mortality ratio of over 10 (6, 54).

Etiological Factors

Relatively rare complex disorders such as AN pose a particular challenge for risk factor research because population-based and longitudinal investigations often identify only a small number of cases (41, 51). Moreover, in the presence of etiological heterogeneity, the identification of a small number of cases reflecting multiple etiological factors renders it particularly challenging to identify risk factors.

Comprehensive reviews on risk factors for eating disorders exist (27). Common risk factors for AN, although not specific to the disorder, are female sex, a history of childhood eating and gastrointestinal problems, prior sexual abuse or other significant adverse experiences, elevated weight and shape concerns, negative self-evaluation, and general psychiatric morbidity (27). Prematurity, smallness for gestational age, and cephalohematoma have been identified as specific risk factors for AN (17). Overall, few longitudinal studies exist in which sufficient numbers of cases have been detected to enable the identification of risk factors for AN. Moreover, it is difficult to differentiate between early symptoms of AN and risk factors (e.g., dieting and high exercise levels). Finally, studies have been unable to explore specificity of risk factors across the eating disorder subtypes, with outcome variables often crossing both diagnostic and threshold boundaries.

Unpacking the Family History Risk Factor

A family history of AN appears to be a risk factor for AN. This observation could be due to genes, environment, or a combination of both. Twin and adoption studies are the main designs by which genetic factors are disentangled from environmental factors in humans. Because there are no adoption studies of AN, we discuss family and twin studies below.

From the perspective of a group of individuals with AN, it is critical to view AN as a complex trait. On average, at a group level, AN results from a mixture of genetic and environmental influences. For AN, "nature versus nurture" is a false dichotomy; it is always "nature and nurture." AN is likely to be complex for a second reason. At the individual level, the pathophysiology of AN is unlikely to be uniform, and any sample of individuals with clinically defined AN is likely to consist of a number of different "types" of illness. Some proportion of individuals may have a highly genetic form of AN, some a highly environmental variant, and, in others, AN may result from interactions between genetic and environmental influences.

Family Studies

The familial nature of AN has been well established. The first-degree relatives of individuals with anorexia nervosa have approximately a tenfold greater lifetime risk of having AN than relatives of unaffected individuals (37, 52, 53). Yet anorexia nervosa does not "breed true" in that there is increased risk for an array of eating disorders in relatives of individuals with anorexia nervosa rather than a disorder-specific pattern of familial aggregation. This reflects the fact that anorexia and bulimia nervosa are indeed not mutually exclusive conditions, with individuals commonly crossing over between anorexic and bulimic presentations (57). Family studies are unable to determine the extent to which the observed familial aggregation is due to genetic or environmental factors.

Twin Studies

Twin studies, which are challenging given the relative rarity of the disorder, have yielded heritability estimates for subthreshold AN in the context of a bivariate twin analysis with major depression [a^2 = 58% (95% CI: 0.33–0.84)] (58), basing analysis on the single question of "Have you ever had AN?" [a^2 = 48% (95% CI: 0.27–0.65)] (35), and broadening the definition of AN syndrome [a^2 = 76% (95% CI: 0.35–0.95)] (34). We recently completed a large twin study on the narrow DSM-IV definition of AN (13) by screening all living, contactable, interviewable, and consenting twins in the Swedish Twin Registry (N = 31,406) born between 1935 and 1958. AN was identified by clinical interview, hospital discharge diagnosis of AN, or cause-of-death certificate. The heritability of narrowly defined DSM-IV AN was estimated to be $a^2 = 0.56$ (95% CI: 0.00–0.87), with the remaining variance attributable to shared environment [$c^2 = 0.05$ (95% CI: 0.00–0.64)] and unique environment [$e^2 = 0.38$ (95% CI: 0.13–0.84)]. Convergence of heritability estimates across populations is encouraging. Evidence of violations of fundamental assumptions of the twin method has not been found (14, 31, 33); however, results are limited to European populations and may not necessarily generalize to world populations.

Molecular Genetic Studies

In the past 30 years, human genetic studies have identified more than 1000 genes responsible for human diseases. These successes have largely been for uncommon diseases whose inheritance follows a classical pattern (e.g., Huntington's disease or cystic fibrosis) or traits for which a more genetically homogeneous subgroup can be isolated for a more common disease (e.g., *BRCA1* and familial breast and ovarian cancer or subforms of type 2 diabetes mellitus). The picture for complex traits more generally has been mixed: Despite an enormous effort to identify genes responsible for numerous critically important human diseases (cancer, cardiovascular disease, metabolic diseases, neuropsychiatric disorders, etc.), a surfeit of reproducible findings is still lacking.

The pattern of findings for AN resembles that of many disorders—initial intriguing findings diminished by the absence of clear-cut replication and definitive identification of causal DNA sequence variation—with the caveat that far fewer studies exist for AN.

Two main study designs are generally employed to attempt to identify genes responsible for complex traits like AN: linkage and association studies. The purpose of a genomewide linkage study for a complex trait like AN is to identify the genomic regions that might harbor predisposing or protective genes. In essence, linkage is a "discovery science" tool that does not require a priori assumptions about the nature and locations of genes involved in the etiology of AN (15, 49). Linkage analysis for complex traits requires a large sample of pedigrees with multiply affected individuals (1). Anonymous genetic markers across the genome are genotyped and used to identify chromosomal regions that may contain etiological genes. Linkage approaches effectively narrow the search space from the entire genome (3 billion base pairs) to one or several chromosomal regions (perhaps 10–30 million base pairs). Genes known to be in these chromosomal regions become positional candidate genes.

Association studies contrast cases with AN to appropriate controls without AN. The usual approach has been to select a set of specific candidate genes thought by the investigator to be involved in the pathophysiology of AN. Historically, unlike linkage studies, prior knowledge has been required in order to conduct an association study—to select candidate genes, to genotype a set of genetic markers, and to compare genotype and haplotype frequencies between cases and controls.

Recently, genotyping technologies have progressed to the point where it is possible (although expensive) to genotype hundreds of thousands of genetic markers in all cases and all controls. A large number of genomewide association studies are likely to be published by the end of 2007, and it will be interesting to see if these produce definitive findings. To our knowledge, no such studies are in progress for AN, and the extant literature for AN is limited to a few genomewide linkage studies and a somewhat larger number of candidate gene association studies that have focused on genes in central pathways known to influence feeding, appetite, and mood.

Linkage Studies of Anorexia Nervosa

Linkage studies for AN (3, 19, 23) have yielded significant results and underscored the importance of detailed phenotyping. A linkage study of a heterogeneous sample of individuals with broadly defined eating disorders yielded no statistically significant findings; however, when the sample was restricted to relative pairs exhibiting the classic restricting AN, it yielded significant evidence for a susceptibility locus on chromosome 1 (23). Additional approaches that enhanced the focus of the linkage analysis by incorporating key behavioral covariates into linkage analyses (19)—drive for thinness and obsessionality—isolated several regions of interest on chromosomes 1, 2, and 13. The chromosome 1 region contained two genes that intersected with pathophysiological theories of the etiology of AN—the serotonin 1D receptor (*HTR1D*) and the delta opioid receptor (*OPRD1*)—and a subsequent association study found significant associations with AN (4).

Further work developed a systematic roadmap for utilizing a rich set of phenotypes for genetic analyses and identified variables that were relevant to eating disorders pathology and had published evidence for heritability. Based on these criteria, six traits were analyzed for linkage. Obsessionality, age at menarche, and a composite anxiety measure displayed features of heritable quantitative traits, such as normal distribution and familial correlation, and thus appeared ideal for quantitative linkage analysis. By contrast, some families showed highly concordant and extreme values for three additional variables—lifetime minimum body mass index (lowest body mass index attained during the course of illness), concern over mistakes, and food-related obsessions—whereas others did not. These distributions are consistent with a mixture of populations, and thus the variables were matched with covariate linkage analysis. Linkage analysis found a number of suggestive signals: obsessionality at 6q21, anxiety at 9p21.3, body mass index at 4q13.1, concern over mistakes at 11p11.2 and 17q25.1, and food-related obsessions at 17q25.1 and 15q26.2.

From the perspective of identifying very strong candidate genes for AN, however, the extant studies do not yet narrow the genomic search space in a highly compelling manner. The three linkage reports for AN (3, 19, 23) have 27 findings at a "suggestive" level and two findings at a "significant" type 1 error level. The latter two findings are both on chromosome 1—a 32 million base pair region from 1p36.13–1p34.2 for restricting AN (23) and a 41 million base pair region from 1q25.q–1q41 for a composite phenotype of AN with drive for thinness and obsessionality. These large genomic regions are located on opposite arms of chromosome 1 and contain 546 genes (perhaps 1.4% of all known genes in the human genome). About half of these genes are known to be expressed in brain. A number of genes in these regions overlap with existing theories of the pathophysiology of AN (*HTR1D*, *HTR6*) or are relevant to feeding behavior or satiety (the cannabinoid receptor *CNR2*) along with multiple genes whose products play roles in potentially relevant neuronal processes (e.g., multiple regulator of G-protein signaling family genes).

It is not clear whether these linkage findings truly contain one or more genes relevant to AN. To our knowledge, there has not yet been a comprehensive fine-mapping study of these regions. Therefore, at present, these findings constitute tentative knowledge—they may contain genes of etiological relevance to AN, or they may represent false signals. Encouragingly, a replication study with an independent sample is nearing completion (W. Kaye, personal communication). A hard replication would be a valuable next step in advancing the field.

Association Studies of Anorexia Nervosa

The volume of genetic association studies along with their specialized terminology can be dizzying to the reader unfamiliar with genetic research. One feature of this work that deserves particular mention is the tendency of significant initial reports not to replicate in subsequent studies (24). This phenomenon has been dubbed the "Proteus effect" (26) and underscores the methodological and statistical challenges of finding a needle in a haystack while dealing with issues of multiple comparisons and uncertain prior probabilities. We briefly review the association studies for AN and discuss challenges in interpreting the literature.

Serotonergic Genes

The serotonin pathway has been studied intensively in anorexia nervosa. It is involved in a broad range of biological, physiological, and behavioral functions (7, 8, 50). Serotonin is involved in body weight regulation, specifically in eating behavior, and has also been implicated in the development of eating disorders (9, 30, 59).

Many small, statistically underpowered association studies on genes belonging to the serotonin pathway have been performed. We recalculated the power of the studies, assuming a dominant model with an allele frequency of 0.10, alpha 0.05, and a relative risk of 2. To obtain a power of 80% under these assumptions, at least 178 cases and 178 controls are required. Only three association studies have been performed that had adequate statistical power to detect an effect (4, 10, 22); results of these studies are listed in the first section of **Table 1**. Two studies focused on the serotonin receptor 1D gene (4, 10). Several serotonin 1D polymorphisms were associated with AN or restrictive AN (4, 10). However, only one single nucleotide polymorphism (SNP), rs674386, was replicated in both studies. The third association study tested whether the rs6311 polymorphism of the serotonin 2A receptor gene was associated with AN (22). This analysis yielded no association. A recent investigation examined four SNPs in HTR1D in 276 women with AN and 768 controls and found evidence of association between two polymorphisms within HTR1D and RAN (10).

Overall, the serotonin 1D gene looks promising, and, notably it is located under the linkage peak for restricting AN (23). However, no hard replications in adequately powered samples have yet been published. Since only one polymorphism was examined in the serotonin 2A receptor gene, no conclusions can be drawn about the involvement of this gene in the etiology of anorexia nervosa.

Dopaminergic Genes

Increased dopaminergic activity has been hypothesized to be involved in many of the major symptoms related to AN. Repulsion to food, weight loss, hyperactivity, menstrual abnormalities (amenorrhea), distortion of body image, and obsessive-compulsive behavior have all been related to dopamine activity (29).

The results of two association studies in AN with genes from the dopamine pathway are presented in the second section of **Table 1**. The COMT gene encodes catechol-*O*-methyltransferase, which catabolizes brain catecholamine neurotransmitters such as dopamine and norepinephrine (2). No association was found between the rs4680 polymorphism located within this gene and AN in a combined transmission disequilibrium test and case-control analysis (20). Several polymorphisms within the dopamine D2 receptor gene were tested for association with AN (5). Association was reported with the purging-type AN for the rs1800497 and rs6278 polymorphisms in a case-control design, and the transmission disequilibrium test yielded preferential transmission for the rs6277 and the rs1799732 polymorphisms.

The dopamine receptor D2 gene remains of interest, although the findings require replication in a large independent sample. For catechol-*O*-methyltransferase, the existing data do not support a role for the rs4680 polymorphism in AN.

Neuropeptides and Feeding Regulation

Three genes involved in neuropeptide and feeding regulation (**Table 1**) have been tested in methodologically adequate association studies: ghrelin (16), hypocretin receptor

Table 1 Candidate gene studies performed by collaborations

Gene	Polymorphism	Phenotype	*N*	*p*-Value[a]	Reference	Note
Serotonin						
Serotonin receptor 1D HTR1D (1p36)	C1080T	AN Controls	196 98	0.01 0.01 (genotype)	(4)	OR 2.63, TDT NS U.S., U.K., and Germany
	A2190G	AN Controls	196 98	NS	(4)	OR 1.37, TDT 0.04 U.S., U.K., and Germany
	T-628C	AN Controls	196 98	NS	(4)	OR 0.72, TDT 0.01 U.S., U.K., and Germany
	T-1123C	AN Controls	196 98	NS	(4)	OR 0.73, TDT 0.02 U.S., U.K., and Germany
Serotonin receptor 2A, HTR2A (13q14)	G-1438A (rs6311)	AN	316 (trios)	NS	(22)	TDT and HHRR, France, Germany, U.K., Italy, and Spain
Catecholamine						
Catechol-*O*-methyltransferase COMT (22q11)	Val-158-Met (rs4680)	AN Controls	266 418	NS	(20)	OR 0.98, TDT NS Austria, Germany, Italy, Slovenia, Spain, and U.K.
Dopamine D2 receptor DRD2 (11q23)	−141→C (rs1799732)	ANr AN purging Controls	108 88 98	NS	(5)	Haplo rs6275 0.013, 0.050 (RAN); Haplo rs6277 0.011; TDT 0.014, haplo TDT (2) rs6275 (1), rs6277 (1) 0.0015 U.S., U.K., and Germany
	T2730C (rs1800498)	ANr AN purging Controls	108 88 98	NS	(5)	TDT NS U.S., U.K., and Germany
	C932G (rs1801028)	ANr AN purging Controls	108 88 98	NS	(5)	TDT NS U.S., U.K., and Germany
	C939T (rs6275)	ANr AN purging Controls	108 88 98	NS	(5)	Haplo rs1799732 0.013, 0.05 (RAN); Haplo rs6278 0.038; Haplo rs1800497 0.021 (RAN); TDT NS U.S., U.K., and Germany

(*Continued*)

Table 1 (*Continued*)

Gene	Polymorphism	Phenotype	N	p-Value[a]	Reference	Note
	C957T (rs6277)	ANr AN purging Controls	108 88 98	NS	(5)	Haplo rs1799732 0.011, TDT 0.0062 U.S., U.K., and Germany
	725 bp 3′ C/T (rs6278)	ANr AN purging Controls	108 88 98	0.042 (genotype PAN)	(5)	Haplo rs6275 0.038 TDT ns U.S., U.K., and Germany
	C10620T (rs1800497)	ANr AN purging Controls	108 88 98	0.045 (genotype PAN)	(5)	Haplo rs6275 0.021 (RAN); TDT ns U.S., U.K., and Germany
Neuropeptide and feeding regulation						
Hypocretin receptor 1 HCRTR1 (1p35)	C114T (rs1056526)	AN Controls	196 98	NS	(4)	Germany, U.K., and U.S.
	A846G	AN Controls	196 98	NS	(4)	Germany, U.K., and U.S.
	A7757G	AN Controls	196 98	NS	(4)	Germany, U.K., and U.S.
	C8793T	AN Controls	196 98	NS	(4)	Germany, U.K., and U.S.
Opioid receptor delta-1 OPRD1 (1p35)	T80G (rs1042114)	AN Controls	196 98	NS	(4)	OR 0.98, TDT NS Germany, U.K., and U.S.
	T8214C (rs536706)	AN Controls	196 98	0.045	(4)	OR 1.46, TDT NS Germany, U.K., and U.S.
	G23340A (rs760589)	AN Controls	196 98	0.046	(4)	OR 0.68, TDT NS Germany, U.K., and U.S.
	A47821G (rs204081)	AN Controls	196 98	0.01 0.03 (genotype)	(4)	OR 0.61, TDT 0.06 Germany, U.K., and U.S.
	A51502T (rs204076)	AN Controls	196 98	NS	(4)	OR 0.70, TDT 0.06 Germany, U.K., and U.S.
Other candidate genes						
Brain-derived neurotrophic factor BDNF (11p13–14)	C-270T	AN unclassified ANr ANbp BN Controls	98 347 308 389 510	NS	(46)	France, Germany, Italy, Spain, and U.K.
		ANr ANbp	219 140	NS	(47)	HRR/TDT Austria, France, Germany, Italy, Slovenia, Spain, and U.K.

(*Continued*)

Table 1 (*Continued*)

Gene	Polymorphism	Phenotype	*N*	*p*-Value[a]	Reference	Note
	Val-66-Met (rs6265)	AN unclassified ANr ANbp BN Controls	98 347 308 389 510	0.0008 (AN versus C; genotype) 0.003 (ANr versus C; genotype) 0.012 (ANbp versus C; genotype) <0.001 (BN versus C; genotype)	(46)	OR AN 1.37 (Met-allele) OR ANr 1.43 (Met-allele) OR ANbp 1.29 (Met-allele) OR BN 1.59 (Met-allele) France, Germany, Italy, Spain, and U.K.
		ANr ANbp	219 140	0.019 (ANr versus C; HRR)	(47)	HRR and TDT Austria, France, Germany, Italy, Slovenia, Spain, and U.K.

[a]*p*-Values are reported for the allele-wise association of the polymorphism, unless stated otherwise.
Abbreviations: AN, anorexia nervosa; ANbp, anorexia nervosa binge/purging; ANr, anorexia nervosa restrictive; BDNF, brain-derived neurotrophic factor; BN, bulimia nervosa; COMT, catechol-*O*-methyltransferase; DRD2, dopamine D2 receptor; HCRTR1, hypocretin receptor 1; HRR, haplotype relative risk; OPRD1, opioid receptor delta-1; TDT, transmission disequilibrium test.

1 (4), and opioid receptor delta-1 (4, 10). No association was found between AN and the ghrelin and hypocretin receptor 1 genes. Despite the use of different polymorphisms, two studies reported associations between the opioid receptor delta-1 gene, AN, and the restrictive subtype of AN. Recently, a third study genotyped six SNPs in OPRD1 and found three SNPs to be associated with both RAN and binge-purge AN (10).

The accumulated data do not support the involvement of ghrelin and hypocretin receptor 1 in the etiology of AN. The involvement of opioid receptor delta-1 should be replicated in an independent sample to confirm the reported association.

Other Candidate Pathways

Brain-derived neurotrophic factor (BDNF) plays an important role in the growth and maintenance of several neuronal systems, serves as a neurotransmitter modulator, and participates in use-dependent plasticity mechanisms, such as learning and memory (36, 56). Physiological and animal models have shown that BDNF induces appetite suppression and body weight reduction (32, 39, 42, 48) and support the hypothesis that alterations in this neurotrophic system and their consequences could determine abnormalities in eating behavior predisposing to eating disorders.

Two European collaboration studies have investigated the association between AN and two polymorphisms located in the gene encoding for BDNF (46, 47). As can be seen in the final section of **Table 1**, the rs6265 polymorphism was associated with AN, especially the restrictive subtype, in both studies. Again, this gene looks promising, although replication is required.

Critical Evaluation of the Genetic Literature

Genetic studies of AN clearly are in an early phase. Compared with many other complex traits, relatively few linkage and association studies have been completed. Most of the association studies were underpowered (type 2 error) and/or suffered from multiple testing (thus increasing type 1 error). Consequently, it is not currently possible to evaluate replication in the literature to determine which findings are true. Researchers need to pay careful attention to published standards, as with association studies in all of biomedicine (38).

What's the Phenotype? Clarifying Phenotypes, Endophenotypes, and Subphenotypes

Although replicated across primarily European populations, a hidden complication may exist in twin and genetic studies of AN. Substantial differences in genetic and environmental contributions to component symptoms of AN suggest that we may be obscuring our ability to detect loci that contribute to risk by focusing on a contrived and heterogeneous condition. Our search for relevant genes may be more effective if we focus on homogeneous and measurable component behaviors rather than on compound syndromes that comprise our DSM categorical definition of AN. We have suggested that there may be distinct sources of familial resemblance for different symptoms of bulimia nervosa, an eating disorder related to AN. As codified in the DSM-IV, binge eating and self-induced vomiting represent more genetically mediated symptoms of bulimia nervosa (44), whereas psychological features, such as placing undue importance on weight as an indicator of self-worth, represent more environmentally mediated symptoms (45). The same may hold true for AN. Thus, our multipart diagnostic syndromes may represent commonly co-occurring mixtures of genetically and environmentally influenced symptoms that also differ by sex. In order to reduce the potential obscuring effects of focusing on compound syndromes, investigators in the future may choose to focus on heritable and homogeneous subphenotypes for AN.

Future Directions and Research Needs

The needs for the future are clear: The genetics of AN needs more and larger studies. Given the current rush to conduct genomewide association studies (a type of case-control association study with >500,000 genetic markers spaced across the genome), it may be possible for AN researchers to avoid the mistakes of the early adopters of this approach. Adequate sample sizes are especially critical for genomewide studies.

The potential payoffs of this line of inquiry are also apparent. The clear-cut identification of the genomic variation that predisposes to AN would likely revolutionize the field by providing researchers and clinicians with a hard finding upon which to base the next generation of research. Moreover, hard findings on AN may be advantageous to the understanding of related psychopathology (e.g., depression, anxiety disorders, and obsessive-compulsive disorder) as well as critical aspects of appetite and weight dysregulation.

LITERATURE CITED

1. Allison DB, Heo M, Schork NJ, Wong SL, Elston RC. 1998. Extreme selection strategies in gene mapping studies of oligogenic quantitative traits do not always increase power. *Hum. Hered.* 48:97–107
2. Axelrod J, Tomchick R. 1958. Enzymatic O-methylation of epinephrine and other catechols. *J. Biol. Chem.* 233:702–5
3. Bacanu S, Bulik C, Klump K, Fichter M, Halmi K, et al. 2005. Linkage analysis of anorexia and bulimia nervosa cohorts using selected behavioral phenotypes as quantitative traits or covariates. *Am. J. Med. Genet. B Neuropsychiatr. Genet.* 139:61–68

4. Bergen AW, van den Bree MBM, Yeager M, Welch R, Ganjei JK, et al. 2003. Candidate genes for anorexia nervosa in the 1p33–36 linkage region: serotonin 1D and delta opioid receptor loci exhibit significant association to anorexia nervosa. *Mol. Psychiatry* 8:397–406
5. Bergen AW, Yeager M, Welch RA, Haque K, Ganjei JK, et al. 2005. Association of multiple DRD2 polymorphisms with anorexia nervosa. *Neuropsychopharmacology* 30:1703–10
6. Birmingham C, Su J, Hlynsky J, Goldner E, Gao M. 2005. The mortality rate from anorexia nervosa. *Int. J. Eat. Disord.* 38:143–46
7. Blundell J. 1984. Systems and interactions: an approach to the pharmacology of eating and hunger. In *Eating and Its Disorders*, ed. AJ Stunkard, E Stellar, pp. 39–65. New York: Raven
8. Blundell JE. 1992. Serotonin and the biology of feeding. *Am. J. Clin. Nutr.* 55:155–59S
9. Brewerton T, Jimerson D. 1996. Studies of serotonin function in anorexia nervosa. *Psychiatr. Res.* 62:31–42
10. Brown K, Bujac S, Mann E, Stubbins M, Blundell J. 2007. Further evidence of association of OPRD1 & HTR1D polymorphisms with susceptibility to anorexia nervosa. *Biol. Psychiatry* 61:367–73
11. Bulik C, Sullivan P, Fear J, Joyce P. 1997. Eating disorders and antecedent anxiety disorders: a controlled study. *Acta Psychiatr. Scand.* 96:101–7
12. Bulik C, Sullivan P, Kendler K. 2000. An empirical study of the classification of eating disorders. *Am. J. Psychiatry* 157:886–95
13. Bulik C, Sullivan P, Tozzi F, Furberg H, Lichtenstein P, Pedersen N. 2006. Prevalence, heritability and prospective risk factors for anorexia nervosa. *Arch. Gen. Psychiatry* 63:305–12
14. Bulik C, Sullivan P, Wade T, Kendler K. 2000. Twin studies of eating disorders: a review. *Int. J. Eat. Disord.* 27:1–20
15. Cardon L, Bell J. 2001. Association study designs for complex diseases. *Nat. Rev. Genet.* 2:91–99
16. Cellini E, Nacmias B, Brecelj-Anderluh M, Badia-Casanovas A, Bellodi L, et al. 2006. Case-control and combined family trios analysis of three polymorphisms in the ghrelin gene in European patients with anorexia and bulimia nervosa. *Psychiatr. Genet.* 16:51–52
17. Cnattingius S, Hultman C, Dahl M, Sparen P. 1999. Very preterm birth, birth trauma, and the risk of anorexia nervosa among girls. *Arch. Gen. Psychiatry* 56:634–38
18. de la Rie SM, Noordenbos G, van Furth EF. 2005. Quality of life and eating disorders. *Qual. Life Res.* 14:1511–22
19. Devlin B, Bacanu S, Klump KL, Bulik C, Fichter M, et al. 2002. Linkage analysis of anorexia nervosa incorporating behavioral covariates. *Hum. Mol. Genet.* 11:689–96
20. Gabrovsek M, Brecelj-Anderluh M, Bellodi L, Cellini E, Di Bella D, et al. 2004. Combined family trio and case-control analysis of the COMT Val158Met polymorphism in European patients with anorexia nervosa. *Am. J. Med. Genet. B Neuropsychiatr. Genet.* 124:68–72
21. Godart N, Flament M, Perdereau F, Jeammet P. 2002. Comorbidity between eating disorders and anxiety disorders: a review. *Int. J. Eat. Disord.* 32:253–70
22. Gorwood P, Ades J, Bellodi L, Cellini E, Collier DA, et al. 2002. The 5-HT(2A)-1438G/A polymorphism in anorexia nervosa: a combined analysis of 316 trios from six European centres. *Mol. Psychiatry* 7:90–94
23. Grice DE, Halmi KA, Fichter MM, Strober M, Woodside DB, et al. 2002. Evidence for a susceptibility gene for anorexia nervosa on chromosome 1. *Am. J. Hum. Genet.* 70:787–92

24. Hirschhorn J, Daly M. 2005. Genome-wide association studies for common diseases and complex traits. *Nat. Rev. Genet.* 6:95–108
25. Hoek H, van Hoeken D. 2003. Review of the prevalence and incidence of eating disorders. *Int. J. Eat. Disord.* 34:383–96
26. Ioannidis J, Trikalinos T. 2005. Early extreme contradictory estimates may appear in published research: the Proteus phenomenon in molecular genetics research and randomized trials. *J. Clin. Epidemiol.* 58:543–49
27. Jacobi C, Hayward C, de Zwaan M, Kraemer H, Agras W. 2004. Coming to terms with risk factors for eating disorders: application of risk terminology and suggestions for a general taxonomy. *Psychol. Bull.* 130:19–65
28. Kaye W, Bulik C, Thornton L, Barbarich BS, Masters K, Price Found. Collab. Group. 2004. Comorbidity of anxiety disorders with anorexia and bulimia nervosa. *Am. J. Psychiatry* 161:2215–21
29. Kaye W, Strober M, Jimerson D. 2004. The neurobiology of eating disorders. In *The Neurobiology of Mental Illness*, ed. D Charney, E Nestler, pp. 1112–28. New York: Oxford Univ. Press
30. Kaye WH. 1997. Anorexia nervosa, obsessional behavior, and serotonin. *Psychopharmacol. Bull.* 33:335–44
31. Kendler KS, Neale MC, Kessler RC, Heath AC, Eaves LJ. 1993. A test of the equal environment assumption in twin studies of psychiatric illness. *Behav. Genet.* 23:21–27
32. Kernie SG, Liebl DJ, Parada LF. 2000. BDNF regulates eating behavior and locomotor activity in mice. *EMBO J.* 19:1290–300
33. Klump KL, Holly A, Iacono WG, McGue M, Willson LE. 2000. Physical similarity and twin resemblance for eating attitudes and behaviors: a test of the equal environments assumption. *Behav. Genet.* 30:51–58
34. Klump KL, Miller KB, Keel PK, McGue M, Iacono WG. 2001. Genetic and environmental influences on anorexia nervosa syndromes in a population-based twin sample. *Psychol. Med.* 31:737–40
35. Kortegaard LS, Hoerder K, Joergensen J, Gillberg C, Kyvik KO. 2001. A preliminary population-based twin study of self-reported eating disorder. *Psychol. Med.* 31:361–65
36. Kuipers S, Bramham C. 2006. Brain-derived neurotrophic factor mechanisms and function in adult synaptic plasticity: new insights and implications for therapy. *Curr. Opin. Drug Discov. Devel.* 9:580–86
37. Lilenfeld L, Kaye W, Greeno C, Merikangas K, Plotnikov K, et al. 1998. A controlled family study of restricting anorexia and bulimia nervosa: comorbidity in probands and disorders in first-degree relatives. *Arch. Gen. Psychiatry* 55:603–10
38. Little J, Bradley L, Bray M, Clyne M, Dorman J, et al. 2002. Reporting, appraising, and integrating data on genotype prevalence and gene-disease associations. *Am. J. Epidemiol.* 156:300–10
39. Lyons WE, Mamounas LA, Ricaurte GA, Coppola V, Reid SW, et al. 1999. Brain-derived neurotrophic factor-deficient mice develop aggressiveness and hyperphagia in conjunction with brain serotonergic abnormalities. *Proc. Natl. Acad. Sci. USA* 96:15239–44
40. Mathers CD, Vos ET, Stevenson CE, Begg SJ. 2000. The Australian Burden of Disease Study: measuring the loss of health from diseases, injuries and risk factors. *Med. J. Aust.* 172:592–96
41. McKnight Investigators. 2003. Risk factors for the onset of eating disorders in adolescent girls: results of the McKnight longitudinal risk factor study. *Am. J. Psychiatry* 160:248–54

42. Pelleymounter M, Cullen M, Wellman C. 1995. Characteristics of BDNF-induced weight loss. *Exp. Neurol.* 131:229–38
43. Pinheiro A, Thornton L, Plotonicov K, Tozzi T, Klump K, et al. 2007. Patterns of menstrual disturbance in eating disorders. *Int. J. Eat. Disord.* In press
44. Reichborn-Kjennerud T, Bulik C, Kendler K, Maes H, Roysamb E, et al. 2003. Gender differences in binge-eating: a population-based twin study. *Acta Psychiatr. Scand.* 108:196–202
45. Reichborn-Kjennerud T, Bulik C, Kendler K, Roysamb E, Tambs K, et al. 2004. Influence of weight on self-evaluation: a population-based study of gender differences. *Int. J. Eat. Disord.* 35:123–32
46. Ribases M, Gratacos M, Fernandez-Aranda F, Bellodi L, Boni C, et al. 2004. Association of BDNF with anorexia, bulimia and age of onset of weight loss in six European populations. *Hum. Mol. Genet.* 13:1205–12
47. Ribases M, Gratacos M, Fernandez-Aranda F, Bellodi L, Boni C, et al. 2005. Association of BDNF with restricting anorexia nervosa and minimum body mass index: a family-based association study of eight European populations. *Eur. J. Hum. Genet.* 13:428–34
48. Rios M, Fan G, Fekete C, Kelly J, Bates B, et al. 2001. Conditional deletion of brain-derived neurotrophic factor in the postnatal brain leads to obesity and hyperactivity. *Mol. Endocrinol.* 15:1748–57
49. Sham P. 1998. *Statistics in Human Genetics*. London: Arnold
50. Simansky KJ. 1996. Serotonergic control of the organization of feeding and satiety. *Behav. Brain Res.* 73:37–42
51. Stice E, Presnell K, Bearman S. 2001. Relation of early menarche to depression, eating disorders, substance abuse, and comorbid psychopathology among adolescent girls. *Dev. Psychol.* 37:608–19
52. Strober M, Freeman R, Lampert C, Diamond J, Kaye W. 2000. Controlled family study of anorexia nervosa and bulimia nervosa: evidence of shared liability and transmission of partial syndromes. *Am. J. Psychiatry* 157:393–401
53. Strober M, Freeman R, Lampert C, Diamond J, Kaye W. 2001. Males with anorexia nervosa: a controlled study of eating disorders in first-degree relatives. *Int. J. Eat. Disord.* 29:263–69
54. Sullivan PF. 1995. Mortality in anorexia nervosa. *Am. J. Psychiatry* 152:1073–74
55. Sullivan PF, Bulik CM, Fear JL, Pickering A. 1998. Outcome of anorexia nervosa. *Am. J. Psychiatry* 155:939–46
56. Thoenen H. 1995. Neurotrophins and neuronal plasticity. *Science* 270:593–98
57. Tozzi F, Thornton L, Klump K, Bulik C, Fichter M, et al. 2005. Symptom fluctuation in eating disorders: correlates of diagnostic crossover. *Am. J. Psychiatry* 162:732–40
58. Wade TD, Bulik CM, Neale M, Kendler KS. 2000. Anorexia nervosa and major depression: shared genetic and environmental risk factors. *Am. J. Psychiatry* 157:469–71
59. Weltzin T, Fernstrom M, Kaye W. 1994. Serotonin and bulimia nervosa. *Nutr. Rev.* 52:399–408
60. Wittchen HU, Nelson CB, Lachner G. 1998. Prevalence of mental disorders and psychosocial impairments in adolescents and young adults. *Psychol. Med.* 28:109–26
61. Wonderlich S, Lilenfeld L, Riso L, Engel S, Mitchell J. 2005. Personality and anorexia nervosa. *Int. J. Eat. Disord.* 37(Suppl.):S68–71

Energy Metabolism During Human Pregnancy

Elisabet Forsum and Marie Löf

Department of Biomedicine and Surgery, Division of Nutrition, Linköping University, S-581 85 Linköping, Sweden; email: elifo@ibk.liu.se, Marie.Lof@ki.se

Annu. Rev. Nutr. 2007. 27:277–92

First published online as a Review in Advance on April 27, 2007

The *Annual Review of Nutrition* is online at http://nutr.annualreviews.org

This article's doi:
10.1146/annurev.nutr.27.061406.093543

0199-9885/07/0821-0277$20.00

Key Words

basal metabolic rate, energy intake, energy requirements, gestation, physical activity

Abstract

This review summarizes information regarding how human energy metabolism is affected by pregnancy, and current estimates of energy requirements during pregnancy are presented. Such estimates can be calculated using either increases in basal metabolic rate (BMR) or increases in total energy expenditure (TEE). The two modes of calculation give similar results for a complete pregnancy but different distributions of energy requirements in the three trimesters. Recent information is presented regarding the effect of pregnancy on BMR, TEE, diet-induced thermogenesis, and physical activity. The validity of energy intake (EI) data recently assessed in well-nourished pregnant women was evaluated using information regarding energy metabolism during pregnancy. The results show that underreporting of EI is common during pregnancy and indicate that additional longitudinal studies, taking the total energy budget during pregnancy into account, are needed to satisfactorily define energy requirements during the three trimesters of gestation.

Contents

INTRODUCTION

EI: energy intake

The requirement for dietary energy is the main factor affecting the amount of food a human being consumes. Therefore, the content of essential nutrients in a diet must be sufficient to cover the needs of a person consuming the amount of this diet corresponding to his or her energy needs. Furthermore, knowledge regarding energy requirements per se is important when providing dietary advice as well as in relation to the understanding of body weight regulation, an area that recently has attracted interest (4). Finally, knowledge regarding human energy metabolism is needed in relation to the increasing prevalence of obesity worldwide (38) and when evaluating the accuracy with which dietary intake can be assessed.

Extensive studies have provided a solid basis of information regarding the energy metabolism in human adults (7), whereas corresponding studies during specific periods of life, such as infancy, childhood, pregnancy, and lactation, are much less prevalent. It is a special concern that studies in pregnant women are comparatively few. Thus, the scientific basis of dietary advice currently provided to pregnant women is considerably weaker than that available to nonpregnant adults. Furthermore, we have very limited possibilities for evaluating the effects of a low or a high energy intake (EI) on the body weight and composition of pregnant women, let alone evaluating how such variations in intake affect the growing fetus. Finally, it is very difficult to evaluate the validity of dietary studies conducted in pregnant women. These limitations are serious, since nutritional factors in utero have been linked to adverse conditions later in life such as obesity (33) and cardiovascular disease (15).

An important reason for the relatively scarce information regarding energy metabolism during pregnancy concerns the difficulties involved when recruiting and investigating pregnant women. For example, to provide reliable assessments regarding the effect of pregnancy on energy metabolism and body composition, studies must be started before conception. Difficulties associated with recruiting women likely to become pregnant in the near future represent a serious problem for studies in this area. Furthermore, pregnancy is a dynamic state characterized by continuously changing conditions. No simple description regarding how pregnancy affects energy metabolism and body composition can therefore be given. Finally, these effects of pregnancy differ considerably among individual women.

ENERGY METABOLISM IN PREGNANT AND NONPREGNANT INDIVIDUALS

The concept of energy balance is fundamental to the understanding of human requirements for dietary energy (7). Thus, intake of food energy must be equal to energy expenditure corrected for any change in body energy stores. A positive energy balance represents the most common situation during pregnancy, but the energy balance of a pregnant woman may also be negative.

As shown in **Figure 1**, human energy expenditure may be divided into components, the so-called partitioning of the total energy expenditure (TEE). It is thus common to divide TEE into basal metabolic rate (BMR), diet-induced thermogenesis (DIT), and energy expended in response to physical activity or activity energy expenditure (AEE).

TEE: total energy expenditure

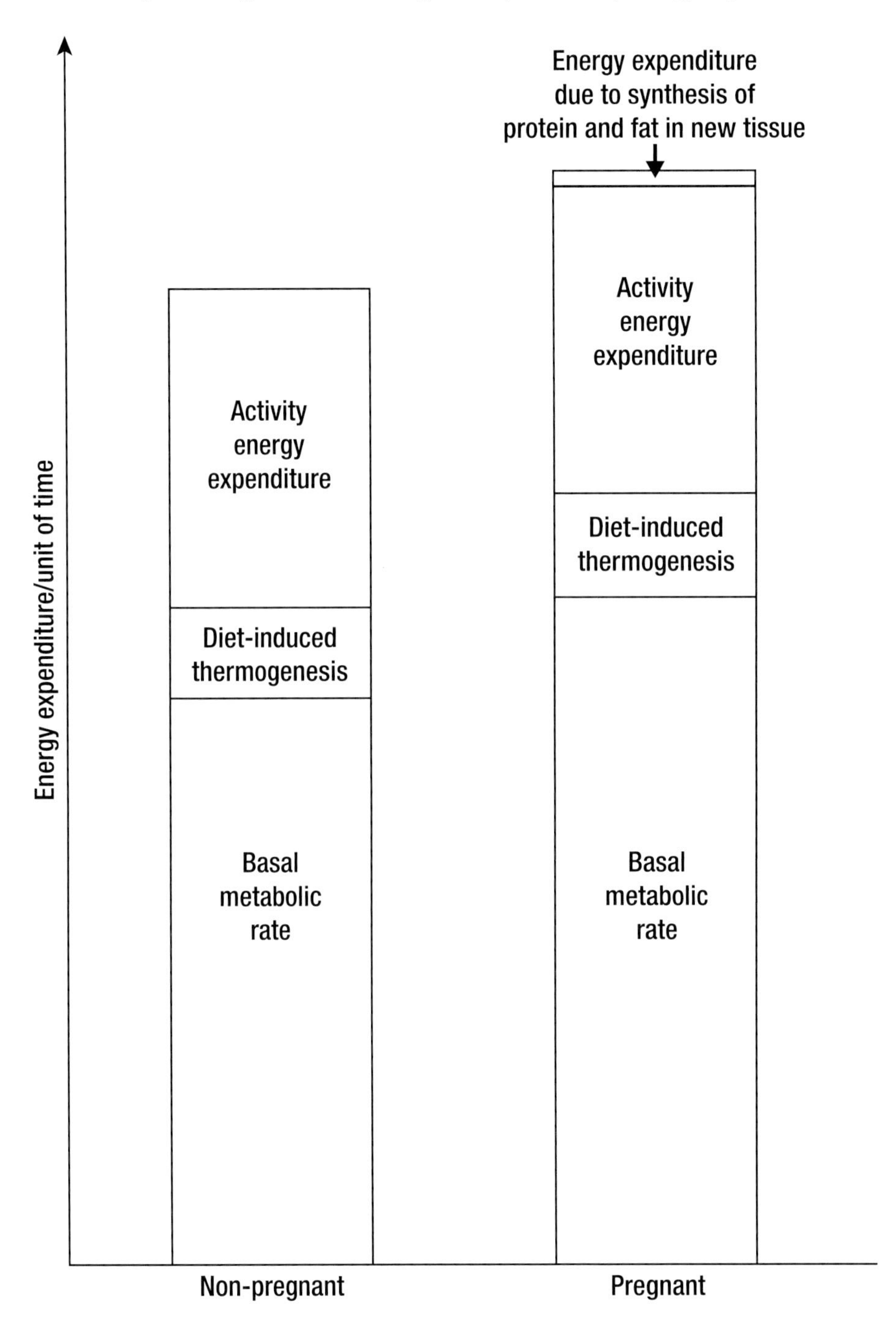

Figure 1

Partitioning of total energy expenditure in nonpregnant versus pregnant subjects.

BMR: basal metabolic rate

DIT: diet-induced thermogenesis

AEE: activity energy expenditure

RMR: resting metabolic rate

FFM: fat-free mass

PAL: physical activity level

MET: metabolic equivalent

For subjects in energy balance, TEE is the sum of these three components. The resting metabolic rate (RMR), which is slightly higher than the BMR, is often measured instead of the BMR (7). The main predictor of BMR (and RMR) is the fat-free mass (FFM) of the body; in contrast, fat mass is poorly related to BMR in healthy, nonpregnant adults (7). As indicated in **Figure 1**, BMR tends to be increased in response to pregnancy. The physiological basis for AEE is the increase in energy expenditure as the result of muscular activity (10). AEE represents the difference between TEE and BMR plus DIT but, since DIT is small, AEE is often assessed as TEE minus BMR. Another important concept is the physical activity level (PAL), which is TEE/BMR or TEE/RMR. Calculating this ratio for specific activities gives so-called MET (metabolic equivalent) values (1, 2). These can be used to calculate the TEE of a human subject over an extended period if the RMR and activity pattern of the subject are known. Prentice et al. (29) reviewed the effect of pregnancy on physical activity, AEE, and PAL and pointed out that changing energy costs of performing specific activities as well as changes in activity patterns must then be considered. Therefore, simple conclusions cannot be reached regarding how AEE is affected by pregnancy. However, PAL values obtained in pregnant women, especially during the second part of pregnancy, are not comparable with PAL values obtained in nonpregnant individuals (29). The reason is that pregnancy is often associated with a comparatively large increase in BMR, whereas the effect of pregnancy on energy expenditure when performing many specific activities tends to be rather small. Therefore, MET values tend to be lower in the pregnant than in the nonpregnant state.

In humans, energy expenditure can be augmented by stimuli other than muscular activity, such as food ingestion (7). DIT refers to the increase in energy expenditure elicited by food consumption and is generally considered to be about 10% of TEE (7, 29). Results regarding the effect of pregnancy on DIT are contradictory (29). Nevertheless, Prentice et al. (29) concluded that "it is reasonable to assume that DIT remains essentially unaltered during pregnancy when expressed as a proportion of energy intake."

The anabolic situation during pregnancy leads to a positive energy balance, with synthesis of new tissue and retention of fat and protein in the mother and in the fetus. The energy needed to synthesize new tissue containing the appropriate amounts of fat and protein consists of two components: the energy in the fat and protein actually retained in the body, and the energy needed to synthesize these compounds, the so-called energy costs of synthesis. As shown in **Figure 1**, TEE during pregnancy should be regarded as the sum of four components: BMR, DIT, AEE, and the energy costs for synthesizing the fat and protein retained.

ENERGY REQUIREMENTS DURING PREGNANCY

Butte & King (8) recently summarized the definition of energy requirements during pregnancy: "The energy requirement of a pregnant woman is the level of energy intake from food that will balance her energy expenditure when the woman has a body size and composition and level of physical activity consistent with good health, and that will allow for the maintenance of economically necessary and socially desirable physical activity. In pregnant women the energy requirement includes the energy needs associated with the deposition of tissue consistent with optimal pregnancy outcome." This definition was recently used to revise the basis for energy requirements during pregnancy (8, 13). In 1985, FAO/WHO/UNU (12) assessed energy requirements during pregnancy on the basis of a theoretical model developed by Hytten (21) with the following inherent assumptions: The prepregnant body weight of the women varied between 60 and 65 kg, the average gestational weight gain was 12.5 kg, retentions of protein and fat during the complete

Table 1 Total energy cost of pregnancy in well-nourished women calculated using two different alternatives[a] (8)

Energy costs	First trimester (kJ/24 h)	Second trimester (kJ/24 h)	Third trimester (kJ/24 h)	Total pregnancy (MJ)
Energy in retained fat and protein (a)	232	876	892	182.6
Efficiency of food energy utilization for fat and protein deposition (b)	48	134	191	34.0
Increment in basal metabolic rate (c)	249	465	1015	157.0
(b + c)	297	599	1206	191.0
Increment in total energy expenditure (d)	100	400	1500	186.0
Energy cost, alternative 1 (a + b + c)	529	1475	2097	373.6
Energy cost, alternative 2 (a + d)	332	1276	2391	368.6

[a]Calculations are based on a gestational weight gain of 13.8 kg.

gestation were 925 g and 3.8 kg, respectively, and the cumulative increase in BMR during the complete pregnancy represented an energy cost of 150 MJ (6, 8, 21). Butte & King (8) revised this model using more recently published data. They found that an average weight gain of 13.8 kg represented a useful basis for assessing energy needs during pregnancy in well-nourished women. Based on their review of the literature, they suggested that retention of 4.3 kg fat and 686 g protein as well as a cumulative increase in BMR of 157 MJ, all during a complete pregnancy, is compatible with optimal reproductive performance in well-nourished women. It is relevant to point out that for fat retention and the increase in BMR, Butte & King (8) arrived at figures in close agreement with those of Hytten (21), whereas their figure for protein retention was lower, 686 g versus 925 g (21). The model developed by Butte & King (8) forms the basis for recent recommendations regarding energy requirements during pregnancy (13). As shown in **Table 1**, these requirements were calculated using two different approaches. Both are based on the assumption that a woman retains 4.3 kg fat and 686 g protein during pregnancy. The first alternative is based on increments in BMR throughout pregnancy. The energy cost of pregnancy is calculated as the energy content in the fat and protein retained, plus the increments in BMR, plus the energy costs of synthesizing the appropriate amounts of fat and protein. The energy costs of synthesis, i.e., the efficiency of food energy utilization for protein and fat deposition, were assumed to be 90% (8). It is also assumed that AEE and DIT are not affected by pregnancy. According to this calculation, the energy cost of a complete pregnancy is 373.6 MJ. In the second alternative, calculations are based on increments in TEE obtained using the doubly labeled water (DLW)-method. This method estimates the TEE during free-living conditions (11), and such estimates will therefore include the energy costs of synthesizing the retained fat and protein as well as any changes in DIT and AEE. Consequently, the energy costs of pregnancy can be calculated as the energy content in the retained fat and protein plus the increment in TEE. Using this alternative, the total energy cost of pregnancy is 368.6 MJ. It is noteworthy that the two alternative calculations produce similar estimates for a complete pregnancy. However, the two alternatives will result in different distributions of energy costs during pregnancy. Thus, in the second approach, a larger proportion of the costs appear in late rather than in early pregnancy. This is important when assessing energy needs of women at different stages of pregnancy. It seems reasonable for such estimates to be based on assessments of TEE in agreement with corresponding estimates for other population groups. For pregnant women, however, the energy retained in the body must also be considered. The main part of this energy is due to retention of body

DLW: doubly labeled water

fat, and it is therefore relevant to note that available data on body fat retention during pregnancy (8) are of different quality for the different trimesters. The best data are available for the second trimester; these are based on several studies, all with rather similar results. Relatively few studies have focused on the first trimester, and results from different studies regarding the third trimester are quite variable.

ENERGY METABOLISM DURING PREGNANCY: RECENT INFORMATION

Basal Metabolic Rate

Butte (6) recently reviewed studies regarding the increase in BMR of well-nourished women during pregnancy. On the basis of results from 261 women in eight studies, it was found that the average cumulative increase in BMR during the complete pregnancy was 157 MJ and that average BMR increased by 4%, 10%, and 24% during the first, second, and third trimesters, respectively (6). Several authors have pointed out that the effect of pregnancy on BMR in different women often varies considerably (8). Prentice et al. (29) compiled results from developed and developing countries regarding the effect of pregnancy on BMR and demonstrated that pregnant women from developing countries increased their BMR to a much smaller extent than did women from developed countries. The increase in BMR during pregnancy may even be negative, i.e., a depression in BMR, especially during the first part of pregnancy. This probably can be attributed in part to the nutritional situation because such a depression in BMR is more common in developing than in affluent countries. However, women in developed countries may also show a depression in BMR during the first part of gestation (13). The physiological basis for this depression is incompletely understood.

Two studies (9, 25) including longitudinal measurements of BMR in well-nourished pregnant women have recently been published. In the study by Löf et al. (25), BMR in 22 healthy Swedish women was measured before, five times during, and after pregnancy. The average increments in BMR were in fair agreement with those described by Butte (6) and also confirmed that many well-nourished women (12 out of 22) decrease their BMR during the first part of gestation; in some women, this decrease persisted into the second half of pregnancy. In the study by Butte et al. (9), the BMR of women with low, normal, and high BMI values before conception was measured before and three times during pregnancy. For women with low and normal BMI values, changes in BMR during pregnancy were in agreement with those previously reported (6), whereas for women with high prepregnant BMI values, increments in BMR were larger.

The increase in BMR during pregnancy is considered to be the result of accelerated tissue synthesis, increased tissue mass, and increased cardiovascular, respiratory, and renal work (21). To understand the basis for the large variation among women in the change in BMR in response to pregnancy, specific studies of appropriate physiological changes during pregnancy are of interest. For example, Butte et al. (9) reported that during pregnancy, changes in BMR were correlated with changes in FFM but not with changes in fat mass. Bronstein et al. (5) found that BMR during pregnancy was correlated with fat mass rather than with FFM, in contrast to the situation in nonpregnant women. Löf et al. (25) observed that BMR was correlated with FFM but not with total body fat in women before pregnancy, although in the same women, significant correlations with both FFM and total body fat were obtained for BMR in gestational weeks 14 and 32. These observations may indicate an increase in the metabolic activity of adipose tissue during pregnancy.

Relatively few studies have aimed at understanding the physiological basis for a depressed BMR during pregnancy. Spanderman et al. (32) investigated circulatory changes during early pregnancy in 12 healthy women and found these changes to be unrelated to changes in BMR. It was concluded that the high-flow, low-resistance circulation that is typical for pregnancy develops independently of concomitant changes in BMR. Löf et al. (25) confirmed and extended those observations. These authors found that increases in BMR correlated with increases in cardiac output in gestational week 32 but not in gestational week 14. Other relevant observations (25) were that serum levels of free triiodothyronine decreased during pregnancy, and decreases in these levels in gestational week 32 were weakly but significantly correlated with increases in BMR. This was suggested to be of potential interest in relation to the regulation of BMR during pregnancy, since this can help to maintain an appropriate metabolic rate, perhaps by counteracting the stimulating effect on energy expenditure associated with a high body-fat content and a large fetus.

In their review from 1996, Prentice et al. (29) used mean values from nine different studies in developed and developing countries, and reported that the cumulative increase in BMR during the complete pregnancy was strongly correlated ($r = 0.75$, $p < 0.001$) with percent body fat of the women before pregnancy. This finding suggests that the nutritional status of women is important regarding the magnitude of the increase in BMR during pregnancy. This statement is supported by data (9) showing that 40% of the variability of the change in BMR during the entire pregnancy could be explained by gestational gains in weight and FFM in combination with BMI and percent body fat before pregnancy. Löf et al. (25) reported that 40% of the variability of the increase in BMR in gestational week 14 could be explained by the increase in body weight in combination with the body fat content before pregnancy. In gestational week 32, as much as 63.7% of the variability of the increase in BMR could be explained by increases in body weight in combination with fetal weight in gestational week 31. Since the increase in body weight during pregnancy and the prepregnant body fat content are both related to the woman's nutritional situation, these data support the statement that the change in BMR during pregnancy is largely a function of maternal nutritional status. However, Kopp-Hoolihan et al. (22) were unable to confirm this statement, possibly because their study had only 10 subjects with a rather small variation in prepregnancy BMI and body fat content.

Total Energy Expenditure and Activity Energy Expenditure

In 1996, Prentice et al. (29) reviewed four studies (5, 14, 18, 19) from developed countries where TEE was assessed using the DLW method in pregnant women. In the recent FAO/WHO/UNU report on human energy requirements (13), three of these (14, 18, 19) and two additional studies (9, 22) were used to calculate the effect of pregnancy on TEE in gestational weeks 30–36. The mean TEE of pregnant women was found to be 11.5 versus 9.9 MJ/24 h for nonpregnant women. When expressed as kJ/kg/24 h, a slightly lower value (160 versus 164) was found at this late stage of pregnancy in comparison with the nonpregnant state. AEE was similar for pregnant and nonpregnant women (4.3 versus 4.2) when expressed in MJ/24 h, but was lower during pregnancy (60 versus 69) when expressed as kJ/kg/24 h.

The FAO/WHO/UNU expert consultation of 1985 (12) suggested that the energy cost of pregnancy could be partly offset by reductions in physical activity. Prentice et al. (29) concluded in 1996 that "about half the energy cost of pregnancy could theoretically be spared by reductions in the physical activity of the mother. However, it is difficult to uncover any patterns that could be described as typical pregnancy-induced behavior. This emphasizes that it cannot be assumed that a high proportion of energy costs of pregnancy are normally or automatically met by reductions in activity." Butte & King (8) did not conclude that available evidence could support a

Table 2 Activity energy expenditure and physical activity level before and during pregnancy

Reference	Subjects	AEE[a] (kJ/24 h)	PAL[a]
(9)	**Low BMI[b] (n = 17)**		
	Prepregnant	3816 ± 954	1.97 ± 0.25
	Gestational week 22	3012 ± 1347	1.72 ± 0.28
	Gestational week 36	2929 ± 1866	1.63 ± 0.33[c]
	Normal BMI[d] (n = 34)		
	Prepregnant	3632 ± 1238	1.84 ± 0.25
	Gestational week 22	3535 ± 1381	1.78 ± 0.28
	Gestational week 36	3146 ± 1347	1.62 ± 0.24[c]
	High BMI[e] (n = 12)		
	Prepregnant	4778 ± 1335	1.96 ± 0.22
	Gestational week 22	3787 ± 1456	1.72 ± 0.25
	Gestational week 36	2900 ± 1682	1.49 ± 0.22[c]
(24)	**BMI 18–39[f] (n = 23)**		
	Prepregnant	5080 ± 1270	1.95 ± 0.24
	Gestational week 14	4940 ± 1070	1.89 ± 0.20
	Gestational week 32	4910 ± 1170	1.72 ± 0.17[g]
(22)	**Normal BMI[h] (n = 10)**		
	Prepregnant	3728 ± 969	–
	Gestational week 8–10	3115 ± 1416	–
	Gestational week 24–26	3625 ± 1174	–
	Gestational week 34–36	4338 ± 1336	–

[a]Values are means ± SD.
[b]BMI = 18.9 ± 0.8 kg/m^2.
[c]Significantly ($p = 0.04$) lower than the corresponding value before pregnancy.
[d]BMI = 22.1 ± 1.5 kg/m^2.
[e]BMI = 28.8 ± 2.6 kg/m^2.
[f]BMI = 24.2 ± 4.8 kg/m^2.
[g]Significantly ($p < 0.001$) lower than the corresponding value before pregnancy.
[h]BMI = 23.1 ± 2.1 kg/m^2.
AEE, activity energy expenditure; BMI, body mass index; PAL, physical activity level.

statement that reductions in physical activity could cover a significant proportion of energy needs during pregnancy, and current recommendations do not take such reductions into account (13). The three longitudinal studies (9, 22, 24) using the DLW method in well-nourished pregnant women that have been published since the review by Prentice et al. in 1996 (29) have all addressed this issue. The results, which are summarized in **Table 2**, show that pregnancy is associated with nonsignificant and quite small changes in AEE, which is in agreement with previously published data. This occurs in spite of the increase in body weight during pregnancy, an increase associated with higher costs of performing many common activities (29). Butte et al. (9) mention that where a nonsignificant decrease in AEE was observed during pregnancy, activity records confirmed a decrease in physical activity, but no data describing this decrease are presented. Kopp-Hoolihan et al. (22) did not report the physical activity patterns of their subjects. Löf & Forsum (24) studied the physical activity patterns of their 23 women using a questionnaire as well as heart-rate recording in a subgroup of 12 of these women. As shown in **Figure 2**, only minor changes in physical activity pattern were observed in gestational weeks 14 and 32 when compared with prepregnancy data. This is in agreement with the results in **Table 2** showing only small and nonsignificant changes in AEE during pregnancy for these women. However, this interpretation is only valid at the group level, and individual women may show highly variable changes in AEE during pregnancy. Data published by Kopp-Hoolihan et al. (22) indicate that there may be considerable variation among women regarding changes in AEE during pregnancy.

Table 2 also shows that in two of the three studies, PAL values decreased significantly during pregnancy. However, as previously noted, PAL values obtained in pregnant women are not comparable with PAL values obtained in nonpregnant individuals (29). The results described above demonstrate that the effect of physical activity on energy metabolism during pregnancy is complex and incompletely understood. For example, Pivarnik et al. (28) have demonstrated that regression lines relating heart rate to oxygen consumption change during pregnancy, which has implications when heart rate is used to assess energy expenditure. This indicates that alterations in the interaction between physical activity and energy expenditure may occur during pregnancy. Further evidence for such alterations was found by Löf & Forsum (24), who assessed relationships between MET values and heart rate in the same women before and during pregnancy. In the resting state (equivalent to performing an activity with a MET value of one), heart rate was 17 beats faster per minute in gestational week 32 when compared with the value before pregnancy, whereas when the women performed an activity with the MET value of 6, heart rate was the same before pregnancy and in gestational week 32. These observations may indicate that the conventional way of assessing BMR is invalid during pregnancy, when such estimates may not represent the BMR component of TEE during physical activity. In this context, it is relevant to note that BMR is usually measured during a short period assuming that the result represents the energy metabolism at complete rest during 24 hours or even several days. It is conceivable that, during pregnancy, the metabolic processes normally considered as included in BMR require less energy during physical activity than they do in the resting state. Such alterations would result in an apparently increased energetic efficiency during exercise. A possible candidate for mediating such an effect is the circulatory changes occurring during pregnancy, as mentioned above. The low-resistance circulation typical for pregnancy may influence energy costs of processes normally considered to be included in BMR measurements. It is quite conceivable that the energy costs of such processes are different for a pregnant woman when she is resting and when she is physically active. This suggestion is of course speculative, and more studies are needed on these and other aspects of interactions between physical activity and energy expenditure during pregnancy.

Diet-Induced Thermogenesis

After the review by Prentice et al. in 1996 (29), Kopp-Hoolihan et al. (22) conducted a longitudinal study of DIT in 10 pregnant women. The results demonstrate the considerable variation among women regarding the effect of pregnancy on DIT. Considering these results, it is hardly surprising that previous studies in this area have been inconclusive. The authors present their findings as part of a strategy by women to balance their energy budget during pregnancy (22).

EVALUATION OF ENERGY INTAKE IN STUDIES CONDUCTED IN PREGNANT WOMEN

Extensive studies in nonpregnant, nonlactating adults have shown that reported EI is often

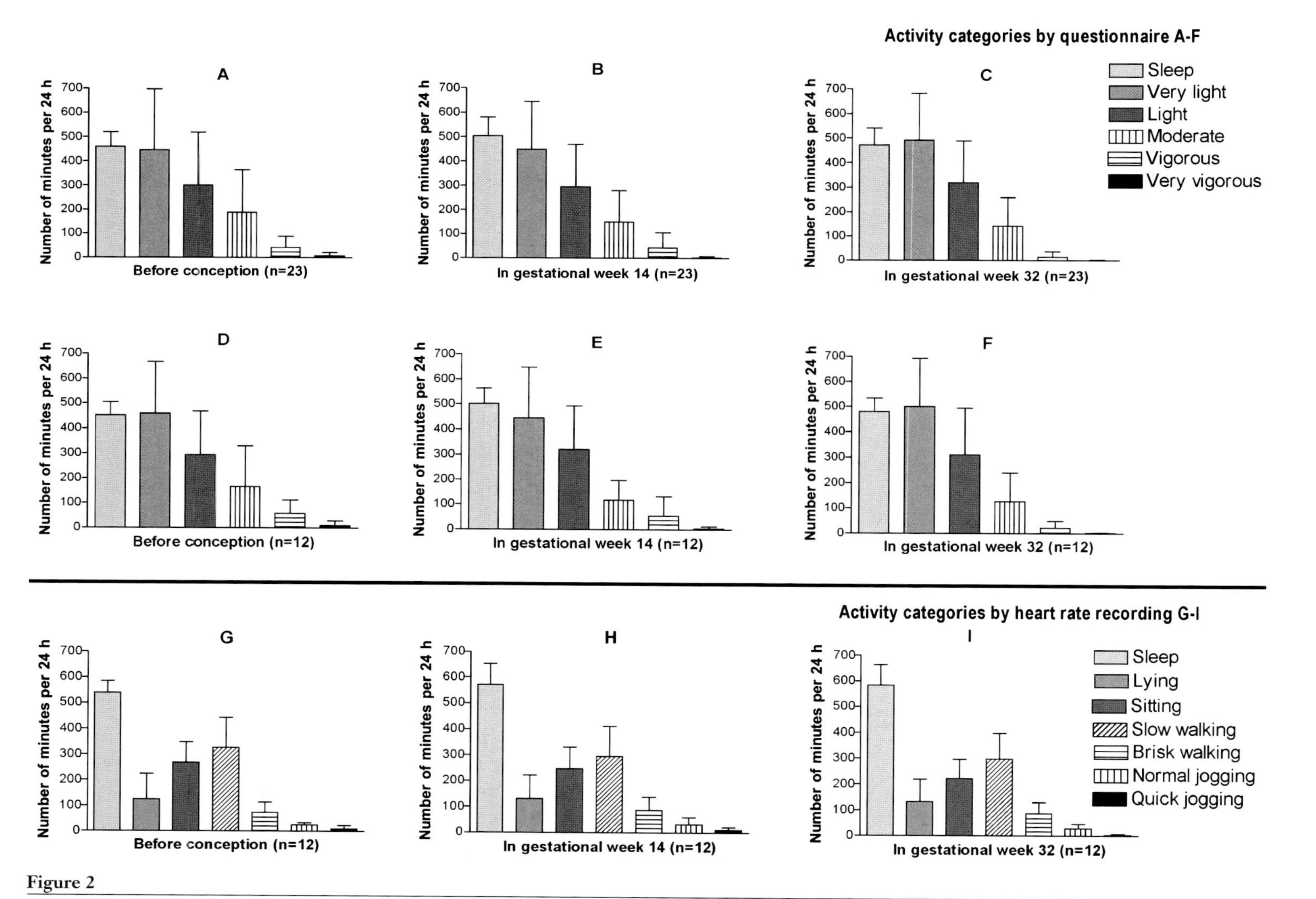

Figure 2

Pattern of physical activity assessed using a questionnaire in 23 women before pregnancy and in gestational weeks 14 and 32 (*A*, *B*, and *C*). On the same measurement occasions, physical activity pattern was also assessed using heart-rate recording in a subgroup of 12 women (*G*, *H*, and *I*). The physical activity pattern for the 12 women assessed using the questionnaire is also shown (*D*, *E*, and *F*) (24).

too low to meet physiological energy requirements (20, 35). Women, overweight individuals, and weight-conscious subjects are especially likely to underreport their EI (20). Furthermore, as pointed out by Prentice et al. (29), a substantial amount of data have been collected regarding EI during pregnancy, with results indicating that the observed increase in EI is too small to meet the energy costs of pregnancy. In 1991, Goldberg et al. (17) published a procedure by which the validity of dietary records could be evaluated. This procedure defined so-called cut-off limits for EI/BMR, thereby providing limits below which EI must be recognized as being incompatible with long-term maintenance of energy balance and survival. This kind of procedure has been widely applied to indicate the quality of dietary reports, including those of pregnant women (16, 30, 37). However, for the following reasons this procedure is not appropriate for pregnant women: First, it assumes that subjects are in energy balance, an assumption that is rarely valid during pregnancy. Second, equations to predict BMR in pregnant women are not available. Finally, there are presently no PAL or MET values for different activities that are appropriate and applicable during pregnancy.

As discussed above, information concerning the energy metabolism of pregnant women obtained by means of the DLW method has recently become available. We propose that this information can be used to formulate a procedure by which the accuracy of EI assessed in pregnant women can be evaluated; an example demonstrating such a procedure is given below. It should be pointed out that the proposed procedure has limitations due to the incomplete data on which it is based. For example, an important shortcoming is that these data are based on longitudinal studies to only a limited extent. However, the proposed procedure would be improved in stride with the further increase in the quantity and quality of available data.

We have based our example on studies reporting the EI of pregnant women that were published after the review by Prentice et al. in 1996 (29). Studies were included if they (*a*) were published on MEDLINE (**http://www.ncbi.nlm.nih.gov/entrez/query.fcgi**) before September 2006; (*b*) reported original data; (*c*) were identified by the search terms "EI" and "pregnant women" or "human pregnancy"; (*d*) were written in English; (*e*) reported an average EI, a mean body weight no later than gestational week 14, and a mean gestational weight gain of 12–14 kg and/or an average birth weight around 3.5 kg; and (*f*) were conducted in developed countries. Seven studies meeting these criteria were identified (3, 22, 26, 27, 31, 34, 36). **Table 3** describes subject characteristics, dietary assessment methods, gestational weeks when diet was assessed, prepregnancy body weight, and reported mean EI for the seven studies. The table also gives expected EI, which was calculated using data on energy metabolism obtained in healthy, well-nourished, nonpregnant women (13), as well as the data on changes in TEE and body energy stores reported for healthy, well-nourished, pregnant women shown in **Table 1**. For the studies presented in **Table 3**, we consider that average reported EI would generally equal the average expected EI.

In five of the studies in **Table 3** (26, 27, 31, 34, 36), reported EI was considerably lower than expected EI (ranging from −15% to −37%). In the study by Antal et al. (3), reported EI differed by +10%, +1%, −9%, and −12% from expected EI in gestational week 12, 20, 30, and 38, respectively. In the study by Kopp-Hoolihan et al. (22), good agreement between reported and expected EI was found in gestational week 9 (−2%), although later in pregnancy reported EI was 21% to 25% lower than expected EI.

Unfortunately, we were only able to review studies from developed countries. Available data regarding changes in energy expenditure and body composition during pregnancy for women in developing countries are much too incomplete to allow a calculation of expected

Table 3 Characteristics of studies, including reported and expected energy intake, conducted in pregnant women from developed countries

Reference	Population	Age of women	N	Dietary assessment method	EI assessed in:	Body weight before pregnancy (kg)	Reported mean EI (MJ/24 h)	Expected mean EI (MJ/24 h)[a]	Reported EI/ Expected EI
(3)	Hungarian women	26	70	Food frequency questionnaire	gw 12, gw 20, gw 30, gw 38	60.7[b]	11.16, 11.15, 10.97, 10.67	10.1, 11.0, 12.1, 12.1	1.10, 1.01, 0.91, 0.88
(36)	Dutch women[c]	28	53	Weighed food records	gw 13	65.8[d]	8.4	10.6	0.79
(31)	British women	28	11,923	Food frequency questionnaire	third trimester	61.6	7.7	12.2	0.63
(22)	American women	29	10	Weighed food records	gw 9, gw 25, gw 35	64.8	8.49, 8.50, 9.34	8.69[e], 11.4[e], 11.8[e]	0.98, 0.75, 0.79
(26)	American women[f]	25	31	Repeated 24-h recalls	third trimester	67.5	9.07	12.8[g]	0.71[h]
(27)	Australian women	29	556	Food frequency questionnaire	first trimester, third trimester	65.9	9.0[i], 9.2[i]	10.6, 12.7	0.85, 0.72
(34)	British women[f]	28	44	Weighed food records	third trimester	61.4	9.26	12.2	0.76

[a]Expected EI = prepregnant TEE plus increment in TEE for first, second, or third trimester and energy content in fat plus protein retained during first, second, and third trimesters calculated as shown in **Table 1**. Prepregnant TEE was prepregnant BMR × prepregnant PAL. BMR was calculated using maternal age and prepregnant body weight as described by FAO/WHO/UNU (13). The prepregnant PAL value was assumed to be 1.68.

[b]Body weight measured in gestational week 12.

[c]This study included two groups of women (intervention and control). The table gives results for controls only.

[d]Body weight measured in gestational week 13.

[e]Expected EI was calculated using data for TEE and body fat retention published by Kopp-Hoolihan et al. (22, 23). In addition, 35 kJ/24 h and 140 kJ/24 h were added to allow for the energy content in retained protein for the second and third trimester, respectively (8).

[f]This study included women with gestational diabetes and healthy controls. The table gives results for healthy controls only.

[g]This value is likely to be too low since the average gestational weight gain of the women was 17.2 kg; i.e., higher than 13.8, the figure for well-nourished women (8).

[h]Reported EI/expected EI is likely to be too high since expected EI is likely to be underestimated (see footnote g).

[i]Median EI.

BMR, basal metabolic rate; EI, energy intake; gw, gestational week; PAL, physical activity level; TEE, total energy expenditure.

EI as was done for well-nourished women. It is important to point out that our calculation of expected EI is based on values from the literature (8, 13). Expected EI may thus be inaccurate also for well-nourished women since it is conceivable that the women in the studies described in **Table 3** may differ from the women examined when energy requirements were established. For example, it may be argued that a prepregnant PAL value of 1.68 is too high for many women. However, using a lower PAL value (i.e., 1.55) to calculate expected EI did not affect the results in **Table 3** in any important way.

The results in **Table 3** support the general conclusion that underreporting is also common during pregnancy. However, the results of Antal et al. (3) and Kopp-Hoolihan et al. (22) showed relatively good agreement between reported and expected EI, especially during early pregnancy. One possible explanation for the results reported by Antal et al. (3) may be that in the 1990s, Hungarian women were not exposed to commercial campaigns idealizing a slender female body to the same extent as were Western women. The longitudinal studies presented in **Table 3** (3, 22, 27) may give the impression that the degree of underreporting increases with advancing pregnancy. A possible explanation could be "measurement fatigue," i.e., the subjects get tired of registering what they eat and therefore tend to record a lower food intake upon repeated reporting. However, Prentice et al. (29) found little evidence for such a phenomenon in pregnant or lactating women. If this explanation can be excluded, the results presented in **Table 3** imply that in late pregnancy, women do not generally cover their physiological energy requirements by means of diet. This can be reconciled with the common contention that in late pregnancy women have difficulty eating large amounts of food. However, it is important to point out that whether this actually is true or not requires further elucidation.

Our example in **Table 3** warrants some comments regarding the common observation that pregnant women tend to report increments in EI that are too low to meet their energy needs. It is possible that part of the reason such intake during the first part of pregnancy has appeared to be too low is because energy needs were previously based on assessments of BMR, whereas low estimate of EI towards the end of pregnancy cannot be explained in this way. It should be pointed out, however, that available information regarding the amount of energy retained in the body or mobilized from energy stores during each of the three trimesters of pregnancy is not only limited in quantity but also lacks a longitudinal aspect concerning the total energy budget during pregnancy. This may be an important consideration; for example, a woman who retains a large amount of fat during the first or second trimester may well use some mobilized fat to cover her physiological energy requirements during the last trimester. Studies considering such longitudinal aspects will be needed to obtain a satisfactory understanding of the energy requirements during pregnancy and to make it possible to evaluate the validity of EI data during pregnancy.

SUMMARY POINTS

1. The effect of pregnancy on energy metabolism varies during the course of pregnancy and differs considerably among women.
2. Energy requirements during pregnancy are calculated using increases in BMR or increases in TEE. The two modes of calculation give similar results for a complete pregnancy but result in different distributions of energy requirements during the three trimesters of pregnancy.

3. The effects of pregnancy on BMR include both stimulation and depression. A depression in BMR is also common in well-nourished women, but its physiological basis is unknown.
4. In pregnant women, MET values for defined activities are often lower than in nonpregnant subjects, especially during the second part of pregnancy. Therefore, the so-called MET system is not applicable during pregnancy.
5. Current knowledge regarding the effect of pregnancy on AEE and physical activity pattern is very incomplete and more studies are needed in this area.
6. Available evidence suggests that the efficiency of energy metabolism during physical activity may be increased during pregnancy. The mechanisms involved are unknown. We suggest that the low-resistance circulation that is typical for pregnancy plays a role in establishing this increased efficiency.
7. Recent data regarding EI during pregnancy support the conclusion that underreporting of EI is also common in pregnant women.
8. Longitudinal studies considering the total energy budget during pregnancy are needed to satisfactorily define energy requirements during the three different trimesters of gestation.

LITERATURE CITED

1. Ainsworth B, Haskell W, Leon A, Jacobs D, Montoye H, et al. 1993. Compendium of physical activities: classification of energy costs of human physical activities. *Med. Sci. Sports Exerc.* 25:71–80
2. Ainsworth B, Haskell W, Whitt M, Irwin M, Swartz A, et al. 2000. Compendium of physical activities: an update of activity codes and MET intensities. *Med. Sci. Sports Exerc.* 32:S498–516
3. Antal M, Regöly-Mérei A, Varsányi H, Biró L, Sági K, et al. 1997. Nutritional survey of pregnant women in Hungary. *Int. J. Vit. Nutr. Res.* 67:115–22
4. Broberger C. 2005. Brain regulation of food intake and appetite: molecules and networks. *J. Int. Med.* 258:301–27
5. Bronstein M, Mak R, King J. 1996. Unexpected relationship between fat mass and basal metabolic rate in pregnant women. *Br. J. Nutr.* 75:659–68
6. Butte N. 2005. Energy requirements during pregnancy and consequences of deviations from requirements on fetal outcome. In *The Impact of Maternal Nutrition on the Offspring. Nestlé Nutrition Workshop Series Pediatric Program*, ed. G Hornstra, R Uauy, X Yang, 55:49–71. Basel, Switzerland: Vevey/S. Karger AG
7. Butte N, Caballero B. 2006. Energy needs: assessment and requirements. In *Modern Nutrition in Health and Disease*, ed. M Shils, M Shike, A Ross, B Caballero, R Cousins, pp. 136–48. Baltimore/Philadelphia: Lippincott Williams & Wilkins. 10th ed.
8. Butte N, King J. 2005. Energy requirements during pregnancy and lactation. *Public Health Nutr.* 8:1010–27
9. Butte N, Wong W, Treuth M, Ellis K, O'Brian Smith E. 2004. Energy requirements during pregnancy based on total energy expenditure and energy deposition. *Am. J. Clin. Nutr.* 79:1078–87

10. Caspersen C, Powell K, Christenson G. 1985. Physical activity, exercise, and physical fitness: definitions and distinctions for health-related research. *Public Health Rep.* 100:126–31
11. Coward W, Cole T. 1991. The doubly labeled water method for the measurement of energy expenditure in humans: risks and benefits. In *New Techniques in Nutritional Research*, ed. R Whitehead, A Prentice, pp. 139–76. San Diego/London: Academic
12. FAO/WHO/UNU Expert Consultation. 1985. Requirements during pregnancy. In *Energy and Protein Requirements. Tech. Rep. Ser. 724*, pp. 84–87. Geneva, Switzerland: WHO
13. FAO/WHO/UNU Expert Consultation. 2004. Human energy requirements. *Food and Nutrition Tech. Rep. Ser. 1*, pp. 53–62. Rome: FAO. 96 pp.
14. Forsum E, Kabir N, Sadurskis A, Westerterp K. 1992. Total energy expenditure of healthy Swedish women during pregnancy and lactation. *Am. J. Clin. Nutr.* 56:334–42
15. Godfrey K, Barker D. 2003. Fetal, infant and childhood growth and adult health. In *Nutrition in Early Life*, ed. J Morgan, J Dickerson, pp. 179–203. Chichester, UK: Wiley-Intersci.
16. Godfrey K, Robinson S, Barker D, Osmond C, Cox V. 1996. Maternal nutrition in early and late pregnancy in relation to placental and fetal growth. *Br. Med. J.* 312:410–14
17. Goldberg G, Black A, Jebb S, Cole T, Murgatroyd P, et al. 1991. Critical evaluation of energy intake data using fundamental principles of energy physiology: 1. Derivation of cut-off limits to identify under-recording. *Eur. J. Clin. Nutr.* 45:569–81
18. Goldberg G, Prentice A, Coward W, Davies HL, Murgatroyd P, et al. 1991. Longitudinal assessment of the components of energy balance in well-nourished lactating women. *Am. J. Clin. Nutr.* 54:788–98
19. Goldberg G, Prentice A, Coward W, Davies HL, Murgatroyd P, et al. 1993. Longitudinal assessment of energy expenditure in pregnancy by the doubly labeled water method. *Am. J. Clin. Nutr.* 57:494–505
20. Hill R, Davies P. 2001. The validity of self-reported energy intake as determined using the doubly labeled water technique. *Br. J. Nutr.* 85:415–30
21. Hytten F. 1980. Nutrition. In *Clinical Physiology in Obstetrics*, ed. F Hytten, G Chamberlain, pp. 163–92. Oxford: Blackwell Sci.
22. Kopp-Hoolihan L, van Loan M, Wong W, King J. 1999. Longitudinal assessment of energy balance in well-nourished, pregnant women. *Am. J. Clin. Nutr.* 69:697–704
23. Kopp-Hoolihan L, van Loan M, Wong W, King J. 1999. Fat mass deposition during pregnancy using a four-component model. *J. Appl. Physiol.* 87:196–202
24. Löf M, Forsum E. 2006. Activity pattern and energy expenditure due to activity before and during pregnancy in healthy Swedish women. *Br. J. Nutr.* 95:296–302
25. Löf M, Olausson H, Boström K, Janerot-Sjöberg B, Sohlström A, et al. 2005. Changes in basal metabolic rate during pregnancy in relation to changes in body weight and composition, cardiac output, insulin-like growth factor I, and thyroid hormones and in relation to fetal growth. *Am. J. Clin. Nutr.* 81:678–85
26. Loosemore E, Judge M, Lammi-Keefe C. 2004. Dietary intake of essential and long-chain polyunsaturated fatty acids in pregnancy. *Lipids* 39:421–24
27. Moore V, Davies M, Willson K, Worsley A, Robinson J. 2004. Dietary composition of pregnant women is related to size of the baby at birth. *J. Nutr.* 134:1820–26
28. Pivarnik J, Stein A, Rivera J. 2002. Effect of pregnancy on heart rate/oxygen consumption calibration curves. *Med. Sci. Sports Exerc.* 34:750–55
29. Prentice A, Spaaij C, Goldberg G, Poppitt S, van Raaij J, et al. 1996. Energy requirements of pregnant and lactating women. *Eur. J. Clin. Nutr.* 50:S82–111

30. Robinson S, Godfrey K, Osmond C, Cox V, Barker D. 1996. Evaluation of a food frequency questionnaire used to assess nutrient intakes in pregnant women. *Eur. J. Clin. Nutr.* 50:302–8
31. Rogers I, Emmett P. 1998. The ALSPAC Study Team. Diet during pregnancy in a population of pregnant women in South West England. *Eur. J. Clin. Nutr.* 52:246–50
32. Spanderman M, Meertens M, van Bussel M, Ekhart T, Peeters L. 2000. Cardiac output increases independently of basal metabolic rate in early human pregnancy. *Am. J. Physiol. Heart Circ. Physiol.* 278:H1585–88
33. Stettler N, Zemel B, Kumanyika S, Stallings V. 2002. Infant weight gain and childhood overweight status in a multicenter cohort study. *Pediatrics* 109:194–99
34. Thomas B, Ghebremeskel K, Lowy C, Crawford M, Offley-Shore B. 2006. Nutrient intake of women with and without gestational diabetes with a specific focus on fatty acids. *Nutrition* 22:230–36
35. Trabulsi J, Schoeller DA. 2001. Evaluation of dietary assessment instruments against doubly labeled water, a biomarker of habitual energy intake. *Am. J. Physiol. Endocrinol. Metab.* 281:E891–99
36. van der Maten G, van Raaij J, Visman L, van der Heijden L, Oosterbaan H, et al. 1997. Low-sodium diet in pregnancy: effects on blood pressure and maternal nutritional status. *Br. J. Nutr.* 77:703–20
37. Winkvist A, Persson V, Hartini T. 2002. Underreporting of energy intake is less common among pregnant women in Indonesia. *Public Health Nutr.* 5:523–29
38. WHO Consultation. 2000. Obesity: preventing and managing the global epidemic. *WHO Tech. Rep. Ser. 894*, Geneva, Switzerland: WHO

Role of Dietary Proteins and Amino Acids in the Pathogenesis of Insulin Resistance

Frédéric Tremblay,[1] Charles Lavigne,[2] Hélène Jacques,[2,3] and André Marette[1,2]

[1]Department of Anatomy & Physiology and Lipid Research Unit, Laval University Hospital Research Center, Québec, Canada, [2]Institute of Nutraceuticals and Functional Foods, and [3]Department of Food Science and Nutrition, Laval University, Québec, Canada; email: andre.marette@crchul.ulaval.ca

Annu. Rev. Nutr. 2007. 27:293–310

First published online as a Review in Advance on April 27, 2007

The *Annual Review of Nutrition* is online at http://nutr.annualreviews.org

This article's doi:
10.1146/annurev.nutr.25.050304.092545

0199-9885/07/0821-0293$20.00

Key Words

obesity, diabetes, cancer, metabolism, signal transduction

Abstract

Dietary proteins and amino acids are important modulators of glucose metabolism and insulin sensitivity. Although high intake of dietary proteins has positive effects on energy homeostasis by inducing satiety and possibly increasing energy expenditure, it has detrimental effects on glucose homeostasis by promoting insulin resistance and increasing gluconeogenesis. Varying the quality rather than the quantity of proteins has been shown to modulate insulin resistance induced by Western diets and has revealed that proteins derived from fish might have the most desirable effects on insulin sensitivity. In vitro and in vivo data also support an important role of amino acids in glucose homeostasis through modulation of insulin action on muscle glucose transport and hepatic glucose production, secretion of insulin and glucagon, as well as gene and protein expression in various tissues. Moreover, amino acid signaling is integrated by mammalian target of rapamycin, a nutrient sensor that operates a negative feedback loop toward insulin receptor substrate 1 signaling, promoting insulin resistance for glucose metabolism. This integration suggests that modulating dietary proteins and the flux of circulating amino acids generated by their consumption and digestion might underlie powerful new approaches to treat various metabolic diseases such as obesity and diabetes.

Contents

INTRODUCTION

Dietary intake of proteins is essential for normal growth and development. In Western societies, protein consumption has increased considerably during the past 50 years and is now thought to exceed by ~80% the recommended dietary intake (43). Although our understanding of fat and carbohydrates as nutrients affecting glucose and energy metabolism has greatly increased in the past two decades, the roles of proteins and amino acids in glucose homeostasis and insulin resistance and the mechanisms behind their effects are still poorly characterized. In this review, we explore the mechanisms by which dietary proteins and amino acids modulate glucose and energy homeostasis in relationship to the pathogenesis of insulin resistance.

DIETARY PROTEINS AND INSULIN RESISTANCE

The popularity of high-protein diets (e.g., Atkins and Montignac) has created a renewed interest in dietary interventions as effective and relatively easy means to achieve significant and sustained body weight loss. Furthermore, it is now well recognized that not only glucose and lipid but also protein metabolism are altered in diabetic states (98). However, the long-term safety and efficacy of high-protein diets are not well documented. This underscores the need for rational and tailored approaches in the clinical management of body weight, as well as insulin resistance and glycemic control in obese prediabetic or diabetic individuals, that involve modulation of both the quantity and quality of proteins from the diet.

High-Protein Diets: Their Effects on Energy Balance

Numerous studies have shown that an increased consumption of dietary proteins results in greater body weight loss (reviewed in 52, 66, 83). What is unclear at this point is whether high-protein diets reduce body weight by reducing energy intake through satiety signal(s) or by increasing energy expenditure. On one hand, some studies support the concept that the consumption of a high-protein diet decreases circulating ghrelin, an orexigenic gut peptide, whereas it increases the concentrations of the anorexic peptides cholecystokinin and glucagon-like peptide 1 (16, 21, 142). On the other hand, however, other studies suggest that the satiety induced by high-protein diets is unrelated to changes in circulating ghrelin (102, 155). Genetic evidence also supports a role for the anorexic peptide YY (Pyy) in protein-mediated reduction in food intake. Indeed, Pyy-null mice are hyperphagic and display obesity in comparison with their wild-type littermates and are insensitive to the satiating effect of dietary proteins (9).

High-protein diets may also promote a negative energy balance by increasing energy expenditure. This has been attributed to the heightened thermal effect of dietary proteins (23%–30%) as compared with that of carbohydrates (5%–10%) and lipids (2%–3%) (106). Dietary proteins may also increase energy expenditure through up-regulation of uncoupling proteins (UCPs) and facultative thermogenesis. Indeed, high-protein intake was recently found to increase UCP-2 in the liver and UCP-1 in brown adipose tissue (115). Changes in UCP-1 and UCP-2 expression were inversely correlated with feeding efficiency and positively correlated with energy expenditure and oxygen consumption (115).

High-Protein Diets: Their Effects on Insulin Resistance and Glycemic Control

Varying the amount of protein not only affects body weight maintenance and feeding behavior, but also insulin secretion and action, thereby regulating glucose homeostasis. Short-term studies in normal or diabetic humans showed that dietary proteins stimulate insulin secretion (2, 46, 114, 122, 138) and reduce glycemia (75, 138). Importantly, consumption of a high-protein diet for six months in healthy nonobese individuals induced a higher glucose-stimulated insulin secretion, increased fasting glucose level, impaired suppression of hepatic glucose output by insulin, and enhanced gluconeogenesis (92). Furthermore, a one-year study in type 1 diabetic patients revealed that consumption of a high-protein diet decreased overall insulin sensitivity while it increased glucose production by the liver (91). Feeding rats with an increasing amount of protein at the expense of carbohydrates was also shown to increase fasting glycemia and the basal rate of endogenous glucose production (124). Furthermore, the assessment of insulin action in these animals, using the euglycemic-hyperinsulinemic clamp technique, revealed that a higher protein intake promotes a state of insulin resistance in peripheral tissues (124). Another study showed that rats fed a high-protein diet for 12 months had lower glycemia but higher insulin levels (136). Finally, it has been proposed that an accelerated pancreas "fatigue" or "failure" due to β-cell apoptosis might be responsible for the higher incidence of diabetes in prediabetic animals fed a high-protein diet (93, 126).

Dietary Proteins Sources and Insulin Resistance

Although high-protein diets might have beneficial effects on body weight and energy homeostasis, their potential long-term consequences on glycemic control, insulin resistance, and renal function limit their appeal for improving energy balance. Varying the source rather than the amount of proteins might represent a safer approach to the treatment of metabolic disorders.

Soy protein. Soy protein is well known for its hypolipidemic and hypocholesterolemic effects in animals and in humans (3). In addition to its effect on serum lipids, soy protein intake can also positively affect glucose homeostasis. For instance, consumption of soy protein, in comparison with casein, reduces fasting insulin and glucose levels in animals (15, 139). Similarly, human studies revealed that ingestion of a soy protein–based meal induces a lower insulin response than that induced following a casein-based meal (67, 125). However, the differential hormonal response following consumption of casein or soy proteins was not observed in another study (20). Incorporation of dietary soy protein was also shown to improve glucose tolerance and insulin sensitivity in rats fed a high-sucrose diet when compared with those fed with casein (87). Although the exact mechanism behind the beneficial effect of soy proteins on glycemic control is not known, it was proposed that a decrease in serum glucagon levels might be involved (87) since glucagon is known to promote hepatic glucose production. Soy protein may also improve insulin sensitivity by increasing insulin signaling in fat and liver since insulin receptor mRNA expression was reported to be increased in the liver and adipose tissues of soy protein–fed rats (72).

Fish protein. It has been known for years that populations from Alaska and Greenland that consume large amounts of fish have a low incidence of type 2 diabetes (39, 84, 104, 105). The beneficial effect of fish consumption was first attributed to fish oil. Although a meta-analysis revealed that intake of as much as 3 g of fish oil per day has no beneficial effect on glycemia in type 2 diabetes (44), consumption of lean fish (24 g/day; providing only ~140 mg of ω-3 fatty acid) was inversely correlated with the incidence of insulin resistance and type 2 diabetes (38). This latter finding was consistent with the hypothesis that a constituent other than lipid was responsible for the beneficial effect of fish consumption on glucose metabolism. Because protein is the most abundant nutrient in lean fish, it was proposed that fish protein could actually be responsible for the beneficial metabolic effects of lean fish consumption. This hypothesis was first tested in rabbits fed purified diets containing as the sole source of protein either casein, soy, or cod protein (12–14). The results showed that consumption of fish protein improved cholesterol transport via high-density lipoprotein (HDL) while reducing triglyceride-rich very-low-density lipoprotein (12–14). Human studies also demonstrated beneficial effects of cod protein consumption on plasma lipid profile by reducing plasma triglycerides in women and increasing HDL_2 cholesterol in men (47, 73, 86, 118).

In addition to their effect on plasma lipids, proteins derived from fish were also shown to affect glucose metabolism and insulin sensitivity. For instance, cod protein–fed rats in comparison to casein-fed animals are protected against the development of insulin resistance and glucose intolerance induced by diabetogenic diets rich in sucrose (87) or in saturated fat (88). These studies further revealed that soy protein can prevent insulin resistance induced by a diet rich in sucrose (87), but it had no beneficial effect on insulin sensitivity when the animals were fed a high-fat diet (88). Prevention of diet-induced insulin resistance by cod protein was related to enhanced insulin-stimulated glucose uptake by skeletal muscles but not by adipose tissues (88). Investigation of the mechanisms behind the insulin sensitization of skeletal muscles revealed that cod protein restored the activation of the phosphoinositide (PI) 3-kinase/Akt pathway and selectively improved GLUT4 translocation to the T-tubules (148), a cell-surface domain thought to mediate the bulk of glucose transport in response to insulin (145). The beneficial effect of cod protein could be recapitulated by incubating cultured skeletal muscle cells with a mixture of amino acids as found in the plasma of rats fed with the fish proteins, indicating that cod protein–derived amino acids can affect muscle insulin sensitivity in a cell-autonomous fashion (88). Importantly, human studies are compatible with the proposition that cod protein exerts beneficial effects on glycemic control. Indeed, it has been reported that postmeal plasma insulin concentrations increased significantly less in six healthy males when they were consuming a cod fillet meal compared with a beefsteak meal (137), suggesting improved insulin sensitivity in the former group. Moreover, a recent study reported that during a test meal in humans (119), cod protein induced a lower insulin/glucose ratio at 120 min and a lower area under the insulin curve as compared with milk protein. The results from the two studies cited above suggest there are decreased insulin secretion and/or higher insulin clearance and sensitivity with lower insulin/glucose ratio when humans are consuming cod protein as compared with other animal sources.

AMINO ACIDS AND INSULIN RESISTANCE

In pioneering studies published several decades ago, Felig et al. (36, 37) were the first to observe that amino acid levels are elevated in the plasma of obese individuals. These findings raised the possibility that amino acids may be involved in the development of obesity-linked and/or diet-induced insulin resistance. Elevated amino acid concentrations have also been detected in the skeletal muscle of diet-induced obese animals, but not in the same tissue of genetically induced obese *fa/fa* rats (61), a finding that suggests that dietary modulation of insulin action in skeletal muscle might directly implicate amino acids. Indeed, the role of amino acids on multiple aspects of glucose metabolism and insulin action has become well recognized. (The various effects of amino acids are schematically represented in **Figure 1** (see color insert); see text below for details and explanations.)

Regulation of Insulin Action and Glucose Metabolism

Studies performed in healthy humans have shown that short-term elevations of plasma amino acids lead to a decreased whole-body glucose disposal under euglycemic and hyperinsulinemic conditions (40, 82, 118, 143). This insulin-resistant state induced by amino acids has been primarily attributed to a reduced peripheral glucose uptake (40, 82, 118). In addition, infusion of the branched-chain amino acid leucine alone was found to impair glucose uptake in humans despite inducing a significant rise in insulin levels (1). The regulatory role of amino acids on skeletal muscle insulin sensitivity in vivo appears to involve a direct action of amino acids on muscle cells. Indeed, the rise of basal and insulin-stimulated glucose transport in ex vivo muscle preparations after prolonged incubation could be prevented by amino acids (50). Furthermore, amino acids acutely inhibit insulin-stimulated glucose transport in muscle cells in vitro (149). The negative effect of amino acids on insulin action in muscle was shown to be associated with inhibitory phosphorylation of insulin receptor substrate-1 (IRS-1) on serine and/or threonine residues and impaired activation of PI 3-kinase (149), a key effector of insulin's metabolic actions that signals to the downstream effectors Akt and atypical protein kinase C ζ/λ (PKC-ζ/λ) (145 and **Figure 2**, see color insert). The negative modulatory effects of amino acids on insulin action have also been demonstrated in cultured hepatocytes (111) and adipocytes (140), and this was also shown to involve dysregulated IRS-1-mediated signaling. Impaired muscle insulin signaling as a consequence of increased amino acid sufficiency was reported in animal and human studies. For instance, oral administration of leucine was found to reduce the duration of PI 3-kinase activation by insulin in rat skeletal muscle (10). Furthermore, a cross-over study in which human subjects were studied twice showed that infusion of amino acids under physiological hyperinsulinemia markedly increased the phosphorylation of IRS-1 on Ser312 and Ser636/639 and completely blunted the activation of PI 3-kinase associated with IRS-1 in skeletal muscle while leaving intact the stimulation of Akt phosphorylation (147).

Another mechanism by which amino acids can negatively affect insulin-stimulated glucose transport was revealed by Traxinger & Marshall (144), who showed that incubation of adipocytes with amino acids under hyperglycemic and hyperinsulinemic conditions promotes a state of insulin resistance. They further found that among all amino acids, glutamine was the most potent at reducing glucose transport through its ability to activate the hexosamine pathway (99). In agreement with a potential role of hexosamine build-up in amino acid–mediated insulin resistance, direct activation of this pathway by glucosamine infusion in animals also induces peripheral insulin resistance and defective postreceptor insulin signaling in muscle (59, 112).

Although amino acids are generally believed to interfere with insulin's ability to increase peripheral glucose uptake, most notably in skeletal muscle, some studies suggest that amino acids might actually be beneficial for one aspect of glucose metabolism, i.e., glycogen synthesis. Indeed, amino acids stimulate glycogen synthesis in human skeletal muscle cells in vitro via phosphorylation and inactivation of GSK-3 and activation of glycogen synthase (5, 116). However, amino acid infusion in humans did not result in the phosphorylation of GSK-3 or activation of glycogen synthase (94). Interestingly, it was recently found that under conditions in which Akt is inhibited, S6K1 can phosphorylate and inactivate GSK-3 (161). The branched-chain amino acids leucine and isoleucine were found to improve glucose tolerance and stimulate glucose uptake in skeletal muscle by mechanisms that might involve enhanced glycogen synthase activity and a greater translocation of glucose transporters GLUT1 and GLUT4 at the plasma membrane (33, 34, 108). This reported effect of leucine (108), however, is at odds with other studies showing a negative effect of leucine on insulin action and muscle glucose uptake (1, 10). In line with a positive role of amino acids in glucose metabolism is the observation that insulin-stimulated GLUT4 translocation in 3T3-L1 adipocytes is positively modulated by the addition of amino acids to the incubation medium (18). Finally, amino acids were also shown to slightly enhance insulin-stimulated Akt phosphorylation in the presence of the PI 3-kinase inhibitor, wortmannin in freshly isolated adipocyte, and in untreated adipose tissue of obese *db/db* mice (62, 63). This latter effect of amino acids is still ill defined but was proposed to be mediated by PDK-1 independently from PI 3-kinase and required the presence of glucose in the incubation medium (63).

Amino acids also play a role in the modulation of hepatic glucose production through direct and indirect mechanisms (35, 80, 81). By acting as substrates (35), amino acids can contribute to gluconeogenesis, endogenous glucose production, and the development of hyperglycemia in humans under conditions where insulin secretion is inhibited by somatostatin (81). Amino acids, through their ability to stimulate glucagon and insulin secretion (41, 110) infused in the absence of somatostatin can directly and indirectly affect gluconeogenesis, in which case glycemia might not be affected because of peripheral glucose uptake (81). Infusion of amino acids can also interfere with the ability of insulin to repress endogenous glucose production when hyperinsulinemia is kept constant (17, 40, 137, 147), although this observation remains controversial (82). In fact, it appears that low peripheral, fasting-like insulinemia is not sufficient to decrease amino acid–induced endogenous glucose production (147), whereas prandial-like hyperinsulinemia is generally sufficient to completely blunt hepatic glucose output (82, 147). Importantly, it has been recently shown that the contribution of gluconeogenesis to hepatic glucose output in obese nondiabetic subjects was associated with their increased postprandial protein catabolism (28). This latter study suggests that an increased flux of amino acids in obesity may be involved in the increased gluconeogenesis observed during the development of insulin resistance with respect to protein metabolism (28).

Amino Acids, Nutrient Sensing, and Insulin Resistance

The notion that amino acids not only serve as metabolic substrates but also are involved in activating and/or modulating signaling pathways has refined our understanding of how proteins from the diet can affect insulin action at the cellular and molecular levels. Early evidence linking amino acids to activation of intracellular signals came from in vitro studies showing amino acid–dependent phosphorylation of ribosomal protein S6 kinase 1 (S6K1) and eIF4E-binding protein 1 (4E-BP1) (54, 111, 153, 158), two effectors of mTOR involved in mRNA translation (60). These effects were found to be fully reversible upon amino acid withdrawal or by exposure to the specific mTOR inhibitor rapamycin (54, 111, 153, 158). These studies were later extended to animals and humans (24, 78, 128, 147). It has been suggested that amino acids activate the mTOR pathway through activation of class III phosphatidylinositol 3-kinase, hVps34 (25, 109). Interestingly, amino acids and insulin act in concert to promote phosphorylation of mTOR effectors (54, 111, 149). Insulin stimulates the mTOR pathway in a PI 3-kinase/Akt-dependent manner, which leads to phosphorylation and destabilization of the tuberous sclerosis 1 and 2 (TSC1/2) complex and enables Rheb-mediated activation of mTOR (reviewed in 60, 90, 133; schematically represented in **Figure 2**). Alternatively, Akt was reported to directly phosphorylate mTOR in vitro (107, 127); however, recent data suggest that S6K1 is responsible for this phosphorylation in cells (29, 64).

Temporal analysis of amino acid–mediated inhibition of glucose transport and activation of the mTOR pathway revealed similar kinetics suggesting that these events might be linked together (149). This idea was first tested in skeletal muscle cells in vitro, where it was observed that amino acid–induced inhibition of insulin-stimulated glucose uptake was completely reversed by the mTOR inhibitor rapamycin (149). It was further revealed that activation of the mTOR pathway by both insulin and amino acids causes insulin resistance by inhibiting PI 3-kinase due to increased serine/threonine phosphorylation of IRS-1 (149), a process known to cause inhibition of downstream signaling (163). Administration of the branched-chain amino acid leucine, a potent activator of mTOR, was shown to decrease the duration of insulin-induced IRS-1-associated PI 3-kinase in rat skeletal muscle (10), whereas mTOR blockade by rapamycin injection had the opposite effect in the mouse (49). This negative feedback loop mediated by the mTOR pathway during amino acid sufficiency (mimicked by leucine alone) was also found to be operative in murine and human adipocytes (58, 140, 147) and in hepatocytes (76).

Increased amino acid availability leads to a rapamycin-sensitive phosphorylation of IRS-1 on Ser307 and Ser636/639 in cultured adipose and muscle cells (27, 146, 147). In addition, overactivation of S6K1 was detected in skeletal muscle biopsies obtained from humans infused with amino acids, and this was associated with increased phosphorylation of IRS-1 on Ser307 and Ser636/639 and impaired PI 3-kinase activity (147). Genetic evidence also supports the role of mTOR and/or S6K1 in mediating inhibitory phosphorylation of IRS-1 on serine and the development of insulin resistance. Deletion of TSC1/2 in mouse embryonic fibroblasts was found to dramatically increase the activation of mTOR/S6K1, causing inhibition of insulin signaling at the level of IRS-1/PI3K/Akt (56, 131). In addition, S6K was found to directly phosphorylate IRS-1 at Ser302, an effect that was proposed to reduce the association of IRS-1 with the insulin receptor (56). The physiological importance of the mTOR/S6K1 pathway in insulin resistance was further highlighted by the findings that its activation was enhanced in obese animals (76, 152) and that S6K1 deficiency in mice protects against diet-induced insulin resistance by preventing, at least in part, phosphorylation of IRS-1 on serine residues and inhibition of Akt phosphorylation (152).

The activation of mTOR by amino acids may also modulate insulin action independently from the negative feedback mechanism toward IRS-1. For instance, modulation of hypothalamic mTOR by leucine was shown to reduce food intake in rats (31). Interestingly, leptin also increased the phosphorylation of S6K1 (31), which suggests that the anorexic effect of leptin might be mediated via the mTOR pathway. Alternatively, the inhibitory effect of leptin on AMPK in the hypothalamus (4, 101) might mediate the activation of S6K1 because AMPK is a negative regulator of mTOR (19, 71, 132). If leptin is able to control the activation of the mTOR pathway in the brain, amino acids can stimulate leptin secretion from white adipocytes by activating the mTOR pathway (96, 123). It should be noted that central sensing of amino acids also occurred in the brain's anterior piriform cortex, where deficiency of essential amino acids affects food selection and feeding behavior (53, 79) in mice by a mechanism that involves the phosphorylation of eukaryotic initiation factor 2-α (eIF2α) by the eIF2α

kinase general control nonderepressible 2 (48, 100).

The role of amino acids as regulators of gene expression and protein synthesis is well documented (reviewed in 74, 78). However, it is unclear how induction of certain genes upon amino acid starvation or increased mRNA translation following amino acid exposure can modulate glucose metabolism and insulin resistance. Of particular interest is the observation that C/EBP homologous protein (CHOP) gene expression is induced in response to amino acid starvation, a process involving the transcription factors ATF2 and ATF4 (6, 23). Indeed, ATF2 and ATF4 can bind to the amino acid response element located in the CHOP promoter (22). CHOP expression has been shown to be down-regulated during adipogenesis while ectopic expression of CHOP prevents the adipocytic conversion of 3T3-L1 cells by interfering with C/EBPα/β expression and function (8, 141). Signaling through the mTOR pathway also plays a crucial role in adipogenesis. Indeed, rapamycin treatment blocks clonal expansion and terminal differentiation of 3T3-L1 and human preadipocytes (11, 45, 159). In addition, mice lacking the mTOR effector 4E-BP1 have reduced fat pad mass, which suggests an important role for translational events in adipose tissue development (150). Furthermore, amino acid–induced activation of mTOR was reported to be important for peroxisome proliferator-activated receptor γ (PPARγ) in 3T3-L1 adipocytes; amino acid withdrawal or rapamycin decreased, whereas adding back amino acids restored PPARγ transcriptional activity (77). Interestingly, the thiazolidinedione troglitazone was shown to reverse the effect of rapamycin or amino acid starvation on PPARγ activity (77). mTOR has also been implicated in the phosphorylation of lipin induced by insulin and amino acids in rat adipocytes (68). Mutation of the lipin gene has been shown to cause lipodystrophy in fatty liver dystrophy mice (113), which suggests an important role of lipin in adipogenesis. Indeed, lipin deficiency in mouse embryonic fibroblasts prevents lipid accumulation and induction of PPARγ and C/EBPα (117). Amino acids were also found to participate in the three-dimensional organization of rat adipocytes into clusters in vitro (42). These data suggest another set of mechanisms by which amino acids might modulate insulin sensitivity in vivo through adipose tissue remodeling, brought about at least in part by the modulation of key adipogenic transcription factors.

Amino Acid Sensing via mTOR: Linking Diabetes and Cancer

Much evidence points toward mTOR as an important checkpoint hub involved in diabetes and cancer (reviewed in 97, 121, 133, 151, 157). Multiple signaling branches converge at the level of mTOR, including LKB1/AMPK, TSC1/2, and PI3K/PTEN/Akt (see **Figure 3**, see color insert). The LKB1/AMPK pathway senses the energy status of the cells and is activated upon elevation of the AMP/ATP ratio (55). Glucose starvation, exercise, and the widely prescribed antidiabetic drug metformin activate LKB1/AMPK, which in turn shuts down ATP-consuming processes such as protein synthesis by inhibiting mTOR activity (71, 132, 134). The LKB1/AMPK signaling pathway is necessary for mediating the glucose-lowering effect of metformin (135, 162) and was recently shown to mediate inhibition of breast cancer cells in vitro (160). These data suggest that inhibition of mTOR via LKB1/AMPK might underlie, at least in part, the beneficial effect of metformin on glucose homeostasis/insulin sensitivity and tumor development. In a similar fashion, the PI3K/PTEN/Akt pathway is involved in both glucose homeostasis and tumor development (32, 51, 89, 133). Mutation of the tumor suppressor PTEN leads to up-regulated Akt and mTOR activities (32, 51, 89, 133). Interestingly, cancer cells in which the PTEN gene is mutated are particularly sensitive to the antiproliferative effect of rapamycin (32, 51, 89, 133). Furthermore,

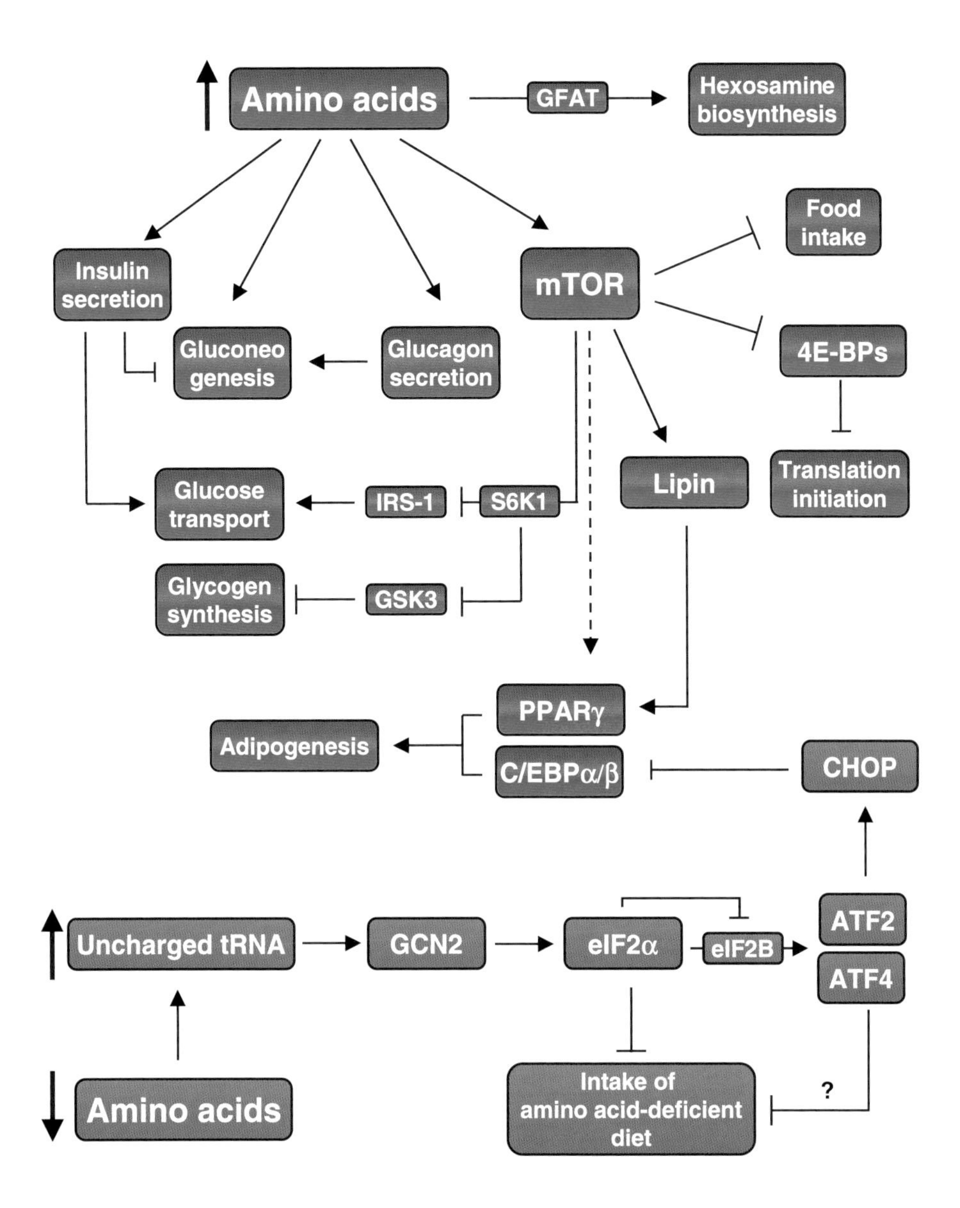

Figure 1

Effects of amino acid sufficiency (*red*) or deficiency (*blue*) on cell signaling and biological processes involved in the pathogenesis of insulin resistance. (See Amino Acids and Insulin Resistance section for details and explanations.)

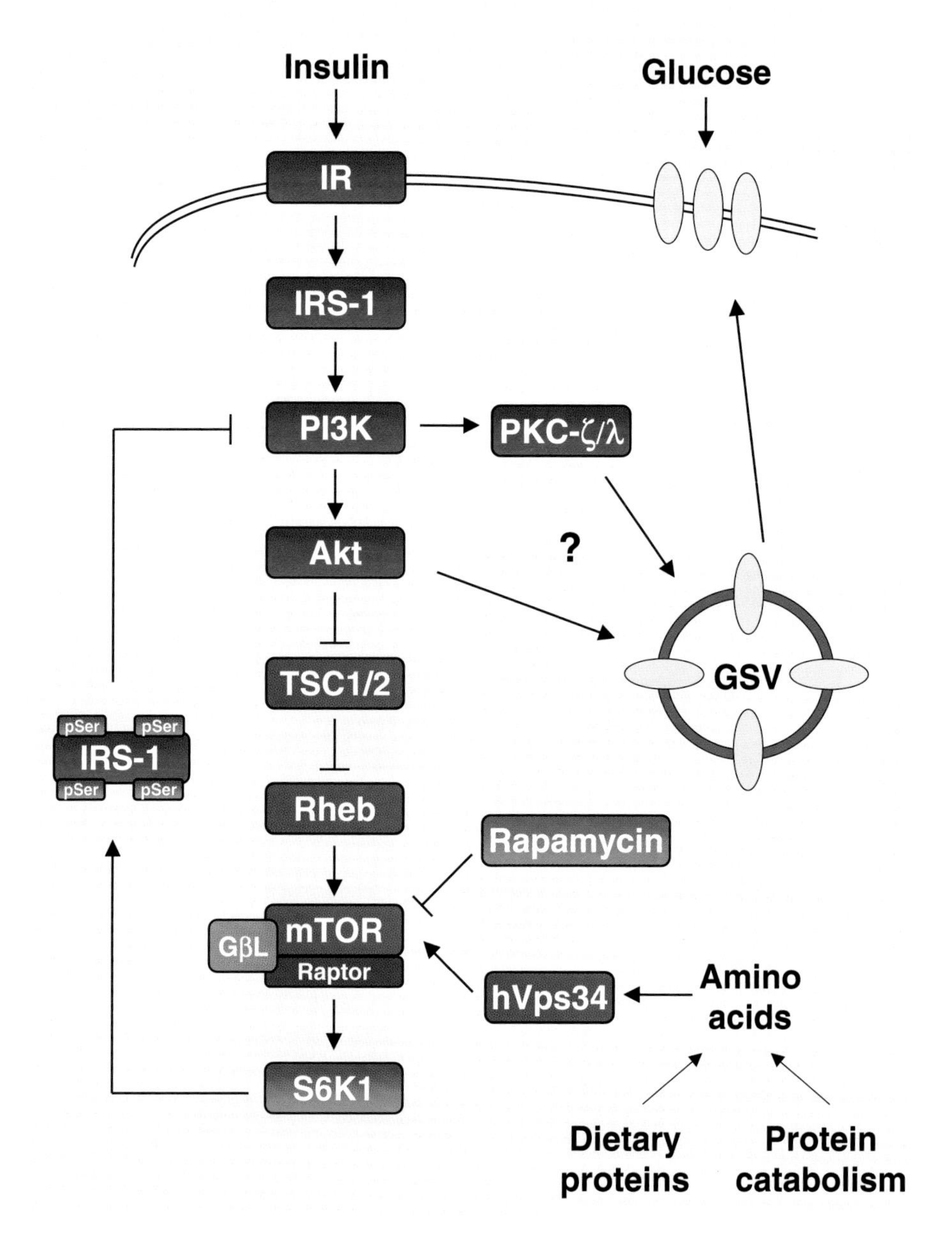

Figure 2

See legend on next page.

Figure 2

Feedback inhibition of IRS-1 signaling mediated by the mammalian target of rapamycin (mTOR). Insulin binds and activates the insulin receptor (IR), which phosphorylates intracellular substrates such as insulin receptor substrate-1 (IRS-1). Upon binding to tyrosyl-phosphorylated IRS-1, the activated phosphatidylinositol 3-kinase (PI3K) relays the signal to both Akt and protein kinase C (PKC)-ζ/λ, which are thought to be involved in glucose transporter 4 translocation and glucose transport stimulated by insulin. Akt can also phosphorylate and destabilize tuberous sclerosis complex (TSC)2, enabling Rheb-mediated mTOR activation. Amino acids can also activate mTOR through hVps34. The rapamycin-sensitive mTORC1 [composed of mTOR, raptor, and G protein β-subunit-like protein (GβL)] requires both insulin and amino acids for mediating full activation of S6K1 and promoting inhibitory phosphorylation of IRS-1 on serine residues. Heavily serine-phosphorylated IRS-1 causes insulin resistance by blocking PI3K signaling.

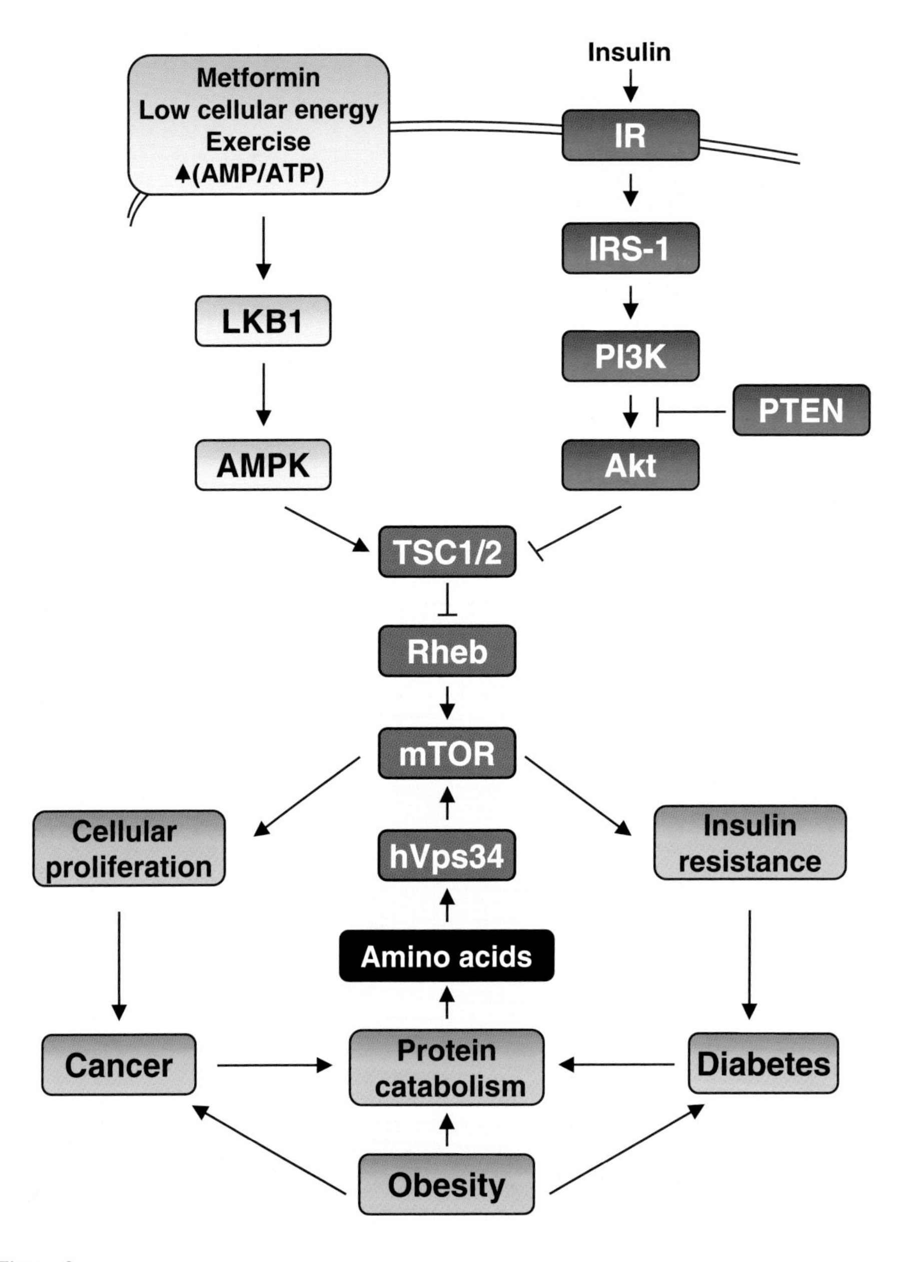

Figure 3

See legend on next page.

Figure 3

Interplay between energy-, hormonal-, and amino acid–sensitive signaling pathways in relationship to the development of cancer and diabetes. LKB1/AMPK activates TSC2, whereas PI3K/PTEN/Akt inhibits TSC2, resulting in the inhibition or activation of Rheb/mTOR, respectively. Amino acids can also activate mTOR via hVps34 independently from the insulin-signaling pathway. Activation of the mTOR pathway increases cellular proliferation and causes insulin resistance, events that are closely linked to the development of cancer and diabetes, respectively. Obesity, which has been shown to be an important risk factor for both cancer and diabetes, can maintain the mTOR pathway activation despite insulin resistance by favoring a constant supply of amino acids via enhanced protein catabolism.

selective deletion of PTEN in muscle or adipose tissue in mice improves both glucose metabolism and insulin sensitivity (85, 156), whereas it was shown to cause hepatocellular carcinomas when selectively deleted from mouse liver (65). The TSC1/TSC2 complex is also involved in the modulation of cell proliferation as well as in the control of insulin action/sensitivity (57, 69, 129). Analysis of mouse embryonic fibroblasts from $TSC2^{-/-}$ mice showed dysregulated mTOR/S6K1 activity as well as hyperphosphorylation and degradation of IRS-1 (56, 130, 131). As an upstream negative regulator of mTOR, the TSC1/2 complex integrates signals from both the LKB1/AMPK and PI3K/PTEN/Akt pathways through phosphorylation events (70, 71). AMPK-mediated phosphorylation of TSC2 enhances its activity, which leads to an effective repression of Rheb/mTOR (71), whereas phosphorylation of TSC2 by Akt destabilizes the complex, allowing for Rheb-mediated activation of mTOR (70).

Because mTOR is exquisitely sensitive to amino acid availability, exogenous as well as endogenous supplies of amino acids are likely to play an important role not only in glucose homeostasis and insulin resistance as described above, but also in tumor development. Furthermore, the observations that amino acids signal to mTOR independently from TSC2 (25, 109) and in synergy with hormonal stimuli (54) strongly suggest that modulation of the quantity as well as the quality of amino acids derived from dietary proteins might have profound and significant effects on chronic diseases associated with insulin resistance and mTOR overactivation such as diabetes, obesity, and cancer. Of significant importance is the observation that through increased protein catabolism in the postabsorptive state, plasma amino acid concentrations are elevated in obese mice and human subjects (28, 35, 37, 154). Recent studies have shown that the mTOR/S6K1 pathway is overactivated in the liver and muscle of high-fat-fed obese rats despite the occurrence of insulin resistance for PI3K/Akt activation (76). The activation of both mTOR and S6K1 by insulin was found to be accelerated in obese rats, in association with increased inhibitory phosphorylation of IRS-1 on Ser636/639 (76). Interestingly, the activities of both enzymes were higher even in the absence of insulin administration (76). One can hypothesize that mTOR and S6K1 are chronically activated because of the elevated and constant flux of amino acids (which activate mTOR independently from the insulin-signaling cascade), thereby worsening their insulin resistance for glucose metabolism, but also possibly promoting tumor development. Indeed, obesity is associated with various forms of cancer in humans, including breast and prostate cancer (26, 95, 120). Increased muscle wasting/cachexia in cancer patients may also contribute to mTOR activation through increased availability of amino acids upon protein catabolism (7, 103). However, some studies indicate that nutritional support of cancer patients with branched-chain amino acids improves nitrogen balance, increases skeletal muscle protein synthesis, and reduces skeletal muscle catabolism (30). Whether such treatment also promotes mTOR-induced insulin resistance in these patients remains unclear. Thus, more work is needed to determine whether amino acid–mediated modulation of mTOR directly plays a role in tumor growth and development.

CONCLUSION

Dietary proteins and amino acids have emerged in recent years as potent modulators of insulin action and glucose metabolism. Amino acids are thought to play a significant role in the pathogenesis of insulin resistance by modulating the endocrine function of the pancreas, acting as gluconeogenic precursors, stimulating hexosamine biosynthesis, or activating the mTOR-signaling pathway. Although activation of the mTOR pathway is increased in liver of obese animals (76, 152) and in amino acid–induced insulin resistance in humans (147), it remains to be determined whether overactivation of mTOR is a common feature of human obesity. How varying the amount or the source of dietary proteins affects the activation of mTOR/S6K1 and the phosphorylation status of IRS-1 under acute and chronic settings is clearly an area of investigation that deserves more attention in relationship to both glucose metabolism and tumor development. Finally, identification of mechanistic links between energy-signaling (LKB1/AMPK) and hormonal-signaling (PI3K/PTEN/Akt) pathways in relationship to amino acid sensing via hVps34 might help define novel nutritional and/or pharmacological approaches for the treatment of diabetes, obesity, and cancer.

LITERATURE CITED

1. Abumrad NN, Robinson RP, Gooch BR, Lacy WW. 1982. The effect of leucine infusion on substrate flux across the human forearm. *J. Surg. Res.* 32:453–63
2. Ahmed M, Nuttall FQ, Gannon MC, Lamusga RF. 1980. Plasma glucagon and alpha-amino acid nitrogen response to various diets in normal humans. *Am. J. Clin. Nutr.* 33:1917–24
3. Anderson JW, Johnstone BM, Cook-Newell ME. 1995. Meta-analysis of the effects of soy protein intake on serum lipids. *N. Engl. J. Med.* 333:276–82
4. Andersson U, Filipsson K, Abbott CR, Woods A, Smith K, et al. 2004. AMP-activated protein kinase plays a role in the control of food intake. *J. Biol. Chem.* 279:12005–8
5. Armstrong JL, Bonavaud SM, Toole BJ, Yeaman SJ. 2001. Regulation of glycogen synthesis by amino acids in cultured human muscle cells. *J. Biol. Chem.* 276:952–56
6. Averous J, Bruhat A, Jousse C, Carraro V, Thiel G, Fafournoux P. 2004. Induction of CHOP expression by amino acid limitation requires both ATF4 expression and ATF2 phosphorylation. *J. Biol. Chem.* 279:5288–97
7. Baracos VE. 2006. Cancer-associated cachexia and underlying biological mechanisms. *Annu. Rev. Nutr.* 26:435–61
8. Batchvarova N, Wang XZ, Ron D. 1995. Inhibition of adipogenesis by the stress-induced protein CHOP (Gadd153). *EMBO J.* 14:4654–61
9. Batterham RL, Heffron H, Kapoor S, Chivers JE, Chandarana K, et al. 2006. Critical role for peptide YY in protein-mediated satiation and body-weight regulation. *Cell Metab.* 4:223–33
10. Baum JI, O'Connor JC, Seyler JE, Anthony TG, Freund GG, Layman DK. 2005. Leucine reduces the duration of insulin-induced PI 3-kinase activity in rat skeletal muscle. *Am. J. Physiol. Endocrinol. Metab.* 288:E86–91
11. Bell A, Grunder L, Sorisky A. 2000. Rapamycin inhibits human adipocyte differentiation in primary culture. *Obes. Res.* 8:249–54
12. Bergeron N, Deshaies Y, Jacques H. 1992a. Dietary fish protein modulates high density lipoprotein cholesterol and lipoprotein lipase activity in rabbits. *J. Nutr.* 122:1731–37
13. Bergeron N, Deshaies Y, Jacques H. 1992b. Factorial experiment to determine influence of fish protein and fish oil on serum and liver lipids in rabbits. *Nutrition* 8:354–58
14. Bergeron N, Jacques H. 1989. Influence of fish protein as compared to casein and soy protein on serum and liver lipids, and serum lipoprotein cholesterol levels in the rabbit. *Atherosclerosis* 78:113–21
15. Beynen AC, West CE, Spaaij CJ, Huisman J, Van Leeuwen P, et al. 1990. Cholesterol metabolism, digestion rates and postprandial changes in serum of swine fed purified diets containing either casein or soybean protein. *J. Nutr.* 120:422–30

16. Blom WA, Lluch A, Stafleu A, Vinoy S, Holst JJ, et al. 2006. Effect of a high-protein breakfast on the postprandial ghrelin response. *Am. J. Clin. Nutr.* 83:211–20
17. Boden G, Tappy L. 1990. Effects of amino acids on glucose disposal. *Diabetes* 39:1079–84
18. Bogan JS, McKee AE, Lodish HF. 2001. Insulin-responsive compartments containing GLUT4 in 3T3-L1 and CHO cells: regulation by amino acid concentrations. *Mol. Cell Biol.* 21:4785–806
19. Bolster DR, Crozier SJ, Kimball SR, Jefferson LS. 2002. AMP-activated protein kinase suppresses protein synthesis in rat skeletal muscle through down-regulated mammalian target of rapamycin (mTOR) signaling. *J. Biol. Chem.* 277:23977–80
20. Bos C, Metges CC, Gaudichon C, Petzke KJ, Pueyo ME, et al. 2003. Postprandial kinetics of dietary amino acids are the main determinant of their metabolism after soy or milk protein ingestion in humans. *J. Nutr.* 133:1308–15
21. Bowen J, Noakes M, Clifton PM. 2006. Appetite regulatory hormone responses to various dietary proteins differ by body mass index status despite similar reductions in ad libitum energy intake. *J. Clin. Endocrinol. Metab.* 91:2913–19
22. Bruhat A, Jousse C, Carraro V, Reimold AM, Ferrara M, Fafournoux P. 2000. Amino acids control mammalian gene transcription: activating transcription factor 2 is essential for the amino acid responsiveness of the CHOP promoter. *Mol. Cell Biol.* 20:7192–204
23. Bruhat A, Jousse C, Wang XZ, Ron D, Ferrara M, Fafournoux P. 1997. Amino acid limitation induces expression of CHOP, a CCAAT/enhancer binding protein-related gene, at both transcriptional and post-transcriptional levels. *J. Biol. Chem.* 272:17588–93
24. Burrin DG, Davis TA. 2004. Proteins and amino acids in enteral nutrition. *Curr. Opin. Clin. Nutr. Metab. Care* 7:79–87
25. Byfield MP, Murray JT, Backer JM. 2005. hVps34 is a nutrient-regulated lipid kinase required for activation of p70 S6 kinase. *J. Biol. Chem.* 280:33076–82
26. Calle EE, Thun MJ. 2004. Obesity and cancer. *Oncogene* 23:6365–78
27. Carlson CJ, White MF, Rondinone CM. 2004. Mammalian target of rapamycin regulates IRS-1 serine 307 phosphorylation. *Biochem. Biophys. Res. Commun.* 316:533–39
28. Chevalier S, Burgess SC, Malloy CR, Gougeon R, Marliss EB, Morais JA. 2006. The greater contribution of gluconeogenesis to glucose production in obesity is related to increased whole-body protein catabolism. *Diabetes* 55:675–81
29. Chiang GG, Abraham RT. 2005. Phosphorylation of mammalian target of rapamycin (mTOR) at Ser-2448 is mediated by p70S6 kinase. *J. Biol. Chem.* 280:25485–90
30. Choudry HA, Pan M, Karinch AM, Souba WW. 2006. Branched-chain amino acid-enriched nutritional support in surgical and cancer patients. *J. Nutr.* 136:314–18S
31. Cota D, Proulx K, Smith KA, Kozma SC, Thomas G, et al. 2006. Hypothalamic mTOR signaling regulates food intake. *Science* 312:927–30
32. Cully M, You H, Levine AJ, Mak TW. 2006. Beyond PTEN mutations: the PI3K pathway as an integrator of multiple inputs during tumorigenesis. *Nat. Rev. Cancer* 6:184–92
33. Doi M, Yamaoka I, Fukunaga T, Nakayama M. 2003. Isoleucine, a potent plasma glucose-lowering amino acid, stimulates glucose uptake in C2C12 myotubes. *Biochem. Biophys. Res. Commun.* 312:1111–17
34. Doi M, Yamaoka I, Nakayama M, Mochizuki S, Sugahara K, Yoshizawa F. 2005. Isoleucine, a blood glucose-lowering amino acid, increases glucose uptake in rat skeletal muscle in the absence of increases in AMP-activated protein kinase activity. *J. Nutr.* 135:2103–8
35. Felig P. 1975. Amino acid metabolism in man. *Annu. Rev. Biochem.* 44:933–55
36. Felig P, Marliss E, Cahill GF Jr. 1969. Plasma amino acid levels and insulin secretion in obesity. *N. Engl. J. Med.* 281:811–16

37. Felig P, Marliss E, Cahill GF Jr. 1970. Are plasma amino acid levels elevated in obesity? *N. Engl. J. Med.* 282:166
38. Feskens EJ, Bowles CH, Kromhout D. 1991. Inverse association between fish intake and risk of glucose intolerance in normoglycemic elderly men and women. *Diabet. Care* 14:935–41
39. Feskens EJ, Kromhout D. 1993. Epidemiologic studies on Eskimos and fish intake. *Ann. N. Y. Acad. Sci.* 683:9–15
40. Flakoll PJ, Wentzel LS, Rice DE, Hill JO, Abumrad NN. 1992. Short-term regulation of insulin-mediated glucose utilization in four-day fasted human volunteers: role of amino acid availability. *Diabetologia* 35:357–66
41. Floyd JCJ, Fajans SS, Conn JW, Knopf RF, Rull J. 1966. Stimulation of insulin secretion by amino acids. *J. Clin. Invest.* 45:1487–502
42. Fox HL, Kimball SR, Jefferson LS, Lynch CJ. 1998. Amino acids stimulate phosphorylation of p70S6k and organization of rat adipocytes into multicellular clusters. *Am. J. Physiol.* 274:C206–13
43. Franz MJ. 2002. Protein and diabetes: much advice, little research. *Curr. Diab. Rep.* 2:457–64
44. Friedberg CE, Janssen MJ, Heine RJ, Grobbee DE. 1998. Fish oil and glycemic control in diabetes. A meta-analysis. *Diabetes Care* 21:494–500
45. Gagnon A, Lau S, Sorisky A. 2001. Rapamycin-sensitive phase of 3T3-L1 preadipocyte differentiation after clonal expansion. *J. Cell Physiol.* 189:14–22
46. Gannon MC, Nuttall FQ, Lane JT, Burmeister LA. 1992. Metabolic response to cottage cheese or egg white protein, with or without glucose, in type II diabetic subjects. *Metabolism* 41:1137–45
47. Gascon A, Jacques H, Moorjani S, Deshaies Y, Brun LD, Julien P. 1996. Plasma lipoprotein profile and lipolytic activities in response to the substitution of lean white fish for other animal protein sources in premenopausal women. *Am. J. Clin. Nutr.* 63:315–21
48. Gietzen DW, Ross CM, Hao S, Sharp JW. 2004. Phosphorylation of eIF2alpha is involved in the signaling of indispensable amino acid deficiency in the anterior piriform cortex of the brain in rats. *J. Nutr.* 134:717–23
49. Gual P, Gremeaux T, Gonzalez T, Marchand-Brustel Y, Tanti JF. 2003. MAP kinases and mTOR mediate insulin-induced phosphorylation of insulin receptor substrate-1 on serine residues 307, 612 and 632. *Diabetologia* 46(11):1532–42
50. Gulve EA, Cartee GD, Holloszy JO. 1991. Prolonged incubation of skeletal muscle in vitro: prevention of increases in glucose transport. *Am. J. Physiol.* 261:154–60
51. Hafen E. 2004. Cancer, type 2 diabetes, and ageing: news from flies and worms. *Swiss. Med. Wkly.* 134:711–19
52. Halton TL, Hu FB. 2004. The effects of high-protein diets on thermogenesis, satiety and weight loss: a critical review. *J. Am. Coll. Nutr.* 23:373–85
53. Hao S, Sharp JW, Ross-Inta CM, McDaniel BJ, Anthony TG, et al. 2005. Uncharged tRNA and sensing of amino acid deficiency in mammalian piriform cortex. *Science* 307:1776–78
54. Hara K, Yonezawa K, Weng QP, Kozlowski MT, Belham C, Avruch J. 1998. Amino acid sufficiency and mTOR regulate p70 S6 kinase and eIF-4E BP1 through a common effector mechanism. *J. Biol. Chem.* 273:14484–94
55. Hardie DG. 2005. New roles for the LKB1→AMPK pathway. *Curr. Opin. Cell Biol.* 17:167–73

56. Harrington LS, Findlay GM, Gray A, Tolkacheva T, Wigfield S, et al. 2004. The TSC1-2 tumor suppressor controls insulin-PI3K signaling via regulation of IRS proteins. *J. Cell Biol.* 166:213–23
57. Harrington LS, Findlay GM, Lamb RF. 2005. Restraining PI3K: mTOR signalling goes back to the membrane. *Trends Biochem. Sci.* 30:35–42
58. Haruta T, Uno T, Kawahara J, Takano A, Egawa K, et al. 2000. A rapamycin-sensitive pathway down-regulates insulin signaling via phosphorylation and proteasomal degradation of insulin receptor substrate-1. *Mol. Endocrinol.* 14:783–94
59. Hawkins M, Hu M, Yu J, Eder H, Vuguin P, et al. 1999. Discordant effects of glucosamine on insulin-stimulated glucose metabolism and phosphatidylinositol 3-kinase activity. *J. Biol. Chem.* 274:31312–19
60. Hay N, Sonenberg N. 2004. Upstream and downstream of mTOR. *Genes Dev.* 18:1926–45
61. Herrero MC, Remesar X, Blade C, Arola L. 1997. Muscle amino acid pattern in obese rats. *Int. J. Obes. Relat. Metab. Disord.* 21:698–703
62. Hinault C, Mothe-Satney I, Gautier N, Lawrence JC Jr, van Obberghen E. 2004. Amino acids and leucine allow insulin activation of the PKB/mTOR pathway in normal adipocytes treated with wortmannin and in adipocytes from db/db mice. *FASEB J.* 18:1894–96
63. Hinault C, Mothe-Satney I, Gautier N, van Obberghen E. 2006. Amino acids require glucose to enhance, through phosphoinositide-dependent protein kinase 1, the insulin-activated protein kinase B cascade in insulin-resistant rat adipocytes. *Diabetologia* 49:1017–26
64. Holz MK, Blenis J. 2005. Identification of S6 kinase 1 as a novel mammalian target of rapamycin (mTOR)-phosphorylating kinase. *J. Biol. Chem.* 280:26089–93
65. Horie Y, Suzuki A, Kataoka E, Sasaki T, Hamada K, et al. 2004. Hepatocyte-specific Pten deficiency results in steatohepatitis and hepatocellular carcinomas. *J. Clin. Invest.* 113:1774–83
66. Hu FB. 2005. Protein, body weight, and cardiovascular health. *Am. J. Clin. Nutr.* 82:242–47S
67. Hubbard R, Kosch CL, Sanchez A, Sabate J, Berk L, Shavlik G. 1989. Effect of dietary protein on serum insulin and glucagon levels in hyper- and normocholesterolemic men. *Atherosclerosis* 76:55–61
68. Huffman TA, Mothe-Satney I, Lawrence JC Jr. 2002. Insulin-stimulated phosphorylation of lipin mediated by the mammalian target of rapamycin. *Proc. Natl. Acad. Sci. USA* 99:1047–52
69. Inoki K, Corradetti MN, Guan KL. 2005. Dysregulation of the TSC-mTOR pathway in human disease. *Nat. Genet.* 37:19–24
70. Inoki K, Li Y, Zhu T, Wu J, Guan KL. 2002. TSC2 is phosphorylated and inhibited by Akt and suppresses mTOR signalling. *Nat. Cell Biol.* 4:648–57
71. Inoki K, Zhu T, Guan KL. 2003. TSC2 mediates cellular energy response to control cell growth and survival. *Cell* 115:577–90
72. Iritani N, Sugimoto T, Fukuda H, Komiya M, Ikeda H. 1997. Dietary soybean protein increases insulin receptor gene expression in Wistar fatty rats when dietary polyunsaturated fatty acid level is low. *J. Nutr.* 127:1077–83
73. Jacques H, Noreau L, Moorjani S. 1992. Effects on plasma lipoproteins and endogenous sex hormones of substituting lean white fish for other animal-protein sources in diets of postmenopausal women. *Am. J. Clin. Nutr.* 55:896–901

74. Jousse C, Averous J, Bruhat A, Carraro V, Mordier S, Fafournoux P. 2004. Amino acids as regulators of gene expression: molecular mechanisms. *Biochem. Biophys. Res. Commun.* 313:447–52
75. Kabadi UM. 1991. Dose-kinetics of pancreatic alpha- and beta-cell responses to a protein meal in normal subjects. *Metabolism* 40:236–40
76. Khamzina L, Veilleux A, Bergeron S, Marette A. 2005. Increased activation of the mammalian target of rapamycin pathway in liver and skeletal muscle of obese rats: possible involvement in obesity-linked insulin resistance. *Endocrinology* 146:1473–81
77. Kim JE, Chen J. 2004. Regulation of peroxisome proliferator-activated receptor-gamma activity by mammalian target of rapamycin and amino acids in adipogenesis. *Diabetes* 53:2748–56
78. Kimball SR, Jefferson LS. 2006. New functions for amino acids: effects on gene transcription and translation. *Am. J. Clin. Nutr.* 83:500–7S
79. Koehnle TJ, Russell MC, Morin AS, Erecius LF, Gietzen DW. 2004. Diets deficient in indispensable amino acids rapidly decrease the concentration of the limiting amino acid in the anterior piriform cortex of rats. *J. Nutr.* 134:2365–71
80. Krebs M. 2005. Amino acid-dependent modulation of glucose metabolism in humans. *Eur. J. Clin. Invest.* 35:351–54
81. Krebs M, Brehm A, Krssak M, Anderwald C, Bernroider E, et al. 2003. Direct and indirect effects of amino acids on hepatic glucose metabolism in humans. *Diabetologia* 46:917–25
82. Krebs M, Krssak M, Bernroider E, Anderwald C, Brehm A, et al. 2002. Mechanism of amino acid-induced skeletal muscle insulin resistance in humans. *Diabetes* 51:599–605
83. Krieger JW, Sitren HS, Daniels MJ, Langkamp-Henken B. 2006. Effects of variation in protein and carbohydrate intake on body mass and composition during energy restriction: a meta-regression. *Am. J. Clin. Nutr.* 83:260–74
84. Kromann N, Green A. 1980. Epidemiological studies in the Upernavik district, Greenland. Incidence of some chronic diseases 1950–1974. *Acta Med. Scand.* 208:401–6
85. Kurlawalla-Martinez C, Stiles B, Wang Y, Devaskar SU, Kahn BB, Wu H. 2005. Insulin hypersensitivity and resistance to streptozotocin-induced diabetes in mice lacking PTEN in adipose tissue. *Mol. Cell Biol.* 25:2498–510
86. Lacaille B, Julien P, Deshaies Y, Lavigne C, Brun LD, Jacques H. 2000. Responses of plasma lipoproteins and sex hormones to the consumption of lean fish incorporated in a prudent-type diet in normolipidemic men. *J. Am. Coll. Nutr.* 19:745–53
87. Lavigne C, Marette A, Jacques H. 2000. Cod and soy proteins compared with casein improve glucose tolerance and insulin sensitivity in rats. *Am. J. Physiol. Endocrinol. Metab.* 278:E491–500
88. Lavigne C, Tremblay F, Asselin G, Jacques H, Marette A. 2001. Prevention of skeletal muscle insulin resistance by dietary cod protein in high fat-fed rats. *Am. J. Physiol. Endocrinol. Metab.* 281:E62–71
89. Lazar DF, Saltiel AR. 2006. Lipid phosphatases as drug discovery targets for type 2 diabetes. *Nat. Rev. Drug Discov.* 5:333–42
90. Li Y, Corradetti MN, Inoki K, Guan KL. 2004. TSC2: filling the GAP in the mTOR signaling pathway. *Trends Biochem. Sci.* 29:32–38
91. Linn T, Geyer R, Prassek S, Laube H. 1996. Effect of dietary protein intake on insulin secretion and glucose metabolism in insulin-dependent diabetes mellitus. *J. Clin. Endocrinol. Metab.* 81:3938–43
92. Linn T, Santosa B, Gronemeyer D, Aygen S, Scholz N, et al. 2000. Effect of long-term dietary protein intake on glucose metabolism in humans. *Diabetologia* 43:1257–65

93. Linn T, Strate C, Schneider K. 1999. Diet promotes beta-cell loss by apoptosis in prediabetic nonobese diabetic mice. *Endocrinology* 140:3767–73
94. Liu Z, Wu Y, Nicklas EW, Jahn LA, Price WJ, Barrett EJ. 2004. Unlike insulin, amino acids stimulate p70S6K but not GSK-3 or glycogen synthase in human skeletal muscle. *Am. J. Physiol. Endocrinol. Metab.* 286:E523–28
95. Lorincz AM, Sukumar S. 2006. Molecular links between obesity and breast cancer. *Endocr. Relat. Cancer* 13:279–92
96. Lynch CJ, Gern B, Lloyd C, Hutson SM, Eicher R, Vary TC. 2006. Leucine in food mediates some of the postprandial rise in plasma leptin concentrations. *Am. J. Physiol. Endocrinol. Metab.* 291:E621–30
97. Mamane Y, Petroulakis E, LeBacquer O, Sonenberg N. 2006. mTOR, translation initiation and cancer. *Oncogene* 25:6416–22
98. Marliss EB, Gougeon R. 2002. Diabetes mellitus, lipidus et. proteinus! *Diabet. Care* 25:1474–76
99. Marshall S, Garvey WT, Traxinger RR. 1991. New insights into the metabolic regulation of insulin action and insulin resistance: role of glucose and amino acids. *FASEB J.* 5:3031–36
100. Maurin AC, Jousse C, Averous J, Parry L, Bruhat A, et al. 2005. The GCN2 kinase biases feeding behavior to maintain amino acid homeostasis in omnivores. *Cell Metab.* 1:273–77
101. Minokoshi Y, Alquier T, Furukawa N, Kim YB, Lee A, et al. 2004. AMP-kinase regulates food intake by responding to hormonal and nutrient signals in the hypothalamus. *Nature* 428:569–74
102. Moran LJ, Luscombe-Marsh ND, Noakes M, Wittert GA, Keogh JB, Clifton PM. 2005. The satiating effect of dietary protein is unrelated to postprandial ghrelin secretion. *J. Clin. Endocrinol. Metab.* 90:5205–11
103. Morley JE, Thomas DR, Wilson MM. 2006. Cachexia: pathophysiology and clinical relevance. *Am. J. Clin. Nutr.* 83:735–43
104. Mouratoff GJ, Carroll NV, Scott EM. 1969. Diabetes mellitus in Athabaskan Indians in Alaska. *Diabetes* 18:29–32
105. Mouratoff GJ, Scott EM. 1973. Diabetes mellitus in Eskimos after a decade. *JAMA* 226:1345–46
106. Nair KS, Halliday D, Garrow JS. 1983. Thermic response to isoenergetic protein, carbohydrate or fat meals in lean and obese subjects. *Clin. Sci. (Lond.)* 65:307–12
107. Nave BT, Ouwens M, Withers DJ, Alessi DR, Shepherd PR. 1999. Mammalian target of rapamycin is a direct target for protein kinase B: identification of a convergence point for opposing effects of insulin and amino-acid deficiency on protein translation. *Biochem. J.* 344:427–31
108. Nishitani S, Takehana K, Fujitani S, Sonaka I. 2005. Branched-chain amino acids improve glucose metabolism in rats with liver cirrhosis. *Am. J. Physiol. Gastrointest. Liver Physiol.* 288:G1292–300
109. Nobukuni T, Joaquin M, Roccio M, Dann SG, Kim SY, et al. 2005. Amino acids mediate mTOR/raptor signaling through activation of class 3 phosphatidylinositol 3OH-kinase. *Proc. Natl. Acad. Sci. USA* 102:14238–43
110. Ohneda A, Parada E, Eisentraut AM, Unger RH. 1968. Characterization of response of circulating glucagon to intraduodenal and intravenous administration of amino acids. *J. Clin. Invest.* 47:2305–22
111. Patti ME, Brambilla E, Luzi L, Landaker EJ, Kahn CR. 1998. Bidirectional modulation of insulin action by amino acids. *J. Clin. Invest.* 101:1519–29

112. Patti ME, Virkamaki A, Landaker EJ, Kahn CR, Yki-Jarvinen H. 1999. Activation of the hexosamine pathway by glucosamine in vivo induces insulin resistance of early postreceptor insulin signaling events in skeletal muscle. *Diabetes* 48:1562–71
113. Peterfy M, Phan J, Xu P, Reue K. 2001. Lipodystrophy in the *fld* mouse results from mutation of a new gene encoding a nuclear protein, lipin. *Nat. Genet.* 27:121–24
114. Peters AL, Davidson MB. 1993. Protein and fat effects on glucose responses and insulin requirements in subjects with insulin-dependent diabetes mellitus. *Am. J. Clin. Nutr.* 58:555–60
115. Petzke KJ, Riese C, Klaus S. 2007. Short-term, increasing dietary protein and fat moderately affect energy expenditure, substrate oxidation and uncoupling protein gene expression in rats. *J. Nutr. Biochem.* In press
116. Peyrollier K, Hajduch E, Blair AS, Hyde R, Hundal HS. 2000. L-leucine availability regulates phosphatidylinositol 3-kinase, p70 S6 kinase and glycogen synthase kinase-3 activity in L6 muscle cells: evidence for the involvement of the mammalian target of rapamycin (mTOR) pathway in the L-leucine-induced up-regulation of system A amino acid transport. *Biochem. J.* 350(Pt. 2):361–68
117. Phan J, Peterfy M, Reue K. 2004. Lipin expression preceding peroxisome proliferator-activated receptor-gamma is critical for adipogenesis in vivo and in vitro. *J. Biol. Chem.* 279:29558–64
118. Pisters PW, Restifo NP, Cersosimo E, Brennan MF. 1991. The effects of euglycemic hyperinsulinemia and amino acid infusion on regional and whole body glucose disposal in man. *Metabolism* 40:59–65
119. Post-Skagegard M, Vessby B, Karlstrom B. 2006. Glucose and insulin responses in healthy women after intake of composite meals containing cod-, milk-, and soy protein. *Eur. J. Clin. Nutr.* 60:949–54
120. Presti JCJ. 2005. Obesity and prostate cancer. *Curr. Opin. Urol.* 15:13–16
121. Reiling JH, Sabatini DM. 2006. Stress and mTORture signaling. *Oncogene* 25:6373–83
122. Remer T, Pietrzik K, Manz F. 1996. A moderate increase in daily protein intake causing an enhanced endogenous insulin secretion does not alter circulating levels or urinary excretion of dehydroepiandrosterone sulfate. *Metabolism* 45:1483–86
123. Roh C, Han J, Tzatsos A, Kandror KV. 2003. Nutrient-sensing mTOR-mediated pathway regulates leptin production in isolated rat adipocytes. *Am. J. Physiol. Endocrinol. Metab.* 284:E322–30
124. Rossetti L, Rothman DL, DeFronzo RA, Shulman GI. 1989. Effect of dietary protein on in vivo insulin action and liver glycogen repletion. *Am. J. Physiol.* 257:E212–19
125. Sanchez A, Hubbard RW. 1991. Plasma amino acids and the insulin/glucagon ratio as an explanation for the dietary protein modulation of atherosclerosis. *Med. Hypotheses* 35:324–29
126. Schneider K, Laube H, Linn T. 1996. A diet enriched in protein accelerates diabetes manifestation in NOD mice. *Acta Diabetol.* 33:236–40
127. Scott PH, Brunn GJ, Kohn AD, Roth RA, Lawrence JC Jr. 1998. Evidence of insulin-stimulated phosphorylation and activation of the mammalian target of rapamycin mediated by a protein kinase B signaling pathway. *Proc. Natl. Acad. Sci. USA* 95:7772–77
128. Shah OJ, Anthony JC, Kimball SR, Jefferson LS. 2000. 4E-BP1 and S6K1: translational integration sites for nutritional and hormonal information in muscle. *Am. J. Physiol. Endocrinol. Metab.* 279:715–29
129. Shah OJ, Hunter T. 2005. Tuberous sclerosis and insulin resistance. Unlikely bedfellows reveal a TORrid affair. *Cell Cycle* 4:46–51

130. Shah OJ, Hunter T. 2006. Turnover of the active fraction of IRS1 involves raptor-mTOR- and S6K1-dependent serine phosphorylation in cell culture models of tuberous sclerosis. *Mol. Cell Biol.* 26:6425–34
131. Shah OJ, Wang Z, Hunter T. 2004. Inappropriate activation of the TSC/Rheb/mTOR/S6K cassette induces IRS1/2 depletion, insulin resistance, and cell survival deficiencies. *Curr. Biol.* 14:1650–56
132. Shaw RJ, Bardeesy N, Manning BD, Lopez L, Kosmatka M, et al. 2004. The LKB1 tumor suppressor negatively regulates mTOR signaling. *Cancer Cell* 6:91–99
133. Shaw RJ, Cantley LC. 2006. Ras, PI(3)K and mTOR signalling controls tumour cell growth. *Nature* 441:424–30
134. Shaw RJ, Kosmatka M, Bardeesy N, Hurley RL, Witters LA, et al. 2004. The tumor suppressor LKB1 kinase directly activates AMP-activated kinase and regulates apoptosis in response to energy stress. *Proc. Natl. Acad. Sci. USA* 101:3329–35
135. Shaw RJ, Lamia KA, Vasquez D, Koo SH, Bardeesy N, et al. 2005. The kinase LKB1 mediates glucose homeostasis in liver and therapeutic effects of metformin. *Science* 310:1642–46
136. Siegel EG, Trapp VE, Wollheim CB, Renold AE, Schmidt FH. 1980. Beneficial effects of low-carbohydrate, high-protein diets in long-term diabetic rats. *Metabolism* 29:421–28
137. Soucy J, Leblanc J. 1999. The effects of a beef and fish meal on plasma amino acids, insulin and glucagon levels. *Nutr. Res.* 19:17–24
138. Spiller GA, Jensen CD, Pattison TS, Chuck CS, Whittam JH, Scala J. 1987. Effect of protein dose on serum glucose and insulin response to sugars. *Am. J. Clin. Nutr.* 46:474–80
139. Sugano M, Ishiwaki N, Nagata Y, Imaizumi K. 1982. Effects of arginine and lysine addition to casein and soya-bean protein on serum lipids, apolipoproteins, insulin and glucagon in rats. *Br. J. Nutr.* 48:211–21
140. Takano A, Usui I, Haruta T, Kawahara J, Uno T, et al. 2001. Mammalian target of rapamycin pathway regulates insulin signaling via subcellular redistribution of insulin receptor substrate 1 and integrates nutritional signals and metabolic signals of insulin. *Mol. Cell Biol.* 21:5050–62
141. Tang QQ, Lane MD. 2000. Role of C/EBP homologous protein (CHOP-10) in the programmed activation of CCAAT/enhancer-binding protein-beta during adipogenesis. *Proc. Natl. Acad. Sci. USA* 97:12446–50
142. Tannous dit EK, Obeid O, Azar ST, Hwalla N. 2006. Variations in postprandial ghrelin status following ingestion of high-carbohydrate, high-fat, and high-protein meals in males. *Ann. Nutr. Metab.* 50:260–69
143. Tessari P, Inchiostro S, Biolo G, Duner E, Nosadini R, et al. 1985. Hyperaminoacidaemia reduces insulin-mediated glucose disposal in healthy man. *Diabetologia* 28:870–72
144. Traxinger RR, Marshall S. 1989. Role of amino acids in modulating glucose-induced desensitization of the glucose transport system. *J. Biol. Chem.* 264:20910–16
145. Tremblay F, Dubois MJ, Marette A. 2003. Regulation of GLUT4 traffic and function by insulin and contraction in skeletal muscle. *Front. Biosci.* 8:d1072–84
146. Tremblay F, Gagnon A, Veilleux A, Sorisky A, Marette A. 2005. Activation of the mammalian target of rapamycin pathway acutely inhibits insulin signaling to Akt and glucose transport in 3T3-L1 and human adipocytes. *Endocrinology* 146:1328–37
147. Tremblay F, Krebs M, Dombrowski L, Brehm A, Bernroider E, et al. 2005. Overactivation of s6 kinase 1 as a cause of human insulin resistance during increased amino acid availability. *Diabetes* 54:2674–84

148. Tremblay F, Lavigne C, Jacques H, Marette A. 2003. Dietary cod protein restores insulin-induced activation of phosphatidylinositol 3-kinase/Akt and GLUT4 translocation to the T-tubules in skeletal muscle of high-fat-fed obese rats. *Diabetes* 52:29–37
149. Tremblay F, Marette A. 2001. Amino acid and insulin signaling via the mTOR/p70 S6 kinase pathway. A negative feedback mechanism leading to insulin resistance in skeletal muscle cells. *J. Biol. Chem.* 276:38052–60
150. Tsukiyama-Kohara K, Poulin F, Kohara M, DeMaria CT, Cheng A, et al. 2001. Adipose tissue reduction in mice lacking the translational inhibitor 4E-BP1. *Nat. Med.* 7:1128–32
151. Um SH, D'Alessio D, Thomas G. 2006. Nutrient overload, insulin resistance, and ribosomal protein S6 kinase 1, S6K1. *Cell Metab.* 3:393–402
152. Um SH, Frigerio F, Watanabe M, Picard F, Joaquin M, et al. 2004. Absence of S6K1 protects against age- and diet-induced obesity while enhancing insulin sensitivity. *Nature* 431:200–5
153. Wang X, Campbell LE, Miller CM, Proud CG. 1998. Amino acid availability regulates p70 S6 kinase and multiple translation factors. *Biochem. J.* 334:261–67
154. Wang X, Hu Z, Hu J, Du J, Mitch WE. 2006. Insulin resistance accelerates muscle protein degradation: activation of the ubiquitin-proteasome pathway by defects in muscle cell signaling. *Endocrinology* 147:4160–68
155. Weigle DS, Breen PA, Matthys CC, Callahan HS, Meeuws KE, et al. 2005. A high-protein diet induces sustained reductions in appetite, ad libitum caloric intake, and body weight despite compensatory changes in diurnal plasma leptin and ghrelin concentrations. *Am. J. Clin. Nutr.* 82:41–48
156. Wijesekara N, Konrad D, Eweida M, Jefferies C, Liadis N, et al. 2005. Muscle-specific Pten deletion protects against insulin resistance and diabetes. *Mol. Cell Biol.* 25:1135–45
157. Wullschleger S, Loewith R, Hall MN. 2006. TOR signaling in growth and metabolism. *Cell* 124:471–84
158. Xu G, Kwon G, Marshall CA, Lin TA, Lawrence JC Jr, McDaniel ML. 1998. Branched-chain amino acids are essential in the regulation of PHAS-I and p70 S6 kinase by pancreatic beta-cells. A possible role in protein translation and mitogenic signaling. *J. Biol. Chem.* 273:28178–84
159. Yeh WC, Bierer BE, McKnight SL. 1995. Rapamycin inhibits clonal expansion and adipogenic differentiation of 3T3-L1 cells. *Proc. Natl. Acad. Sci. USA* 92:11086–90
160. Zakikhani M, Dowling R, Fantus IG, Sonenberg N, Pollak M. 2006. Metformin is an AMP kinase-dependent growth inhibitor for breast cancer cells. *Cancer Res.* 66:10269–73
161. Zhang HH, Lipovsky AI, Dibble CC, Sahin M, Manning BD. 2006. S6K1 regulates GSK3 under conditions of mTOR-dependent feedback inhibition of Akt. *Mol. Cell* 24:185–97
162. Zhou G, Myers R, Li Y, Chen Y, Shen X, et al. 2001. Role of AMP-activated protein kinase in mechanism of metformin action. *J. Clin. Invest.* 108:1167–74
163. Zick Y. 2001. Insulin resistance: a phosphorylation-based uncoupling of insulin signaling. *Trends Cell Biol.* 11:437–41

Effects of Brain Evolution on Human Nutrition and Metabolism

William R. Leonard,[1] J. Josh Snodgrass,[2] and Marcia L. Robertson[1]

[1]Department of Anthropology, Northwestern University, Evanston, Illinois 60208,
[2]Department of Anthropology, University of Oregon, Eugene, Oregon 97403;
email: w-leonard1@northwestern.edu

Annu. Rev. Nutr. 2007. 27:311–27

First published online as a Review in Advance on April 17, 2007

The *Annual Review of Nutrition* is online at http://nutr.annualreviews.org

This article's doi:
10.1146/annurev.nutr.27.061406.093659

0199-9885/07/0821-0311$20.00

Key Words

encephalization, hominin, diet quality, body composition, *Homo erectus*

Abstract

The evolution of large human brain size has had important implications for the nutritional biology of our species. Large brains are energetically expensive, and humans expend a larger proportion of their energy budget on brain metabolism than other primates. The high costs of large human brains are supported, in part, by our energy- and nutrient-rich diets. Among primates, relative brain size is positively correlated with dietary quality, and humans fall at the positive end of this relationship. Consistent with an adaptation to a high-quality diet, humans have relatively small gastrointestinal tracts. In addition, humans are relatively "undermuscled" and "over fat" compared with other primates, features that help to offset the high energy demands of our brains. Paleontological evidence indicates that rapid brain evolution occurred with the emergence of *Homo erectus* 1.8 million years ago and was associated with important changes in diet, body size, and foraging behavior.

Contents

INTRODUCTION

Encephalization: brain size in relation to body size. In general, primates are more encephalized than other mammals

RMR: resting metabolic rate

GI: gastrointestinal

Over the past 20 years, the evolution of human nutritional requirements has received ever greater attention among both anthropologists and nutritional scientists (3, 21, 28, 29, 35, 48, 49, 86). Increasingly, we have come to understand that many of the key features that distinguish humans from other primates (e.g., our bipedal form of locomotion and large brain sizes) have important implications for our distinctive nutritional needs (3, 47, 50). The most important of these is our high levels of encephalization (large brain:body mass). The energy demands (kcal/g/min) of brain and other neural tissues are extremely high—approximately 16 times that of skeletal muscle (37, 43). Consequently, the evolution of large brain size in the human lineage came at a very high metabolic cost.

Despite the fact that humans have much larger brains per body weight in comparison with other primates or terrestrial mammals, the resting energy demands for the human body are no more than for any other mammal of the same size (48, 49). The consequence of this paradox is that humans allocate a much larger share of their daily energy budget to "feed their brains." Brain metabolism accounts for ~20% to 25% of resting metabolic rate (RMR) in an adult human body. This is far more than the 8% to 10% observed in other primate species and still more than the 3% to 5% allocated to the brain by other (nonprimate) mammals (49).

The disproportionately large allocation of our energy budget to brain metabolism has important implications for our dietary needs. This review draws on both analyses of living primate species and the human fossil record to examine the avenues through which humans have adapted to the metabolic demands of greater encephalization. We begin by considering the energy demands associated with large brain size in modern humans relative to other primates and nonprimate mammals. Next we examine comparative dietary data for modern human groups and other primate species to evaluate the influence that variation in relative brain size has on dietary patterns among modern primates. We then turn to an examination of the human fossil record to examine when and under what conditions in our evolutionary past key changes in brain size and diet likely took place. Finally, we explore how the evolution of large human brains was likely accommodated by differential changes in the relative sizes of other organs [e.g., muscle, fat, and gastrointestinal (GI) tract]. The high metabolic costs of our large brains appear to play a strong hand in shaping distinctive aspects of human growth and development.

COMPARATIVE PERSPECTIVES ON BRAIN SIZE, BODY SIZE, DIET, AND METABOLIC RATE

Table 1 presents comparative data on RMR, brain size, body size, and diet for living humans and nonhuman primates (from 51). Primates, as a group, are similar to other mammals in having RMRs that scale to approximately three-fourths power of body mass (see 44). **Figure 1** (see color insert) presents the relationship of RMR (kcal/day) and body

Table 1 Comparative data on resting metabolic rate (RMR; kcal/day), body mass (kg), brain mass (g), and diet quality (DQ) in 41 primate species[a]

Species	Metabolic data		Brain data		DQ
	RMR (kcal/d)	Body mass (kg)	Brain mass (g)	Body mass (kg)	
Alouatta palliata	231.9	4.670	51	6.400	136
Aotus trivirgatus	52.4	1.020	16	0.850	177.5
Arctocebus calabarensis	15.2	0.206	7.2	0.323	327.5
Callithrix geoffroyi	27.0	0.225	7.6	0.280	235
Callithrix jacchus	22.8	0.356	7.6	0.280	235
Cebuella pygmaea	10.1	0.105	4.5	0.140	249.5
Cercopithecus mitis	407.7	8.500	76	6.500	201.5
Cercocebus torquatus	196.2	4.000	104	7.900	234
Cheirogaleus medius	22.7	0.300	3.1	0.177	
Colobus guereza	357.9	10.450	73	7.000	126
Erythrocebus patas	186.9	3.000	118	8.000	
Eulemur fulvus	42.0	2.397	25.2	2.397	129
Euoticus elegantulus	25.1	0.260	7.2	0.274	230
Galago moholi	13.9	0.155			
Galago senegalensis	18.1	0.215	4.8	0.186	278
Galagoides demidoff	6.3	0.058	3.4	0.081	305
Homo sapiens	1400.0	53.500	1295	53.500	263
Hylobates lar	123.4	1.900	102	6.000	181
Lemur catta	45.1	2.678	25.6	2.678	166
Leontopithecus rosalia	51.1	0.718			
Lepilemur ruficaudatus	27.6	0.682	7.6	0.682	149
Loris tardigradus	14.8	0.284	6.6	0.322	327.5
Macaca fascicularis	400.9	7.100	74	5.500	200
Macaca fuscata	485.4	9.580	84	5.900	223
Macaca mulatta	231.9	5.380	110	8.000	159
Microcebus murinus	4.9	0.054	1.8	0.054	
Nycticebus coucang	32.4	1.380	12.5	0.800	
Otolemur crassicaudatus	47.6	0.950	10.3	0.850	195
Otolemur garnettii	47.8	1.028	275		
Pan troglodytes	581.9	18.300	420	46.000	178
Papio anubis	342.9	9.500	205	26.000	207
Papio cynacephalus	668.9	14.300	195	19.000	184
Papio papio	297.3	6.230	190	18.000	
Papio ursinus	589.3	16.620	190	18.000	189.5
Perodicticus potto	41.3	1.000	14	1.150	190
Pongo pygmaeus	569.1	16.200	370	55.000	172.5
Propithecus verreauxi	86.8	3.080	26.7	3.480	200
Saguinus geoffroyi	50.5	0.500	10	3.800	263
Saimiri sciureus	68.8	0.850	22	6.800	323
Tarsius syrichta	8.9	0.113	350		
Varecia variegata	69.9	3.512	34.2	3.512	

[a]Data sources: References 8, 40, 42, 49, 58, 69, 70, 72, 79, and 85.

Scaling (allometry): the change in size on biological measure with respect to another biological measure (often body size)

DQ: diet quality

mass (kg) for humans and the 40 other primate species from **Table 1**. It is clear that humans conform to the general primate scaling relationship between RMR and body weight, having RMRs that fall within 2% of the value predicted from the general primate relationship. The implication of this is that humans allocate a much larger share of our daily energy budget for brain metabolism than do other species.

The disproportionately high energy costs of our large brains are evident in **Figure 2** (see color insert), which shows the scaling relationship between brain weight (grams) and RMR for humans and 35 other primate species (from **Table 1**) and 22 nonprimate mammalian species. The solid line denotes the best-fit regression for nonhuman primate species, and the dashed line denotes the best-fit regression for the nonprimate mammals. The slopes of the two regressions are similar (0.94 primates, 0.90 mammals; n.s.), whereas the y-intercepts are significantly different (−0.377 primates, −0.832 mammals; $P < 0.01$). Thus, at a given metabolic rate, primates have systematically larger brain sizes than those of other mammals, and humans, in turn, have larger brain sizes than do other primates. As a group, primates have brains that are approximately three times the size of brains of other mammals. Human brain sizes are some three times those of other primates.

The large allocation of our energy budget to brain metabolism raises the question of how humans are nutritionally able to accommodate the metabolic demands of our large brains. Recent work suggests that important dimensions of human nutritional biology are associated with the high energy demands of our large brains. It appears that humans consume diets that are denser in energy and nutrients in comparison with diets of other primates of similar size. Recent studies have shown that modern human foraging populations typically derive more than half of their dietary energy intake from animal foods, although considerable variation in diets exists (20, 41). In comparison, modern great apes obtain much of their diet from low-quality plant foods. Gorillas derive more than 80% of their diet from fibrous foods such as leaves and bark (69). Even among common chimpanzees (*Pan troglodytes*), only about 5% to 10% of calories are derived from vertebrate animal foods (62, 78, 84). Field studies indicate that meat is a desirable and prized food item for many primate species. The low rates of consumption reflect the limited ability of chimpanzees and other primates to obtain large and consistent quantities of vertebrate foods because of high foraging costs (61). That is, the time and energy associated with pursuing game animals appear to be prohibitively high for most large-bodied primates.

Comparative dietary analyses of living primate species (including humans) are shown in **Figure 3** (see color insert), which plots dietary quality (DQ) as function of body mass (kg) for 33 different primate species (from **Table 1**). The DQ index was developed by Sailer et al. (72) and quantifies the energy and nutrient density of the diet based on the relative proportions of structural plant parts (***s***; e.g., leaves, stem, bark), reproductive plant parts (***r***; e.g., fruits, flowers), and animal foods (***a***; vertebrates and invertebrates):

$$DQ = s + 2r + 3.5a$$

The index ranges from a minimum of 100 (a diet of all leaves and/or structural plant parts) to 350 (a diet of all animal material).

Figure 3 shows that an inverse relationship exists between DQ and body mass ($r = -0.59$ total sample, −0.68 nonhuman primates only; $P < 0.001$). This tendency of larger primates to feed on lower-quality diets is something that is observed in other mammals (10, 39) and appears to be a consequence of the scaling relationship between energy requirements and body mass. As noted in **Figure 1**, the scaling coefficient between RMR and mass is less than one, implying that larger primates have proportionally lower metabolic rates than smaller ones. Large primates such as gorillas (*Gorilla gorilla*) and orangutans (*Pongo pygmaeus*) have high total energy requirements but relatively low mass-specific needs (e.g., kcal/kg/day). They fulfill their energy needs by feeding on foods that are abundant but low in quality (e.g., leaves and foliage). Conversely, small animals [e.g., the pygmy marmoset (*Cebuella pygmaea*)] have low total energy requirements but very high mass-specific needs. They typically subsist on foods that are rich in calories and nutrients but relatively limited in abundance (e.g., saps, gums, and insects).

Humans, however, have substantially higher-quality diets than would be expected for a primate of our size. Note that the average diet for modern human foragers (based on dietary data from five modern human foraging populations; see 49) falls substantially above the regression line. Overall, the staple foods for *all* human societies are much more nutritionally dense than those of other large-bodied primates. This higher-quality diet for humans relative to other large-bodied primates means that we need to eat a smaller volume of food to get the energy and nutrients we require.

Figure 4 (see color insert) shows relative brain size versus relative dietary quality for the 33 different primate species from **Figure 3**. Relative brain size for each species is measured as the standardized residual (z-score) from the primate brain versus body mass regression, and relative DQ is measured as the residual from the DQ versus body mass regression. There is a strong positive relationship ($r = 0.63$; $P < 0.001$) between the amount of energy allocated to the brain and the caloric and nutrient density of the diet. Across all primates, larger brains require higher-quality diets. Humans fall at the positive extremes for both parameters, having the largest relative brain size ($z = +3.27$) and the highest quality diet ($z = +2.05$). Thus, the large, metabolically expensive human brain is partially offset by the consumption of an energy-dense and nutrient-rich diet. This relationship implies that the evolution of larger hominin brains would have necessitated the adoption of a sufficiently high-quality diet (including meat and energy-rich fruits) to support the increased metabolic demands of greater encephalization.

The relative size and morphology of the human GI tract also reflect our high-quality diet. Most large-bodied primates have expanded large intestines (colons), an adaptation to fibrous, low-quality diets (59). Humans, on the other hand, have small gut volumes for our size, with relatively enlarged small intestines and a smaller colon (3, 53, 75).

The enlarged colons of most large-bodied primates permits fermentation of low-quality plant fibers, allowing for extraction of additional energy in the form of volatile fatty acids (60, 63). In contrast, the GI morphology of humans (small colon and relatively enlarged small intestine) is more similar to a carnivore and reflects an adaptation to an easily digested, nutrient-rich diet (52, 53, 81).

Together, these comparative data suggest that the dramatic expansion of brain size over the course of human evolution likely would have required the consumption of a diet that was more concentrated in energy and nutrients than is typically the case for most large primates. This does not imply that dietary change was the driving force behind major brain expansion during human evolution. Rather, the available evidence indicates that a sufficiently high-quality diet was probably a necessary condition for supporting the metabolic demands associated with evolving larger hominin brains.

Hominin: living humans and our fossil ancestors that lived after the last common ancestor between humans and apes

EVOLUTIONARY CHANGES IN BRAIN SIZE AND DIET

Trends in the Hominin Brain Size, Body Size, and Tooth Size

Over the past four million years, average brain size in the hominin lineage has more than tripled, increasing from approximately 400 cm^3 in the earliest australopithecines to 1300–1400 cm^3 in modern humans (57). However, the rates of evolutionary change in brain size have been highly variable over this

Table 2 Geological ages (millions of years ago), brain size (cm^3), estimated male and female body weights (kg), and postcanine tooth surface areas (mm^2) for selected fossil hominid species

Species	Geological age (mya)	Brain size (cm^3)	Body weight		Postcanine tooth surface area (mm^2)
			Male (kg)	Female (kg)	
A. afarensis	3.9–3.0	438	45	29	460
A. africanus	3.0–2.4	452	41	30	516
A. boisei	2.3–1.4	521	49	34	756
A. robustus	1.9–1.4	530	40	32	588
Homo habilis (sensu strictu)	1.9–1.6	612	37	32	478
H. erectus (early)	1.8–1.5	863	66	54	377
H. erectus (late)	0.5–0.3	980	60	55	390
H. sapiens	0.4–0.0	1350	58	49	334

All data, except for *Homo erectus*, from (57). Early *H. erectus* brain size is the average of African specimens as presented in (56), Indonesian specimens from (5), and Georgian specimens from (31, 32). Data for late *H. erectus* are from (55).

period. Human evolution has been characterized by periods of slow increases in brain size alternating with periods of dramatic change. The human fossil record indicates that the first substantial burst of evolutionary change in hominin brain size occurred about 2.0 to 1.7 million years ago (mya) and was associated with the emergence and evolution of early members of our own genus, *Homo*.

Table 2 presents data on evolutionary changes in hominin brain size (cm^3), estimated adult male and female body mass (kg), and posterior tooth area (mm^2) (data from 5, 31, 32, 55–57). Hominin body masses were estimated from measurements of weight-bearing joint surfaces using predictive equations derived from a diverse skeletal sample of modern humans (see 54). Posterior tooth areas are the summed surface areas of the premolar and molar teeth (57).

The australopithecines showed only modest brain size evolution from about 430 to 530 cm^3 over more than two million years (from about 4 to 1.5 mya). With the evolution of the genus *Homo* there were substantial increases in encephalization, with brain sizes of over 600 cm^3 in *Homo habilis* (at 1.9 to 1.6 mya) and 800 to 900 cm^3 in early members of *Homo erectus* (at 1.8 to 1.5 mya). Although body sizes also increase with *H. erectus*, the changes in brain size are disproportionately greater than those in body mass. Thus, the level of encephalization we find with *H. erectus* is greater than that seen among any living nonhuman primate species today (49).

Australopithecus: genus of early hominins that existed in Africa between 4 and 1.2 mya

The changes in the craniofacial and dental anatomy of *H. erectus* suggest that these forms were consuming different foods from those consumed by its australopithecine relatives. During the evolution of the australopithecines, the total surface area of the grinding teeth increased dramatically from 460 mm^2 in *Australopithecus afarensis* to 756 mm^2 in *A. boisei*. In contrast, with the emergence of early *Homo* at approximately 2 mya, we see marked reductions in the posterior dentition. Postcanine tooth surface area is 478 mm^2 in *H. habilis* and 377 mm^2 in early *H. erectus*.

H. erectus also shows substantial reductions in craniofacial and mandibular robusticity relative to the australopithecines (91). Yet, despite having smaller teeth and jaws, *H. erectus* was a much bigger animal than the australopithecines, being humanlike in its stature, body mass, and body proportions (54, 55, 57, 71). Together, these features indicate that early *H. erectus* was consuming a richer, more calorically dense diet with less low-quality fibrous plant material. How the diet might have changed with the emergence of *H. erectus* is examined in the following section.

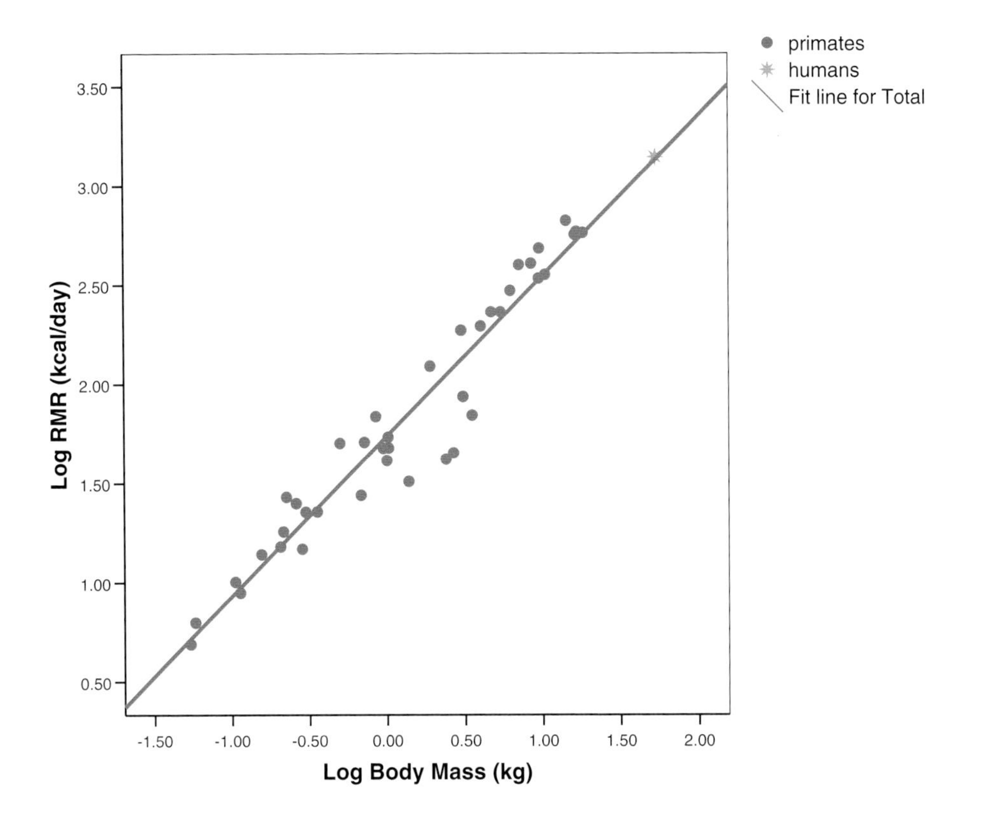

Figure 1

Log-Log plot of resting metabolic rate (RMR; kcal/day) versus body mass (kg) for 41 species of primates (including humans). Humans conform to the general primate scaling relationship [$RMR = 55(Wt^{0.81})$]. Adapted from Reference 51.

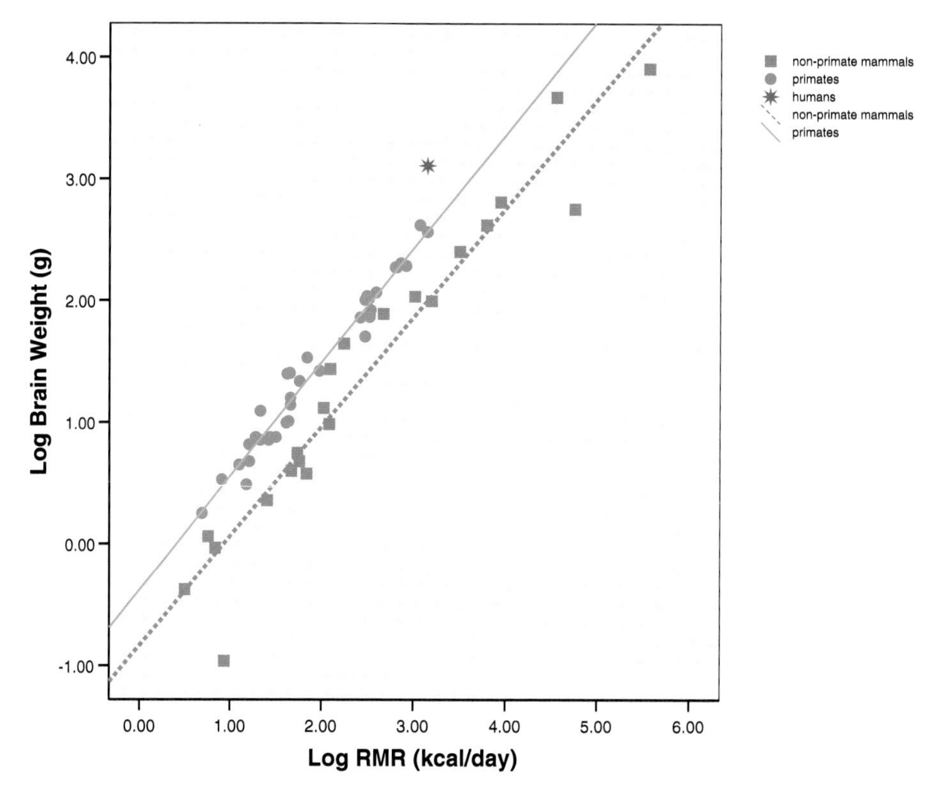

Figure 2

Log-Log plot of brain weight (BW; g) versus resting metabolic rate (RMR) (kcal/day) for humans, 35 other primate species, and 22 species of nonprimate mammals. The primate regression line (*solid*) is elevated systematically and significantly above the nonprimate mammal regression (*dashed*) (y-intercepts = −0.377primates, −0.832mammals; $P < 0.01$). The scaling relationships for nonprimate mammals are $BW = 0.14 (RMR^{0.90})$; primates, $BW = 0.42 (RMR^{0.94})$. Thus, for a given RMR, primates have brain sizes that are approximately three times those of other mammals, and humans have brains that are three times those of other primates.

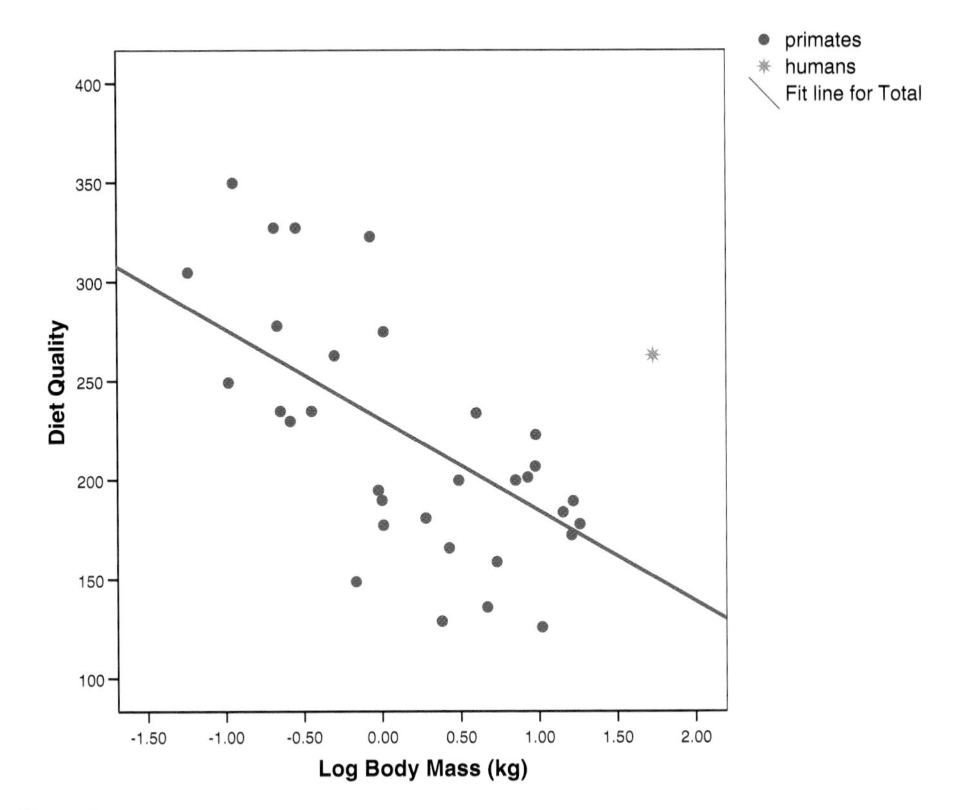

Figure 3

Plot of diet quality (DQ) versus log-body mass for 33 primate species. DQ is inversely related to body mass ($r = -0.59$ total sample, -0.68 nonhuman primates only; $P < 0.001$), indicating that smaller primates consume relatively higher-quality diets. Humans have systematically higher-quality diets than predicted for their size.

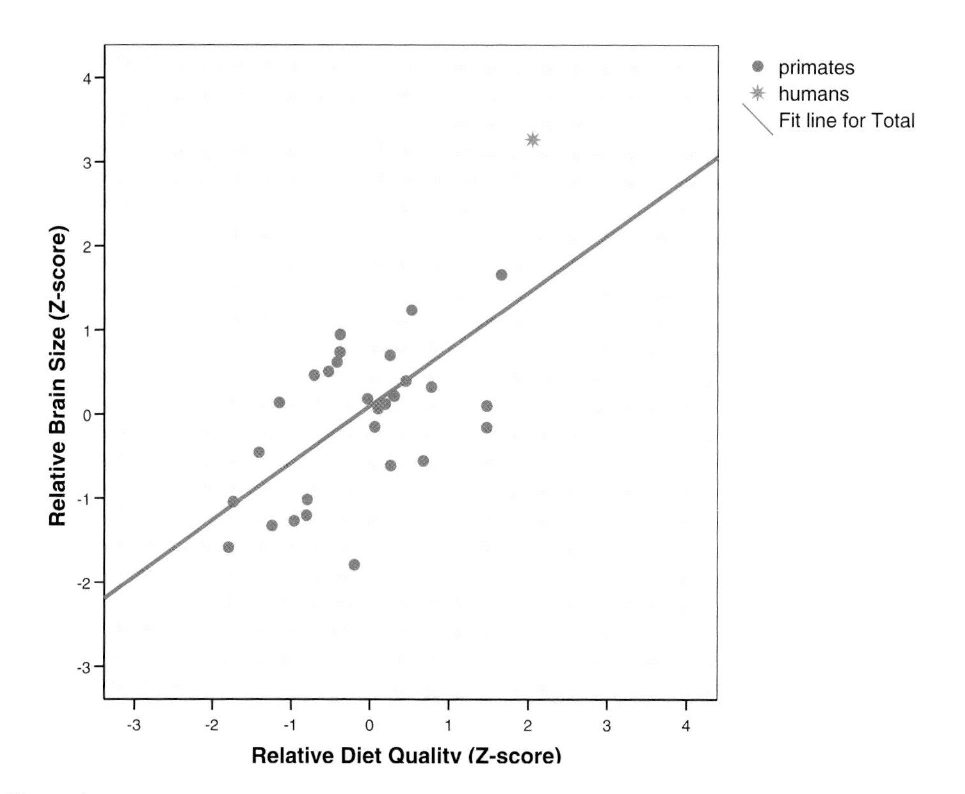

Figure 4

Plot of relative brain size versus relative diet quality for 33 primate species. Primates with higher-quality diets for their size have relatively larger brain size ($r = 0.63$; $P < 0.001$). Humans represent the positive extremes for both measures, having large brain:body size and a substantially higher-quality diet than would be expected for their size.

Dietary Changes Associated with Brain Evolution in Early *Homo*

Increasing evidence suggests that the evolution of early *Homo*, particularly *H. erectus*, was associated with important changes in foraging patterns and dietary consumption compared with earlier hominin species. Recent analyses of dental microwear and stable carbon isotope levels of tooth enamel indicate that the australopithecines consumed a seasonally variable diet composed of both plant (e.g., fruits, seeds, grasses, and tubers) and some animal foods (76, 77, 83). Earlier interpretations of the so-called "robust" australopithecines (*A. robustus* and *A. boisei*)—with their massive jaws, robust faces, and large molar teeth—viewed these species as being dietary specialists that subsisted largely on seeds, nuts, and other hard objects common to the African savanna. However, the isotopic analyses now show that their diets were likely broader and more varied than previously thought (76, 77, 87). The consumption by australopithecines of limited quantities of animal foods (including invertebrates) is suggested by analogies with living primates (especially chimpanzees) and supported by stable isotope studies and association with putative bone tools likely used for termite extraction (7).

Paleontological and archaeological evidence indicates modest dietary change in earliest *Homo* (i.e., *H. habilis*); this species likely incorporated more animal foods in its diet, although the relative amounts obtained through hunting compared with scavenging are debated (12, 13, 36, 65). Evidence for dietary change in this species can be seen in the reduced masticatory functional complex (e.g., posterior tooth size); dental reduction in *H. habilis* reversed successive increases in cheek tooth size among the australopithecines (57). Technological advancements, such as the development of Oldowan industry tools, allowed easier processing of vertebrate carcasses and increased access to meat as well as energy- and nutrient-rich marrow and brains (74).

The evolution of *H. erectus* appears to be a major adaptive shift in human evolution. With the emergence of *H. erectus* in East Africa 1.8 mya we find (*a*) marked increases in brain and body size, (*b*) reductions of posterior tooth size and craniofacial robusticity, (*c*) the evolution of humanlike limb proportions, and (*d*) important changes in foraging/subsistence behavior (2, 4, 91, 92). These changes occurred within the context of large-scale climatic shifts (88, 95). The environment was becoming much drier, resulting in declines in forested areas and an expansion of open woodlands and grasslands (14, 26, 68, 95). Such a transformation of the African landscape would have strongly influenced the distribution of food resources for our hominin ancestors, making animal foods more abundant and thus an increasingly attractive food resource (9, 65). Using modern tropical ecosystems as our reference, we have found that although savanna/grasslands have much lower net primary (energetic) productivity than do woodlands (4050 versus 7200 kcal/m^2/yr), the level of herbivore productivity in savannas is almost three times that of the woodlands (10.2 versus 3.6 kcal/m^2/yr) (50). Thus, fundamental changes in ecosystem structure 2.0 to 1.8 mya appear to have resulted in a net increase in the energetic abundance of grazing mammals (e.g., ungulates) on the E. African landscape. Such an increase would have offered an opportunity for hominins with sufficient behavioral and technological capability to exploit those resources.

Oldowan: the first stone tool technology in the human fossil record, characterized by simple flakes and choppers. First evident approximately 2.5 mya

The archeological record provides evidence that this occurred with *H. erectus*, as this species is associated with stone tools and the development of the first rudimentary hunting and gathering economy. Meat does appear to have been more common in the diet of *H. erectus* than it was in the australopithecines. *H. erectus* likely acquired mammalian carcasses through both hunting and confrontational scavenging (i.e., allowing other animal hunters to make the kill and then chasing them away from the carcass) (18, 65). In addition, the archaeological evidence

Acheulean: stone tool industry of the early and middle Pleistocene characterized by hand axes and cleavers. First evident 1.6 to 1.4 mya, associated with early *Homo*

DHA: docosahexaenoic acid

AA: arachidonic acid

indicates that butchered animals were transported back to a central location (home base) where the resources were shared within foraging groups (18, 36, 66, 67). Increasingly sophisticated stone tools (i.e., the Acheulean industry) emerged approximately 1.6 to 1.4 mya, improving the ability of these hominins to process animal and plant materials (6). These changes in diet and foraging behavior would not have turned our hominin ancestors into carnivores; however, the addition of even modest amounts of meat to the diet (10% to 20% of dietary energy) combined with the sharing of resources that is typical of hunter-gatherer groups would have significantly increased the quality and stability of the diet of *H. erectus*.

Cordain and colleagues (22) have noted that beyond the energetic benefits, greater consumption of animal foods would have provided increased levels of key fatty acids that would have been necessary for supporting the rapid hominin brain evolution. Mammalian brain growth is dependent upon sufficient amounts of two long-chain polyunsaturated fatty acids: docosahexaenoic acid (DHA) and arachidonic acid (AA) (22, 24). Because the composition of all mammalian brain tissue is similar with respect to these two fatty acids, species with higher levels of encephalization have greater requirements for DHA and AA (24). It also appears that mammals have a limited capacity to synthesize these fatty acids from dietary precursors. Consequently, dietary sources of DHA and AA were likely limiting nutrients that constrained the evolution of larger brain size in many mammalian lineages (23, 24).

Cordain and colleagues (22) have demonstrated that wild plant foods available on the African savanna (e.g., tubers, nuts) contain, at most, trace amounts of AA and DHA, whereas muscle tissue and organ meat of wild African ruminants provide moderate to high levels of these key fatty acids. As shown in **Table 3**, brain tissue is a rich source of both AA and DHA, whereas liver and muscle tissues are good sources of AA and moderate sources of DHA. Other good sources of AA and DHA are freshwater fish and shellfish (17, 22, 24). Cunnane and colleagues (17, 25) have suggested that the major increases in hominin encephalization were associated with systematic use of aquatic (marine, riverine, or lacustrian) resources. However, there is little archeological evidence for the systematic use of aquatic resources until much later in human evolution (45).

An alternative strategy for increasing dietary quality in early *Homo* has been proposed by Wrangham and colleagues (93, 94). These authors argue that the controlled use of fire for cooking allowed early *Homo* to improve the nutritional density of their diet. They note that the cooking of savanna tubers and other plant foods would have served to both soften them and increase their energy/nutrient bioavailability. In their raw form, the starch in roots and tubers is not absorbed in the small intestine and is passed through the body as nondigestible carbohydrate (30, 82). However, when heated, the

Table 3 Energy (kcal), fat (g), protein (g), arachidonic acid (AA), and docosahexaenoic acid (DHA) contents of African ruminant, fish, and wild plant foods per 100 grams. Data derived from (22)

Food item	Energy (kcal)	Fat (g)	Protein (g)	AA (mg)	DHA (mg)
African ruminant (brain)	126	9.3	9.8	533	861
African ruminant (liver)	159	7.1	22.6	192	41
African ruminant (muscle)	113	2.1	22.7	152	10
African ruminant (fat)	745	82.3	1.0	20–180	trace
African fish	119	4.5	18.8	270	549
Wild tuber/roots	96	0.5	2.0	0	0
Mixed wild plants	129	2.8	4.1	0	0

starch granules swell and are disrupted from the cell walls. This process, known as gelatinization, makes the starch much more accessible to breakdown by digestive enzymes (34). Thus, cooking increases the nutritional quality of tubers by making more of the carbohydrate energy available for biological processes.

Although cooking, which served to increase dietary digestibility and quality, is clearly an important innovation in hominin evolution, there is very limited evidence for the controlled use of fire by hominins before 1.5 mya (11, 15, 64). The more widely held view is that the use of fire and cooking did not occur until later in human evolution, at 200,000 to 250,000 years ago (80, 90). Moreover, nutritional analyses of wild tubers used by modern foraging populations (e.g., 16, 73, 89) suggest that the energy content of these resources is markedly lower than that of animal foods, even after cooking (22). Unlike animal foods, tubers are also devoid of both DHA and AA (22; see **Table 3**). Consequently, major questions remain about whether cooking and the heavy reliance on roots and tubers were important forces for promoting rapid brain evolution with the emergence of early *Homo*.

Overall, the available evidence seems to best support a mixed dietary strategy in early *Homo* that involved the consumption of larger amounts of animal foods in comparison with the australopithecines. Ungar and colleagues (87) recently suggested that early *Homo* likely pursued a flexible and versatile subsistence strategy that would have allowed them to adapt to the patchy and seasonally variable distribution of food resources on the African savanna. They note that such a model is more plausible than are ones proposing heavy reliance on one particular type of resource (e.g., meat or tubers). This is indeed true; however, what appears to be happening with early *Homo*—especially with *H. erectus*—is the development of a more stable and effective way of extracting resources from the environment. The increase in dietary quality and stability was likely achieved partly through changes in diet composition (22, 49) and partly through social and behavioral changes like food sharing and perhaps division of foraging tasks (36, 38, 41). This greater nutritional stability provided a critical foundation for fueling the energy demands of larger brain sizes.

BRAIN EVOLUTION AND HUMAN BODY COMPOSITION

In addition to improvements in dietary quality, the increased metabolic cost of larger brain size in human evolution also appears to have been supported by changes in body composition. Humans allocate a substantially larger share of their daily energy budget to their brains than do other primates or other mammals, which implies that the size and metabolic demands of certain other organs/organ systems may be relatively reduced in humans compared with other species. Thus, the critical question is, which organs have been reduced or altered in their relative size over the course of human evolution to compensate for the expansion of brain size?

Analyses of human and primate body composition offer possible answers to this question. Aiello (1) and Aiello & Wheeler (3) have argued that the increased energy demands of the human brain were accommodated by the reduction in size of the GI tract. Since the intestines are similar to the brain in having very high energy demands (so-called expensive tissues), the reduction in size of the large intestines of humans relative to other primates is thought to provide the necessary energy "savings" required to support elevated brain metabolism. Aiello & Wheeler (3) have shown that among a sample of 18 primate species (including humans), increased brain size was associated with reduced gut size. However, recent analyses by Snodgrass et al. (75) have failed to demonstrate significant differences in GI size between primates and nonprimate mammals that are predicted from the expensive tissue hypothesis. Thus, while it is clear that humans have relatively small GI sizes for their body mass, questions remain about the extent to which reductions in GI size helped to balance the increased metabolic costs associated with expansion of brain size during the course of human evolution. The reduced GI size in humans instead may be the direct consequence of improvements in DQ over the course of human evolution.

Leonard and colleagues (51) and Kuzawa (46) have suggested that differences in muscle and fat mass between humans and other primates may also account for variation in the budgeting of metabolic energy. Relative to other primates and other mammals, humans have lower levels of muscle mass and higher levels of body fatness (46, 51, 65). The relatively high levels of adiposity in humans have two important metabolic implications for brain metabolism. First, because fat has lower energy requirements than that of muscle tissue, replacing muscle mass with fat mass results in energy savings that can be allocated to the brain. Additionally, fat provides a ready source of stored energy that can be drawn upon during periods of limited food availability. Consequently, the higher levels of body fat in humans may also help to support larger brain size by providing stored energy to buffer against environmental fluctuations in nutritional resources.

The importance of body fat is particularly notable in human infants, which have both high brain-to-body weight ratios and high levels of body fatness (46). **Table 4** shows age-related changes in body weight (kg), brain weight (g), fatness (%), RMR (kcal/day), and percent of RMR allocated to the brain for humans from birth to adulthood. We see that in infants, brain metabolism accounts for upward of 60% of RMR. Human infants are also considerably fatter than infants of other mammalian species (46). Body fatness in human infants is approximately 15% to 16% at birth, and continues to increase to 25% to 26% during the first 12 to 18 months of postnatal growth. Fatness then declines to about 15% by early childhood (27). Thus, during early human growth and development, it appears that body fatness is highest during the periods of the greatest metabolic demand of the brain.

It is likely that fundamental changes in body composition (i.e., the relative sizes of different organ systems) during the course of hominin evolution allowed for the expansion of brain size without substantial increases in the total energy demands for the body. At present, we do not know which alterations were the most critical for accommodating brain expansion. Variation in body composition both within and between primate species is still not well understood. Our knowledge of variation in body composition among humans is based largely on data from populations of the industrialized world. Consequently, more and better data on interspecific and ontogenetic variation in primate and human body composition are necessary to further resolve these issues.

Table 4 Body weight (kg), brain weight (g), percent body fat (%), resting metabolic rate (RMR; kcal/day), and percent of RMR allocated to brain metabolism (BrMet, %) for humans from birth to adulthood[a]

Age	Body weight (kg)	Brain weight (g)	Body fat (%)	RMR (kcal/day)	BrMet (%)
Newborn	3.5	475	16	161	87
3 months	5.5	650	22	300	64
18 months	11.0	1045	25	590	53
5 years	19.0	1235	15	830	44
10 years	31.0	1350	15	1160	34
Adult male	70.0	1400	11	1800	23
Adult female	50.0	1360	20	1480	27

[a]All data are from (37), except for percent body fat data for children 18 months and younger, which are from (27).

New imaging techniques such as magnetic resonance imaging and positron emission tomography scans offer the potential to directly explore variation in organ weight and organ-specific energy demands in living humans and primates. For example, Gallagher et al. (33) recently used magnetic resonance imaging technology to measure how differences in organ weights contribute to ethnic differences in RMRs among living humans. These authors demonstrated that the significant differences in RMR between their African American and Euro-American samples could be accounted for by differences in the summed weight of the most metabolically expensive organs (liver, heart, spleen, kidneys, and brain). Similarly, Chugani (19) utilized positron emission tomography scans to quantify changes in glucose utilization in the human brain from birth to adulthood. His findings suggest that the extremely high metabolic costs of brain metabolism characteristic of early human life (as outlined in **Table 4**) may extend further into childhood than previously realized. Together, these studies highlight the potential use of new imaging techniques for better understanding how interspecific variation in body composition contributes to differences in metabolic rate.

CONCLUSIONS

The evolution of large human brain size has had important implications for the nutritional biology of our species. Our large brains are energetically expensive, yet, paradoxically, our overall metabolic requirements are similar to those of any comparably sized mammal. As a consequence, humans expend a relatively larger proportion of their resting energy budget on brain metabolism than do other primates or nonprimate mammals.

Comparative analyses of primate dietary patterns indicate that the high costs of large human brains are supported, in part, by diets that are relatively rich in energy and other nutrients. Among living primates, the relative proportion of metabolic energy allocated to the brain is positively correlated with dietary quality. Humans fall at the positive end of this relationship, having both a very high-quality diet and a large brain.

Greater encephalization also appears to have consequences for other aspects of body composition, most notably the GI mass, muscularity, and adiposity. Relative to other primates, human have smaller GI tracts and a relatively reduced colon. This type of gut is consistent with adaptation to a diet that is relatively high in energy and nutrients and is easy to digest.

In addition, humans appear to be relatively undermuscled (i.e., less skeletal muscle) and over fat compared with other primates of similar size. The relatively high levels of adiposity in humans are particularly notable in infancy. These greater levels of body fatness and reduced levels of muscle mass allow human infants to accommodate the growth of their large brains in two important ways: (*a*) by having a ready supply of stored energy to feed the brain and (*b*) by reducing the total energy costs of the rest of the body.

The human fossil record indicates that major changes in both brain size and diet occurred in association with the emergence of early members of the genus *Homo* between 2.0 and 1.7 mya in Africa. With the evolution of early *H. erectus* 1.8 mya, we find evidence of an important adaptive shift—the evolution of the first hunting and gathering economy, characterized by greater consumption of animal foods, transport of food resources to home bases, and sharing of food within social groups. *H. erectus* was humanlike in body size and proportions and had a brain size beyond that seen in nonhuman primates, approaching the range of modern humans. In addition, the reduced size of the face and grinding teeth of *H. erectus*, coupled with its more sophisticated tool technology, suggest that these hominins were consuming a higher-quality and more stable diet that would have helped to fuel the increases in brain size. Consequently, although dietary change was not the prime force responsible for the evolution of large human brain size, improvements in dietary quality appear to have been a necessary condition for promoting encephalization in the human lineage.

Further research is needed to better understand the nature of the dietary changes that took place with emergence of *Homo*. In addition, the application of new biomedical imaging techniques offers the potential to directly explore how intra- and interspecific variation in body composition may contribute to variation in metabolic rates.

SUMMARY POINTS

1. Our large brains are energetically expensive, yet paradoxically our overall metabolic requirements are similar to those of any comparably sized mammal. Consequently, humans expend a relatively larger proportion of their resting energy budget on brain metabolism than do other primates or nonprimate mammals.
2. Comparative analyses of living primate species show that the relative proportion of metabolic energy allocated to the brain is positively correlated with dietary quality. Humans fall at the positive end of this relationship, having both a very high-quality diet and a large brain. This suggests that large human brains are supported, in part, by diets that are relatively rich in energy and other nutrients.
3. Compared with other primates, humans have smaller overall gastrointestinal tracts with a relatively reduced colon. This type of gut is consistent with adaptation to a diet that is relatively high in energy and nutrients and is easy to digest.
4. Humans have relatively lower levels of muscularity and higher levels of adiposity than do other primates of similar size. High levels of adiposity in humans are particularly notable in infancy. Greater body fatness and lower muscle mass allow human infants to accommodate the growth of their large brains by having a ready supply of stored energy, reducing the total energy costs of the rest of the body.
5. The human fossil record indicates that major changes in both brain size and diet occurred in association with the emergence of early members of the genus *Homo* between 2.0 and 1.7 mya in Africa. With the evolution of early *H. erectus* 1.8 mya, we find evidence of an important adaptive shift—the evolution of the first hunting and gathering economy, characterized by greater consumption of animal foods, transport of food resources to home bases, and sharing of food within social groups. Improvements in diet quality with *H. erectus* appear to have been important for fueling rapid rates of encephalization.
6. Consumption of more animal foods with early *Homo* was likely important for providing high levels of key long-chain polyunsaturated fatty acids (docosahexaenoic acid and arachidonic acid) that are necessary for brain growth.

ACKNOWLEDGMENTS

We are grateful to S.C. Antón and C.W. Kuzawa for discussions about this research.

LITERATURE CITED

1. **Aiello LC. 1997. Brains and guts in human evolution: the expensive tissue hypothesis. *Braz. J. Genet.* 20:141–48**

1. Posits that the high metabolic costs of large human brains have been partially offset by the reductions in the size of our gastrointestinal tracts.

2. Aiello LC, Key C. 2002. Energetic consequences of being a *Homo erectus* female. *Am. J. Hum. Biol.* 14:551–65
3. Aiello LC, Wheeler P. 1995. The expensive-tissue hypothesis: the brain and the digestive system in human and primate evolution. *Curr. Anthropol.* 36:199–221
4. Antón SC. 2003. A natural history of *Homo erectus*. *Yrbk. Phys. Anthropol.* 46:126–70
5. Antón SC, Swisher CC III. 2001. Evolution of cranial capacity in Asian *Homo erectus*. In *A Scientific Life: Papers in Honor of Dr. T. Jacob*, ed. E Indriati, pp. 25–39. Yogyakarta, Indonesia: Bigraf
6. Asfaw B, Beyene Y, Suwa G, Walter RC, White TD, et al. 1992. The earliest Acheulean from Konso-Gardula. *Nature* 360:732–35
7. Backwell LR, d'Errico F. 2001. Evidence of termite foraging by Swartkrans early hominids. *Proc. Nat. Acad. Sci. USA* 98:1358–63
8. Bauchot R, Stefan H. 1969. Encephalisation et niveau evolutif ches les simiens. *Mammalia* 33:225–75
9. Behrensmeyer K, Todd NE, Potts R, McBrinn GE. 1997. Late Pliocene faunal turnover in the Turkana basin, Kenya and Ethiopia. *Science* 278:1589–94
10. Bell RH. 1971. A grazing ecosystem in the Serengeti. *Sci. Am.* 225(1):86–93
11. Bellomo RV. 1994. Methods of determining early hominid behavioral activities associated with the controlled use of fire at FxJj 20 Main, Koobi Fora. *J. Hum. Evol.* 27:173–95
12. Blumenschine RJ. 1987. Characteristics of the early hominid scavenging niche. *Curr. Anthropol.* 28:383–407
13. Blumenschine RJ, Cavallo JA, Capaldo SD. 1994. Competition for carcasses and early hominid behavioral ecology: a case study and conceptual framework. *J. Hum. Evol.* 27:197–213
14. Bobe R, Behrensmeyer AK. 2002. Faunal change, environmental variability and late Pliocene hominin evolution. *J. Hum. Evol.* 42:475–97
15. Brain CK, Sillen A. 1988. Evidence from the Swartkrans cave for the earliest use of fire. *Nature* 336:464–66
16. Brand-Miller JC, Holt SHA. 1998. Australian aboriginal plant foods: a consideration of their nutritional composition and health implications. *Nutr. Res. Rev.* 11:5–23
17. Broadhurst CL, Cunnane SC, Crawford MA. 1998. Rift Valley lake fish and shellfish provided brain-specific nutrition for early Homo. *Br. J. Nutr.* 79:3–21
18. Bunn HT. 2006. Meat made us human. In *Evolution of the Human Diet: The Known, the Unknown, and the Unknowable*, ed. PS Unger, pp. 191–211. New York: Oxford Univ. Press
19. Chugani HT. 1998. A critical period of brain development: studies of cerebral glucose utilization with PET. *Prevent. Med.* 27:184–88
20. Cordain L, Brand-Miller J, Eaton SB, Mann N, Holt SHA, Speth JD. 2000. Plant to animal subsistence ratios and macronutrient energy estimations in world-wide hunter-gatherer diets. *Am. J. Clin. Nutr.* 71:682–92
21. Cordain L, Eaton SB, Sebastian A, Mann N, Lindberg S, et al. 2005. Origins and evolution of the Western diet: health implications for the 21st century. *Am. J. Clin. Nutr.* 81:341–54
22. Cordain L, Watkins BA, Mann NJ. 2001. Fatty acid composition and energy density of foods available to African hominids. *World Rev. Nutr. Diet.* 90:144–61
23. Crawford MA. 1992. The role of dietary fatty acids in biology: their place in the evolution of the human brain. *Nutr. Rev.* 50:3–11
24. Crawford MA, Bloom M, Broadhurst CL, Schmidt WF, Cunnane SC, et al. 1999. Evidence for unique function of docosahexaenoic acid during the evolution of the modern human brain. *Lipids* 34:S39–47

25. Cunnane SC, Crawford MA. 2003. Survival of the fattest: fat babies were the key to evolution of the large human brain. *Comp. Biochem. Physiol. A* 136:17–26

26. deMenocal PB. 2004. African climate change and faunal evolution during the Pliocene-Pleistocene. *Earth Planet. Sci. Lett.* 220:3–24

27. Dewey KG, Heinig MJ, Nommsen LA, Peerson JM, Lonnerdal B. 1993. Breast-fed infants are leaner than formula-fed infants at 1 year of age: the Darling Study. *Am. J. Clin. Nutr.* 52:140–45

28. Eaton SB. 2006. The ancestral human diet: What was it and should it be a paradigm for contemporary nutrition? *Proc. Nutr. Soc.* 65:1–6

29. Eaton SB, Konner MJ. 1985. Paleolithic nutrition: a consideration of its nature and current implications. *New Engl. J. Med.* 312:283–89

30. Englyst KN, Englyst HN. 2005. Carbohydrate bioavailability. *Br. J. Nutr.* 94:1–11

31. Gabunia L, Vekua A, Lordkipanidze D, Swisher CC, Ferring R, et al. 2000. Earliest Pleistocene cranial remains from Dmanisi, Republic of Georgia: taxonomy, geological setting, and age. *Science* 288:1019–25

32. Gabunia L, Antón SC, Lordkipanidze D, Vekua A, Justus A, Swisher CC III. 2001. Dmanisi and dispersal. *Evol. Anthropol.* 10:158–70

33. Gallagher D, Albu J, He Q, Heshka S, Boxt L, et al. 2006. Small organs with a high metabolic rate explain lower resting energy expenditure in African American than in white adults. *Am. J. Clin. Nutr.* 83:1062–67

34. García-Alonso A, Goñi I. 2000. Effect of processing on potato starch: in vitro availability and glycemic index. *Nahrung* 44:19–22

35. Garn SM, Leonard WR. 1989. What did our ancestors eat? *Nutr. Rev.* 47:337–45

36. Harris JWK, Capaldo S. 1993. The earliest stone tools: their implications for an understanding of the activities and behavior of late Pliocene hominids. In *The Use of Tools by Human and Nonhuman Primates*, ed. A Berthelet, J Chavaillon, pp. 196–220. Oxford: Oxford Sci.

37. Holliday MA. 1986. Body composition and energy needs during growth. In *Human Growth: A Comprehensive Treatise, Volume 2*, ed. F. Falkner, JM Tanner, pp. 101–17. New York: Plenum. 2nd ed.

38. Isaac GL. 1978. Food sharing and human evolution: archaeological evidence from the Plio-Pleistocene of East Africa. *J. Anthropol. Res.* 34:311–25

39. Jarman PJ. 1974. The social organization of antelope in relation to their ecology. *Behaviour* 58:215–67

40. Jerison HJ. 1973. *The Evolution of the Brain and Intelligence*. New York: Academic

41. Kaplan H, Hill K, Lancaster J, Hurtado AM. 2000. A theory of life history evolution: diet, intelligence and longevity. *Evol. Anthropol.* 9:156–85

42. Kappeler PM. 1996. Causes and consequences of life-history variation among strepsirhine primates. *Am. Nat.* 148:868–91

43. Kety SS. 1957. The general metabolism of the brain in vivo. In *Metabolism of the Central Nervous System*, ed. D Richter, pp. 221–37. New York: Pergamon

44. Kleiber M. 1961. *The Fire of Life*. New York: Wiley

45. Klein RG. 1999. *The Human Career: Human Biological and Cultural Origins*. Chicago: Univ. Chicago Press. 2nd ed.

46. Kuzawa CW. 1998. Adipose tissue in human infancy and childhood: an evolutionary perspective. *Yrbk. Phys. Anthropol.* 41:177–209

47. Leonard WR. 2002. Food for thought: dietary change was a driving force in human evolution. *Sci. Am.* 287(6):106–15

29. One of the first papers to consider human nutrition from an evolutionary perspective. Argues that many of today's common diseases stem from diets that differ from those of our prehistoric ancestors.

46. Demonstrates the adaptive value of body fat in human infants for buffering against disease and supporting the high energetic costs of large, growing brains.

47. Uses an energetics approach for understanding major trends in human evolution, such as bipedality, encephalization, and the expansion of hominins from Africa.

48. Leonard WR, Robertson ML. 1992. Nutritional requirements and human evolution: a bioenergetics model. *Am. J. Hum. Biol.* 4:179–95
49. Leonard WR, Robertson ML. 1994. Evolutionary perspectives on human nutrition: the influence of brain and body size on diet and metabolism. *Am. J. Hum. Biol.* 6:77–88
50. Leonard WR, Robertson ML. 1997. Comparative primate energetics and hominid evolution. *Am. J. Phys. Anthropol.* 102:265–81
51. Leonard WR, Robertson ML, Snodgrass JJ, Kuzawa CW. 2003. Metabolic correlates of hominid brain evolution. *Comp. Biochem. Physiol. A* 135:5–15
52. **Martin RD. 1989. *Primate Origins and Evolution: A Phylogenetic Reconstruction.* Princeton, NJ: Princeton Univ. Press**

52. Synthesizes research on primate and human evolution, drawing on a rich body of comparative data on primate biology.

53. Martin RD, Chivers DJ, MacLarnon AM, Hladik CM. 1985. Gastrointestinal allometry in primates and other mammals. In *Size and Scaling in Primate Biology*, ed. WL Jungers, pp. 61–89. New York: Plenum
54. McHenry HM. 1992. Body size and proportions in early hominids. *Am. J. Phys. Anthropol.* 87:407–31
55. McHenry HM. 1994a. Tempo and mode in human evolution. *Proc. Natl. Acad. Sci. USA* 91:6780–86
56. McHenry HM. 1994b. Behavioral ecological implications of early hominid body size. *J. Hum. Evol.* 27:77–87
57. McHenry HM, Coffing K. 2000. Australopithecus to Homo: transformations in body and mind. *Annu. Rev. Anthropol.* 29:125–46
58. McNab BK, Wright PC. 1987. Temperature regulation and oxygen consumption in the Philippine tarsier *Tarsius syrichta*. *Physiol. Zool.* 60:596–600
59. Milton K. 1987. Primate diets and gut morphology: implications for hominid evolution. In *Food and Evolution: Toward a Theory of Human Food Habits*, ed. M Harris, EB Ross, pp. 93–115. Philadelphia, PA: Temple Univ. Press
60. **Milton K. 1993. Diet and primate evolution. *Sci. Am.* 269(2):86–93**

60. Examines the evolution of primate and human diets, drawing on comparative studies of primate ecology.

61. Milton K. 1999. A hypothesis to explain the role of meat-eating in human evolution. *Evol. Anthropol.* 8:11–21
62. Milton K. 2003. The critical role played by animal source foods in human (*Homo*) evolution. *J. Nutr.* 133:3886–92S
63. Milton K, Demment MW. 1988. Digestion and passage kinetics of chimpanzees fed high- and low-fiber diets and comparison with human data. *J. Nutr.* 118:1082–88
64. Pennisi E. 1999. Did cooked tubers spur the evolution of big brains?*Science* 283:2004–5
65. Plummer T. 2004. Flaked stones and old bones: biological and cultural evolution at the dawn of technology. *Yrbk. Phys. Anthropol.* 47:118–64
66. Potts R. 1988. *Early Hominid Activities at Olduvai*. New York: Aldine
67. Potts R. 1998. Environmental hypotheses of hominin evolution. *Yrbk. Phys. Anthropol.* 41:93–136
68. Reed K. 1997. Early hominid evolution and ecological change through the African Plio-Pleistocene. *J. Hum. Evol.* 32:289–322
69. Richard AF. 1985. *Primates in Nature*. New York: Freeman
70. Rowe N. 1996. *The Pictorial Guide to Living Primates.* New York: Pogonias
71. Ruff CB, Trinkaus E, Holliday TW. 1997. Body mass and encephalization in Pleistocene Homo. *Nature* 387:173–76
72. Sailer LD, Gaulin SJC, Boster JS, Kurland JA. 1985. Measuring the relationship between dietary quality and body size in primates. *Primates* 26:14–27

73. Schoeninger MJ, Bunn HT, Murray SS, Marlett JA. 2001. Nutritional composition of some wild plant foods and honey used by Hadza foragers of Tanzania. *J. Food Comp. Anal.* 14:3–13
74. Semaw S, Rogers MJ, Quade J, Renne PR, Butler RF, et al. 2003. 2.6-million-year-old stone tools and associated bones from OGS-6 and OGS-7, Gona, Afar, Ethiopia. *J. Hum. Evol.* 45:169–77
75. Snodgrass JJ, Leonard WR, Robertson ML. 2007. Energetics of encephalization in early hominids. In *The Evolution of Hominid Diets: Integrating Approaches to the Study of Palaeolithic Subsistence*, ed. M Richards, JJ Hublin. New York: Springer. In press
76. Sponheimer M, Lee-Thorp J, de Ruiter DJ, Codron D, Codron J, et al. 2005. Hominins, sedges, and termites: new carbon isotope data from Sterkfontein valley and Kruger National Park. *J. Hum. Evol.* 48:301–12
77. Sponheimer M, Passey BH, de Ruiter DJ, Guatelli-Steinberg D, Cerling TE, Lee-Thorp JA. 2006. Isotopic evidence for dietary variability in the early hominin *Paranthropus robustus*. *Science* 314:980–82
78. Stanford CB. 1996. The hunting ecology of wild chimpanzees: implications for the evolutionary ecology of Pliocene hominids. *Am. Anthropol.* 98:96–113
79. Stephan H, Frahm H, Baron G. 1981. New and revised data on volumes of brain structures in insectivores and primates. *Folia Primatol.* 35:1–29
80. Straus LG. 1989. On early hominid use of fire. *Curr. Anthropol.* 30:488–91
81. Sussman RW. 1987. Species-specific dietary patterns in primates and human dietary adaptations. In *Evolution of Human Behavior: Primate Models*, ed. W Kinzey, pp. 151–79. Albany, NY: SUNY Press
82. Tagliabue A, Raben A, Heijnen ML, Duerenberg P, Pasquali E, Astrup A. 1995. The effect of raw potato starch on energy expenditure and substrate oxidation. *Am. J. Clin. Nutr.* 61:1070–75
83. Teaford MF, Ungar PS. 2000. Diet and the evolution of the earliest human ancestors. *Proc. Natl. Acad. Sci. USA* 97:13506–11
84. Teleki G. 1981. The omnivorous diet and eclectic feeding habits of the chimpanzees of Gombe National Park. In *Omnivorous Primates*, ed. RSO Harding, G Teleki, pp. 303–43. New York: Columbia Univ. Press
85. Thompson SD, Power ML, Rutledge CE, Kleiman DG. 1994. Energy metabolism and thermoregulation in the golden lion tamarin (*Leontopithecus rosalia*). *Folia Primatol.* 63:131–43
86. **Ungar PS, ed. 2007. *Evolution of the Human Diet: The Known, the Unknown, and the Unknowable*. New York: Oxford Univ. Press**
87. Ungar PS, Grine FE, Teaford MF. 2006. Diet in early *Homo*: a review of the evidence and a new model of adaptive versatility. *Annu. Rev. Anthropol.* 35:209–28
88. Vrba ES. 1995. The fossil record of African antelopes relative to human evolution. In *Paleoclimate and Evolution, With Emphasis on Human Origins*, ed. ES Vrba, GH Denton, TC Partridge, LH Burkle, pp. 385–424. New Haven, CT: Yale Univ. Press
89. Wehmeyer AS, Lee RB, Whiting M. 1969. The nutrient composition and dietary importance of some vegetable foods eaten by the !Kung bushmen. *S. Afr. Med. J.* 95:1529–30
90. Weiner S, Qunqu X, Goldberg P, Liu J, Bar-Yosef O. 1998. Evidence for the use of fire at Zhoukoudian, China. *Science* 281:251–53
91. Wolpoff MH. 1999. *Paleoanthropology*. Boston: McGraw-Hill. 2nd ed.
92. Wood B, Collard M. 1999. The human genus. *Science* 284:65–71

86. Provides an authoritative overview of research on human nutritional evolution from the fields of paleontology, archaeology, primatology and comparative human biology.

93. Wrangham RW, Conklin-Brittain NL. 2003. Cooking as a biological trait. *Comp. Biochem. Physiol. A Mol. Integr. Physiol.* 136:35–46
94. Wrangham RW, Jones JH, Laden G, Pilbeam D, Conklin-Brittain NL. 1999. The raw and the stolen: cooking and the ecology of human origins. *Curr. Anthropol.* 40:567–94
95. Wynn JG. 2004. Influence of Plio-Pleistocene aridification on human evolution: evidence from paleosols from the Turkana Basin, Kenya. *Am. J. Phys. Anthropol.* 123:106–18

Splanchnic Regulation of Glucose Production

John Wahren and Karin Ekberg

Department of Molecular Medicine and Surgery, Karolinska Institute, SE-171 77 Stockholm, Sweden; email: john.wahren@ki.se

Annu. Rev. Nutr. 2007. 27:329–45

First published online as a Review in Advance on April 27, 2007

The *Annual Review of Nutrition* is online at http://nutr.annualreviews.org

This article's doi:
10.1146/annurev.nutr.27.061406.093806

0199-9885/07/0821-0329$20.00

Key Words

glycogenolysis, gluconeogenesis, exercise, starvation, diabetes

Abstract

The liver plays a key role for the maintenance of blood glucose homeostasis under widely changing physiological conditions. In the overnight fasted state, breakdown of hepatic glycogen and synthesis of glucose from lactate, amino acids, glycerol, and pyruvate contribute about equally to hepatic glucose production. Postprandial glucose uptake by the liver is determined by the size of the glucose load reaching the liver, the rise in insulin concentration, and the route of glucose delivery. Hepatic glycogen stores are depleted within 36 to 48 hours of fasting, but gluconeogenesis continues to provide glucose for tissues with an obligatory glucose requirement. Glucose output from the liver increases during exercise; during short-term intensive exertion, hepatic glycogenolysis is the primary source of extra glucose for skeletal muscle, and during prolonged exercise, hepatic gluconeogenesis becomes gradually more important in keeping with falling insulin and rising glucagon levels. Type 1 diabetes is accompanied by diminished hepatic glycogen stores, augmented gluconeogenesis, and increased basal hepatic glucose production in proportion to the severity of the diabetic state. The hyperglycemia of type 2 diabetes is in part caused by an overproduction of glucose from the liver that is secondary to accelerated gluconeogenesis.

Contents

INTRODUCTION

The liver plays a key role in the maintenance of blood glucose homeostasis. It releases glucose in the fasted state and it takes up and stores some of the glucose ingested in meals. In so doing, the liver ensures an even and predictable supply of glucose to the extrahepatic tissues, primarily the brain. The liver is able to release glucose to the circulation from its glycogen stores and it has the capacity to take up the 3-carbon fragments lactate, pyruvate, glycerol, and amino acids and convert these to glucose. Hence, hepatic gluconeogenesis and glycogenolysis are the two processes responsible for hepatic glucose production. A dynamic equilibrium between the two serves to maintain blood glucose levels within a narrow range under widely changing physiological conditions.

NMRS: nuclear magnetic resonance spectroscopy

The central role of the liver in blood glucose regulation was first identified by the French physiologist Claude Bernard, who documented that the liver is capable of producing glucose even in the absence of intestinal absorption. He discovered that carbohydrates could be stored in the liver as a polysaccharide, which he named "glycogen." He could also demonstrate that the liver continues to release glucose even after depletion of its glycogen stores, thus demonstrating that hepatic glucose production is possible via pathways other than the breakdown of glycogen. The experimental work was presented during the years 1848–1860 (96), but it took many decades before the significance of Bernard's observations was recognized.

Claude Bernard's studies were based on direct blood sampling from the hepatic blood vessels in dogs. Current development of techniques involving isotopic tracer dilution methods and nuclear magnetic resonance spectroscopy (NMRS) have made it possible to assess hepatic glucose and glycogen metabolism in animals and noninvasively in humans in a variety of physiological situations and in specific disorders, thereby providing improved insight into the metabolic regulation. This review summarizes recent findings on the regulation of splanchnic glucose exchange in the overnight and prolonged fasted state, during physical exercise, and in diabetes.

BASAL SPLANCHNIC GLUCOSE PRODUCTION

In the morning, after an overnight fast absorption of nutrients from the intestine is completed, plasma insulin and glucagon concentrations have returned to their basal levels and body fuel consumption is matched by the release of endogenous substrates from storage depots. The major source of energy is free fatty acids (FFAs), but the body continues to consume glucose at rates of 8–10 g/hour. The brain and the tissues with an obligatory need for glucose account for more than half of this amount (16). This rate of glucose consumption cannot be supported by the small pool of circulating glucose (4–5 g). The liver adapts to this situation by switching from postprandial glucose uptake and storage to postabsorptive production of glucose. In the overnight fasted state, the liver is the dominating source of glucose production, even though there is also a small contribution from the kidneys (36). Basal glucose output from the splanchnic area in healthy subjects amounts to approximately 0.8 mmol/min or 10 μmoles $\cdot$ min^{-1} $\cdot$ kg^{-1} (36, 108).

Glycogenolysis

Hepatic glycogenolysis contributes substantially to the liver's glucose output after an overnight fast. Even though the energy content of the hepatic glycogen stores is small in comparison with the body's daily energy requirements, it is evident that liver glycogen is essential for blood glucose homeostasis in the postabsorptive state. Thus, direct determinations of liver glycogen concentrations in biopsy material (81) and ^{13}C-NMRS measurements of hepatic glycogen during the postabsorptive phase (12–24 hours) show that liver glycogen decreases linearly at rates corresponding to approximately 40% of the simultaneous whole body glucose turnover (97). During continued fasting, hepatic glycogenolysis decreases gradually, and the glycogen stores are almost completely exhausted after 48 hours (**Figure 1**, see color insert) (81, 97).

Gluconeogenesis

The rapid depletion of hepatic glycogen during the postabsorptive and early fasting period underscores the importance of gluconeogenesis from nonglucose precursors for the maintenance of blood glucose homeostasis. Our understanding of the quantitative contribution by gluconeogenesis to total glucose production has until recently been limited because of methodological problems. Early estimates of hepatic gluconeogenesis were based on arterial-hepatic venous catheterization and balance measurements in healthy subjects. These indicated a relative contribution of gluconeogenesis to splanchnic glucose output in the postabsorptive state of maximally 35% (**Figure 2**, see color insert) (42, 108, 109). It should be recognized, however, that such estimates do not take into account splanchnic glucose utilization, nor extrahepatic splanchnic exchange or intrahepatic precursor supply (10). The balance technique estimates seem low in comparison with determinations of gluconeogenesis based on the difference between ^{13}C-NMRS-measured rates of hepatic glycogen breakdown and glucose turnover rates estimated by tracer dilution methodology, which indicate a gluconeogenic contribution of 50% to 65% (91, 97). Isotope tracing techniques using ^{14}C-lactate or ^{14}C-acetate have also been employed, but these are limited by inadequate labeling of the intracellular precursor pool or significant extrahepatic metabolism of the tracer (67, 99). Mass isotopomer distribution analysis (MIDA) using ^{13}C-glycerol has been employed for estimation of enrichment of the glucose precursor pool (52), but it now appears that this method is limited by hepatic heterogeneity in the metabolism of glycerol (64).

The above limitations in the determination of gluconeogenesis are avoided by the deuterated water technique (65, 66). With this method, the relative contribution of gluconeogenesis to whole-body glucose production can be estimated from the ratio of ^{2}H enrichment at carbon 5 over that at carbon 2 of plasma glucose after the ingestion of ^2H_2O. This approach is based on the observation that all glucose molecules exchange hydrogens between body water and those at carbon 5 of glucose during gluconeogenesis and additional hydrogens at carbon 2 during both

FFAs: free fatty acid

MIDA: mass isotopomer distribution analysis

gluconeogenesis and glycogenolysis. This technique indicates a contribution of gluconeogenesis, including any renal component, to glucose turnover ranging from 47% to 53% at 12–16 hours of fasting in healthy subjects (**Figure 1**) (17, 66). Support for the validity of the deuterated water technique is obtained from the finding that after more than 42 hours of fasting, when the hepatic glycogen stores are almost completely exhausted, gluconeogenesis as estimated by this method accounts for 93 ± 6% of glucose turnover (17). In view of these findings, it is now widely believed that glycogenolysis and gluconeogenesis each contribute approximately 50% of glucose turnover in healthy subjects in the postabsorptive state.

Regulatory Aspects

Insulin is a primary regulator of hepatic glucose production, even though basal glucagon levels are required to support glucose output in the overnight fasted state (111). Insulin acts directly on the liver by binding to hepatic insulin receptors and activating insulin-signaling pathways. Small changes in portal insulin concentrations effectively modulate hepatic glycogenolysis as evident from studies in dogs (103) and in healthy subjects (40). Hepatic glycogenolysis and gluconeogenesis show differential sensitivities to changes in insulin concentration: even small increases effectively inhibit glycogenolysis (**Figure 3**, see color insert), whereas substantial increments in insulin levels are required for inhibition of gluconeogenesis (21, 40). It has, however, been observed in obese subjects that suppression of glucose production in response to insulin infusion can occur even when the estimated portal insulin concentration does not increase (92), which suggests that insulin may inhibit glucose production also by indirect mechanisms. This may occur by insulin-induced inhibition of adipose tissue lipolysis that reduces both FFA levels and glycerol availability for gluconeogenesis. Likewise, insulin inhibits muscle proteolysis, resulting in further reduction of gluconeogenic precursor supply. Insulin also exerts inhibitory effects on pancreatic α-cells, resulting in reduced glucagon levels (57). Finally, studies in mice suggest that insulin action in the brain may play a role in the regulation of hepatic glucose output (82). A schematic representation of insulin's direct and indirect influence on hepatic glucose output is presented in **Figure 4** (see color insert). It is now widely accepted that both direct and indirect effects of insulin are involved in the regulation of hepatic glucose output (1, 20), but the relative contributions of the two mechanisms have been controversial. Recent studies examining the effects of portal venous, systemic venous, and carotid arterial insulin infusion provide compelling evidence that the direct effects of insulin are dominant in overnight-fasted dogs and that indirect effects of insulin via the brain are of minor importance (35).

Extrahepatic Splanchnic Tissues

Besides the liver, only the kidney is recognized as being capable of gluconeogenesis. Recently, however, gluconeogenic capacity has been proposed also for the small intestine of the rat (77, 78). Gluconeogenic enzyme activities are expressed by the intestinal mucosa of rats and mice (95). Tracer dilution studies indicate ongoing simultaneous glucose production and utilization by the small intestine during starvation and diabetes (77). Attempts to identify the precursor for intestinal gluconeogenesis have indicated that glutamine and glycerol carbon may be incorporated into glucose by the intestine (26). The results from experiments in small rodents are not unequivocal and have recently been challenged (73). Studies using stable isotopes have failed to demonstrate the presence of measurable intestinal gluconeogenesis in fasting piglets (15). Moreover, arterial-portal venous concentration differences for glucose and gluconeogenic precursors in humans do not indicate net intestinal glucose synthesis (10). Thus, the interesting concept of intestinal

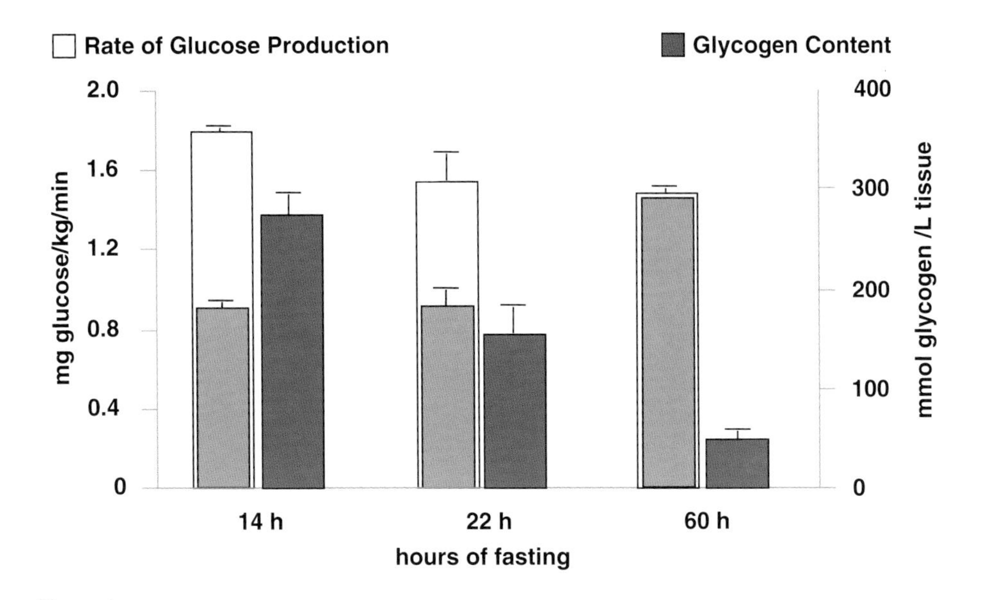

Figure 1

Rates of whole-body glucose production (*yellow*) and gluconeogenesis (*green*) as well as hepatic glycogen content (*red*) after 14, 22, and 60 hours of fasting. Adapted from (17, 66, 97).

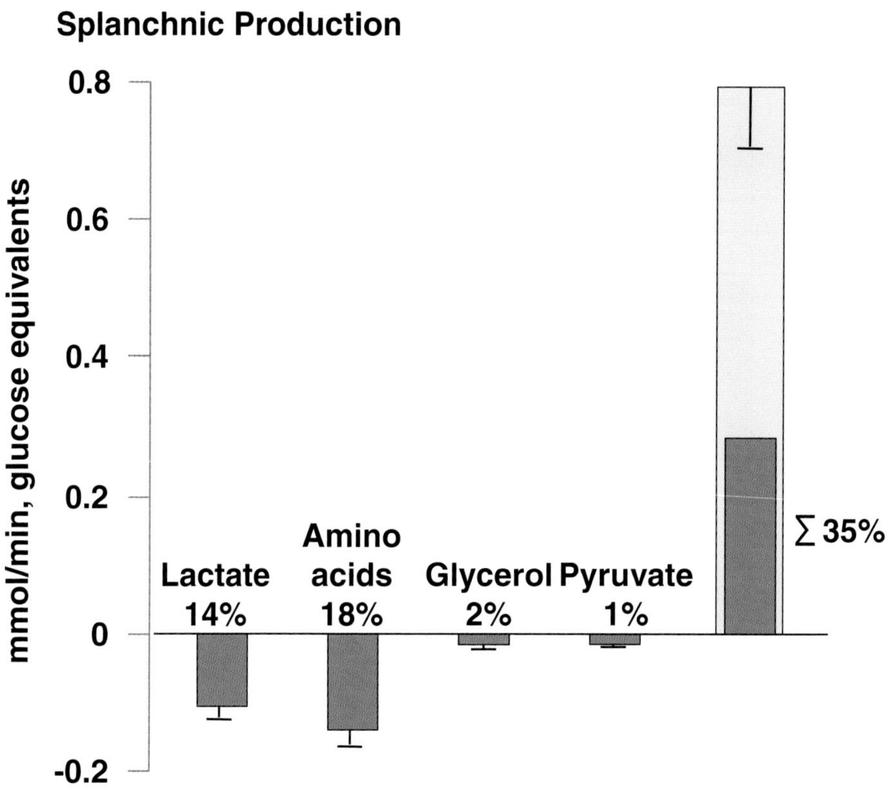

Figure 2

Rates of splanchnic glucose production (*yellow*) and gluconeogenic precursor uptake (*green*) in the overnight fasted state in healthy subjects. Adapted from (4, 42, 108, 109).

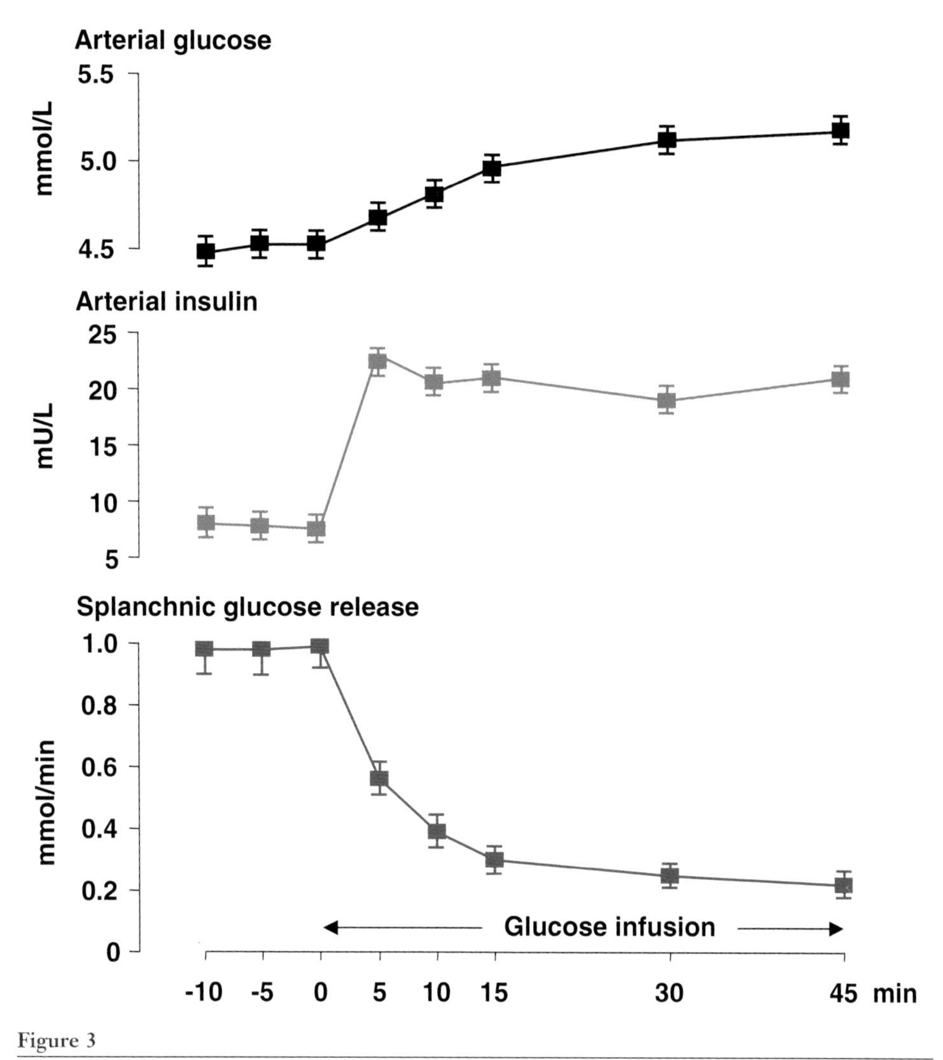

Figure 3

Arterial glucose and insulin concentrations and splanchnic glucose output in the basal state and during intravenous glucose administration (0.8 mmol/min) in healthy subjects. Data from (40).

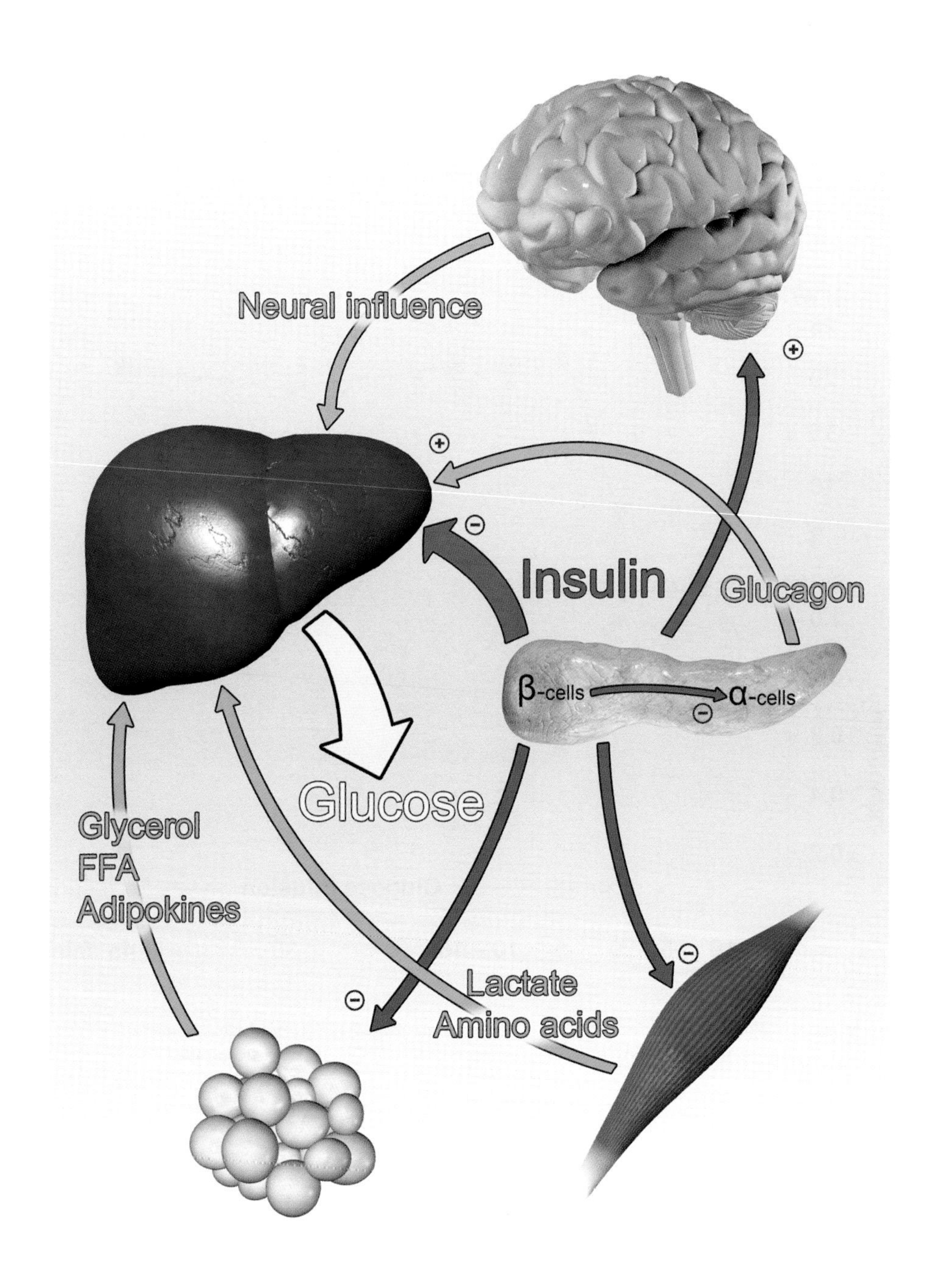

Figure 4

Schematic presentation of insulin's direct and indirect inhibitory effects on hepatic glucose production.

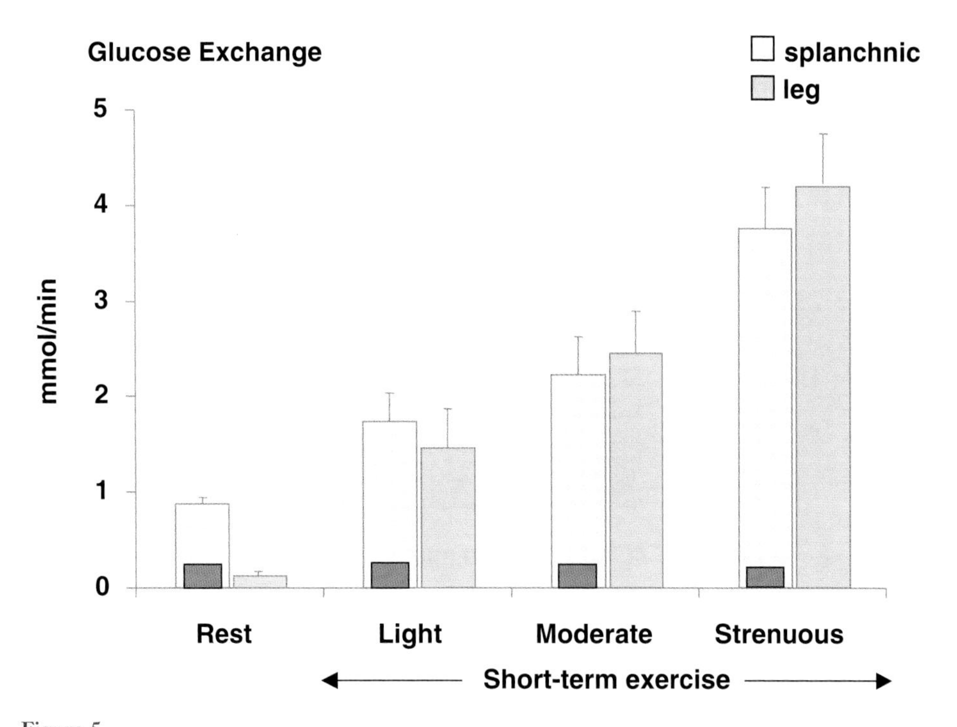

Figure 5

Splanchnic (*yellow*) and leg (*gray*) glucose exchange during short-term exercise of varying intensity in healthy subjects. Gluconeogenesis, evaluated as the sum of gluconeogenic precursor uptake by the splanchnic area, is indicated in green. Data from (108).

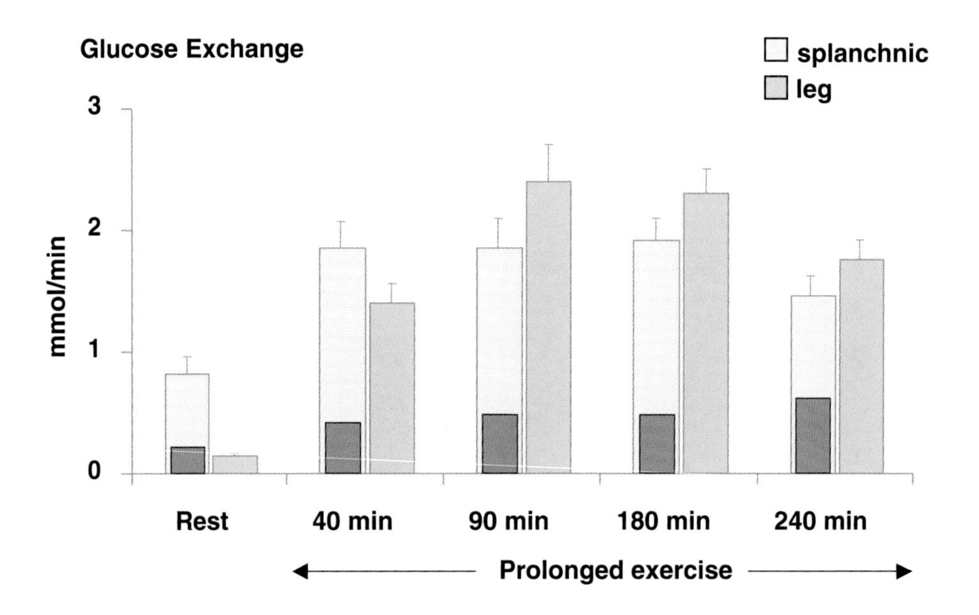

Figure 6

Splanchnic (*yellow*) and leg (*gray*) glucose exchange during prolonged exercise. Gluconeogenesis, evaluated as the sum of gluconeogenic precursor uptake by the splanchnic area, is indicated in green. Data from (4).

gluconeogenesis does not appear tenable on the basis of available evidence.

SPLANCHNIC GLUCOSE DISPOSAL

The liver's localization and its vascular anatomy make it ideally suited to regulate the flux of nutrients to the systemic circulation. It is also the only organ capable of both producing and assimilating substantial net amounts of glucose. Several studies have now established that the liver takes up approximately one third of an oral glucose load; muscle adipose tissue and the noninsulin-dependent tissues together account for the other two thirds (43, 76). Following ingestion of glucose, insulin and glucose levels rise, hepatic glucose output is suppressed, and net splanchnic glucose uptake can proceed at high rates (25–30 μmoles $\cdot$ min^{-1} $\cdot$ kg^{-1}) (14, 43). Direct determinations of hepatic glycogen concentrations following ingestion of a glucose load using ^{13}C-NMRS confirm a marked increase in glycogen synthesis; hepatic glycogen deposition at 5 h after a glucose load accounts for 23% to 26% of the ingested glucose (7, 8). Studies of glycogen metabolism during infusion of ^{13}C-glucose in healthy subjects have revealed that hepatic synthesis and degradation of glycogen occur simultaneously under conditions of net glycogen breakdown (71). The observations indicate that glycogen may regulate its own rate of breakdown and that hepatic glycogen turnover may be a factor in limiting the accumulation of liver glycogen. Hepatic glycogen accumulation during normal eating behavior has also been examined. Liver glycogen was found to gradually increase following ingestion of three consecutive mixed meals with 5 h intervals, indicating that hepatic glycogenolysis may be limited during the daytime, with glucose absorbed from meals accounting for the dominating part of whole-body glucose turnover while net hepatic glycogenolysis contributes to glucose production primarily during the night (55).

Varying results have been obtained in the estimation of the extent of suppression of hepatic glucose production following ingestion of an oral glucose load. Using tracer infusion and arterial-hepatic venous balance measurements in healthy subjects, suppression of hepatic glucose production has been estimated at 28% to 55% compared with basal levels (59, 75). The variability may partly be explained by the absence of steady state conditions after oral glucose ingestion, resulting in changes in glucose-specific activity. A new approach has been developed that is based on variable tracer infusion rates and results in relatively stable tracee/tracer ratios (105, 106). The findings using this technique indicate that 65% to 80% of the basal glucose production is suppressed at one hour after a mixed meal, which underscores the importance of this factor in the disposal of oral carbohydrates.

Hormonal Regulation of Hepatic Glucose Uptake

Glucose has the ability to modulate its own metabolism by the liver. Thus, there is a close relationship between the net balance of glucose across the liver and the ambient glucose concentration independent of any change in insulin concentration (101). When insulin and glucagon are at basal levels, hyperglycemia results in modest suppression of net release of glucose from the liver, and supraphysiological hyperglycemia (>12 mmol/L) is required to achieve a substantial rate of hepatic glucose uptake (29, 85, 104). This autoregulation by glucose is influenced by insulin, since the ability of the liver to respond to variations in glucose concentration is impaired in insulin-deficient states and ameliorated by insulin administration (27). Insulin stimulates glucose uptake by the liver, but physiological hyperinsulinemia by itself is relatively ineffective in promoting net hepatic glucose uptake. In healthy subjects, only modest rates of glucose uptake were evident in the presence of insulin levels greater than 500 pmol/L and euglycemia (29, 32). Similarly, pharmacological concentrations of insulin (>12000 pmol/L) were required to achieve a substantial increase in net hepatic glucose uptake in the presence of euglycemia, as evident from studies in dogs (74). Glucagon concentrations tend to decrease following carbohydrate ingestion (76). Somatostatin-induced selective glucagon deficiency with simultaneous insulin replacement results in reduced basal hepatic glucose output but not in augmented hepatic glucose uptake after a glucose load (102). Likewise, lower-than-basal glucagon concentrations in dogs made hyperinsulinemic and hyperglycemic were not accompanied by increased hepatic glucose uptake compared with basal glucagon under the same conditions (53). Thus, there is no evidence to indicate that a decrease in glucagon concentrations is of importance for glucose uptake by the liver after oral glucose intake.

Route of Glucose Delivery

Oral ingestion of a carbohydrate load in comparison with systemic glucose infusion in healthy subjects results in substantially higher rates of hepatic glucose uptake (29). This increase is achieved by augmented splanchnic fractional extraction of glucose after oral compared with systemic glucose administration (44), a finding initially attributed to a gut-derived factor (31). Subsequent studies have demonstrated, however, that intraportal infusion of glucose in dogs elicits similar rates of hepatic glucose uptake, as observed after oral glucose administration (6, 56), rendering an incretin contribution unlikely. The enhancement of hepatic glucose uptake with portal infusion was found to be correlated to the arterial-portal venous concentration difference for glucose and has been referred to as the portal signal (2). In fact, the influence of this signal is such that if insulin concentrations and glucose load to the liver are maintained constant, portal as compared with systemic glucose administration results in a 2- to 2.5-fold greater hepatic glucose uptake (79, 85). Further studies have shown that the portal signal also affects nonhepatic tissues; it mediates suppression of glucose uptake by skeletal muscle (47) and stimulates insulin release from the pancreas (34), thereby further enhancing hepatic glycogen accumulation after an oral glucose load.

Much experimental work has been undertaken to elucidate the mechanism underlying the portal signal. Surgical denervation of the liver totally blocks the enhancement of hepatic glucose uptake following portal glucose delivery (3), indicating neural mediation of the portal signal. Glucose-sensitive neurons have been demonstrated in the portal vein, and their discharge rate is proportional to the portal vein glucose concentration (80), suggesting a role in mediating the portal glucose signal. Cooling of the vagus nerves, which interrupts the efferent parasympathetic firing, had no effect on hepatic glucose uptake in the presence of the portal signal (58), indicating that parasympathetic signaling is not involved in the transmission of the portal signal. Instead, recent evidence suggests that sympathetic efferents may be of importance in the regulation of hepatic glucose uptake by exerting a basal inhibitory influence that limits glucose uptake in response to systemic glucose administration (33). It may then be hypothesized that the portal signal leads to removal of a sympathetic inhibitory influence on the liver, which in turn allows hepatic glucose uptake to increase. Whether removal of sympathetic tone to the liver is accompanied by a stimulatory signal will require further evaluation.

Hepatic Glucose Uptake in the Postexercise Period

It is well known that muscle glucose uptake and glycogen synthesis are enhanced in the postexercise period. Important alterations in glucose metabolism occur also within the splanchnic area. Thus, the efficiency with which oral carbohydrate is made available to the systemic circulation is increased during the postexercise period as a consequence of both accelerated intestinal absorption (88) and a shift in the partitioning of the absorbed glucose, resulting in a larger fraction escaping hepatic retention (51, 70). Nevertheless, net hepatic glucose uptake after exercise and oral ingestion of glucose is substantially increased (45). This phenomenon appears unrelated to any change in the portal signal, since its effectiveness in stimulating hepatic glucose uptake after portal glucose administration is similar in the basal and postexercise states (46). Exercise-induced changes in insulin and glucagon are not required for the postexercise enhancement of hepatic glucose uptake (87), and other, possibly intrinsic, hepatic mechanisms will have to be examined. However, irrespective of the exact mechanism involved, it is apparent that the above observations provide an additional physiological argument for advocating the benefits of physical exercise in individuals at risk of developing type 2 diabetes, particularly in view of the hepatic insulin resistance in this disorder (28, 89).

SPLANCHNIC GLUCOSE OUTPUT DURING FASTING

A series of well-coordinated hormonal and metabolic adjustments serve to ensure adequate supply of substrates to body tissues during periods of food deprivation. Blood glucose falls slightly when fasting extends beyond the first 12 hours after ingestion of a meal and reaches a new steady state level approximately 10% to 20% lower than before. This is accompanied by a reduction in insulin and rise in glucagon concentrations. Adipose tissue lipolysis is stimulated by the hormonal changes, resulting in increased availability and tissue utilization of FFA. As the period of fasting extends beyond 24–48 hours, there is augmented hepatic FFA uptake and acceleration of ketogenesis. The concentrations of betahydroxybutyrate and acetoacetate in plasma rise gradually and may in 2–3 weeks have risen as much as 100-fold above prefasting levels. The lipid-derived substrates FFA and ketoacids become the dominating fuels for most tissues, contributing substantially also to the supply of fuel for the brain. For a recent review of the metabolic adaptation to starvation, see (16).

Fasting for 12 to 60 Hours

A continued supply of glucose during fasting is essential for the function of specific tissues. The brain requires glucose during the early phase of fasting, but as food deprivation continues and ketoacid availability increases, there is a gradual shift toward utilization of ketoacids, particularly betahydroxybutyrate by the brain, with a correspondingly diminished but not abolished need for glucose (84). Bone marrow, renal medulla, red blood cells, and peripheral nerves are all tissues with an obligatory requirement for glucose unable to utilize FFA or ketoacids. As a consequence, a minimum rate of glucose production has to be maintained throughout the period of fasting. This is achieved by continued hepatic glucose production supported by a gradually increasing component of renal gluconeogenesis. The contribution from hepatic glycogenolysis, accounting for 50% in the overnight fasted state, decreases progressively during the first 12–40 hours of fasting and then ceases altogether (**Figure 1**) (81, 97). Gluconeogenesis, primarily derived from the liver, continues during 12–40 hours of fasting at approximately the same rate as in the overnight fasted state (17, 19, 66) and shows a modest increase at 60 hours (36). Since glycogenolysis decreases during progressive fasting, it follows that the relative contribution by gluconeogenesis to total glucose production increases gradually and accounts for $93 \pm 2\%$ after 60 hours of fasting (36). Several factors contribute to the sustained or even augmented rates of gluconeogenesis during fasting. The arterial concentration and splanchnic uptake of glycerol increase, secondary to augmented lipolysis (9). Uptake of glucogenic amino acids tends to rise due to increased fractional extraction, which overrides the effect of falling arterial concentrations (36, 37). Finally, a distinct component of renal gluconeogenesis is detectable after

60 hours of fasting, accounting for 20% to 25% of whole-body glucose turnover (11, 36).

max VO_2: maximal pulmonary oxygen uptake

Prolonged (Five to Six Weeks) Fasting

The liver and the kidneys show further metabolic adjustments when fasting continues beyond 60 hours. In the prolonged fasted state, hepatic glucose output derived from gluconeogenesis is further decreased, as indicated by reduced net splanchnic glucose output and diminished urinary urea excretion (84). The attenuation of hepatic gluconeogenesis is an important step in the sparing of body protein during prolonged starvation, which is essential for survival. It results from diminished presentation of amino acids, primarily alanine, to the liver, while splanchnic fractional extraction is unchanged (39). The elevated levels of ketoacids during fasting have been suggested as an important regulating factor in the reduction of muscle proteolysis during fasting (100). Administration of exogenous alanine results in a prompt hyperglycemic response, suggesting that provision of gluconeogenic precursor substrate is the rate-limiting step in the control of hepatic gluconeogenesis in prolonged starvation (38). The increased levels of ketoacids are accompanied by a need to balance their urinary loss of ammonium cation excretion. Renal ammoniagenesis, accounting for approximately 40% of total nitrogen excretion in prolonged fasting, is tightly coupled to renal gluconeogenesis, which explains why renal gluconeogenesis may account for as much as 45% of total glucose production in prolonged fasting (83).

GLUCOSE PRODUCTION DURING PHYSICAL EXERCISE

It has been more than 100 years since it was demonstrated that glucose uptake increases by contracting muscle (18). The magnitude of the exercise-induced rise in glucose utilization during, for example, leg exercise, indicates that the turnover of the blood glucose pool must increase substantially. Since the arterial glucose concentration is maintained or even increased during heavy exercise, one can conclude that the augmented peripheral glucose utilization must be accompanied by continuous and matching repletion of the blood glucose pool. Although the kidney has the capacity to synthesize glucose, direct measurements show that there is very little or no renal glucose output during exercise (108). The liver is the only other tissue capable of significant glucose production, and it can be concluded that augmented hepatic glucose output is the primary source of the increased glucose available to exercising muscle.

It is primarily the intensity and duration of the exercise that determine the magnitude of the rise in glucose output and the relative contributions from glycogenolysis and gluconeogenesis (**Figure 5**, see color insert). During light bicycle or treadmill exercise of short duration (20–30 minutes), glucose output rises by 50% to 100%; during moderate to heavy exercise it may increase 2 to 5 fold (108), as determined by either arterial-hepatic venous balance technique (108) or isotope tracer methods (5). Low- to moderate-intensity exercise [~30% maximal pulmonary oxygen uptake (max VO_2)] lasting several hours is accompanied by an initial rise in glucose output by 50% to 100% to a level that is sustained for several hours and then gradually decreases (4). During more strenuous (>60% max VO_2) and long-lasting exercise, glucose utilization by working muscle may outstrip glucose production, resulting in gradual development of hypoglycemia (**Figure 6**, see color insert) (107).

Hepatic glycogenolysis accelerates in direct proportion to the intensity of the exercise during work of short to intermediate duration (<60 minutes) as estimated both from NMRS measurements (90) and arterial-hepatic venous balance measurements (108). Particularly during strenuous exercise, augmented hepatic glycogenolysis is the dominating source of increased glucose production

(108). With prolonged exercise, the contribution from glycogenolysis decreases gradually, in keeping with diminished hepatic glycogen stores, and the contribution from gluconeogenesis become greater. The rate of hepatic gluconeogenesis during exercise has been estimated primarily on the basis of splanchnic uptake of glucose precursors. Measurements show that splanchnic precursor uptake increases by 50% to 100% during mild to moderate exercise, mostly because of augmented availability and uptake of lactate (108), but total splanchnic glucose output rises more, so that the fractional contribution by gluconeogenesis becomes smaller than in the basal state. During prolonged exercise, splanchnic precursor uptake increases severalfold as a result of augmented precursor availability and splanchnic fractional extraction, resulting primarily in increased lactate and glycerol uptake (4). In addition, there is evidence to suggest that intrahepatic mechanisms more efficiently channel glucose precursors to glucose during exercise (113). Thus, during prolonged exercise, gluconeogenesis may account for as much as 30% to 40% of total glucose output (4).

It should be remembered, however, that estimates of hepatic gluconeogenesis based on precursor uptake during exercise are based on several assumptions; extrahepatic splanchnic metabolism of glucose and precursors is considered negligible and intrahepatic conversion of the gluconeogenic precursors is assumed to be fully efficient. Other methods for estimation of hepatic gluconeogenesis during exercise have been employed. The results using MIDA- and NMRS-based estimates support the contention that hepatic gluconeogenesis increases with exercise (90, 107), but quantitative interpretation of the data is complicated by the methodological difficulties discussed above. In summary, it may be concluded that both hepatic glycogenolysis and gluconeogenesis contribute importantly to the body's remarkable ability to maintain blood glucose homeostasis over a wide range of exercise intensities and durations.

Regulatory Aspects

Several hormonal changes that accompany the onset of physical exercise serve to regulate splanchnic release of glucose. The plasma insulin concentration, which decreases with light exercise, decreases even more so during heavy work (108), thereby increasing the liver's sensitivity to the effects of glucagon (68). Glucagon levels are largely unchanged during mild to moderate exercise but rise in response to either strenuous or prolonged work (4, 41), particularly if a degree of hypoglycemia ensues. It should be recognized that the liver is exposed to more marked changes in glucagon concentration during exercise—because of the portal venous drainage of the pancreas—than is reflected by the systemic concentrations of the hormone. In addition, hepatic blood flow is known to decrease during exercise. Thus, if hepatic blood flow decreases by 50% during exercise (108), then a doubling of the glucagon concentration in the portal vein would be expected even if secretion rates did not change. Research in humans and dogs involving clamp studies, pharmacological blockage, and replacement infusions of insulin and glucagon have demonstrated that the exercise-induced reciprocal changes in the two glucoregulatory hormones account for a major proportion of the increase in hepatic glucose output by augmenting glycogenolysis and stimulating both glucose precursor extraction and their intrahepatic conversion to glucose (22, 111, 114).

Factors other than altered levels of insulin and glucagon have also been suggested to be of importance for the exercise-induced rise in glucose production (24). Plasma concentrations of adrenaline and noradrenalin markedly increase during exercise (60, 98). Yet, despite a close relationship between exercise-induced changes in glucose output and catecholamine levels, several studies using a variety of experimental techniques have failed to establish causality (23, 25, 54). Likewise, neither pharmacological blockade of the sympathetic innervation of the liver and the adrenals nor surgical denervation of the liver, as in humans with a liver transplant, result in marked effects on the exercise-induced increment in glucose output (61, 62, 112). Thus, it appears that although glucagon and insulin are of primary importance for the accurate regulation of hepatic glucose production during exercise, other and yet undetermined factors may also contribute.

SPLANCHNIC GLUCOSE PRODUCTION IN DIABETES

Type 1 Diabetes

The metabolic alterations observed in type 1 diabetes primarily reflect the degree to which there is an absolute or relative deficiency of insulin. Mild insulin deficiency can be expected to result in diminished ability to replenish the stores of carbohydrates and other fuels. With major insulin deficiency, not only is postprandial carbohydrate accumulation hampered, but excessive mobilization of endogenous substrates also occurs, resulting in hyperglycemia, hyperaminoacidemia, and elevated FFA levels. In keeping with these considerations, net splanchnic glucose production in patients with type 1 diabetes, who were studied after an overnight fast and without having received their morning dose of insulin, was similar or slightly augmented compared with controls (109, 110). Splanchnic uptake of gluconeogenic precursors was increased as a consequence of augmented fractional extraction in the case of lactate and amino acids. Hepatic gluconeogenesis, estimated from splanchnic precursor uptake, was 60% greater in the patients compared with controls (109). Direct determinations of hepatic glycogen using ^{13}C-NMRS in mildly insulin-deficient type 1 patients have indicated reduced glycogen levels and diminished rates of glycogenolysis (8, 90). Both defects of glycogen metabolism improved substantially after restoration of near-normal levels of insulin and blood glucose (7). In agreement with these observations, gluconeogenesis determined by the deuterated water technique has been found to be in the normal range in well-controlled type 1 patients (13). Hepatic glucose uptake and glycogen repletion after carbohydrate ingestion is reduced in type 1 diabetes (8, 55), resulting in excessive entry of glucose into the systemic circulation, in part caused by insufficient suppression of hepatic glucose output (86). Again, intensive insulin therapy and achievement of good blood glucose control restored normal postprandial suppression of hepatic glucose production (86) and net hepatic glucose assimilation after glucose ingestion (7). These observations emphasize that optimal metabolic control in type 1 diabetes ensures adequate postprandial hepatic glycogen accumulation despite systemic, as distinct from portal, delivery of insulin.

Type 2 Diabetes

The abnormal glucose homeostasis in type 2 diabetes is a consequence of several metabolic alterations: defective insulin secretion, insulin resistance involving muscle, liver, and adipose tissue, and abnormal splanchnic glucose metabolism. Only the latter factor is discussed here. The potential role of augmented basal glucose production from the liver in the pathogenesis of hyperglycemia in type 2 diabetes has been much discussed, and measurements of glucose production have yielded varying results [for a review see (93)]. When the diversity of the patient population, the experimental conditions, and techniques of measurement are carefully considered, the combined evidence supports the view that there is a direct relationship between hepatic glucose production in type 2 diabetes patients and fasting blood glucose levels (30, 94). An excessive rate of glucose production may thus be an important factor contributing to the elevated fasting glucose levels in patients with poor metabolic control (30).

The augmented flux of glucose from the liver in type 2 diabetes can derive from accelerated glycogenolysis, gluconeogenesis, or both. The hepatic glycogen store and rates of glycogenolysis have been estimated using ^{13}C-NMRS techniques and were found to be reduced in type 2 patients with relatively poor metabolic control (72) and similar to that of healthy subjects in type 2 patients with good metabolic control (49). Hepatic gluconeogenesis, on the other hand, is reported to be increased in proportion to the severity of the diabetic state and the reduction in hepatic glycogen stores, both in absolute and relative terms (12, 49, 72). In this context, it is noted that an important component of the therapeutic effect of peroxisome proliferator-activated receptor-γ activating agents, such as thiazolidinediones, on the fasting blood glucose level is exerted by reducing the gluconeogenic flux in type 2 diabetic subjects (48).

Elevated plasma insulin levels after an overnight fast together with varying degrees of hyperglycemia are characteristic features in subjects with type 2 diabetes. Since hyperinsulinemia together with elevated levels of glucose are potent inhibitors of hepatic glucose output in healthy subjects (**Figure 3**) (40, 103), it can be concluded that there is hepatic resistance to the action of both insulin and glucose in type 2 patients (28) and that this defect becomes more pronounced with increasing severity of the diabetic state (50). Consequently, ingestion of glucose or a mixed meal leads to excessive and prolonged hyperglycemia in type 2 diabetes, which in part can be attributed to diminished net hepatic glucose uptake and failure to adequately suppress glucose production (63, 105). Thus, a reduced efficiency of the splanchnic tissues to take up glucose after oral ingestion is an important contributing factor in the impaired glucose tolerance of type 2 diabetes.

Finally, although Claude Bernard was unable to identify the pathogenic mechanisms underlying the development of diabetes, primarily due to lack of knowledge of the existence of insulin, much of his original work applies to normal physiology and to the forms of diabetes that we now distinguish as type 1 and type 2 (69). Bernard's fundamental contributions in the middle of the nineteenth century proved a rational basis for subsequent discoveries to build on.

LITERATURE CITED

1. Ader M, Bergman R. 1990. Peripheral effects of insulin dominates suppression of fasting hepatic glucose production. *Am. J. Physiol. Endocrinol. Metab.* 258:E1020–32
2. Adkins B, Myers S, Hendrick G, Stevenson R, Williams P, Cherrington A. 1987. Importance of the route of intravenous glucose delivery to hepatic glucose balance in the conscious dog. *J. Clin. Invest.* 79:557–65
3. Adkins-Marshall B, Pagliassotti M, Asher J, Connolly C, Neal D, et al. 1992. Role of hepatic nerves in response of liver to intraportal glucose delivery in dogs. *Am. J. Physiol. Endocrinol. Metab.* 262:E679–86
4. Ahlborg G, Felig P, Hagenfeldt L, Hendler R, Wahren J. 1974. Substrate turnover during prolonged exercise in man. Splanchnic and leg metabolism of glucose, free fatty acids, and amino acids. *J. Clin. Invest.* 53:1080–90
5. Bergeron R, Kjaer M, Simonsen L, Bulow J, Galbo H. 1999. Glucose production during exercise in humans: a-hv balance and isotopic-tracer measurements compared. *J. Appl. Physiol.* 87:111–15
6. Bergman R, Beir J, Hourigan P. 1982. Intraportal glucose infusion matched to oral glucose absorption. Lack of evidence for "gut factor" involvement in hepatic glucose storage. *Diabetes* 31:27–35
7. Bischof M, Bernroider E, Krssak M, Krebs M, Stingl H, et al. 2002. Hepatic glycogen metabolism in type 1 diabetes after long-term near normoglycemia. *Diabetes* 51:49–54

8. Bischof M, Krssak M, Krebs M, Bernroider E, Stingl H, et al. 2001. Effects of short-term improvement of insulin treatment and glycemia on hepatic glycogen metabolism in type 1 diabetes. *Diabetes* 50:392–98
9. Björkman O, Eriksson L. 1983. Splanchnic glucose metabolism during leg exercise in 60-hour fasted human subjects. *Am. J. Physiol. Endocrinol. Metab.* 245:E443–48
10. Björkman O, Eriksson L, Nyberg B, Wahren J. 1990. Gut exchange of glucose and lactate in basal state and after oral glucose ingestion in postoperative patients. *Diabetes* 39:747–51
11. Björkman O, Felig P, Wahren J. 1980. The contrasting responses of splanchnic and renal glucose output to gluconeogenic substrates and to hypoglucagonemia in 60-h fasted humans. *Diabetes* 29:610–16
12. Boden G, Chen X, Stein T. 2001. Gluconeogenesis in moderately and severely hyperglycemic patients with type 2 diabetes mellitus. *Am. J. Physiol. Endocrinol. Metab.* 280:E23–30
13. Boden G, Cheung P, Homko C. 2003. Effects of acute insulin excess and deficiency on gluconeogenesis and glycogenolysis in type 1 diabetes. *Diabetes* 52:133–37
14. Bratusch-Marrain P, Waldhäusl W, Gasic S, Korn A, Nowotny P. 1980. Oral glucose tolerance test: effect of different glucose loads on splanchnic carbohydrate and substrate metabolism in healthy man. *Metabolism* 29:289–95
15. Burrin D, Lambert B, Stoll B, Guan X. 2005. Gastrointestinal gluconeogenesis is absent in the 36-hour fasted piglet. *FASEB J.* 19:A1675
16. Cahill G. 2006. Fuel metabolism in starvation. *Annu. Rev. Nutr.* 26:1–22
17. Chandramouli V, Ekberg K, Schumann WC, Kalhan SC, Wahren J, Landau BR. 1997. Quantifying gluconeogenesis during fasting. *Am. J. Physiol. Endocrinol. Metab.* 273:E1209–15
18. Chauveau M, Kaufmann M. 1887. Experiments to determine the nutritive and respiratory coefficient of activity in resting and working muscles. *C. R. Acad. Sci.* 104:1126–32
19. Chen X, Iqbal N, Boden G. 1999. The effects of free fatty acids on gluconeogenesis and glycogenolysis in normal subjects. *J. Clin. Invest.* 103:365–72
20. Cherrington A. 2005. The role of hepatic insulin receptors in the regulation of glucose production. *J. Clin. Invest.* 115:1136–39
21. Chiasson J, Liljenquist J, Finger F, Lacy W. 1976. Differential sensitivity of glycogenolysis and gluconeogenesis to insulin infusion in dogs. *Diabetes* 25:283–91
22. Cocker R, Kjaer M. 2005. Glucoregulation during exercise. *Sports Med.* 35:575–83
23. Coker R, Krishna M, Lacy D, Bracy D, Wasserman D. 1997. Role of hepatic alpha- and beta-adrenergic receptor stimulation on hepatic glucose production during heavy exercise. *Am. J. Physiol. Endocrinol. Metab.* 273:E831–38
24. Coker R, Simonsen L, Bulow J, Wasserman DH, Kjaer M. 2001. Stimulation of splanchnic glucose production during exercise in humans contains a glucagon-independent component. *Am. J. Physiol. Endocrinol. Metab.* 280:E918–27
25. Connolly C, Steiner K, Stevenson R, Neal D, Williams P, et al. 1991. Regulation of glucose metabolism by norepinephrine in conscious dogs. *Am. J. Physiol. Endocrinol. Metab.* 261:E764–72
26. Croset M, Rajas F, Zitoun C, Hurot J, Montano S, Mithieux G. 2001. Rat small intestine is an insulin-sensitive gluconeogenic organ. *Diabetes* 50:740–46
27. Davidson M. 1981. Autoregulation by glucose of hepatic glucose balance: permissive effect of insulin. *Metabolism* 30:279–84
28. DeFronzo R, Ferrannini E, Hendler R, Felig P, Wahren J. 1983. Regulation of splanchnic and peripheral glucose uptake by insulin and hyperglycemia in man. *Diabetes* 32:35–45

29. DeFronzo R, Ferrannini E, Hendler R, Wahren J, Felig P. 1978. Influence of hyperinsulinemia, hyperglycemia and the route of glucose administration on splanchnic glucose exchange. *Proc. Natl. Acad. Sci. USA* 75:5173–77
30. DeFronzo R, Ferrannini E, Simonson D. 1989. Fasting hyperglycemia in noninsulin-dependent diabetes mellitus: contributions of excessive hepatic glucose production and impaired tissue glucose uptake. *Metabolism* 38:387–95
31. DeFronzo R, Ferrannini E, Wahren J, Felig P. 1978. Lack of gastrointestinal mediator of insulin action in maturity-onset diabetes. *Lancet* 18:1077–79
32. DeFronzo RA, Ferrannini E. 1987. Regulation of hepatic glucose metabolism in humans. *Diabet. Metab. Rev.* 3:415–59
33. Dicostanzo C, Dardevet D, Neal D, Lautz M, Allen E, et al. 2006. Role of the hepatic sympathetic nerves in the regulation of net hepatic glucose uptake and the mediation of the portal glucose signal. *Am. J. Physiol. Endocrinol. Metab.* 290:E9–16
34. Dunning B, Moore M, Ikeda T, Neal D, Scott M, Cherrington AD. 2002. Portal glucose infusion exerts an incretin effect associated with changes in pancreatic neural activity in conscious dogs. *Metabolism* 51:1324–30
35. Edgerton D, Lautz M, Scott M, Everett C, Stettler K, et al. 2006. Insulin's direct effect on the liver dominates the control of hepatic glucose production. *J. Clin. Invest.* 116:302–4
36. Ekberg K, Landau BR, Wajngot A, Chandramouli V, Efendic S, et al. 1999. Contributions by kidney and liver to glucose production in the postabsorptive state and after 60 h of fasting. *Diabetes* 48:292–98
37. Eriksson LS, Olsson M, Bjorkman O. 1988. Splanchnic metabolism of amino acids in healthy subjects: effect of 60 hours of fasting. *Metabolism* 37:1159–62
38. Felig P, Marliss E, Owen O, Cahill G. 1969. Blood glucose and gluconeogenesis in fasting man. *Arch. Intern. Med.* 123:293–98
39. Felig P, Owen OE, Wahren J, Cahill GF Jr. 1969. Amino acid metabolism during prolonged starvation. *J. Clin. Invest.* 48:584–94
40. Felig P, Wahren J. 1971. Influence of endogenous insulin secretion on splanchnic glucose and metabolism in man. *J. Clin. Invest.* 50:1702–11
41. Felig P, Wahren J, Haendler R, Ahlborg G. 1972. Plasma glucagon levels in exercising man. *New Engl. J. Med.* 287:184–85
42. Felig P, Wahren J, Raf L. 1973. Evidence of interorgan amino-acid transport by blood cells in humans. *Proc. Natl. Acad. Sci. USA* 70:1775–79
43. Ferrannini E, Björkman O, Reichard GJ, Pilo A, Olsson M, et al. 1985. The disposal of an oral glucose load in healthy subjects. A quantitative study. *Diabetes* 34:580–88
44. Ferrannini E, Wahren J, Felig P, DeFronzo R. 1980. The role of fractional glucose extraction in the regulation of splanchnic glucose metabolism in normal and diabetic man. *Metabolism* 29:28–35
45. Galasetti P, Coker R, Lacy D, Cherrington A, Wasserman D. 1999. Prior exercise increases net hepatic glucose uptake during a glucose load. *Am. J. Physiol. Endocrinol. Metab.* 276:E1022–29
46. Galasetti P, Koyama Y, Coker R, Lacy D, Cherrington A, Wasserman D. 1999. Role of a negative arterial-portal venous glucose gradient in the postexercise state. *Am. J. Physiol. Endocrinol. Metab.* 277:E1038–45
47. Galasetti P, Shoita M, Zinker B, Wasserman D, Cherrington A. 1998. A negative arterial-portal venous glucose gradient decreases skeletal muscle glucose uptake. *Am. J. Physiol. Endocrinol. Metab.* 275:E101–11

48. Gastaldelli A, Miyazaki Y, Pettiti M, Santini E, Ciociaro D, et al. 2006. The effect of rosiglitazone on the liver: decreased gluconeogenesis in patients with type 2 diabetes. *J. Clin. Endocrinol. Metab.* 91:806–12
49. Gastaldelli A, Toschi E, Pettiti M, Frascerra S, Quinones-Galvan A, et al. 2001. Effect of physiological hyperinsulinemia on gluconeogenesis in nondiabetic subjects and in type 2 diabetic patients. *Diabetes* 50:1807–12
50. Groop L, Bonadonna R, DelPrato S, Ratheiser K, Zyck K, et al. 1989. Glucose and free fatty acid metabolism in noninsulin-dependent diabetes mellitus. Evidence for multiple sites of insulin resistance. *J. Clin. Invest.* 84:205–13
51. Hamilton K, Gibbons F, Bracy D, Lacy D, Cherrington A, Wasserman D. 1996. Effect of prior exercise on the partitioning of an intestinal glucose load between splanchnic bed and skeletal muscle. *J. Clin. Invest.* 98:125–35
52. Hellerstein MK, Neese RA. 1992. Mass isotopomer distribution analysis: a technique for measuring biosynthesis and turnover of polymers. *Am. J. Physiol. Endocrinol. Metab.* 263:E988–1001
53. Holste L, Connolly C, Moore M, Neal D, Cherrington A. 1997. Physiological changes in circulating glucagon after hepatic glucose disposition during portal glucose delivery. *Am. J. Physiol. Endocrinol. Metab.* 273:E488–96
54. Howlett K, Balbo H, Lorentsen J, Bergeron R, Zimmerma-Belsing T, et al. 1999. Effect of adrenaline on glucose kinetics during exercise in adrenalectomised humans. *J. Physiol.* 519:911–21
55. Hwang JH, Perseghin G, Rothman DL, Cline GW, Magnusson I, et al. 1995. Impaired net hepatic glycogen synthesis in insulin-dependent diabetic subjects during mixed meal ingestion. A ^{13}C nuclear magnetic resonance spectroscopy study. *J. Clin. Invest.* 95:783–87
56. Ishida T, Chap Z, Chou J, Lewis R, Hartley C, et al. 1983. Differential effects of oral, peripheral intravenous, and intraportal glucose on hepatic glucose uptake and insulin and glucagon extraction in conscious dogs. *J. Clin. Invest.* 72:590–601
57. Ishihara H, Maechler P, Gjinovci A, Herrera P, Wollheim C. 2003. Islet beta-cell secretion determines glucagon release from neighboring alpha-cells. *Nat. Cell Biol.* 5:330–35
58. Jackson P, Pagliassotti M, Shoita M, Neal D, Cardin S, Cherrington A. 1997. Effects of vagal blockade on the counterregulatory response to insulin-induced hypoglycemia in the dog. *Am. J. Physiol. Endocrinol. Metab.* 273:E1178–88
59. Kelley D, Mokan M, Veneman T. 1994. Impaired postprandial glucose utilization in noninsulin dependent diabetes mellitus. *Metabolism* 43:1549–57
60. Kjaer M. 1998. Adrenal medulla and exercise training. *Eur. J. Appl. Physiol.* 77:195–99
61. Kjaer M, Engfred K, Fernandez A, Secher N, Galbo H. 1993. Regulation of hepatic glucose production during exercise in humans: role of sympathoadrenergic activity. *Am. J. Physiol. Endocrinol. Metab.* 265:E275–83
62. Kjaer M, Keiding S, Engfred K, Rasmussen K, Sonne B, et al. 1995. Glucose homeostasis during exercise in humans with a liver or kidney transplant. *Am. J. Physiol. Endocrinol. Metab.* 268:E636–44
63. Krssak M, Brehm A, Bernroider E, Anderwald C, Nowotny P, et al. 2004. Alterations in postprandial hepatic glycogen metabolism in type 2 diabetes. *Diabetes* 53:3048–56
64. Landau BR, Fernandez CA, Previs SF, Ekberg K, Chandramouli V, et al. 1995. A limitation in the use of mass isotopomer distributions to measure gluconeogenesis in fasting humans. *Am. J. Physiol. Endocrinol. Metab.* 269:E18–26
65. Landau BR, Wahren J, Chandramouli V, Schumann WC, Ekberg K, Kalhan SC. 1995. Use of ^2H_2O for estimating rates of gluconeogenesis. Application to the fasted state. *J. Clin. Invest.* 95:172–78

66. Landau BR, Wahren J, Chandramouli V, Schumann WC, Ekberg K, Kalhan SC. 1996. Contributions of gluconeogenesis to glucose production in the fasted state. *J. Clin. Invest.* 98:378–85
67. Large V, Soloviev M, Brunengraber H, Beylot M. 1995. Lactate and pyruvate isotopic enrichments in plasma and tissues of postabsorptive and starved rats. *Am. J. Physiol. Endocrinol. Metab.* 268:E880–88
68. Lins P, Wajngot A, Adamson U, Vranic M, Efendic S. 1983. Minimal increase in glucagon levels enhance glucose production in man with partial hypoinsulinemia. *Diabetes* 32:633–36
69. Lippi D, Caleri D, Bucalossi A, Rotella C. 1994. The role of liver in glucose homeostasis in type 2 diabetes: the modernity of Claude Bernard's studies. *Diabet. Metab. Rev.* 10:63–74
70. Maehlum S, Felig P, Wahren J. 1978. Splanchnic glucose and muscle glycogen metabolism after glucose feeding during postexercise recovery. *Am. J. Physiol. Endocrinol. Metab.* 235:E255–60
71. Magnusson I, Rothman DL, Jucker B, Cline GW, Shulman RG, Shulman GI. 1994. Liver glycogen turnover in fed and fasted humans. *Am. J. Physiol. Endocrinol. Metab.* 266:E796–803
72. Magnusson I, Rothman DL, Katz LD, Shulman RG, Shulman GI. 1992. Increased rate of gluconeogenesis in type II diabetes mellitus. A ^{13}C nuclear magnetic resonance study. *J. Clin. Invest.* 90:1323–27
73. Martin G, Ferrier B, Conjard A, Martin M, Nazaret R, et al. 2007. Glutamine gluconeogenesis in the small intestine of 72h-fasted adult rats is undetectable. *Biochem. J.* 401:465–73
74. McGuinness OP, Meyers S, Neal D, Cherrington AD. 1990. Chronic hyperinsulinemia decreases insulin action but not insulin sensitivity. *Metabolism* 39:931–37
75. McMahon M, Marsh H, Rizza R. 1989. Effects of basal insulin supplementation on disposition of mixed meal in obese patients with NIDDM. *Diabetes* 38:291–303
76. Meyer C, Dostou J, Welle S, Gerich J. 2002. Role of human liver, kidney, and skeletal muscle in postprandial glucose homeostasis. *Am. J. Physiol. Endocrinol. Metab.* 282:E419–27
77. Mithieux G, Bady I, Gautier A, Croset M, Rajas F, Zitoun C. 2004. Induction of control genes in intestinal gluconeogenesis is sequential during fasting and maximal diabetes. *Am. J. Physiol. Endocrinol. Metab.* 286:E370–75
78. Mithieux G, Rajas F, Gautier-Stein A. 2004. A novel role for glucose 6-phosphatase in the small intestine in the control of glucose homeostasis. *J. Biol. Chem.* 279:44231–34
79. Myers S, Biggers D, Neal D, Cherrington A. 1991. Intraportal glucose delivery enhances the effects of hepatic glucose load on net hepatic glucose uptake in vivo. *J. Clin. Invest.* 88:158–67
80. Niijima A. 1982. Glucose-sensitive afferent nerve fibres in the hepatic branch of the vagus nerve in the guinea-pig. *J. Physiol.* 332:315–23
81. Nilsson L, Hultman E. 1973. Liver glycogen in man—the effect of total starvation or a carbohydrate-poor diet followed by carbohydrate refeeding. *Scand. J. Clin. Lab. Invest.* 32:325–30
82. Obici S, Zhang B, Karkansias G, Rossetti L. 2002. Hypothalamic insulin signaling is required for inhibition of glucose production. *Nat. Med.* 8:1376–82
83. Owen OE, Felig P, Morgan AP, Wahren J, Cahill GF Jr. 1969. Liver and kidney metabolism during prolonged starvation. *J. Clin. Invest.* 48:574–83
84. Owen OE, Morgan AP, Kemp HG, Sullivan JM, Herrera MG, Cahill GF Jr. 1967. Brain metabolism during fasting. *J. Clin. Invest.* 46:1589–95

85. Pagliassotti M, Holste L, Moore M, Neal D, Cherrington A. 1996. Comparison of the time course of insulin and the portal signal on hepatic glucose and glycogen metabolism in the conscious dog. *J. Clin. Invest.* 97:81–91
86. Pehling G, Tessari P, Gerich J, Haymond M, Service F, Rizza R. 1984. Abnormal meal carbohydrate disposition in insulin-dependent diabetes. Relative contributions of endogenous glucose production and initial splanchnic uptake and effect of intensive insulin therapy. *J. Clin. Invest.* 74:985–91
87. Pencek R, James F, Lacy D, Jabbour K, Williams P, et al. 2004. Exercise-induced changes in insulin and glucagon are not required for enhanced hepatic glucose uptake after exercise but influence the fate of glucose within the liver. *Diabetes* 53:3041–47
88. Pencek R, Koyama Y, Lacy D, James F, Fueger P, et al. 2003. Prior exercise enhances passive absorption of intraduodenal glucose. *J. Appl. Physiol.* 95:1132–38
89. Petersen K, Dufour S, Befroy D, Lehrke D, Hendler R, Shulman G. 2005. Reversal of nonalcoholic hepatic steatosis, hepatic insulin resistance, and hyperglycemia by moderate weight reduction in patients with type 2 diabetes. *Diabetes* 54:603–8
90. Petersen K, Price T, Bergeron R. 2004. Regulation of net hepatic glycogenolysis and gluconeogenesis during exercise: impact of type 1 diabetes. *J. Clin. Endocrinol. Metab.* 89:4656–64
91. Petersen KF, Price T, Cline GW, Rothman DL, Shulman GI. 1996. Contribution of net hepatic glycogenolysis to glucose production during the early postprandial period. *Am. J. Physiol. Endocrinol. Metab.* 270:E186–91
92. Prager R, Wallace P, Olefsky J. 1987. Direct and indirect effects of insulin to inhibit hepatic glucose output in obese subjects. *Diabetes* 36:607–11
93. Radziuk J, Pye E. 2002. Quantitation of basal endogenous glucose production in type II diabetes: importance of the volume distribution. *Diabetologia* 45:1053–84
94. Radziuk J, Pye S. 2003. Tracer-determined glucose fluxes in healthy and type 2 diabetes: basal conditions. *Best Pract. Res. Clin. Endocrinol. Metab.* 17:323–42
95. Rajas F, Croset M, Zitoun C, Montano S, Mithieux G. 2000. Induction of PEPCK gene expression in insulinopenia in rat small intestine. *Diabetes* 49:1165–68
96. Robin E. 1979. *Claude Bernard and the Internal Milieu. A Memorial Symposium.* New York: Marcel Dekker
97. Rothman DL, Magnusson I, Katz LD, Shulman RG, Shulman GI. 1991. Quantitation of hepatic glycogenolysis and gluconeogenesis in fasting humans with ^{13}C NMR. *Science* 254:573–76
98. Savard G, Richter E, Strange S, Kiens B, Christensen N, Saltin B. 1989. Norepinephrine spillover from skeletal muscle during exercise in humans: role of muscle mass. *Am. J. Physiol. Heart Circ. Physiol.* 257:H1812–18
99. Schumann WC, Magnusson I, Chandramouli V, Kumaran K, Wahren J, Landau BR. 1991. Metabolism of [2-14C]acetate and its use in assessing hepatic Krebs cycle activity and gluconeogenesis. *J. Biol. Chem.* 266:6985–90
100. Sherwin R, Hendler R, Felig P. 1975. Effect of ketone infusion on amino acid and nitrogen metabolism in man. *J. Clin. Invest.* 55:1382–90
101. Shulman G, Lacy W, Liljenquist J, Keller U, Williams P, Cherrington A. 1980. Effect of glucose, independent of changes in insulin and glucagon secretion, on alanine metabolism in the conscious dog. *J. Clin. Invest.* 65:496–505
102. Shulman G, Liljenquist J, Williams P, Lacy W. 1978. Glucose disposal during insulinopenia in somatostatin-treated dogs. The roles of glucose and glucagon. *J. Clin. Invest.* 62:487–91

103. Sindelar D, Balcom J, Chu C, Neal D, Cherrington A. 1996. A comparison of the effects of selective increases in peripheral or portal insulin on hepatic glucose production in the conscious dog. *Diabetes* 45:1594–604
104. Sindelar D, Chu C, Venson P, Donahue E, Neal D, Cherrington D. 1998. Basal hepatic glucose production is regulated by the portal vein insulin concentration. *Diabetes* 47:523–29
105. Singhal P, Caumo A, Carey P, Cobelli C, Taylor R. 2002. Regulation of endogenous glucose production after a mixed meal in type 2 diabetes. *Am. J. Physiol. Endocrinol. Metab.* 283:E275–83
106. Taylor R, Magnusson I, Rothman DL, Cline GW, Caumo A, et al. 1996. Direct assessment of liver glycogen storage by ^{13}C nuclear magnetic resonance spectroscopy and regulation of glucose homeostasis after a mixed meal in normal subjects. *J. Clin. Invest.* 97:126–32
107. Trimmer J, Schwarz JM, Casazza G, Horning M, Rodriguez N, Brooks G. 2002. Measurement of gluconeogenesis in exercising men by mass isotopomer distribution analysis. *J. Appl. Physiol.* 93:233–41
108. Wahren J, Felig P, Ahlborg G, Jorfeldt L. 1971. Glucose metabolism during leg exercise in man. *J. Clin. Invest.* 50:2715–25
109. Wahren J, Felig P, Cerasi E, Luft R. 1972. Splanchnic and peripheral glucose and amino acid metabolism in diabetes mellitus. *J. Clin. Invest.* 51:1870–78
110. Wahren J, Hagenfeldt L, Felig P. 1975. Splanchnic and leg exchange of glucose, amino acids, and free fatty acids during exercise in diabetes mellitus. *J. Clin. Invest.* 55:1303–14
111. Wasserman D, Spalding J, Lacy D, Colburn C, Goldstein R, Cherrington A. 1989. Glucagon is a primary controller of hepatic glycogenolysis and gluconeogenesis during muscular work. *Am. J. Physiol. Endocrinol. Metab.* 77:E108–17
112. Wasserman D, Williams P, Lacy D, Bracy D, Cherrington A. 1990. Hepatic nerves are not essential to the increase in hepatic glucose production during muscular work. *Am. J. Physiol. Endocrinol. Metab.* 259:E195–203
113. Wasserman D, Williams P, Lacy D, Green D, Cherrington A. 1988. Importance of intrahepatic mechanisms to gluconeogenesis from alanine during exercise and recovery. *Am. J. Physiol. Endocrinol. Metab.* 254:E518–25
114. Wolfe R, Nadel E, Shaw J, Stephenson L, Wolfe M. 1986. Role of changes in insulin and glucagon in glucose homeostasis in exercise. *J. Clin. Invest.* 77:900–7

Vitamin E Regulatory Mechanisms

Maret G. Traber

Linus Pauling Institute, Department of Nutrition and Exercise Science, Oregon State University, Corvallis, Oregon 97331; email: maret.traber@oregonstate.edu

Annu. Rev. Nutr. 2007. 27:347–62

First published online as a Review in Advance on April 17, 2007

The *Annual Review of Nutrition* is online at http://nutr.annualreviews.org

This article's doi:
10.1146/annurev.nutr.27.061406.093819

0199-9885/07/0821-0347$20.00

Key Words

α-tocopherol, carboxy ethyl hydroxy chroman (CEHC), α-tocopherol transfer protein, vitamin E metabolism, tocopherol omega hydrolase, human vitamin E deficiency

Abstract

Dietary and supplemental vitamin E is absorbed and delivered to the liver, but of the various antioxidants with vitamin E activity, only α-tocopherol is preferentially recognized by the α-tocopherol transfer protein (α-TTP) and is transferred to plasma, while the other vitamin E forms (e.g., γ-tocopherol or tocotrienols) are removed from the circulation. Hepatic α-TTP is required to maintain plasma and tissue α-tocopherol concentrations. The liver is the master regulator of the body's vitamin E levels in that it not only controls α-tocopherol concentrations, but also appears to be the major site of vitamin E metabolism and excretion. Vitamin Es are metabolized similarly to xenobiotics; they are initially ω-oxidized by cytochrome P450s, undergo several rounds of β-oxidation, and then are conjugated and excreted. As a result of these various mechanisms, liver α-tocopherol and other vitamin E concentrations are closely regulated; thus, any potential adverse vitamin E effects are limited.

Contents

INTRODUCTION

Vitamin E was discovered in 1922, when Evans & Bishop (28) reported that rats fed rancid fat resorbed their fetuses during early pregnancy. The description of vitamin E deficiency in humans almost 60 years later then led the way to our understanding that the liver controls vitamin E with respect to the form and amounts of the vitamin. This review seeks to outline these major regulatory steps, show areas where consensus has been reached with respect to vitamin E trafficking, and emphasize areas that remain undeciphered with respect to regulatory mechanisms.

ROO: peroxyl radicals

ROOH: lipid hydroperoxides

VITAMIN E BIOAVAILABILITY PARADOX

In general, the term "vitamin E" includes four tocopherols and four tocotrienols (designated as α-, β-, γ-, and δ-) found in food. Unlike other nutrients, the body cannot interconvert these forms. Moreover, although these vitamin Es have similar antioxidant activities, only α-tocopherol meets human vitamin E requirements (30). Interestingly, the U.S. diet contains as much as ten times the concentration of γ-tocopherol, yet the body has ten times the concentration of α-tocopherol. Thus, the importance of bioavailability and the factors that determine vitamin E bioavailability are critical for understanding the mechanisms for regulation.

Vitamin E Antioxidant Activity

Vitamin E's antioxidant function is that of a peroxyl radical scavenger that terminates chain reactions of oxidation of polyunsaturated fatty acids (PUFAs) (18). When lipid hydroperoxides (ROOH) are oxidized to peroxyl radicals (ROO·), as could occur in the presence of free metals such as iron or copper, the ROO· react faster with α-tocopherol (Vit E-OH) than with PUFAs (17):

In the presence of vitamin E:

$$\text{ROO}\cdot + \text{Vit E-OH} \rightarrow \text{ROOH} + \text{Vit E-O}\cdot$$

In the absence of vitamin E:

$$\text{ROO}\cdot + \text{RH} \rightarrow \text{ROOH} + \text{R}\cdot$$

$$\text{R}\cdot + O_2 \rightarrow \text{ROO}\cdot$$

In this way, α-tocopherol acts as a chain-breaking antioxidant, preventing the further auto-oxidation of PUFAs in membranes or lipoproteins.

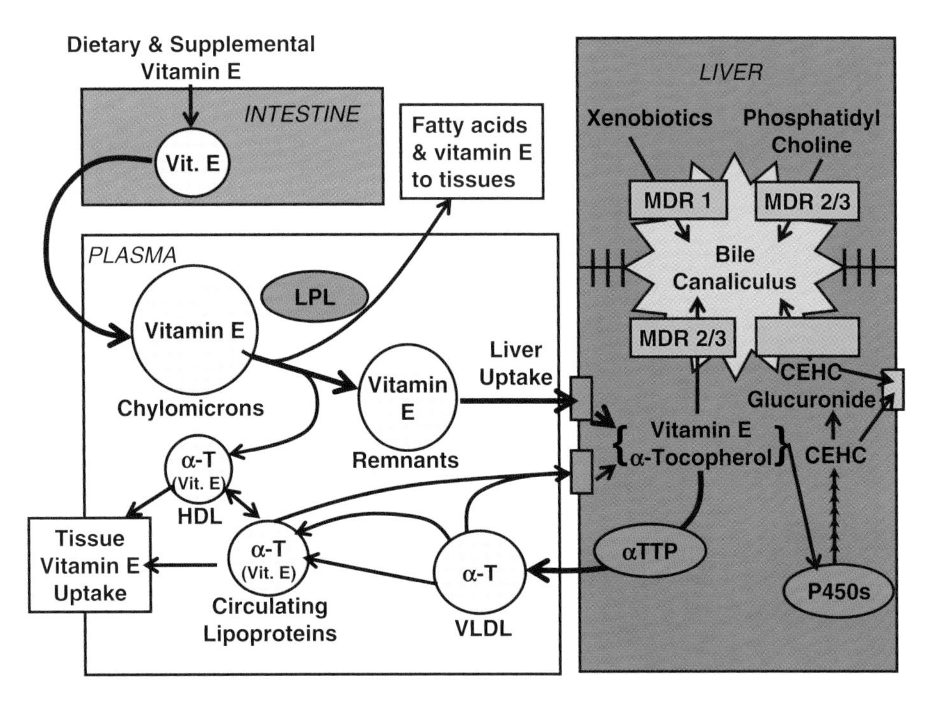

Figure 1

All forms of vitamin E are absorbed in the intestine (*gray*) and secreted into the circulation in chylomicrons. Lipoprotein lipase (lpl) hydrolyzes the chylomicron triglyceride and transfers fatty acids, as well as vitamin E, to tissues. During the formation of chylomicron remnants in the plasma compartment (*yellow*), some of the vitamin E is transferred to high-density lipoproteins (HDLs) and subsequently to other lipoproteins. The chylomicron remnants are taken up by the liver, where the α-tocopherol transfer protein (α-TTP) salvages α-tocopherol (α-T) from the lysosomal degradation pathway and returns it to the circulating lipoproteins, principally very-low-density lipoproteins (VLDLs). During lipoprotein catabolism in the circulation, α-T is redistributed among the various lipoproteins. Lipoproteins are taken up by the liver (and peripheral tissues) by various receptors (*blue rectangles*), and thus tocopherols are delivered to tissues by this process. In the liver, excess α-T and other vitamin E forms can be excreted into bile via the multidrug-resistance gene products (MDR 2/3), e.g., p-glycoprotein [ATP-binding cassette (ABC) and other transporters; *orange rectangles*]. Excess vitamin E is also metabolized by a cytochrome P450 (CYP)-mediated process to carboxy ethyl hydroxy chromans (CEHCs) that can be glucuronidated (or sulfated) and excreted in bile or urine. High α-T concentrations in the liver up-regulate various xenobiotic pathways, including CYP3A and MDR1.

The tocopheroxyl radical (Vit E-O·) reacts with vitamin C or other hydrogen donors, such as thiols (104), especially glutathione (58, 69, 80, 81), returning vitamin E to its reduced state (16).

$$\text{Vit E-O}\cdot + \text{AH} \rightarrow \text{Vit E-OH} + \text{A}\cdot$$

Importantly, this interaction between vitamins E and C has been demonstrated in humans; cigarette smokers have faster vitamin E turnover that can be normalized by vitamin C supplementation (13, 15).

Vitamin E in the Human Diet

All naturally occurring vitamin E forms, as well as those of synthetic *all rac*-α-tocopherol, have relatively similar antioxidant activities, so why does the body prefer the natural stereoisomeric *RRR*-α-tocopherol as its form of vitamin E? Lack of various dietary vitamin E forms does not appear to be the answer. The richest dietary sources of vitamin E are edible vegetable oils (79). These oils contain all four homologs: α-, β-, γ-, and δ-tocopherols in varying proportions. Nonetheless, because α-tocopherol is present in appreciable amounts only in foods such as nuts (almonds), some seeds (sunflower), and vegetable oils (olive), obtaining sufficient vitamin E to meet requirements appears to be challenging for most Americans. Estimates of dietary vitamin E intakes suggest that 90% of men and 96% of women in the United States do not consume the recommended amounts of vitamin E (63) [estimated average requirement 12 mg α-tocopherol (30)].

Most Americans eat a diet that is relatively high in soybean oil. This vegetable oil contains approximately 70 mg γ-tocopherol per 100 g oil, but only about 7 mg α-tocopherol (26). Nonetheless, the plasma contains primarily α-tocopherol; how does this occur?

Basis for the Preference for α-Tocopherol

Regulatory steps in absorption. All of the various vitamin E forms are absorbed apparently to the same extent, and perhaps tocotrienols even better than tocopherols (106). There is limitation in vitamin E absorption if there is inadequate fat intake (14). Vitamin E is a fat-soluble vitamin and requires biliary and pancreatic secretions in order to form micelles for uptake by the intestine. Moreover, chylomicron secretion is also required for transport from the intestine to the circulation. However, none of these steps apparently exerts a preference for one form of vitamin E over another (102).

Despite the relative paucity of α-tocopherol in the diet, it is surprising that the fractional absorption of vitamin E is relatively limited. Estimates in humans of the percentage of a dose of vitamin E absorbed range from 68%, using the collection of fecal radioactivity after administration of radioactive vitamin E (55), to 33% from plasma concentrations following administration of deuterium-labeled vitamin E (14). These data demonstrate our lack of knowledge about vitamin E absorption. We do not know how vitamin E enters the intestinal cell, how it moves through the cell, or how it is incorporated into chylomicrons. Given that absorption of cholesterol, a molecule with similar hydrophobicity to α-tocopherol, is regulated by ATP-binding cassette family transporters (ABC transporters) (7), it seems likely that there may be very specific mechanisms for the regulation of vitamin E absorption that have not yet been described.

Liver—the master regulator. Once vitamin E is absorbed and taken up by the liver, the regulation of the forms and the concentrations appears to take place (**Figure 1**, see color insert). It is not clear which lipoprotein receptors are involved in vitamin E uptake by the liver, but since all lipoproteins transport vitamin E, all lipoprotein receptors could hypothetically take up vitamin E–containing lipoproteins (95). Specifically, involvement of the low-density lipoprotein (LDL), high-density lipoprotein (HDL), and

αTTP: α-Tocopherol transfer protein. A liver cytosolic protein critical for the maintenance of plasma α-tocopherol concentrations

scavenger receptors modulates vitamin E uptake by various cells (4, 33, 65, 93, 98).

Plasma α-tocopherol concentrations in humans range from 11 to 37 μmol/L, whereas γ-tocopherol concentrations are roughly 2 to 5 μmol/L, and tocotrienol concentrations are less than 1 μmol/L, even in subjects supplemented with tocotrienols (70). When plasma lipids are taken into account, the lower limits of normal are 1.6 μmol α-tocopherol/mmol lipid (sum of cholesterol and triglycerides) or 2.5 μmol α-tocopherol/mmol cholesterol (97). The liver is responsible for the disposition, metabolism, and excretion of vitamin E. It does this through (*a*) the α-tocopherol transfer protein that returns α-tocopherol to the plasma, (*b*) the excretion of excess vitamin E into the bile, and (*c*) the metabolism of vitamin E. These topics are explored further in the following sections.

α-TOCOPHEROL TRANSFER PROTEIN

The major regulatory mechanism for controlling plasma α-tocopherol concentrations is the α-tocopherol transfer protein (α-TTP). α-TTP has been isolated and its cDNA sequences reported from a variety of species including human, mouse, rat, dog, and cow (see Entrez retrieval system, National Center for Biotechnology Information). α-TTP has been crystallized and the α-tocopherol-binding pocket identified (59, 62). Interestingly, the structure has a hinge and a cover that entraps α-tocopherol in the binding pocket. α-TTP has differing affinities for various forms of vitamin E with *RRR*-α-tocopherol = 100%, β-tocopherol = 38%, γ-tocopherol = 9%, δ-tocopherol = 2%, α-tocopherol acetate = 2%, α-tocopherol quinone = 2%, *SRR*-α-tocopherol = 11%, α-tocotrienol = 12%, or trolox = 9% (37). Thus, the affinity of α-TTP for vitamin E forms is one of the critical determinants for their plasma concentrations (37).

The human protein has 94% homology to the rat protein and some homology to the retinaldehyde-binding protein in the retina and to sec14, a phospholipid transfer protein (1). The human α-TTP gene is located at the 8q13.1–13.3 region of chromosome 8 (1, 25).

α-TTP expression was first reported in hepatocytes (108). α-TTP mRNA has also been detected in rat brain, spleen, lung, and kidney (38) and in mouse liver and adrenals, but is low or undetectable in mouse cerebral cortex, lungs, heart, and spleen (32). α-TTP protein has been detected in human brain (22). Furthermore, α-TTP is present in pregnant mouse uterus and human placenta (41, 42). Muller-Schmehl et al. (64) reported that concentrations of placental α-TTP mRNA were second only to those in the liver. The reports of uterine and placental α-TTP emphasize the importance of vitamin E during pregnancy and emphasize that the fetal resorption test (54) is not likely to be dependable for assessing bioavailability for various forms of vitamin E because any trace amounts of α-tocopherol present in the test vitamin E would be preferentially taken up by α-TTP to protect the uterus and placenta.

CRAL-TRIO Family

The CRAL-TRIO family is a small group of lipid-binding proteins, including the cellular retinaldehyde binding protein (CRALBP), α-TTP, yeast phosphatidylinositol transfer protein (Sec14p), and supernatant protein factor (SPF), a protein involved in cholesterol biosynthesis (73). CRAL-TRIO members can bind α-tocopherol, but only α-TTP had sufficient affinity for α-tocopherol to serve as a physiological α-tocopherol transfer protein (73). Human SPF also reportedly complexes with *RRR*-α-tocopheryl quinone, the two-electron α-tocopherol oxidation product (91). However, at present, it appears that only α-TTP serves as a regulator of plasma and tissue α-tocopherol concentrations (73).

α-TTP Function

The mechanism by which α-TTP facilitates secretion of α-tocopherol from the liver into the plasma has not been fully described. In general, triglyceride-rich (chylomicrons and VLDL) and low-density lipoproteins carrying vitamin E are taken up by the liver via receptor-mediated endocytosis, delivering vitamin E to multivesicular bodies. Horiguchi et al. (36) suggest that α-TTP acquires α-tocopherol from the endosomes, and then this α-TTP-α-tocopherol complex moves to the plasma membrane, where α-TTP releases α-tocopherol to the membrane to be acquired by lipoproteins, e.g., nascent VLDL. The ATP-binding cassette protein A1 (ABCA1) in endosomes could play a role in this process since ABCA1 can also transfer α-tocopherol (71). Thus, ABCA1 could enrich the outer membrane of the endocytic vesicles with α-tocopherol; then α-TTP could preferentially remove *RRR*-α-tocopherol from the outer leaflet of the endosomal membrane for transfer to the plasma membrane. It remains to be clarified as to whether ABCA1 participates in α-tocopherol transfer directly to and from α-TTP, as was suggested by Horiguchi et al. (36), or if some other proteins are also involved in hepatic α-tocopherol trafficking.

CAUSES OF HUMAN VITAMIN E DEFICIENCY

The importance of α-TTP function in determining human vitamin E status was elucidated when patients with vitamin E deficiency caused by defects in the α-TTP were described, as discussed further below. Overt vitamin E deficiency occurs only rarely in humans. Most often, vitamin E deficiency had been described as a symptom secondary to fat malabsorption. α-Tocopherol deficiency causes both peripheral neuropathy (103) and increased erythrocyte hemolysis (45).

Ataxia with Vitamin E Deficiency

Genetic defects in α-TTP are associated with a characteristic syndrome, ataxia with vitamin E deficiency [AVED, previously called familial isolated vitamin E (FIVE) deficiency]. AVED patients have neurologic abnormalities, which are similar to those of patients with Friedreich's ataxia (5, 6). The symptoms are characterized by a progressive peripheral neuropathy with a specific dying back of the large caliber axons of the sensory neurons, which results in ataxia (86).

AVED: ataxia with vitamin E deficiency

Retinitis pigmentosa is also a symptom associated with vitamin E deficiency, and the defect in the α-TTP gene in patients with AVED has been described (57, 107). Importantly, vitamin E supplementation stops or slows the progression of retinitis pigmentosa in these patients (107).

Fat Malabsorption Syndromes

Vitamin E deficiency secondary to fat malabsorption occurs because vitamin E absorption requires biliary and pancreatic secretions. Children with cholestatic liver disease, who have impaired secretion of bile into the small intestine, have severe fat malabsorption (82). Neurologic abnormalities, which appear as early as the second year of life, become irreversible if the vitamin E deficiency is uncorrected (82–84).

Children with cystic fibrosis can also become vitamin E deficient because the impaired secretion of pancreatic digestive enzymes causes steatorrhea and vitamin E malabsorption, even when pancreatic enzyme supplements are administered orally (41). More severe vitamin E deficiency occurs if bile secretion is impaired (23, 27, 87, 90).

It should be emphasized that any disorder that causes chronic fat malabsorption, including chronic diarrhea in children, can lead to vitamin E deficiency. Thus, poor intake of nutrients generally could lead to vitamin E deficiency if the fat malabsorption is sufficiently severe and the child has low body stores.

Genetic Defects in Lipoprotein Synthesis

Studies of patients with hypobetalipoproteinemia or abetalipoproteinemia (low to

RDA: recommended dietary allowance

nondetectable circulating chylomicrons, VLDL, or LDL) have demonstrated that lipoproteins containing apolipoprotein B are necessary for effective absorption and plasma vitamin E transport (77). These patients have steatorrhea from birth because of the impaired ability to absorb dietary fat, which also contributes to their poor vitamin E status. Clinical features also include retarded growth, acanthocytosis, retinitis pigmentosa, and a chronic progressive neurological disorder with ataxia. Clinically, both hypobetalipoproteinemic or abetalipoproteinemic subjects become vitamin E deficient and develop a characteristic neurologic syndrome—a progressive peripheral neuropathy—if they are not given large vitamin E supplements (approximately 10 g per day) (77, 99). Despite low plasma concentrations, adipose tissue α–tocopherol concentrations reach normal levels in patients given large (10 g/day) vitamin E doses (99). These findings emphasize the difficulty of assessing vitamin E status in patients with abnormal plasma lipid concentrations. Tissue concentrations can be altered, but the plasma vitamin E concentrations reflect the abnormal circulating lipid levels (85).

Severe Malnutrition

Hepatic α-TTP is required to maintain normal plasma α-tocopherol concentrations (72). It is, therefore, not surprising that vitamin E–deficiency symptoms have been reported in children with severely limited food intake, which not only might be limiting in vitamin E, but also limiting in the dietary protein necessary to synthesize α-TTP. Kalra et al. (43) reported that 100 patients with protein energy malnutrition (PEM) had low plasma α-tocopherol concentrations (8 μmol/L or less) and low α-tocopherol/lipid ratios, as well as neurologic abnormalities characteristic of vitamin E deficiency. With 6 weeks vitamin E supplementation, not only were the subjects' circulating α-tocopherol levels normalized, but there was also improvement in their neurologic abnormalities (44). This pair of reports clearly identifies vitamin E deficiency as a cause of the PEM neurologic syndrome (43, 44). In general, the degree to which vitamin E deficiency is associated with kwashiorkor and/or marasmus is not clear because fat malabsorption has been reported as a confounding factor during recovery from extreme malnutrition (66).

HUMAN VITAMIN E EXCESS

It has been estimated that 35 million Americans take vitamin E supplements (31). Although the vitamin E recommended dietary allowance (RDA) is 15 mg of *RRR*-α-tocopherol, vitamin E supplements are available in doses of 100 to 1000 international units (IU) (mg *dl* α-tocopheryl acetate). The Institute of Medicine's Food and Nutrition Board set the upper tolerance level (UL) for α-tocopherol at 1000 mg [1100 IU synthetic (*all rac*); 1500 IU natural (*RRR*)] per day using data from studies in rats (30). No clinical trial has shown that any dose of vitamin E supplements causes adverse side effects in healthy people (34).

Vitamin E Supplements and Mortality

Within the past five years, a vitamin E intervention trial suggested adverse vitamin E effects in patients taking antihyperlipidemic drug therapy. The intervention study was a three-year, double-blind trial of antioxidants (vitamins E and C, β-carotene, and selenium) or placebos in 160 subjects taking both simvastatin and niacin (12, 20). Simvastatin is a 3-hydroxy-3-methylglutaryl coenzyme A (HMG-CoA) reductase inhibitor that is widely utilized in the treatment of hypercholesterolemia. In subjects taking antioxidants, the drugs provided less of a benefit in raising HDL cholesterol than was expected (20).

A widely cited meta-analysis comparing 19 clinical trials has suggested that supplemental vitamin E may increase the risk of death due to any cause (61). This analysis has been criticized for a variety of reasons, especially since simpler meta-analysis models did not report finding statistical significance of an effect of vitamin E supplements on all-cause mortality (3, 10, 19, 24, 35, 40, 48, 51, 56, 60, 76). However, the Heart Outcomes Prevention Evaluation Study Extension (HOPE-TOO) trial has reported a higher risk of heart failure and hospitalization for heart failure in cardiovascular disease patients taking vitamin E supplements (400 IU/day) for seven years compared with a placebo group (53). There were no differences with respect to primary outcomes of cancer incidence, cancer deaths, or major cardiovascular events and deaths in this study. To date, no vitamin E–related mechanism for the increased rate of heart failure has been described. This is an important area of study because identification of the mechanism for adverse vitamin E effects (if any exist) is clearly needed to be able to set upper limits for vitamin E intakes.

Vitamin E and Decreasing Chronic Disease Risk

Several studies have reported that vitamin E supplements are associated with decreased risk of various chronic diseases. The Women's Health Study, a ten-year prevention trial in normal, healthy women 45 years and older, found that 600 IU vitamin E taken every other day significantly decreased cardiovascular mortality by 24% and in women over 65 by 49% (49). Additionally, in hypercholesterolemic (78) and in heart transplant patients (29), supplementation with both vitamins E and C slowed atherosclerotic progression in intimal thickness of coronary and carotid arteries. The Cache County Study reported that antioxidant use (vitamin E >400 IU and vitamin C >500 mg) was associated with reduced Alzheimer disease prevalence and incidence in the elderly (109). Regular vitamin E supplement use for ten years or more was associated with a lower risk of dying of amyotrophic lateral sclerosis (ALS, or Lou Gehrig's disease) (2). Again, these reports of beneficial vitamin E effects encourage the use of vitamin E supplements and highlight the need for furthering our understanding of vitamin E metabolism.

CEHC: carboxyethyl hydroxychroman

HEPATIC VITAMIN E REGULATION

Dietary vitamin E is absorbed and delivered to the liver, but only α-tocopherol is preferentially recognized by α-TTP and transferred to plasma, as discussed above. The fate of hepatic vitamin E is just beginning to be studied, and it is apparent that there are large gaps in our knowledge about hepatic vitamin E trafficking and its mechanisms to regulate vitamin E concentrations (**Figure 1**).

Vitamin E Metabolism

Unlike other fat-soluble vitamins, vitamin E is not accumulated; thus, excretion and metabolism likely are important steps in regulation. Vitamin E metabolites are tail-shortened, carboxylated forms of vitamin E with intact head groups that are derived from tocopherols and tocotrienols, respectively (9, 52). Both α-CEHC [2,5,7,8-tetramethyl-2-(2′-carboxyethyl)-6-hydroxychroman] and γ-CEHC [2,7,8-trimethyl-2-(2′carboxyethyl)-6-hydroxychroman] are readily detected in plasma (50); δ-CEHC was the first of the metabolites reported (21).

Vitamin Es are metabolized similarly to xenobiotics (8) in that they are initially ω-oxidized by cytochrome P450s (CYPs), they undergo several steps of β-oxidation, and then they are conjugated and excreted in urine (11) or bile (46). The ω-oxidation of α- and γ-tocopherols has been shown to be carried out by CYP 4F2 (88), but CYP 3A may also be involved (8, 9, 39, 74). Following β-oxidation, CEHCs are sulfated or glucuronidated (75, 89, 92). Xenobiotic transporters are likely candidates for mediating hepatic CEHC excretion because

CEHCs are found in plasma, urine, and bile. Additionally, α-tocopherol alone has been demonstrated to be excreted into bile via the multidrug-resistance gene product, MDR2 (p-glycoprotein) (68), an ATP-binding cassette phospholipid transporter that facilitates biliary phospholipid excretion.

Vitamin E Kinetics

The rates of α-tocopherol entering or leaving the plasma are dependent on absorption, delivery to tissues, and excretion (**Figure 1**). The apparent half-life of *RRR*-α-tocopherol in plasma of normal subjects is approximately 48 h (100), up to 60 h (15), whereas that of *SRR*-α-tocopherol is only 15 h (100). This relatively fast turnover of 2*S*-α-tocopherol is also accompanied by increased metabolism (96). The relatively fast disappearance of the 2*S*-α-tocopherols means that by 48 h nearly 90% of the 2*S* forms have been removed from the plasma, while 50% of the 2*R* forms remain. Remarkably, the rate of γ-tocopherol disappearance from the plasma is similar to that of *SRR*-α-tocopherol, about 15 h (50). Moreover, this fast γ-tocopherol turnover is also accompanied by a fast disappearance of γ-CEHC (50). These kinetic studies emphasize that vitamin E forms other than α-tocopherol are rapidly removed from the body while α-tocopherol concentrations are maintained.

Vitamin E Disposition and Excretion

α-Tocopherol compared with γ-tocopherol (50), as well as synthetic, *all rac*-α-tocopherol compared with natural, *RRR*-α-tocopherol (96), is preferentially metabolized, a finding that suggests that forms of vitamin E that are not actively transported to the plasma by α-TTP are metabolized. However, if the vitamin E is not salvaged from the endosomal-lysosomal pathway that leads to biliary excretion mediated by p-glycoprotein (68), it is not obvious how the vitamin E is diverted to be metabolized. Regulation of hepatic vitamin E trafficking is an important area for further study.

Hepatic Vitamin E Regulation in Rodents

Although all forms of vitamin E are absorbed, the liver preferentially secretes α- but not γ-tocopherol into plasma. Therefore, to assess the fate of dietary γ-tocopherol, mice that do or do not express α-TTP (*Ttpa*$^{-/-}$, $^{+/-}$, and $^{+/+}$ mice) were fed for five weeks diets that contained either γ-tocopherol (550 mg γ-tocopherol/kg diet or 60 mg γ-tocopherol/kg diet), a vitamin E–deficient diet, or a control diet [30 mg α-tocopherol/kg diet (101)]. The two γ-tocopherol diets also contained about 3% α-tocopherol. Irrespective of genotype after a 12 h fast, the liver γ-tocopherol concentrations in mice fed the highest γ-tocopherol diets were no higher than the α-tocopherol concentrations of wild-type mice fed chow diets. Remarkably, the other tissues did not contain high γ-tocopherol concentrations. To determine the fate of γ-tocopherol, mechanisms of hepatic metabolism were assessed in the mice. Cyp4F protein, suggested to be the tocopherol ω-hydroxylase (88), did not vary between any of the dietary groups. (Note: In rats and humans, CYP protein nomenclature is capitalized; in mice, only the first letter is capitalized.) Hepatic Cyp3a protein concentrations correlated with hepatic α-tocopherol, but not γ-tocopherol concentrations. Similarly, hepatic Cyp3a mRNA increased in mice fed α-tocopherol compared with mice fed a tocotrienol-containing diet (47). Apparently, α-tocopherol modulates a subset of CYP enzymes, thereby increasing its own metabolism and preventing accumulation of "excess" α-tocopherol or other forms of vitamin E.

To evaluate the role of metabolism in protection against excess accumulation of α-tocopherol, studies were undertaken in rats that were injected subcutaneously with 0.5 g α-tocopherol (100 mg/kg body weight) over the course of 18 days (67). In addition to α-tocopherol and α-CEHC, hepatic α-tocopherol intermediate metabolites, 13′-OH-α-tocopherol and 5′-α-CMBHC (5′-α-carboxy-methyl-butyl-hydroxy-chromanol), were measured. By the third day of injections, liver concentrations of α-tocopherol had increased 40- to 75-fold, α-CEHC had increased ~100-fold, 13′-OH-α-tocopherol had increased 20-fold, and 5′-α-CMBHC, which was undetectable prior to α-tocopherol supplementation, had increased to 1.0 nmol/g tissue. These data demonstrate that excess liver α-tocopherol leads to increases of its own metabolites. At the same time, hepatic protein levels of CYP3A, CYP2B, and CYP2C, but not CYP4F, doubled and remained increased over the 18 days of daily α-tocopherol injections despite continuously decreasing α-tocopherol concentrations after day nine (67). Importantly, after nine days hepatic MDR1 protein concentrations increased and this increase in MDR1 corresponded with the decrease in hepatic α-tocopherol levels (67). These data suggest that MDR1 mediates the biliary excretion of α-tocopherol; however, biliary tocopherol concentrations were not measured, so this hypothesis requires further experimentation for confirmation.

The preceding studies used rats given daily injections of vitamin E such that over the course of the study more than 0.5 g had been injected into each rat. Such extraordinary increases in hepatic α-tocopherol concentrations are not likely to be observed in humans taking vitamin E supplements. Therefore, it is noteworthy that in the mice fed dietary vitamin E increases in Cyp 3A were also observed. These data suggest that the interactions of vitamin E metabolism and xenobiotic metabolism may occur in human liver (94).

SUMMARY AND PERSPECTIVES

It is apparent from the discussion above that there are several gaps in our knowledge about the regulation of vitamin E concentrations. Although it is clear that there is an overwhelming preference for α-tocopherol by the various regulatory mechanisms, the reason for this preference is controversial and remains undetermined. Largely, differences observed in cell culture are not dependent upon most of the various regulatory mechanisms described in this review and, thus, various spurious effects can occur and need confirmation in vivo.

The preference for α-tocopherol in vivo is largely accomplished by the action of α-TTP, whose absence in humans causes vitamin E deficiency. Presumably, α-TTP salvages α-tocopherol from the lysosomal degradation pathway and, ultimately, biliary excretion. However, the precise steps by which α-TTP accomplishes this feat are unknown.

γ-Tocopherol serves as an example of the fate of non-α-tocopherols. Promptly upon absorption in humans, γ-tocopherol is metabolized to γ-CEHC (50). Cell culture studies recapitulate this process in that in cells given equal amounts of α- and γ-tocopherols, a 100-fold excess of γ-CEHC is produced (8, 9). Thus, it is clear that the body actively metabolizes forms of vitamin E other than α-tocopherol.

There are several unknowns concerning metabolism. Although the liver has been demonstrated to contain elevated vitamin E metabolites, other tissues may also be capable of vitamin E metabolism; however, other sites have not been documented. Moreover, the various intracellular locations of vitamin E metabolism and the specific xenobiotic systems involved in catabolism, conjugation, and excretion have not been identified. Additionally, the means by which these steps are regulated have not been elucidated. Given the importance of vitamin E for protection against chronic disease mortality (105) and the propensity of the public for the use of vitamin E supplements, as well as the likelihood that some of the observed abnormal findings in trials that combine pharmacologic agents and vitamin E supplements result in vitamin E–drug interactions (12), it is clear that further studies in vitamin E–regulatory mechanisms are needed.

LITERATURE CITED

1. Arita M, Sato Y, Miyata A, Tanabe T, Takahashi E, et al. 1995. Human alpha-tocopherol transfer protein: cDNA cloning, expression and chromosomal localization. *Biochem. J.* 306:437–43
2. Ascherio A, Weisskopf MG, O'Reilly EJ, Jacobs EJ, McCullough ML, et al. 2005. Vitamin E intake and risk of amyotrophic lateral sclerosis. *Ann. Neurol.* 57:104–10
3. Baggott JE. 2005. High-dosage vitamin E supplementation and all-cause mortality. *Ann. Intern. Med.* 143:155–56; author reply 156–58
4. Balazs Z, Panzenboeck U, Hammer A, Sovic A, Quehenberge O, et al. 2004. Uptake and transport of high-density lipoprotein (HDL) and HDL-associated alpha-tocopherol by an in vitro blood-brain barrier model. *J. Neurochem.* 89:939–50
5. **Ben Hamida C, Doerflinger N, Belal S, Linder C, Reutenauer L, et al. 1993. Localization of Friedreich ataxia phenotype with selective vitamin E deficiency to chromosome 8q by homozygosity mapping. *Nat. Genet.* 5:195–200**
6. Ben Hamida M, Belal S, Sirugo G, Ben Hamida C, Panayides K, et al. 1993. Friedreich's ataxia phenotype not linked to chromosome 9 and associated with selective autosomal recessive vitamin E deficiency in two inbred Tunisian families. *Neurology* 43:2179–83
7. Berge KE, Tian H, Graf GA, Yu L, Grishin NV, et al. 2000. Accumulation of dietary cholesterol in sitosterolemia caused by mutations in adjacent ABC transporters. *Science* 290:1771–75
8. Birringer M, Drogan D, Brigelius-Flohe R. 2001. Tocopherols are metabolized in HepG2 cells by side chain omega-oxidation and consecutive beta-oxidation. *Free Radic. Biol. Med.* 31:226–32
9. Birringer M, Pfluger P, Kluth D, Landes N, Brigelius-Flohe R. 2002. Identities and differences in the metabolism of tocotrienols and tocopherols in HepG2 cells. *J. Nutr.* 132:3113–18
10. Blatt DH, Pryor WA. 2005. High-dosage vitamin E supplementation and all-cause mortality. *Ann. Intern. Med.* 143:150–51; author reply 156–58
11. Brigelius-Flohé R, Traber MG. 1999. Vitamin E: function and metabolism. *FASEB J.* 13:1145–55
12. Brown BG, Zhao XQ, Chait A, Fisher LD, Cheung MC, et al. 2001. Simvastatin and niacin, antioxidant vitamins, or the combination for the prevention of coronary disease. *N. Engl. J. Med.* 345:1583–92
13. **Bruno RS, Leonard SW, Atkinson JK, Montine TJ, Ramakrishnan R, et al. 2006. Faster vitamin E disappearance in smokers is normalized by vitamin C supplementation. *Free Radic. Biol. Med.* 40:689–97**
14. Bruno RS, Leonard SW, Park SI, Zhao Y, Traber MG. 2006. Human vitamin E requirements assessed with the use of apples fortified with deuterium-labeled α-tocopheryl acetate. *Am. J. Clin. Nutr.* 83:299–304
15. Bruno RS, Ramakrishnan R, Montine TJ, Bray TM, Traber MG. 2005. α-Tocopherol disappearance is faster in cigarette smokers and is inversely related to their ascorbic acid status. *Am. J. Clin. Nutr.* 81:95–103
16. Buettner GR. 1993. The pecking order of free radicals and antioxidants: lipid peroxidation, alpha-tocopherol, and ascorbate. *Arch. Biochem. Biophys.* 300:535–43
17. Burton GW, Doba T, Gabe EJ, Hughes L, Lee FL, et al. 1985. Autoxidation of biological molecules. 4. Maximizing the antioxidant activity of phenols. *J. Am. Chem. Soc.* 107:7053–65

First demonstration that vitamin E deficiency in humans could be caused by a genetic defect.

Demonstrated for first time in humans that oxidative stress in cigarette smokers causes increased vitamin E disappearance that can be ameliorated by supplementation with vitamin C.

18. Burton GW, Traber MG. 1990. Vitamin E: antioxidant activity, biokinetics, and bioavailability. *Annu. Rev. Nutr.* 10:357–82
19. Carter T. 2005. High-dosage vitamin E supplementation and all-cause mortality. *Ann. Intern. Med.* 143:155; author reply 156–58
20. Cheung MC, Zhao XQ, Chait A, Albers JJ, Brown BG. 2001. Antioxidant supplements block the response of HDL to simvastatin-niacin therapy in patients with coronary artery disease and low HDL. *Arterioscler Thromb. Vasc. Biol.* 21:1320–26
21. Chiku S, Hamamura K, Nakamura T. 1984. Novel urinary metabolite of d-delta-tocopherol in rats. *J. Lipid Res.* 25:40–48
22. Copp RP, Wisniewski T, Hentati F, Larnaout A, Ben Hamida M, Kayden HJ. 1999. Localization of alpha-tocopherol transfer protein in the brains of patients with ataxia with vitamin E deficiency and other oxidative stress related neurodegenerative disorders. *Brain Res.* 822:80–87
23. Cynamon HA, Milov DE, Valenstein E, Wagner M. 1988. Effect of vitamin E deficiency on neurologic function in patients with cystic fibrosis. *J. Pediatr.* 113:637–40
24. DeZee KJ, Shimeall W, Douglas K, Jackson JL. 2005. High-dosage vitamin E supplementation and all-cause mortality. *Ann. Intern. Med.* 143:153–54; author reply 156–58
25. Doerflinger N, Linder C, Ouahchi K, Gyapay G, Weissenbach J, et al. 1995. Ataxia with vitamin E deficiency: refinement of genetic localization and analysis of linkage disequilibrium by using new markers in 14 families. *Am. J. Hum. Genet.* 56:1116–24
26. Eitenmiller R, Lee J. 2004. *Vitamin E: Food Chemistry, Composition, and Analysis*. New York: Marcel Dekker. 530 pp.
27. Elias E, Muller DPR, Scott J. 1981. Association of spinocerebellar disorders with cystic fibrosis or chronic childhood cholestasis and very low serum vitamin E. *Lancet* ii:1319–21
28. Evans HM, Bishop KS. 1922. On the existence of a hitherto unrecognized dietary factor essential for reproduction. *Science* 56:650–51
29. Fang JC, Kinlay S, Beltrame J, Hikiti H, Wainstein M, et al. 2002. Effect of vitamins C and E on progression of transplant-associated arteriosclerosis: a randomised trial. *Lancet* 359:1108–13
30. Food and Nutrition Board, Institute of Medicine. 2000. *Dietary Reference Intakes for Vitamin C, Vitamin E, Selenium, and Carotenoids*. Washington, DC: Natl. Acad. Press. 529 pp.
31. Ford ES, Ajani UA, Mokdad AH. 2005. Brief communication: the prevalence of high intake of vitamin E from the use of supplements among U.S. adults. *Ann. Intern. Med.* 143:116–20
32. Gohil K, Godzdanker R, O'Roark E, Schock BC, Kaini RR, et al. 2004. Alpha-tocopherol transfer protein deficiency in mice causes multi-organ deregulation of gene networks and behavioral deficits with age. *Ann. N.Y. Acad. Sci.* 1031:109–26
33. Gurusinghe A, de Niese M, Renaud JF, Austin L. 1988. The binding of lipoproteins to human muscle cells: binding and uptake of LDL, HDL, and alpha-tocopherol. *Muscle Nerve* 11:1231–39
34. Hathcock JN, Azzi A, Blumberg J, Bray T, Dickinson A, et al. 2005. Vitamins E and C are safe across a broad range of intakes. *Am. J. Clin. Nutr.* 81:736–45
35. Hemila H. 2005. High-dosage vitamin E supplementation and all-cause mortality. *Ann. Intern. Med.* 143:151–52; author reply 156–58
36. **Horiguchi M, Arita M, Kaempf-Rotzoll DE, Tsujimoto M, Inoue K, Arai H. 2003. pH-dependent translocation of alpha-tocopherol transfer protein (alpha-TTP) between hepatic cytosol and late endosomes. *Genes Cells* 8:789–800**

Reports on studies that began to elucidate the mechanism by which α-tocopherol is transferred from the liver to the plasma.

37. Hosomi A, Arita M, Sato Y, Kiyose C, Ueda T, et al. 1997. Affinity for alpha-tocopherol transfer protein as a determinant of the biological activities of vitamin E analogs. *FEBS Lett.* 409:105–8
38. Hosomi A, Goto K, Kondo H, Iwatsubo T, Yokota T, et al. 1998. Localization of alpha-tocopherol transfer protein in rat brain. *Neurosci. Lett.* 256:159–62
39. Ikeda S, Tohyama T, Yamashita K. 2002. Dietary sesame seed and its lignans inhibit 2,7,8-trimethyl-2(2′-carboxyethyl)-6-hydroxychroman excretion into urine of rats fed gamma-tocopherol. *J. Nutr.* 132:961–66
40. Jialal I, Devaraj S. 2005. High-dosage vitamin E supplementation and all-cause mortality. *Ann. Intern. Med.* 143:155; author reply 156–58
41. Kaempf-Rotzoll DE, Horiguchi M, Hashiguchi K, Aoki J, Tamai H, et al. 2003. Human placental trophoblast cells express alpha-tocopherol transfer protein. *Placenta* 24:439–44
42. Kaempf-Rotzoll DE, Igarashi K, Aoki J, Jishage K, Suzuki H, et al. 2002. Alpha-tocopherol transfer protein is specifically localized at the implantation site of pregnant mouse uterus. *Biol. Reprod.* 67:599–604
43. Kalra V, Grover J, Ahuja GK, Rathi S, Khurana DS. 1998. Vitamin E deficiency and associated neurological deficits in children with protein-energy malnutrition. *J. Trop. Pediatr.* 44:291–95
44. Kalra V, Grover JK, Ahuja GK, Rathi S, Gulati S, Kalra N. 2001. Vitamin E administration and reversal of neurological deficits in protein-energy malnutrition. *J. Trop. Pediatr.* 47:39–45
45. Kayden HJ, Silber R, Kossmann CE. 1965. The role of vitamin E deficiency in the abnormal autohemolysis of acanthocytosis. *Trans. Assoc. Am. Physicians* 78:334–42
46. Kiyose C, Saito H, Kaneko K, Hamamura K, Tomioka M, et al. 2001. Alpha-tocopherol affects the urinary and biliary excretion of 2,7,8-trimethyl-2 (2′-carboxyethyl)-6-hydroxychroman, gamma-tocopherol metabolite, in rats. *Lipids* 36:467–72
47. Kluth D, Landes N, Pfluger P, Muller-Schmehl K, Weiss K, et al. 2005. Modulation of Cyp3a11 mRNA expression by alpha-tocopherol but not gamma-tocotrienol in mice. *Free Radic. Biol. Med.* 38:507–14
48. Krishnan K, Campbell S, Stone WL. 2005. High-dosage vitamin E supplementation and all-cause mortality. *Ann. Intern. Med.* 143:151; author reply 156–58
49. Lee IM, Cook NR, Gaziano JM, Gordon D, Ridker PM, et al. 2005. Vitamin E in the primary prevention of cardiovascular disease and cancer: the Women's Health Study: a randomized controlled trial. *JAMA* 294:56–65
50. Leonard SW, Paterson E, Atkinson JK, Ramakrishnan R, Cross CE, Traber MG. 2005. Studies in humans using deuterium-labeled α- and γ-tocopherol demonstrate faster plasma γ-tocopherol disappearance and greater γ-metabolite production. *Free Radic. Biol. Med.* 38:857–66
51. Lim WS, Liscic R, Xiong C, Morris JC. 2005. High-dosage vitamin E supplementation and all-cause mortality. *Ann. Intern. Med.* 143:152; author reply 156–58
52. Lodge JK, Ridlington J, Vaule H, Leonard SW, Traber MG. 2001. α- and γ-Tocotrienols are metabolized to carboxyethyl-hydroxychroman (CEHC) derivatives and excreted in human urine. *Lipids* 36:43–48
53. Lonn E, Bosch J, Yusuf S, Sheridan P, Pogue J, et al. 2005. Effects of long-term vitamin E supplementation on cardiovascular events and cancer: a randomized controlled trial. *JAMA* 293:1338–47
54. Machlin LJ, Gabriel E, Brin M. 1982. Biopotency of alpha-tocopherols as determined by curative myopathy bioassay in the rat. *J. Nutr.* 112:1437–40

55. MacMahon MT, Neale G. 1970. The absorption of alpha-tocopherol in control subjects and in patients with intestinal malabsorption. *Clin. Sci.* 38:197–210
56. Marras C, Lang AE, Oakes D, McDermott MP, Kieburtz K, et al. 2005. High-dosage vitamin E supplementation and all-cause mortality. *Ann. Intern. Med.* 143:152–53; author reply 156–58
57. Matsuya M, Matsumoto H, Chiba S, Kashiwagi M, Kasahara M. 1994. A sporadic case of essential vitamin E deficiency manifested by sensory-dominant polyneuropathy and retinitis pigmentosa. *Brain Nerve (Tokyo)* 46:989–94
58. McCay PB. 1985. Vitamin E: interactions with free radicals and ascorbate. *Annu. Rev. Nutr.* 5:323–40
59. Meier R, Tomizaki T, Schulze-Briese C, Baumann U, Stocker A. 2003. The molecular basis of vitamin E retention: structure of human alpha-tocopherol transfer protein. *J. Mol. Biol.* 331:725–34
60. Meydani SN, Lau J, Dallal GE, Meydani M. 2005. High-dosage vitamin E supplementation and all-cause mortality. *Ann. Intern. Med.* 143:153; author reply 156–58
61. Miller ER, Paston-Barriuso R, Dalal D, Riemersma RA, Appel LJ, Guallar E. 2005. Meta-analysis: high-dosage vitamin E supplementation may increase all-cause mortality. *Ann. Intern. Med.* 142:37–46
62. Min KC, Kovall RA, Hendrickson WA. 2003. Crystal structure of human α-tocopherol transfer protein bound to its ligand: implications for ataxia with vitamin E deficiency. *Proc. Natl. Acad. Sci. USA* 100:14713–18
63. Moshfegh A, Goldman J, Cleveland L. 2005. *What We Eat in America, NHANES 2001–2002: Usual Nutrient Intakes from Food Compared to Dietary Reference Intakes.* Washington, DC: U.S. Dept. Agric., Agric. Res. Serv.
64. Muller-Schmehl K, Beninde J, Finckh B, Florian S, Dudenhausen JW, et al. 2004. Localization of alpha-tocopherol transfer protein in trophoblast, fetal capillaries' endothelium and amnion epithelium of human term placenta. *Free Radic. Res.* 38:413–20
65. Munteanu A, Taddei M, Tamburini I, Bergamini E, Azzi A, Zingg JM. 2006. Antagonistic effects of oxidized low density lipoprotein and alpha-tocopherol on CD36 scavenger receptor expression in monocytes: involvement of protein kinase B and peroxisome proliferator-activated receptor-gamma. *J. Biol. Chem.* 281:6489–97
66. Murphy JL, Badaloo AV, Chambers B, Forrester TE, Wootton SA, Jackson AA. 2002. Maldigestion and malabsorption of dietary lipid during severe childhood malnutrition. *Arch. Dis. Child* 87:522–25
67. Mustacich DJ, Leonard SW, Devereaux MW, Sokol RJ, Traber MG. 2006. α-Tocopherol regulation of hepatic cytochrome P450s and ABC transporters. *Free Radic. Biol. Med.* 41:1069–78
68. Mustacich DJ, Shields J, Horton RA, Brown MK, Reed DJ. 1998. Biliary secretion of alpha-tocopherol and the role of the mdr2 P-glycoprotein in rats and mice. *Arch. Biochem. Biophys.* 350:183–92
69. Niki E. 1987. Antioxidants in relation to lipid peroxidation. *Chem. Phys. Lipids* 44:227–53
70. O'Byrne D, Grundy S, Packer L, Devaraj S, Baldenius K, et al. 2000. Studies of LDL oxidation following alpha-, gamma-, or delta-tocotrienyl acetate supplementation of hypercholesterolemic humans. *Free Radic. Biol. Med.* 29:834–45
71. Oram JF, Vaughan AM, Stocker R. 2001. ATP-binding cassette transporter A1 mediates cellular secretion of alpha-tocopherol. *J. Biol. Chem.* 276:39898–902

72. Ouahchi K, Arita M, Kayden H, Hentati F, Ben Hamida M, et al. 1995. Ataxia with isolated vitamin E deficiency is caused by mutations in the alpha-tocopherol transfer protein. *Nat. Genet.* 9:141–45
73. Panagabko C, Morley S, Hernandez M, Cassolato P, Gordon H, et al. 2003. Ligand specificity in the CRAL-TRIO protein family. *Biochemistry* 42:6467–74
74. Parker RS, Sontag TJ, Swanson JE. 2000. Cytochrome P4503A-dependent metabolism of tocopherols and inhibition by sesamin. *Biochem. Biophys. Res. Commun.* 277:531–34
75. Pope SA, Burtin GE, Clayton PT, Madge DJ, Muller DP. 2002. Synthesis and analysis of conjugates of the major vitamin E metabolite, alpha-CEHC. *Free Radic. Biol. Med.* 33:807–17
76. Possolo AM. 2005. High-dosage vitamin E supplementation and all-cause mortality. *Ann. Intern. Med.* 143:154; author reply 156–58
77. Rader DJ, Brewer HB. 1993. Abetalipoproteinemia—new insights into lipoprotein assembly and vitamin-E metabolism from a rare genetic disease. *JAMA* 270:865–69
78. Salonen RM, Nyyssonen K, Kaikkonen J, Porkkala-Sarataho E, Voutilainen S, et al. 2003. Six-year effect of combined vitamin C and E supplementation on atherosclerotic progression: the Antioxidant Supplementation in Atherosclerosis Prevention (ASAP) Study. *Circulation* 107:947–53
79. Sheppard AJ, Pennington JAT, Weihrauch JL. 1993. Analysis and distribution of vitamin E in vegetable oils and foods. In *Vitamin E in Health and Disease*, ed. L Packer, J Fuchs, pp. 9–31. New York: Marcel Dekker
80. Sies H, Murphy ME. 1991. Role of tocopherols in the protection of biological systems against oxidative damage. *Photochem. Photobiol.* 8:211–24
81. Sies H, Stahl W, Sundquist AR. 1992. Antioxidant functions of vitamins (vitamins E and C, beta-carotene, and other carotenoids). *Ann. N.Y. Acad. Sci.* 669:7–20
82. Sokol RJ. 1993. Vitamin E deficiency and neurological disorders. In *Vitamin E in Health and Disease*, ed. L Packer, J Fuchs, pp. 815–49. New York: Marcel Dekker
83. Sokol RJ, Heubi JE, Butler-Simon N, McClung HJ, Lilly JR, Silverman A. 1987. Treatment of vitamin E deficiency during chronic childhood cholestasis with oral d-α-tocopheryl polyethylene glycol 1000 succinate (TPGS). I. Intestinal absorption, efficacy and safety. *Gastroenterology* 93:975–85
84. Sokol RJ, Heubi JE, Iannaccone S, Bove KE, Harris RE, Balistreri WF. 1983. The mechanism causing vitamin E deficiency during chronic childhood cholestasis. *Gastroenterology* 85:1172–82
85. Sokol RJ, Heubi JE, Iannaccone ST, Bove KE, Balistreri WF. 1984. Vitamin E deficiency with normal serum vitamin E concentrations in children with chronic cholestasis. *N. Engl. J. Med.* 310:1209–12
86. Sokol RJ, Kayden HJ, Bettis DB, Traber MG, Neville H, et al. 1988. Isolated vitamin E deficiency in the absence of fat malabsorption—familial and sporadic cases: characterization and investigation of causes. *J. Lab. Clin. Med.* 111:548–59
87. Sokol RJ, Reardon MC, Accurso FJ, Stall C, Narkewicz M, et al. 1989. Fat-soluble-vitamin status during the first year of life in infants with cystic fibrosis identified by screening of newborns. *Am. J. Clin. Nutr.* 50:1064–71
88. Sontag TJ, Parker RS. 2002. Cytochrome P450 omega-hydroxylase pathway of tocopherol catabolism: novel mechanism of regulation of vitamin E status. *J. Biol. Chem.* 277:25290–96

89. Stahl W, Graf P, Brigelius-Flohe R, Wechter W, Sies H. 1999. Quantification of the alpha- and gamma-tocopherol metabolites 2,5,7,8-tetramethyl-2-(2′-carboxyethyl)-6-hydroxychroman and 2,7,8-trimethyl-2-(2′-carboxyethyl)-6-hydroxychroman in human serum. *Anal. Biochem.* 275:254–59
90. Stead RJ, Muller DPR, Matthews S, Hodson ME, Batten JC. 1986. Effect of abnormal liver function on vitamin E status and supplementation in adults with cystic fibrosis. *Gut* 27:714–18
91. Stocker A, Baumann U. 2003. Supernatant protein factor in complex with RRR-alpha-tocopherylquinone: a link between oxidized vitamin E and cholesterol biosynthesis. *J. Mol. Biol.* 332:759–65
92. Swanson JE, Ben RN, Burton GW, Parker RS. 1999. Urinary excretion of 2,7,8-trimethyl-2-(beta-carboxyethyl)-6-hydroxychroman is a major route of elimination of gamma-tocopherol in humans. *J. Lipid Res.* 40:665–71
93. Teupser D, Thiery J, Seidel D. 1999. Alpha-tocopherol down-regulates scavenger receptor activity in macrophages. *Atherosclerosis* 144:109–15
94. Traber MG. 2004. Vitamin E, nuclear receptors and xenobiotic metabolism. *Arch. Biochem. Biophys.* 423:6–11
95. Traber MG. 2005. Vitamin E. In *Modern Nutrition in Health and Disease*, ed. ME Shils, JA Olson, M Shike, AC Ross, pp. 396–411. Baltimore, MD: Lippincott, Williams & Wilkins
96. Traber MG, Elsner A, Brigelius-Flohe R. 1998. Synthetic as compared with natural vitamin E is preferentially excreted as alpha-CEHC in human urine: studies using deuterated alpha-tocopheryl acetates. *FEBS Lett.* 437:145–48
97. Traber MG, Jialal I. 2000. Measurement of lipid-soluble vitamins—further adjustment needed? *Lancet* 355:2013–14
98. Traber MG, Kayden HJ. 1984. Vitamin E is delivered to cells via the high affinity receptor for low-density lipoprotein. *Am. J. Clin. Nutr.* 40:747–51
99. Traber MG, Rader D, Acuff R, Brewer HB, Kayden HJ. 1994. Discrimination between *RRR*- and *all rac*-α-tocopherols labeled with deuterium by patients with abetalipoproteinemia. *Atherosclerosis* 108:27–37
100. Traber MG, Ramakrishnan R, Kayden HJ. 1994. Human plasma vitamin E kinetics demonstrate rapid recycling of plasma *RRR*-α-tocopherol. *Proc. Natl. Acad. Sci. USA* 91:10005–8
101. Traber MG, Siddens LK, Leonard SW, Schock B, Gohil K, et al. 2005. α-Tocopherol modulates Cyp3a expression, increases γ-CEHC production and limits tissue γ-tocopherol accumulation in mice fed high α-tocopherol diets. *Free Radic. Biol. Med.* 38:773–85
102. Traber MG, Sies H. 1996. Vitamin E in humans: demand and delivery. *Annu. Rev. Nutr.* 16:321–47
103. Traber MG, Sokol RJ, Ringel SP, Neville HE, Thellman CA, Kayden HJ. 1987. Lack of tocopherol in peripheral nerves of vitamin E-deficient patients with peripheral neuropathy. *N. Engl. J. Med.* 317:262–65
104. Wefers H, Sies H. 1988. The protection by ascorbate and glutathione against microsomal lipid peroxidation is dependent on vitamin E. *Eur. J. Biochem.* 174:353–57
105. Wright ME, Lawson KA, Weinstein SJ, Pietinen P, Taylor PR, et al. 2006. Higher baseline serum vitamin E concentrations are associated with lower total and cause-specific mortality in the Alpha-Tocopherol, Beta-Carotene Cancer Prevention Study. *Am. J. Clin. Nutr.* 84:1200–7

106. Yap SP, Yuen KH, Wong JW. 2001. Pharmacokinetics and bioavailability of alpha-, gamma- and delta-tocotrienols under different food status. *J. Pharm. Pharmacol.* 53:67–71

107. Yokota T, Shiojiri T, Gotoda T, Arai H. 1996. Retinitis pigmentosa and ataxia caused by a mutation in the gene for the α-tocopherol-transfer protein. *N. Engl. J. Med.* 335:1769–70

108. Yoshida H, Yusin M, Ren I, Kuhlenkamp J, Hirano T, et al. 1992. Identification, purification and immunochemical characterization of a tocopherol-binding protein in rat liver cytosol. *J. Lipid Res.* 33:343–50

109. Zandi PP, Anthony JC, Khachaturian AS, Stone SV, Gustafson D, et al. 2004. Reduced risk of Alzheimer disease in users of antioxidant vitamin supplements: the Cache County Study. *Arch. Neurol.* 61:82–88

Observes not only ataxia due to vitamin E deficiency, but also retinitis pigmentosa, in humans with a defective α-TTP gene.

Epigenetic Epidemiology of the Developmental Origins Hypothesis

Robert A. Waterland[1] and Karin B. Michels[2]

[1]Department of Pediatrics, USDA Children's Nutrition Research Center, Baylor College of Medicine, Houston, Texas; email: waterland@bcm.edu

[2]Department of Obstetrics, Gynecology and Reproductive Biology, Obstetrics and Gynecology Epidemiology Center, Brigham and Women's Hospital, Harvard Medical School, Boston, Massachusetts

Annu. Rev. Nutr. 2007. 27:363–88

First published online as a Review in Advance on April 27, 2007

The *Annual Review of Nutrition* is online at http://nutr.annualreviews.org

This article's doi: 10.1146/annurev.nutr.27.061406.093705

0199-9885/07/0821-0363$20.00

Key Words

chromatin, DNA methylation, epigenomics, metabolic imprinting, nutrition

Abstract

Extensive human epidemiologic and animal model data indicate that during critical periods of prenatal and postnatal mammalian development, nutrition and other environmental stimuli influence developmental pathways and thereby induce permanent changes in metabolism and chronic disease susceptibility. The biologic mechanisms underlying this "developmental origins hypothesis" are poorly understood. This review focuses on the likely involvement of epigenetic mechanisms in the developmental origins of health and disease (DOHaD). We describe permanent effects of transient environmental influences on the developmental establishment of epigenetic gene regulation and evidence linking epigenetic dysregulation with human disease. We propose a definition of "epigenetic epidemiology" and delineate how this emerging field provides a basis from which to explore the role of epigenetic mechanisms in DOHaD. We suggest strategies for future human epidemiologic studies to identify causal associations between early exposures, long-term changes in epigenetic regulation, and disease, which may ultimately enable specific early-life interventions to improve human health.

Contents

INTRODUCTION

The developmental origins hypothesis (37) proposes that during critical periods of prenatal and postnatal mammalian development, nutrition and other environmental stimuli influence developmental pathways and thereby induce permanent changes in metabolism and chronic disease susceptibility. Although extensive human epidemiologic and animal model data support this thesis (65, 70, 120), the underlying biologic mechanisms are poorly understood. This review focuses on the likely involvement of epigenetic mechanisms in the developmental origins of health and disease (DOHaD). Epigenetic dysregulation causes human disease; animal model data demonstrating that transient environmental influences during development alter the establishment of epigenetic gene regulation underscore the likely role of epigenetic mechanisms in DOHaD.

DOHaD: developmental origins of health and disease

As much as to review existing literature, the overall goal of this article is to delineate the parameters of epigenetic epidemiology. We propose a definition of epigenetic epidemiology, compare this new field with the relatively established discipline of genetic epidemiology, and review human studies illustrating the potential of epigenetic epidemiology. Finally, we suggest strategies for future human epidemiologic studies aimed at identifying causal associations between early environmental exposures and long-term changes in epigenetic regulation and disease. Without such studies, potential opportunities to improve human health by specific nutritional interventions targeted to early life will go unrealized.

THE DEVELOPMENTAL ORIGINS HYPOTHESIS

Awareness of the importance of the intrauterine environment for lifelong health and disease emerged as recently as 40 years ago. The seminal observations of Rose (97) described a family pattern of coronary heart disease (CHD), stillbirth, and infant mortality. Forsdahl (33) was the first to geographically correlate infant mortality with cardiovascular disease (CVD). The hypothesis that CVD originates in utero was subsequently investigated extensively by Barker and colleagues (1). Barker & Osmond (3) found high rates of death due to CHD in areas with high neonatal mortality in England and Wales and proposed that intrauterine deprivation was an important mediator. Retrospective studies of women and men born in Hertfordshire, United Kingdom, found an inverse association between birth weight and adult CHD mortality, supporting this hypothesis (82). Numerous studies subsequently documented associations between low birth weight and increased incidence of heart disease (93), hypertension (61), and type 2 diabetes (40), as well as relevant markers such as abnormal glucose-insulin metabolism (40) and serum cholesterol concentrations (2).

Parallel to the advancement of the Barker thesis, which centered around CHD, hypertension, and type 2 diabetes, a similar hypothesis arose around the fetal origins of cancer. In 1990, Trichopoulos (110) proposed that breast cancer may originate in utero. Indeed, high birth weight is associated with an increase in breast cancer risk (71, 72). Childhood leukemia and testicular cancer have also been related to high birth weight (43). Intrauterine exposure to high levels of growth hormones was initially proposed as an underlying mechanism, increasing both birth weight and cellular proliferation, setting the stage for cancer in later life. Recently, a unifying concept has linked mechanisms for the developmental origins of cardiovascular diseases, cancer, and other chronic diseases (72).

Various terminologies have been proposed to describe biological phenomena relevant to DOHaD. Lucas (65) proposed the term "programming" to refer to permanent or long-term effects of a stimulus or insult at a critical or sensitive period. Barker (1) referred to the fetal origins hypothesis. Realization that developmental plasticity extends into the postnatal period (120) led to a change in nomenclature to the developmental origins hypothesis (37). Waterland & Garza (120) proposed the term "metabolic imprinting" to describe adaptive responses to specific nutritional conditions early in life that occur during limited periods of sensitivity and persist to adulthood. Moreover, metabolic imprinting describes phenomena in which both the exposure and outcome are specific and measurable and exhibit a dose-response or threshold relation. These refinements were intended to focus attention on specific biologic phenomena appropriate for mechanistic characterization.

Most human epidemiologic studies of DOHaD have used birth weight as an indicator of fetal nutrition and intrauterine growth. Although birth weight is easily obtainable, it is a crude measure of intrauterine events and is affected by an array of factors. Moreover, birth weight is likely an inappropriate target for preventive measures aiming to optimize early development during diverse critical periods. We now have the capability to design epidemiologic studies to test potential molecular mechanisms of metabolic imprinting. Given the potential for metabolic imprinting via nutritional influences on epigenetic gene regulation (116), it is timely to consider the epigenetic epidemiology of DOHaD, which focuses on the thesis that early environmental influences induce epigenetic variation and thereby permanently affect metabolism and chronic disease risk. We begin our discussion of epigenetic epidemiology by introducing the meaning and mechanisms of epigenetics.

Epigenetic epidemiology: the study of the associations between epigenetic variation and risk of disease

EPIGENETIC GENE REGULATION: HERITABLE CHANGES IN GENE EXPRESSION POTENTIAL

Most of our cells contain the same DNA—our entire genome—yet gene expression varies dramatically among different tissues. Epigenetic mechanisms establish and maintain this tissue- and cell-type-specific gene expression. The term "epigenetics" was coined by Conrad Waddington several decades ago to describe the study of "the interactions between genes and their products which bring phenotype into being" (48, 114). By Waddington's definition, virtually all development is epigenetic. Indeed, as epigenetics has become increasingly popular in recent years, some

Genomic imprinting: an epigenetic phenomenon resulting in gene expression depending upon parent-of-origin

researchers have begun to use the term very broadly.

A clear definition of "epigenetic" is essential in developing a framework for the study of epigenetic epidemiology. Epigenetics is now understood as the study of heritable changes in gene expression that are not caused by changes in DNA sequence (94). We support the adoption of a further refinement recently advanced by Jaenisch & Bird (50): Rather than heritable changes in gene expression, epigenetics encompasses heritable changes in gene expression potential. This subtle distinction is critical; cell-specific gene expression is not cell-autonomous but rather responds to various extracellular signals (e.g., paracrine, endocrine, and nutrient). Thus, epigenetic mechanisms determine not only constitutive gene expression but also the potential to appropriately alter gene expression in response to extracellular signals. This focus on gene expression potential also distinguishes bona fide epigenetic changes from expression changes that, although sustained through mitosis, are actually induced by extracellular signals.

An area of intense interest in epigenetic epidemiology is the potential for epigenetic inheritance to convey the effects of environmental exposures transgenerationally (83). All epigenetic mechanisms are mitotically heritable, enabling the maintenance of cell-type specific gene expression as cells proliferate throughout life. Epigenetic mechanisms may also be meiotically heritable, potentiating transgenerational epigenetic inheritance (13). The best-characterized examples of such transgenerational epigenetic inheritance in mammals are genomically imprinted genes, which are expressed preferentially from either the maternally or paternally inherited allele (91). Genomically imprinted genes have evolved molecular mechanisms to convey epigenetic information across generations. (Note: "Imprinting" here describes genomic imprinting, not metabolic imprinting.) Transgenerational epigenetic inheritance has also been widely demonstrated in plants (92) and at specific nonimprinted genes in mammals (75).

As with the term "epigenetics" itself, the term "epigenetic inheritance" loses its utility if given too broad a scope. In a recent review on epigenetic epidemiology, Jablonka (47) proposed that epigenetic inheritance encompasses all phenomena in which the transgenerational transmission of phenotypic variation occurs without variation in DNA base sequence, including "reconstruction of developmental and behavioral legacies." Although a useful starting point, that definition does not distinguish innate from acquired phenotypic traits. For example, transgenerational perpetuation of language does not occur by epigenetic inheritance. In our view, transgenerational epigenetic inheritance must be reserved to describe actual transmission of epigenetic information across generations.

Clearly, not all developmental plasticity is epigenetic. Rats born to mothers fed a low-protein diet during pregnancy exhibit reductions in vascularization in the endocrine pancreas, with lifelong consequences for glucose homeostasis (18, 103). The hormone leptin plays a critical role in stimulating development of neural projections in the mouse hypothalamus; ob/ob mice (lacking endogenous leptin expression) show permanent deficits in hypothalamic innervation. Transient leptin treatment of ob/ob mice during the early postnatal period stimulates appropriate hypothalamic development, permanently normalizing food intake (8). In both examples, early environmental influences appear to perturb morphological rather than epigenetic development, inducing permanent changes in organ structure and adult metabolism. Nonetheless, epigenetic mechanisms are likely to underlie many examples of metabolic imprinting (123).

EPIGENETIC MECHANISMS

Epigenetic gene regulation requires molecular mechanisms that encode information in addition to the DNA base sequence and can be propagated through mitosis and meiosis.

Our current understanding of epigenetic gene regulation involves three classes of molecular mechanisms: DNA methylation, histone modifications, and DNA-binding proteins. Although RNA interference contributes to epigenetic regulation in plants and lower organisms, its role in mammalian epigenetic regulation remains unclear (5). Epigenetic mechanisms have recently been reviewed in several excellent articles (50, 60, 62); we therefore provide only a brief overview here.

DNA methylation is the best-characterized epigenetic mechanism. In mammals, DNA methylation occurs almost exclusively at cytosines within cytosine-guanine dinucleotides (CpGs) (the "p" denotes the intervening phosphate group), converting cytosine to 5-methylcytosine. Because of the palindromic nature of CpG dinucleotides, a CpG on one DNA strand always pairs with a CpG on the complementary strand (**Figure 1**). Following DNA replication, the DNA methyltransferase 1 (DNMT1) maintenance methylase restores the original pattern of CpG methylation in the daughter strands (**Figure 1**), providing a simple mechanism for the perpetuation of epigenetic information in proliferating cells. CpG methylation regulates gene expression by affecting the binding of methylation-sensitive DNA-binding proteins and interacting with various modifications of the histone proteins that regulate DNA accessibility (50, 60). Although CpG methylation is generally correlated with gene silencing, methylation-sensitive DNA-binding proteins enable CpG methylation to regulate diverse effects on transcription (50).

Nuclear DNA is packaged with histone proteins in a highly complex and dynamic structure called chromatin. Chromatin conformation is differentially regulated in different cell types by a dizzying array of modifications to lysine residues in the tails of histone proteins: acetylation, methylation, phosphorylation, ubiquitination, and sumoylation (84). The vast potential information content of these permutations led to the suggestion that a histone code (analogous to the genetic code) exists in differentiated cells to dictate locus-specific transcriptional competence (51). The code currently defies decryption, however, and appears increasingly intractable as novel histone modifications are discovered and characterized. Since histones are thought to completely detach from the DNA during

CpG: cytosine-guanine dinucleotide

DNA methyltransferase 1 (DNMT1): the "maintenance methylase" responsible for restoring methylation at hemimethylated CpG sites following DNA replication

Chromatin: the dynamic assembly of genomic DNA and histone proteins. The structural unit of chromatin is the nucleosome: approximately 250 bp of DNA wrapped around an octamer of histone proteins

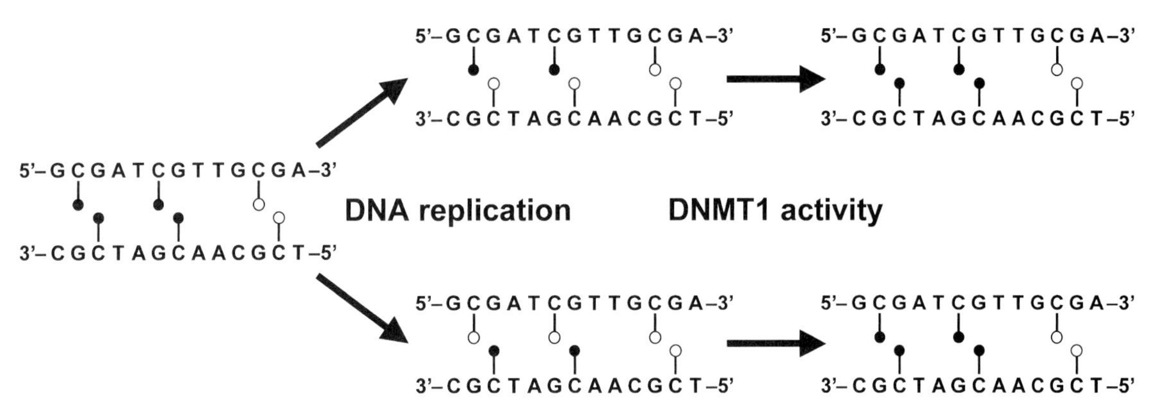

Figure 1

The mechanism for maintenance of site-specific CpG methylation patterns through DNA replication. A short region of DNA is shown; the filled and empty "lollipops" represent methylated and unmethylated CpG sites. Following DNA replication, the newly synthesized strands are unmethylated, resulting in hemimethylation. By preferentially methylating hemimethylated sites, the DNMT1 maintenance methylase restores the original pattern of CpG methylation that existed in the parent DNA molecule. CpG, cytosine-guanine dinucleotide; DNMT1, DNA methyltransferase 1.

DNA replication, it also remains unknown how regional patterns of histone modifications are maintained through mitosis.

The least recognized epigenetic mechanism is feed-forward autoregulation by transcription factors (95). Transcription factor proteins regulate gene expression by binding to recognition sequences within gene promoters. Transcription factors that activate their own gene promoter can perpetuate their expression through cell division. MyoD, an important transcription factor in muscle development, functions in this manner (80). During division of a cell in which *MyoD* has been transcriptionally activated, MyoD protein is partitioned to both daughter nuclei, perpetuating its own transcription while also regulating that of other genes. Thus, contrary to the popular notion that all epigenetic mechanisms involve covalent modification of DNA or histone proteins, autoregulatory transcription factors clearly enable mitotic and potentially meiotic heritability of gene expression potential.

These various mechanisms function in an orchestrated, mutually reinforcing manner to maintain the epigenetic states of differentiated cells throughout life (**Figure 2**). For example, various histone modifications can promote regional CpG methylation, CpG methylation can stimulate specific histone modifications, and the methyl-binding protein MeCP2 appears to facilitate histone deacetylation (50).

EPIGENETIC EPIDEMIOLOGY: CHALLENGES AND OPPORTUNITIES

We define epigenetic epidemiology as the study of the associations between epigenetic variation and risk of disease. Because of genetic-epigenetic interactions, epigenetic epidemiology cannot be completely separated

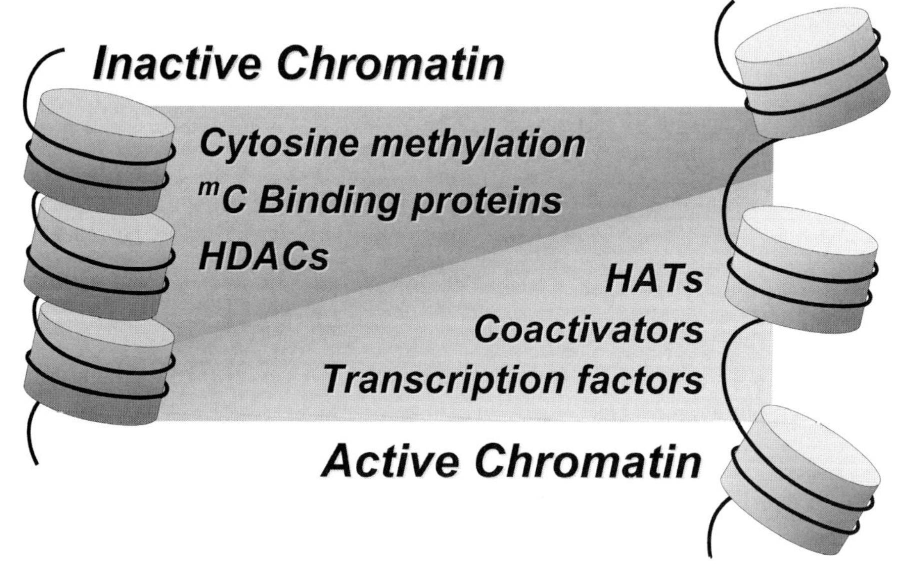

Figure 2

Regional chromatin conformation and transcriptional activity is dynamically regulated by a combination of interacting epigenetic mechanisms. Chromatin is DNA wrapped around nucleosomes, which are composed of histone proteins. Chromatin can exist in either a compact, inactive state or an open, transcriptionally active state. The specific combination of activating and inactivating epigenetic modifications at a genomic locus determines transcriptional competence. ^{m}C, methylcytosine; HATs, histone acetyltransferases; HDACs, histone deacetylases.

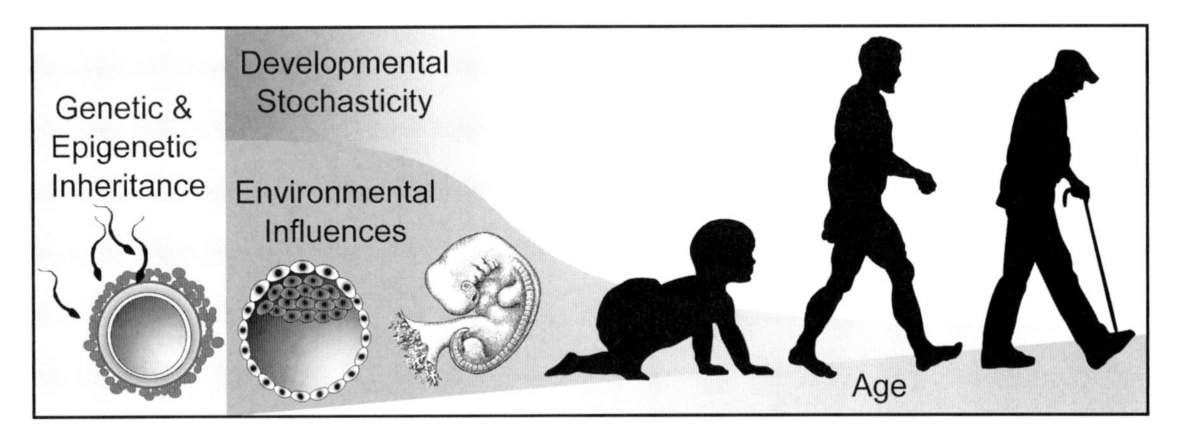

Figure 3

Sources of interindividual epigenetic variation that can contribute to human disease. In addition to genetic and epigenetic inheritance, stochasticity affects the developmental establishment of epigenetic regulation. Environmental influences on epigenetics are likely to be most important during prenatal and early postnatal development, when epigenetic mechanisms undergo establishment and maturation. Cumulative errors in maintenance of epigenetic information will contribute to interindividual epigenetic variation with age.

from genetic epidemiology (7). Nonetheless, it is useful to compare the nascent field of epigenetic epidemiology with the established discipline of genetic epidemiology. Genetic epidemiology focuses on the role of inherited genes in disease etiology; aside from de novo mutations, all genetic variation is inherited. Conversely, epigenetic variation has many sources: genetic and epigenetic inheritance, developmental stochasticity, environmental influences (during development and throughout life), and aging (**Figure 3**) (7, 128). Whereas the starting point for studies of genetic epidemiology is evidence of heritability of disease risk (20), the starting point in epigenetic epidemiology is evidence that interindividual epigenetic variation affects disease risk.

The cornerstone approaches of genetic epidemiology are family-based genetic linkage studies that scan the genome for associations of specific haplotypes with disease, and population-based association studies, in which genetic variation at candidate genes is related to disease (20). Family-based studies are not likely to be of general utility in epigenetic epidemiology. Transgenerational epigenetic inheritance is, in most cases, probably a minor component of interindividual epigenetic variability, and even when familial clustering of epigenotype is detected (11, 101), it will be difficult to determine if it is caused by a genotype-epigenotype interaction (76), shared environment, or epigenetic inheritance. Family-based studies will, however, be critical in epigenetic epidemiology related to genomic imprinting, in which disease risk will depend upon parent of origin. Population-based association studies will be most useful for characterizing relations between epigenetic variability and disease.

Studying monozygotic (MZ) and dizygotic twins to estimate genetic heritability of disease is a classic approach in genetic epidemiology. Twin studies are also an important tool in epigenetic epidemiology: disease discordance within (genetically identical) MZ twin pairs provides support for an epigenetic etiology (85, 132). Just as developmental epigenetics has a stochastic component, so do other developmental processes. Hence, not all phenotypic differences between MZ twins reflect epigenetic differences. Toward understanding the role of epigenetics in DOHaD, studies of

MZ: monozygotic

CpG islands: CpG-rich regions often located at gene promoters

MZ twins may be misleading. Animal studies indicate that effects of maternal nutrition on developmental epigenetics often occur in the preimplantation embryo (122). Before implantation, two twins share the exact same oviduct environment. Thus, although differential placentation and partitioning of placental blood flow often results in discordant nutrient supply within MZ twin pairs, this environmental influence may occur too late to induce systemic epigenetic differences between the twins.

Whereas genetic epidemiology is focused on variation in DNA sequence, epigenetic epidemiology will eventually grapple with the full complexity of interacting epigenetic modifications. Initial studies of epigenetic epidemiology will focus on CpG methylation. Site-specific and regional changes in CpG methylation are often highly correlated with gene expression (27, 50), allowing CpG methylation to serve as an indicator of locus-specific epigenetic regulation. CpG methylation is a relatively simple variable; on a single allele, each CpG site is either methylated or not. Percent methylation within a population of alleles can be measured with high precision (124). Further, CpG methylation is very stable and only small quantities of DNA are required to measure it, so even samples stored for a long time and/or available in limited quantities can be assayed for this epigenetic modification.

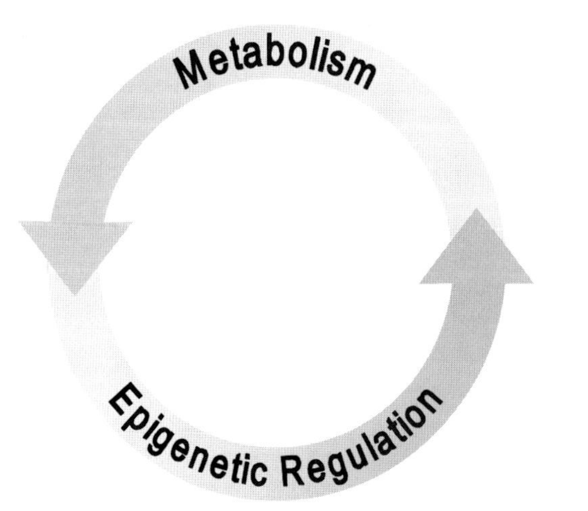

Figure 4

Modeling of epigenetic-environmental interactions will be complicated by the interactions between metabolism and epigenetic regulation.

Modeling the role of environment will be more challenging in epigenetic as compared to genetic epidemiology. Although researchers often discuss "gene-environment interactions," in most cases they are referring to effects of environment or behavior on the probability that a specific genetic variant will result in disease. The other side of the "interaction"—environment altering genotype—is relatively rare. In epigenetic epidemiology, however, true epigenetic-environment interactions are commonplace. Environment can modify the disease risk associated with a specific epigenotype and also has the vast potential to actually change epigenotype (29, 123). Further, whereas the epigenetic epidemiology of DOHaD will focus on the ability of early nutrition to influence DNA methylation, causing persistent changes in metabolism, it is clear that metabolism will also feed back to affect DNA methylation and potentially other epigenetic modifications (**Figure 4**) (111).

In investigating candidate genes for an epigenetic relation with disease, the specific genomic regions of interest will be more diverse than in genetic epidemiology. Whereas changes in DNA sequence will usually affect health and disease by altering protein function, epigenetic changes will usually affect transcription rather than protein function. Characterization of epigenetic regulatory regions will therefore be a component of epigenetic epidemiology. Many studies of epigenetic regulation have focused on CpG islands, CpG-rich regions often found at gene promoters (55). Recent studies, however, indicate that CpG methylation in intragenic and intergenic regions is critical to tissue-specific gene expression (12, 28, 59). Our ability to predict the genomic region(s) at which epigenetic modifications contribute to gene-specific transcriptional regulation remains rudimentary.

The inherent tissue-specificity of epigenetic gene regulation adds yet another level of complexity to epigenetic compared to genetic epidemiology. Each individual has only one genotype, but innumerable epigenotypes. Whereas a DNA sample from peripheral blood leukocytes enables us to obtain information about a genetic variant that predisposes to neurodegenerative disease, the epigenetic regulation of this gene may differ markedly between leukocytic and neuronal DNA. Early nutritional influences on epigenetic regulation may likewise be tissue-specific (119).

Clearly, investigators launching epigenetic epidemiologic studies of DOHaD face daunting challenges. However, given the accumulating data linking epigenetic dysregulation to human disease (25, 52, 96), we cannot ignore animal model data showing that subtle environmental influences during development cause persistent changes in epigenetic gene regulation (29, 123). It is of critical public health importance to determine if similar phenomena occur in humans. Recent epigenetic epidemiologic studies show that the challenges are not insurmountable.

EPIGENETIC EPIDEMIOLOGY: EPIGENETIC VARIATION AND HUMAN DISEASE

Assisted Reproduction and Epigenetic Disease

Inappropriate epigenetic reprogramming during early embryonic development can lead to human disease (50). Assisted reproductive technologies (ART), first introduced three decades ago and now accounting for 1%–3% of births in Western countries, may affect epigenetic reprogramming. The most commonly used ART are in vitro fertilization and intracytoplasmic sperm injection. ART-conceived babies are at increased risk for intrauterine growth retardation, low birth weight (24, 102), and, paradoxically, fetal overgrowth. Developmental syndromes associated with aberrant genomic imprinting are more common in children conceived with ART than in naturally conceived children (41). Beckwith-Wiedemann syndrome has been reported to be nine times more common in infants conceived through in vitro fertilization (19). In the small case studies available, all children with Angelman syndrome conceived by ART exhibited hypomethylation of the imprinting control center on the maternal copy of chromosome 15q, in striking contrast with the 3% of Angelman cases associated with this epigenetic abnormality in normally conceived children (15, 81).

ART: assisted reproductive technologies

The direction of causality underlying the associations between ART and epigenetic disease, however, has been questioned (78). In addition to the potential for ART to induce epigenetic changes, these associations could result from extant epigenetic irregularities in the oocyte causing both infertility and epigenetic dysregulation in the offspring (78). Furthermore, most evidence linking ART to imprinting errors comes from case reports and small case-control studies. Nonetheless, all ART involves in vitro culture of the early embryo from the time of fertilization until introduction into the uterus, and animal model data indicate that the artificial environment during this critical period may affect epigenetic reprogramming (57, 58). Conception by ART is becoming increasingly common, and ART programs are extending the period of in vitro culture to optimize implantation rates. Clearly, systematic large-scale studies of the effects of ART on epigenetic regulation and human disease are warranted (78).

Interindividual Epigenetic Variation

An excellent way to identify genomic regions that may contribute to epigenetic disease is to catalog those showing substantial interindividual epigenetic variation. Holliday (44) recently asserted, "[I]f the methylation was variable between individuals, it would probably not be important." To the contrary, only if methylation of important genes differs between individuals can individual variation in methylation contribute to variation in disease? Population studies of interindividual epigenetic variation are therefore an important part of epigenetic epidemiology.

The Human Epigenome Project aims to "analyze DNA methylation in the regulatory regions of all known genes in most major cell types and their diseased variants" (88). In a pilot project that profiled DNA methylation of the 3.8 Mb major histocompatibility locus, methylation was analyzed in several human tissues, with multiple samples from different individuals for all tissues. Almost half of the amplicons analyzed showed substantial interindividual variation in methylation in at least one tissue (88). A recent study examining the potential for transgenerational epigenetic inheritance (32) used CpG methylation arrays to identify interindividual variation in DNA methylation at several human disease genes in sperm samples from 46 men.

In a study of 48 three-generation families (680 individuals total), Sandovici et al. (101) demonstrated substantial interindividual variation in allelic methylation at the *IGF2/H19* and *IGF2R* imprinted loci in peripheral blood DNA. Interestingly, familial clustering of allelic methylation suggested a genetic component to this epigenetic variation. Temporal changes in individuals over periods up to 20 years indicated influences of environment and aging. A later study on the same population reported dramatic interindividual variation in methylation at specific *Alu* elements (100). *Alu* are short retrotransposon elements present at over a million copies in the human genome. Because of their ability to cause epigenetic dysregulation of neighboring genes (127), interindividual epigenetic variation at retrotransposons could have important implications for human disease.

Together, these studies demonstrate considerable interindividual variation in locus-specific DNA methylation. Loci implicated in human disease are promising candidates for epigenetic association studies. Data are generally lacking, however, regarding potential tissue-specificity of interindividual epigenetic variation.

Epigenetic Discordance in Monozygotic Twins

MZ twins are often discordant for common diseases (85); epigenetic differences provide a potential explanation. In a study of lymphocyte DNA from 40 MZ twin pairs, Fraga et al. (34) employed sophisticated epigenomic approaches to identify loci showing differential DNA methylation within twin pairs. Many of the regions of discordant methylation corresponded to *Alu* sequences, corroborating the findings of Sandovici et al. (100). Highlighting differences between 3-year-old and 50-year-old twin pairs, Fraga et al. (34) concluded that most epigenetic differences between MZ twins are not present in childhood but instead arise over the lifetime. This conclusion is unwarranted, however, since only two 3-year-old twin pairs were studied. Indeed, a study of buccal DNA from twelve 5-year-old MZ twin pairs with discordant birth weights found considerable twin-twin discordance of CpG methylation at the gene encoding catechol-o-methyltransferase (a gene implicated in psychopathology) (73). Notably, birth weight was not associated with catechol-o-methyltransferase methylation, underscoring our previous point that differences in placentation and placental partitioning that result in birth weight differentials among MZ twins may occur too late to affect systemic establishment of epigenetic marks.

Epigenetic differences among MZ twins discordant for disease provide support for the hypothesis that stochastic differences in the establishment of epigenetic gene regulation can lead to human disease. Beckwith-Wiedemann syndrome is a developmental syndrome caused by genetic and epigenetic alterations in an imprinted region on human chromosome 11 (126). Loss of allele-specific methylation and associated biallelic expression of the genomically imprinted gene *LIT1* is the most common epigenetic alteration associated with Beckwith-Wiedemann syndrome. In skin fibroblast DNA of five MZ twin pairs discordant for Beckwith-Wiedemann syndrome, every affected twin, but no unaffected twin, showed these epigenetic alterations (126). A recent study examined a single MZ twin pair discordant for a caudal duplication anomaly (79). Because of the similarity of the phenotype to that of *Axin Fused* mice, the investigators focused on the human *AXIN1* gene. In DNA from peripheral blood, the *AXIN1* promoter-region CpG island was significantly hypermethylated in the affected twin relative to the unaffected twin. There was lower and individually variable methylation at this region in peripheral blood DNA of healthy control individuals.

Epigenetic Epidemiology of Cancer

Epigenetic epidemiology has been applied in the field of cancer epigenetics. One example relates to epigenetic dysregulation of the insulin-like growth factor 2 (*IGF2*) gene in colon cancer. *IGF2* is a genomically imprinted gene usually expressed in humans only from the paternally inherited allele. A population-based study of peripheral blood DNA from 262 Japanese individuals demonstrated that loss of imprinting (LOI, manifesting as biallelic expression of *IGF2*) occurs in 10% of normal adults (99). In a cross-sectional study of 172 patients undergoing colonoscopy, Cui et al. (17) found that, relative to patients with no personal or family history of colorectal cancer, those with a family history of colorectal cancer had a fivefold elevated odds ratio for *IGF2* LOI in peripheral blood, and those diagnosed with colorectal cancer had a 20-fold elevated odds ratio. These results, if confirmed, suggest that *IGF2* LOI in peripheral blood lymphocytes can serve as an indicator of colorectal cancer risk (17). However, since *IGF2* LOI was assessed concurrently with cancer status, temporality of *IGF2* LOI and cancer development cannot be established; systemic LOI could be a consequence of the disease. An epidemiologic study of the same individuals (16) assessed various environmental exposures (cigarette smoking, alcohol ingestion, and intake of several nutrients) but found none associated with *IGF2* LOI. These findings do not exclude the possibility that environmental factors acting during a critical period of development affect *IGF2* LOI (53).

Loss of imprinting (LOI): a change in the expression ratio of a genomically imprinted gene away from monoallelic expression. Loss of imprinting can occur either by up-regulation of the normally silenced allele or preferential silencing of the normally expressed allele

Age, Genetics, and Environment

Age, genetics, and environment all interact to affect epigenetic regulation. One of the earliest studies that can be characterized as epigenetic epidemiology investigated the role of aging in hypermethylation of the estrogen receptor (ER) gene (46). In 39 healthy control individuals age 20–90, ER CpG island methylation in colonic DNA increased linearly with age ($R^2 = 0.50$). Since ER hypermethylation is found in almost all colorectal tumors, these data suggest that ER hypermethylation could contribute to the increased risk of colorectal cancer with age (46). A population-based study of Italian adults explored the combined effects of plasma folate status and a common polymorphism (C677T) in 5,10-methylenetetrahydrofolate reductase on global DNA methylation (35). In a comparison of 187 C/C and 105 T/T individuals, plasma folate concentrations were directly related to global DNA methylation only in T/T individuals (35). Also, plasma homocysteine concentration in T/T individuals was markedly elevated and correlated inversely with global DNA methylation. Plasma homocysteine was also related to epigenetic alterations in a smaller study of men with severe hyperhomocysteinemia (45). Leukocyte DNA was significantly hypomethylated in hyperhomocysteinemic men relative to controls. In a subset of seven men informative for a polymorphism in the imprinted *H19* gene, the three with the highest plasma homocysteine concentrations all showed aberrant biallelic expression. In every case, monoallelic *H19* expression was restored after eight weeks of daily supplementation with pharmacological levels of 5-methyltetrahydrofolate (45).

Metastable epialleles: alleles at which the developmental establishment of epigenotype occurs stochastically, resulting in wide interindividual variation in DNA methylation

Together, these seminal studies illustrate the potential of epigenetic epidemiology. In these studies of select human populations, significant interindividual epigenetic variation at specific loci has been demonstrated and, in many cases, linked to disease. Epigenetic epidemiology of DOHaD will seek to quantify interindividual epigenetic variation that is both induced by early environmental exposures and associated with risk of chronic disease.

EARLY ENVIRONMENTAL INFLUENCES ON EPIGENETIC REGULATION

Our understanding of the specific mechanisms by which epigenetic gene regulation is first established during mammalian differentiation is fairly rudimentary. Of the various epigenetic mechanisms, developmental changes in DNA methylation are best characterized. Shortly after fertilization, the genome of the early embryo undergoes massive demethylation. Except for specific regions that escape this erasure, the genome of the preimplantation embryo is completely hypomethylated, correlating with its pluripotency (74, 89). Starting around the time of implantation, as the embryo develops into a fetus, lineage-specific re-establishment of DNA methylation occurs, ostensibly restricting the gene expression and developmental fate of differentiating tissues (74, 89).

The intuitive assertion that DNA methylation functions as a component of cellular memory to maintain the differentiated state of mammalian tissues has, however, been controversial. It has been proposed that whereas DNA methylation functions in specialized epigenetic phenomena such as genomic imprinting, X-chromosome inactivation, and silencing of retrotransposons, its role in differentiation and tissue-specific gene expression is unclear (115). Evidence for such a role is now accumulating. Studies of mice engineered with an inducible transgene capable of protecting neighboring sequences from de novo methylation during development indicate that establishment of DNA methylation in the early embryo is critical to setting up the epigenetic profile of open versus closed chromatin states (42). The tissue-specific expression of various genes has been correlated with their tissue-specific hypomethylation. Ehrlich (27) recently reviewed the literature on this topic and employed rigorous criteria to identify mammalian genes at which differentiation-associated DNA methylation controls expression. Genes expressed specifically in diverse tissues including testis, myometrium, liver, brain, and leukocytes show tissue-specific hypomethylation that appears both necessary and sufficient for expression (27). Recent studies of tissue-specific CpG methylation on a genomewide scale suggest an explanation for the failure of many studies to correlate DNA methylation with cellular differentiation. Whereas most previous studies focused on methylation in gene promoter regions, these recent epigenomic analyses indicate that tissue-specific methylation in intragenic regions often contributes to tissue-specific gene expression (12, 104).

Once established during development, epigenetic mechanisms are in most cases maintained with high fidelity throughout life. During development, however, the massive loss and subsequent re-establishment of DNA methylation in the embryo and fetus likely comprise diverse critical periods during which environmental stimuli can affect epigenetic regulation (123). We propose that environmental influences on the developmental establishment of DNA methylation occur via two general mechanisms: (*a*) by affecting the supply of dietary methyl donors and/or activity of DNA methyltransferases to induce either hyper- or hypomethylation at metastable epialleles (see below) or (*b*) by altering transcriptional activity of specific genes during ontogenic periods when DNA methylation is being established (**Figure 5**).

Most genomic regions undergo developmentally programmed establishment of epigenetic regulation and show little interindividual variability in DNA methylation. Conversely, at regions referred to as metastable epialleles (86), developmental establishment of DNA methylation occurs probabilistically, resulting in dramatic interindividual differences in epigenetic regulation. Nutritional influences on developmental epigenetics were first suggested by studies of the *viable yellow agouti* (A^{vy}) metastable epiallele. The murine A^{vy} mutation resulted from transposition of an IAP retrotransposon upstream of the *agouti* gene, which regulates the production of yellow pigment in fur. Spontaneous variation in CpG methylation of the A^{vy} IAP causes dramatic variation in coat color and other phenotypes among genetically identical A^{vy}/a mice (75). [The *nonagouti* (*a*) allele encodes a nonfunctional *agouti* transcript and therefore does not contribute to phenotypic variation of A^{vy}/a mice.] Wolff et al. (130) found that supplementing mouse dams with the dietary methyl donors and cofactors folic acid, vitamin B_{12}, betaine, and choline shifts the coat color distribution of their A^{vy}/a offspring from yellow to brown, suggesting hypermethylation of the A^{vy} IAP. It was later confirmed that maternal supplementation affects coat color of A^{vy}/a offspring by inducing hypermethylation at A^{vy} (122). The effect of maternal supplementation on establishment of A^{vy} epigenotype apparently occurs prior to gastrulation (122). Interestingly, supplementation of dams with the soy phytoestrogen genistein before and during pregnancy induced offspring A^{vy} hypermethylation comparable to that caused by methyl donor supplementation (22).

Recent studies in *Axin Fused* ($Axin^{Fu}$) mice indicate that epigenetic lability to early nutrition is a general characteristic of metastable epialleles. The $Axin^{Fu}$ metastable epiallele resulted from an IAP insertion into Axin intron 6 and causes a kinky tail phenotype. Similar to A^{vy}, spontaneous variability in CpG methylation at $Axin^{Fu}$ confers dramatic phenotypic variation among isogenic $Axin^{Fu}/+$ mice (87). Maternal supplementation with methyl donors reduces the incidence of tail kinks in $Axin^{Fu}/+$ offspring by inducing hypermethylation at $Axin^{Fu}$ (119), indicating that developmental establishment of DNA methylation at metastable epialleles is, in general, labile to maternal diet. In studies of another *agouti* metastable epiallele (A^{iapy}), haploinsufficiency for the maintenance DNA methyltransferase Dnmt1 (36) shifted the coat-color distribution of A^{iapy}/a mice toward yellow (hypomethylated). Hence, any environmental exposure during early embryonic development that affects either the substrate availability or enzymatic activity of Dnmt1 will likely influence the establishment of DNA methylation at metastable epialleles, inducing permanent changes in gene expression (**Figure 5*A***).

The second general mechanism for early environmental influences on epigenetic regulation potentially encompasses a much broader range of both environmental stimuli and responsive genes. The model states that during limited ontogenic periods when de novo DNA methylation occurs, genes that are actively transcribed in specific cells are protected from hypermethylation (**Figure 5*B***). There is extensive support for this model. Active promoters in CpG island-containing transgenes faithfully remain hypomethylated, but lose their immunity to hypermethylation if promoter function is impaired (9). In cultured cells with a transgene containing binding sites for the inducible metal-responsive transcription factor, induction of this transcription factor caused activation of transgene expression that persisted after the withdrawal of the induction stimulus, showing that transcriptional activation prevents epigenetic silencing (108). Such observations led Bird (6) to propose that, by preventing de novo hypermethylation, the transcriptional activity of embryonic promoters is imprinted for the duration of that somatic lifetime.

This model predicts that any early nutritional or environmental stimulus that alters transcriptional activity when DNA methylation is undergoing developmental changes could result in permanent alterations in epigenetic regulation and related phenotypes.

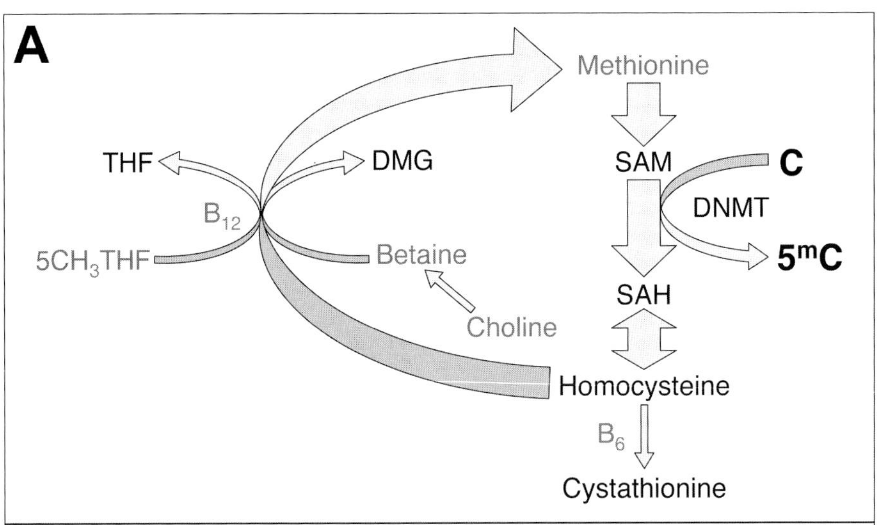
A
Methionine
THF
DMG
SAM
C
DNMT
B12
5CH3THF
Betaine
5mC
SAH
Choline
Homocysteine
B6
Cystathionine

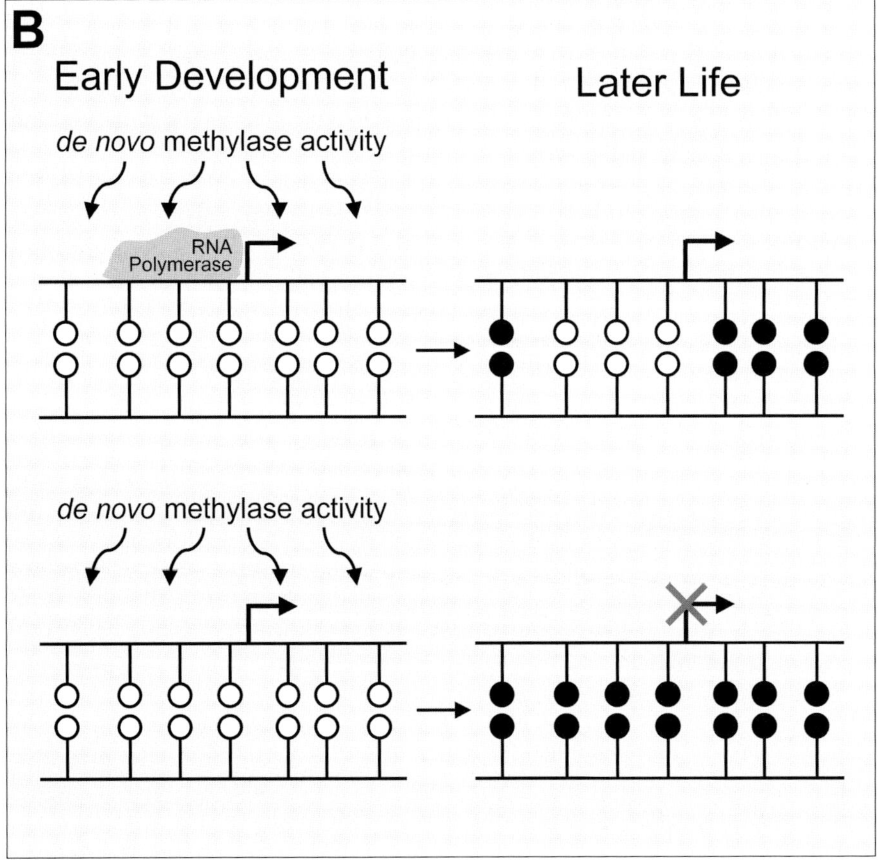
B
Early Development
Later Life
de novo methylase activity
RNA
Polymerase
de novo methylase activity

Studies relating maternal caregiving behavior to epigenetic changes at the rat glucocorticoid receptor (GR) promoter support this model (125). In an inbred strain of rats, there is wide natural variation in the amount of time that dams spend nursing, licking, and grooming their pups. Meaney and colleagues (125) found that the level of maternal care during the suckling period permanently changes offspring physiology and behavior by affecting the ontogeny of methylation at specific CpG sites in the GR promoter. In the hippocampus, a key CpG site in the GR promoter is completely unmethylated just before birth, and then becomes hypermethylated on the first postnatal day (P1). The period from P1 to P6 is a critical window for establishment of CpG methylation and transcriptional regulation of GR in the hippocampus: Methylation at the critical CpG site is almost completely gone by P6 in pups suckled by high-caregiving dams but remains permanently elevated in those suckled by more apathetic dams (125). These observations indicate that high maternal care in the early postnatal period activates GR transcription, inducing permanent GR hypomethylation. This hypomethylation, in turn, causes permanent derepression of GR transcription (125).

Several other examples illustrate that environmental influences during development can induce changes in DNA methylation and epigenetic regulation, but it is unclear whether these effects occur by mass action at metastable epialleles or through transcriptionally mediated effects on the establishment of DNA methylation. In perhaps the earliest such study, Reik et al. (90) transplanted female pronuclei into recipient eggs of a different genotype, allowed the mice to develop to adulthood, and compared hepatic gene expression in these "nucleocytoplasmic hybrids" with that of sham-manipulated control animals. The nucleocytoplasmic hybrids were genetically identical to the control mice, differing only in the cytoplasm to which the early embryonic genome was exposed. Nevertheless, substantial differences in gene expression and CpG methylation in adult liver were induced by this early environmental exposure (90).

More recently, dietary protein restriction of pregnant rats was shown to induce DNA hypomethylation and increased expression of GR and peroxisome proliferator-activated receptor alpha in the livers of offspring at weaning, and these epigenetic changes were completely prevented if the protein-restricted diet was supplemented with folic acid (63). Similarly, dietary choline deficiency during mouse fetal development induced hypomethylation of *Cdkn3* in specific regions of the hippocampus, correlating with increased expression of Kap, the kinase-associated phosphatase encoded by *Cdkn3* (77). Neither of these studies determined whether the epigenetic alterations induced by maternal diet persist to adulthood.

Figure 5

Potential mechanisms for environmental influences on developmental establishment of DNA methylation. (*A*) Nutritional or other stimuli that affect either the efficiency of one-carbon metabolism or the activity of DNMT1 could alter the developmental establishment of DNA methylation at metastable epialleles. Flux through the transmethylation/remethylation pathway is dependent upon nutrients including folate, vitamins B_{12} and B_6, choline, betaine, and methionine. (*B*) Transcriptional activity during critical developmental periods can impair de novo methylation. Any nutritional or other environmental exposure that activates gene transcription during periods of de novo CpG methylation can permanently imprint transcriptional competence by preventing hypermethylation. (Methylated CpG sites are shown as filled "lollipops.") Although a gene promoter region is shown here, similar effects could occur at any genomic region contributing to transcriptional regulation, such as a distal enhancer. $5CH_3THF$, 5-methyl tetrahydrofolate; CpG, cytosine-guanine dinucleotide; DNMT, DNA methyltransferase; SAH, s-adenosylhomocysteine; SAM, s-adenosylmethionine.

Together, these data from animal models indicate that nutrition and other environmental stimuli during development can affect the establishment and/or maturation of epigenetic mechanisms, causing persistent changes in gene expression. Hence, to the extent that epigenetic dysregulation contributes to the etiology of diseases most commonly associated with DOHaD—cardiovascular disease, type 2 diabetes, cancer, and obesity—epigenetic mechanisms may provide a critical link between early environment and adult disease.

EPIGENETIC DYSREGULATION AND HUMAN DISEASE

The role of epigenetic dysregulation in human disease has been reviewed extensively (25, 52, 96). We therefore summarize only the most salient points here. Because the epigenetic basis of several rare developmental diseases is well-established (25), we focus on chronic diseases most often considered in the DOHaD paradigm.

Cancer

A hallmark of tumorigenesis is the coexistence of genomewide hypomethylation and hypermethylation of CpG islands in the promoters of specific genes (26). Promoter-region CpG island hypermethylation associated with inappropriate transcriptional silencing is the most frequently documented epigenetic alteration in tumors. Nearly half of the tumor suppressor genes that cause familial cancer when mutated also undergo epigenetic silencing in sporadic forms of cancer (54). For example, hypermethylation of the mismatch repair gene *MLH1* is associated with tumors exhibiting microsatellite instability, and hypermethylation of the breast cancer gene *BRCA1* is found in 10%–15% of women with nonfamilial breast cancer (54).

Epigenetic dysregulation of genomic imprinting is also implicated in cancer. *IGF2* LOI occurs in several childhood cancers, including a large proportion of Wilms' tumor (30), and in various adult cancers (25). Recent studies suggest that systemic *IGF2* LOI may serve as an indicator of colorectal cancer risk (17). An epigenetic progenitor model of cancer (30) recently highlighted the potential importance of polyclonal epigenetic disruption of stem cells via alterations of tumor progenitor genes including *IGF2*.

As most studies in cancer epigenetics have been cross-sectional, it remains unclear whether the epigenetic dysregulation in tumor tissue or in peripheral blood is a cause or an effect of tumorigenesis. A causal role for *IGF2* LOI was recently supported by a mouse model: Induction of *Igf2* LOI enhanced susceptibility to gastrointestinal cancer (98). Studies of families with strong family histories of cancer have identified apparent germline epimutations in the mismatch repair genes *MLH1* (107) and *MSH2* (11). It is possible, however, that the familial clustering of aberrant epigenetic regulation at these loci is mediated by genetic variation. Regardless of whether they reflect true transgenerational epigenetic inheritance, these epimutations appear to induce carcinogenesis as do genetic mutations at the same loci. Nested case-control studies, in which tissue specimens are collected well before cancer diagnosis, are warranted to determine temporality of the association of epigenetic dysregulation and cancer.

Cardiovascular Disease

CVD, in particular CHD, is now the leading cause of death worldwide, accounting for 27% of deaths in industrialized countries and 21% of deaths in developing countries (64). With genetics explaining less than 5% of CHD, adult lifestyle factors and epigenetics likely explain most of the variation (129). The most obvious link between epigenetics and cardiovascular disease is hyperhomocysteinemia. The basis for the association of hyperhomocysteinemia with cardiovascular disease is unknown, but since elevated homocysteine concentrations can impair one-carbon metabolism and DNA methylation, epigenetic mechanisms have been postulated (10). Aberrant DNA methylation (both hypo- and hypermethylation) secondary to nutritional factors has been implicated as an early step in atherogenesis (66, 134).

Type 2 Diabetes

An article proposing DNA methylation profiling in diabetes reviewed indirect evidence that epigenetic dysregulation contributes to type 2 diabetes (68). A recent data-mining analysis of more than 12 million Medline records (133) identified epigenetic factors among the strongest statistical associations to type 2 diabetes. The most direct evidence implicating epigenetic dysregulation in human diabetes is from studies of transient neonatal diabetes (TND), a rare form of diabetes that presents within the first few days after birth and, although normally resolving within one year, often recurs later in life. Two studies recently showed that infants with sporadic TND show aberrant methylation at several imprinted genes in peripheral blood leukocytes (21, 67). Effects of parental and grandparental nutrition on diabetes risk in humans has been reported, suggesting transgenerational inheritance of epigenetic alterations that affect diabetes susceptibility (56, 83). Several animal models showing persistent effects of prenatal and early postnatal nutrition on endocrine pancreas function and gene expression suggest an epigenetic basis (112, 121).

Obesity

Prader-Willi syndrome is a developmental syndrome that causes hyperphagic obesity, hypogonadism, and characteristic facial features (38). Whereas the disease most commonly results from genetic abnormalities in an imprinted region of chromosome 15, some sporadic cases result from aberrant epigenetic silencing of that region, providing a clear example of epigenetic dysregulation causing human obesity. Genomewide parent-of-origin linkage analyses suggest that maternally imprinted loci in chromosome regions 10p12 (23) and 2q37 (39) also influence human obesity. Moreover, imprinted genes affect the development of the hypothalamus, which plays a central role in regulating energy homeostasis (14).

Animal models provide further illustrations that epigenetic dysregulation can cause obesity (117). When mice are cloned, they have normal birth weights but often develop adult-onset obesity (109). A similar phenomenon, termed "large offspring syndrome," appears to be related to epigenetic dysregulation in cloned sheep (135). A^{vy} mice provide another animal model of epigenetically based obesity. Agouti protein binds antagonistically to the melanocortin 4 receptor in the hypothalamus. A^{vy}/a mice with A^{vy} hypomethylation therefore develop not only yellow coats but also hyperphagic obesity (131).

Overall, direct evidence for an involvement of epigenetic dysregulation in human cardiovascular disease, type 2 diabetes, and obesity is scant. This contrasts markedly with the compelling body of literature implicating epigenetic dysregulation in human cancer. Compared with these other diseases, however, demonstrating an epigenetic basis for cancer is relatively straightforward. Much of the data implicating epigenetic dysregulation in cancer was obtained by examining epigenetic mechanisms in tumor tissue and adjacent normal tissue. Hence, in cancer, the tissue showing epigenetic dysregulation is both easily identifiable and readily obtainable. The other diseases of greatest relevance to DOHaD are more complex and can result from dysregulation in multiple interacting tissues. As demonstrated by the success of cancer epigenetics, however, any disease with a genetic basis is also likely to have an epigenetic basis. The potential tissue-specificity of epigenetic regulation (and dysregulation) will be the major obstacle to epigenetic epidemiology of DOHaD.

EPIGENETIC EPIDEMIOLOGY OF DOHaD: SUGGESTIONS FOR FUTURE STUDIES

The definition of metabolic imprinting (120) was proposed to guide mechanistic studies into the developmental origins hypothesis. Accordingly, several characteristics of metabolic imprinting are instructive to the design of epidemiologic studies testing the hypothesis that environmental influences on developmental epigenetics contribute to health and disease in humans. A key characteristic of metabolic imprinting is the need to distinguish fundamental mechanisms of metabolic memory, "primary imprints," from secondary physiological alterations that arise in response to primary imprints. The fundamental nature of epigenetic regulatory mechanisms makes them logical primary imprint marks. Demonstrating that the epigenetic regulation of a specific gene in adulthood is correlated with some prenatal exposure does not, however, prove that the epigenetic change serves as a primary imprint. Primary imprint marks must be present directly after the imprinting period as well as in adulthood (120). Hence, incorporating a test of temporality into epigenetic epidemiologic studies will aid in the identification of epigenetically based primary imprint marks. This proposal is most practical in follow-up studies of cohorts in which tissues were collected during early life.

The critical-window nature of metabolic imprinting (120) should also be considered in epigenetic epidemiologic studies of DOHaD. For example, epidemiologic studies seeking to identify systemic epigenetic alterations should focus on periconceptional environmental exposures, since epigenetic alterations occurring in the very early embryo are most likely to be propagated to diverse tissues. Conversely, exposures occurring during late gestation or postnatally are more likely to induce tissue-specific epigenetic changes.

The potential tissue-specificity of epigenetic regulation raises the question of what tissues should be collected in epigenetic epidemiologic studies. Many studies have banked DNA isolated from peripheral blood leukocytes (PBLs), but PBLs represent only one germ layer of the early embryo. Because the different germ layers (endoderm, mesoderm, and ectoderm) are epigenetically divergent, it will be useful to collect tissues representing these different embryonic lineages. Since DNA methylation can be analyzed using very small quantities of DNA, it is feasible to noninvasively collect sufficient quantities of human tissues representing different germ lineages. Buccal cells and hair follicles contain ectodermal DNA. PBLs are of mesodermal origin. Obtaining endodermal tissue in large-scale studies of healthy individuals will pose the greatest challenge. One possible approach, assessing DNA methylation in colonocyte DNA isolated from human stool, was recently validated (4).

Identifying interindividual epigenetic variability that occurs systemically will simplify studies of epigenetic epidemiology because DNA methylation in easily obtainable tissues will correlate with that in tissues of physiological relevance. Here, metastable epialleles are of great interest. In addition to their definitive epigenetic variability among different individuals, metastable epialleles generally exhibit little tissue-specificity in DNA methylation (119, 122). Hence, if metastable epialleles of pathophysiological relevance can be identified in humans, these would be obvious loci at which to focus initial epigenetic epidemiologic studies related to DOHaD. Perhaps the best such candidate metastable epiallele in humans is *IGF2* (99). *IGF2* and other genes found to exhibit epigenetic variation among individuals, such as polymorphic *Alu*s (100) and *IGF2R* (101), should be evaluated to determine if their interindividual epigenetic variability occurs systemically.

Even if specific metastable epialleles exhibit epigenetic variation that appears unrelated to human disease, they may be useful as epigenetic biomarkers, enabling a retrospective measure of environmental exposures during development. One of the greatest weaknesses of DOHaD has been the reliance upon birth weight as a proxy for fetal nutritional status. Many factors influence birth weight; the effect of maternal nutrition is relatively minor and occurs mainly in the last trimester (106). Just as the coat color of A^{vy} mice may be used as an epigenetic biosensor to gauge the hypermethylating effects of various diets (118), human metastable epialleles may provide a sensitive retrospective indicator of genomic methylating capacity during embryonic development. Such alleles therefore may be used as sentry loci to select individuals likely to have experienced conditions in utero that could predispose to aberrant epigenetic regulation at multiple loci.

Prospective studies testing for effects of maternal nutrition on DNA methylation of offspring would benefit from the validation of robust biomarkers for maternal one-carbon metabolism. Because moderate folate depletion can induce genomewide DNA methylation (49), genomic methylation may be used as an integrative biomarker of methyl donor nutrition (69). Studies, for example, could determine if maternal periconceptional genomic methylation predicts methylation at specific loci in her offspring. Plasma metabolites related to maternal one-carbon metabolism will also be useful. Because s-adenosylmethionine (SAM) and s-adenosylhomocysteine (SAH) are the substrate and product, respectively, of methyltransferase reactions, it has been proposed that the SAM:SAH ratio can be used as a methylation index to identify individuals with high or low capacity for DNA methylation (113). Because SAM does not readily cross the plasma membrane, however, each mammalian cell must synthesize its own SAM from circulating methionine or homocysteine (31). This could explain why dietary exposures that perturb the SAM:SAH ratio often cause paradoxical changes in DNA methylation (111). Homocysteine, which is in equilibrium with SAH (a product inhibitor of methyltransferases), is a key metabolite in mammalian one-carbon metabolism and readily crosses the plasma membrane. Circulating homocysteine therefore shows promise as a systemic indicator of transmethylation capacity (111). Importantly, gene-nutrient interactions will likely complicate the interpretation of all these potential biomarkers. For example, the previously discussed studies of the 5,10-methylenetetrahydrofolate reductase C677T polymorphism (35) suggest that genomic methylation may serve as an effective biomarker for folate status only in T/T individuals.

Most previous studies of epigenetic epidemiology have taken a candidate gene approach. Technologies are rapidly being developed, however, to scan the genome for locus-specific variation in DNA methylation and other epigenetic modifications (12, 59, 104). Once such epigenomic tools are widely available, they will dramatically accelerate the discovery of human loci at which epigenetic regulation is correlated with early environmental exposures.

Perhaps the most pressing research need related to the epigenetic epidemiology of DOHaD is to improve our understanding of the mechanisms by which epigenetic dysregulation contributes to CVD, type 2 diabetes, and obesity. Controlled experiments in animal models will be essential to identify the critical developmental periods, specific tissues, and genomic loci in which epigenetic alterations are induced, affecting metabolic processes and lifelong disease susceptibility. In addition to mouse models, it will be important to extend studies of comparative epigenetics and pathophysiology into more closely related species, including nonhuman primates. The knowledge gained will enable the formulation of specific hypotheses that can be tested in human studies of epigenetic epidemiology.

CONCLUSION

DNA is not destiny. The stochasticity of mammalian development enables one genotype to result in a wide range of phenotypes. Early nutrition may influence this developmental plasticity to induce metabolic imprinting in humans, with worldwide implications for public health and nutrition policy (105). Overcoming the daunting challenges presented by the epigenetic epidemiology of DOHaD will enable crucial advancements in our understanding of the long-term effects of early nutrition in humans.

SUMMARY POINTS

1. Epigenetic mechanisms are likely to play an important role in the developmental origins of health and disease.
2. Transient environmental influences during development can permanently alter epigenetic gene regulation resulting in metabolic imprinting affecting disease susceptibility.
3. Epigenetic mechanisms include CpG methylation, histone modifications, and autoregulatory DNA-binding proteins.
4. Epigenetic dysregulation is found in developmental diseases and cancer and probably affects cardiovascular disease, diabetes, and obesity.
5. Epigenetic epidemiology provides a basis for future studies of early life exposures, epigenetic mechanisms, and adult disease.
6. Epigenomics will accelerate the discovery of human loci at which epigenetic regulation is correlated with early environmental exposures.
7. Research in animal models is needed to better understand the role of epigenetic dysregulation in disease.

ACKNOWLEDGMENTS

We gratefully acknowledge Jeff Holly, Hannah Landecker, Lanlan Shen, and Lane Strathearn for substantive comments on the manuscript, and Adam Gillum for assistance in developing the figures. RAW is supported by NIH grant 5K01DK070007, research grant #5-FY05-47 from the March of Dimes Birth Defects Foundation, and USDA CRIS #6250-51000-049. KBM is supported in part by research grant R21CA128382 from the National Cancer Institute.

LITERATURE CITED

1. Barker DJ. 1995. Fetal origins of coronary heart disease. *BMJ* 311:171–74
2. Barker DJ, Martyn CN, Osmond C, Hales CN, Fall CH. 1993. Growth in utero and serum cholesterol concentrations in adult life. *BMJ* 307:1524–27
3. Barker DJ, Osmond C. 1986. Infant mortality, childhood nutrition, and ischaemic heart disease in England and Wales. *Lancet* 1(8489):1077–81
4. Belshaw NJ, Elliott GO, Williams EA, Bradburn DM, Mills SJ, et al. 2004. Use of DNA from human stools to detect aberrant CpG island methylation of genes implicated in colorectal cancer. *Cancer Epidemiol. Biomarkers Prev.* 13:1495–501
5. Bernstein E, Allis CD. 2005. RNA meets chromatin. *Genes Dev.* 19:1635–55
6. Bird A. 2002. DNA methylation patterns and epigenetic memory. *Genes Dev.* 16:6–21
7. Bjornsson HT, Fallin MD, Feinberg AP. 2004. An integrated epigenetic and genetic approach to common human disease. *Trends Genet.* 20:350–58
8. Bouret SG, Draper SJ, Simerly RB. 2004. Trophic action of leptin on hypothalamic neurons that regulate feeding. *Science* 304:108–10

9. Brandeis M, Frank D, Keshet I, Siegfried Z, Mendelsohn M, et al. 1994. Sp1 elements protect a CpG island from de novo methylation. *Nature* 371:435–38
10. Castro R, Rivera I, Blom HJ, Jakobs C, Tavares de Almeida I. 2006. Homocysteine metabolism, hyperhomocysteinaemia and vascular disease: an overview. *J. Inherit. Metab. Dis.* 29:3–20
11. Chan TL, Yuen ST, Kong CK, Chan YW, Chan AS, et al. 2006. Heritable germline epimutation of MSH2 in a family with hereditary nonpolyposis colorectal cancer. *Nat. Genet.* 38:1178–83
12. Ching TT, Maunakea AK, Jun P, Hong C, Zardo G, et al. 2005. Epigenome analyses using BAC microarrays identify evolutionary conservation of tissue-specific methylation of SHANK3. *Nat. Genet.* 37:645–51
13. Chong S, Whitelaw E. 2004. Epigenetic germline inheritance. *Curr. Opin. Genet. Dev.* 14:692–96
14. Constancia M, Kelsey G, Reik W. 2004. Resourceful imprinting. *Nature* 432:53–57
15. Cox GF, Burger J, Lip V, Mau UA, Sperling K, et al. 2002. Intracytoplasmic sperm injection may increase the risk of imprinting defects. *Am. J. Hum. Genet.* 71:162–64
16. Cruz-Correa M, Cui H, Giardiello FM, Powe NR, Hylind L, et al. 2004. Loss of imprinting of insulin growth factor II gene: a potential heritable biomarker for colon neoplasia predisposition. *Gastroenterology* 126:964–70
17. Cui H, Cruz-Correa M, Giardiello FM, Hutcheon DF, Kafonek DR, et al. 2003. Loss of IGF2 imprinting: a potential marker of colorectal cancer risk. *Science* 299:1753–55
18. Dahri S, Reusens B, Remacle C, Hoet JJ. 1995. Nutritional influences on pancreatic development and potential links with non-insulin-dependent diabetes. *Proc. Nutr. Soc.* 54:345–56
19. DeBaun MR, Niemitz EL, Feinberg AP. 2003. Association of in vitro fertilization with Beckwith-Wiedemann syndrome and epigenetic alterations of LIT1 and H19. *Am. J. Hum. Genet.* 72:156–60
20. Dekker MC, van Duijn CM. 2003. Prospects of genetic epidemiology in the 21st century. *Eur. J. Epidemiol.* 18:607–16
21. Diatloff-Zito C, Nicole A, Marcelin G, Labit H, Marquis E, et al. 2007. Genetic and epigenetic defects at the 6q24 imprinted locus in a cohort of 13 patients with transient neonatal diabetes: new hypothesis raised by the finding of a unique case with hemizygous deletion in the critical region. *J. Med. Genet.* 44:31–37
22. Dolinoy DC, Weidman JR, Waterland RA, Jirtle RL. 2006. Maternal genistein alters coat color and protects Avy mouse offspring from obesity by modifying the fetal epigenome. *Environ. Health Perspect.* 114:567–72
23. Dong C, Li WD, Geller F, Lei L, Li D, et al. 2005. Possible genomic imprinting of three human obesity-related genetic loci. *Am. J. Hum. Genet.* 76:427–37
24. Doyle P, Beral V, Maconochie N. 1992. Preterm delivery, low birthweight and small-for-gestational-age in liveborn singleton babies resulting from in-vitro fertilization. *Hum. Reprod.* 7:425–28
25. Egger G, Liang G, Aparicio A, Jones PA. 2004. Epigenetics in human disease and prospects for epigenetic therapy. *Nature* 429:457–63
26. Ehrlich M. 2002. DNA methylation in cancer: too much, but also too little. *Oncogene* 21:5400–13
27. Ehrlich M. 2003. Expression of various genes is controlled by DNA methylation during mammalian development. *J. Cell. Biochem.* 88:899–910
28. Fazzari MJ, Greally JM. 2004. Epigenomics: beyond CpG islands. *Nat. Rev. Genet.* 5:446–55

29. Feil R. 2006. Environmental and nutritional effects on the epigenetic regulation of genes. *Mutat. Res.* 600:46–57
30. Feinberg AP, Ohlsson R, Henikoff S. 2006. The epigenetic progenitor origin of human cancer. *Nat. Rev. Genet.* 7:21–33
31. Finkelstein JD. 1998. The metabolism of homocysteine: pathways and regulation. *Eur. J. Pediatr.* 157(Suppl.)2:S40–44
32. Flanagan JM, Popendikyte V, Pozdniakovaite N, Sobolev M, Assadzadeh A, et al. 2006. Intra- and interindividual epigenetic variation in human germ cells. *Am. J. Hum. Genet.* 79:67–84
33. Forsdahl A. 1977. Are poor living conditions in childhood and adolescence an important risk factor for arteriosclerotic heart disease? *Br. J. Prev. Soc. Med.* 31:91–95
34. Fraga MF, Ballestar E, Paz MF, Ropero S, Setien F, et al. 2005. Epigenetic differences arise during the lifetime of monozygotic twins. *Proc. Natl. Acad. Sci. USA* 102:10604–9
35. Friso S, Choi SW, Girelli D, Mason JB, Dolnikowski GG, et al. 2002. A common mutation in the 5,10-methylenetetrahydrofolate reductase gene affects genomic DNA methylation through an interaction with folate status. *Proc. Natl. Acad. Sci. USA* 99:5606–11
36. Gaudet F, Rideout WM, Meissner A, Dausman J, Leonhardt H, Jaenisch R. 2004. Dnmt1 expression in pre- and postimplantation embryogenesis and the maintenance of IAP silencing. *Mol. Cell. Biol.* 24:1640–48
37. Gluckman PD, Hanson MA. 2004. Developmental origins of disease paradigm: a mechanistic and evolutionary perspective. *Pediatr. Res.* 56:311–17
38. Goldstone AP. 2004. Prader-Willi syndrome: advances in genetics, pathophysiology and treatment. *Trends Endocrinol. Metab.* 15:12–20
39. Guo YF, Shen H, Liu YJ, Wang W, Xiong DH, et al. 2006. Assessment of genetic linkage and parent-of-origin effects on obesity. *J. Clin. Endocrinol. Metab.* 91:4001–5
40. Hales CN, Barker DJ, Clark PM, Cox LJ, Fall C, et al. 1991. Fetal and infant growth and impaired glucose tolerance at age 64. *BMJ* 303:1019–22
41. Hansen M, Kurinczuk JJ, Bower C, Webb S. 2002. The risk of major birth defects after intracytoplasmic sperm injection and in vitro fertilization. *N. Engl. J. Med.* 346:725–30
42. Hashimshony T, Zhang J, Keshet I, Bustin M, Cedar H. 2003. The role of DNA methylation in setting up chromatin structure during development. *Nat. Genet.* 34:187–92
43. Hjalgrim LL, Westergaard T, Rostgaard K, Schmiegelow K, Melbye M, et al. 2003. Birth weight as a risk factor for childhood leukemia: a meta-analysis of 18 epidemiologic studies. *Am. J. Epidemiol.* 158:724–35
44. Holliday R. 2005. DNA methylation and epigenotypes. *Biochemistry (Mosc.)* 70:500–4
45. Ingrosso D, Cimmino A, Perna AF, Masella L, De Santo NG, et al. 2003. Folate treatment and unbalanced methylation and changes of allelic expression induced by hyperhomocysteinaemia in patients with uraemia. *Lancet* 361:1693–99
46. Issa JP, Ottaviano YL, Celano P, Hamilton SR, Davidson NE, Baylin SB. 1994. Methylation of the oestrogen receptor CpG island links ageing and neoplasia in human colon. *Nat. Genet.* 7:536–40
47. Jablonka E. 2004. Epigenetic epidemiology. *Int. J. Epidemiol.* 33:929–35
48. Jablonka E, Lamb MJ. 2002. The changing concept of epigenetics. *Ann. NY Acad. Sci.* 981:82–96
49. Jacob RA, Gretz DM, Taylor PC, James SJ, Pogribny IP, et al. 1998. Moderate folate depletion increases plasma homocysteine and decreases lymphocyte DNA methylation in postmenopausal women. *J. Nutr.* 128:1204–12
50. Jaenisch R, Bird A. 2003. Epigenetic regulation of gene expression: how the genome integrates intrinsic and environmental signals. *Nat. Genet.* 33(Suppl.):245–54

51. Jenuwein T, Allis CD. 2001. Translating the histone code. *Science* 293:1074–80
52. Jiang YH, Bressler J, Beaudet AL. 2004. Epigenetics and human disease. *Annu. Rev. Genomics Hum. Genet.* 5:479–510
53. Jirtle RL. 2004. IGF2 loss of imprinting: a potential heritable risk factor for colorectal cancer. *Gastroenterology* 126:1190–93
54. Jones PA, Baylin SB. 2002. The fundamental role of epigenetic events in cancer. *Nat. Rev. Genet.* 3:415–28
55. Jones PA, Takai D. 2001. The role of DNA methylation in mammalian epigenetics. *Science* 293:1068–70
56. Kaati G, Bygren LO, Edvinsson S. 2002. Cardiovascular and diabetes mortality determined by nutrition during parents' and grandparents' slow growth period. *Eur. J. Hum. Genet.* 10:682–88
57. Khosla S, Dean W, Brown D, Reik W, Feil R. 2001. Culture of preimplantation mouse embryos affects fetal development and the expression of imprinted genes. *Biol. Reprod.* 64:918–26
58. Khosla S, Dean W, Reik W, Feil R. 2001. Culture of preimplantation embryos and its long-term effects on gene expression and phenotype. *Hum. Reprod. Update* 7:419–27
59. Khulan B, Thompson RF, Ye K, Fazzari MJ, Suzuki M, et al. 2006. Comparative isoschizomer profiling of cytosine methylation: the HELP assay. *Genome Res.* 16:1046–55
60. Lande-Diner L, Cedar H. 2005. Silence of the genes—mechanisms of long-term repression. *Nat. Rev. Genet.* 6:648–54
61. Law CM, Shiell AW. 1996. Is blood pressure inversely related to birth weight? The strength of evidence from a systematic review of the literature. *J. Hypertens.* 14:935–41
62. Li E. 2002. Chromatin modification and epigenetic reprogramming in mammalian development. *Nat. Rev. Genet.* 3:662–73
63. Lillycrop KA, Phillips ES, Jackson AA, Hanson MA, Burdge GC. 2005. Dietary protein restriction of pregnant rats induces and folic acid supplementation prevents epigenetic modification of hepatic gene expression in the offspring. *J. Nutr.* 135:1382–86
64. Lopez AD, Mathers CD, Ezzati M, Jamison DT, Murray CJ. 2006. Global and regional burden of disease and risk factors, 2001: systematic analysis of population health data. *Lancet* 367:1747–57
65. Lucas A. 1991. Programming by early nutrition in man. *Ciba Found. Symp.* 156:38–50
66. Lund G, Andersson L, Lauria M, Lindholm M, Fraga MF, et al. 2004. DNA methylation polymorphisms precede any histological sign of atherosclerosis in mice lacking apolipoprotein E. *J. Biol. Chem.* 279:29147–54
67. Mackay DJ, Boonen SE, Clayton-Smith J, Goodship J, Hahnemann JM, et al. 2006. A maternal hypomethylation syndrome presenting as transient neonatal diabetes mellitus. *Hum. Genet.* 120:262–69
68. Maier S, Olek A. 2002. Diabetes: a candidate disease for efficient DNA methylation profiling. *J. Nutr.* 132:2440–43S
69. Mason JB. 2003. Biomarkers of nutrient exposure and status in one-carbon (methyl) metabolism. *J. Nutr.* 133(Suppl.)3:941–47S
70. McMillen IC, Robinson JS. 2005. Developmental origins of the metabolic syndrome: prediction, plasticity, and programming. *Physiol. Rev.* 85:571–633
71. Michels KB, Trichopoulos D, Robins JM, Rosner BA, Manson JE, et al. 1996. Birthweight as a risk factor for breast cancer. *Lancet* 348:1542–46
72. Michels KB, Xue F. 2006. Role of birthweight in the etiology of breast cancer. *Int. J. Cancer* 119:2007–25

73. Mill J, Dempster E, Caspi A, Williams B, Moffitt T, Craig I. 2006. Evidence for monozygotic twin (MZ) discordance in methylation level at two CpG sites in the promoter region of the catechol-O-methyltransferase (COMT) gene. *Am. J. Med. Genet. B Neuropsychiatr. Genet.* 141:421–25
74. Morgan HD, Santos F, Green K, Dean W, Reik W. 2005. Epigenetic reprogramming in mammals. *Hum. Mol. Genet.* 14(Spec. No. 1):R47–58
75. Morgan HD, Sutherland HG, Martin DI, Whitelaw E. 1999. Epigenetic inheritance at the agouti locus in the mouse. *Nat. Genet.* 23:314–18
76. Murrell A, Heeson S, Cooper WN, Douglas E, Apostolidou S, et al. 2004. An association between variants in the IGF2 gene and Beckwith-Wiedemann syndrome: interaction between genotype and epigenotype. *Hum. Mol. Genet.* 13:247–55
77. Niculescu MD, Craciunescu CN, Zeisel SH. 2006. Dietary choline deficiency alters global and gene-specific DNA methylation in the developing hippocampus of mouse fetal brains. *FASEB J.* 20:43–49
78. Niemitz EL, Feinberg AP. 2004. Epigenetics and assisted reproductive technology: a call for investigation. *Am. J. Hum. Genet.* 74:599–609
79. Oates NA, van Vliet J, Duffy DL, Kroes HY, Martin NG, et al. 2006. Increased DNA methylation at the AXIN1 gene in a monozygotic twin from a pair discordant for a caudal duplication anomaly. *Am. J. Hum. Genet.* 79:155–62
80. Olson EN, Klein WH. 1994. bHLH factors in muscle development: dead lines and commitments, what to leave in and what to leave out. *Genes Dev.* 8:1–8
81. Orstavik KH, Eiklid K, van der Hagen CB, Spetalen S, Kierulf K, et al. 2003. Another case of imprinting defect in a girl with Angelman syndrome who was conceived by intracytoplasmic semen injection. *Am. J. Hum. Genet.* 72:218–19
82. Osmond C, Barker DJ, Winter PD, Fall CH, Simmonds SJ. 1993. Early growth and death from cardiovascular disease in women. *BMJ* 307:1519–24
83. Pembrey ME, Bygren LO, Kaati G, Edvinsson S, Northstone K, et al. 2006. Sex-specific, male-line transgenerational responses in humans. *Eur. J. Hum. Genet.* 14:159–66
84. Peterson CL, Laniel MA. 2004. Histones and histone modifications. *Curr. Biol.* 14:R546–51
85. Petronis A. 2006. Epigenetics and twins: three variations on the theme. *Trends Genet.* 22:347–50
86. Rakyan VK, Blewitt ME, Druker R, Preis JI, Whitelaw E. 2002. Metastable epialleles in mammals. *Trends Genet.* 18:348–51
87. Rakyan VK, Chong S, Champ ME, Cuthbert PC, Morgan HD, et al. 2003. Transgenerational inheritance of epigenetic states at the murine Axin(Fu) allele occurs after maternal and paternal transmission. *Proc. Natl. Acad. Sci. USA* 100:2538–43
88. Rakyan VK, Hildmann T, Novik KL, Lewin J, Tost J, et al. 2004. DNA methylation profiling of the human major histocompatibility complex: a pilot study for the human epigenome project. *PLoS Biol.* 2:e405
89. Reik W, Dean W, Walter J. 2001. Epigenetic reprogramming in mammalian development. *Science* 293:1089–93
90. Reik W, Romer I, Barton SC, Surani MA, Howlett SK, Klose J. 1993. Adult phenotype in the mouse can be affected by epigenetic events in the early embryo. *Development* 119:933–42
91. Reik W, Walter J. 2001. Genomic imprinting: parental influence on the genome. *Nat. Rev. Genet.* 2:21–32
92. Richards EJ. 2006. Inherited epigenetic variation—revisiting soft inheritance. *Nat. Rev. Genet.* 7:395–401

93. Rich-Edwards JW, Stampfer MJ, Manson JE, Rosner B, Hankinson SE, et al. 1997. Birth weight and risk of cardiovascular disease in a cohort of women followed up since 1976. *BMJ* 315:396–400
94. Riggs AD, Martienssen RA, Russo VE. 1996. Introduction. In *Epigenetic Mechanisms of Gene Regulation*, ed. VE Russo, RA Martienssen, AD Riggs, pp. 1–4. Plainview, NY: Cold Spring Harbor Lab. Press
95. Riggs AD, Porter TN. 1996. Overview of epigenetic mechanisms. In *Epigenetic Mechanisms of Gene Regulation*, ed. VE Russo, RA Martienssen, AD Riggs, pp. 29–46. Plainview, NY: Cold Spring Harbor Lab. Press
96. Robertson KD. 2005. DNA methylation and human disease. *Nat. Rev. Genet.* 6:597–610
97. Rose G. 1964. Familial patterns in ischaemic heart disease. *Br. J. Prev. Soc. Med.* 18:75–80
98. Sakatani T, Kaneda A, Iacobuzio-Donahue CA, Carter MG, de Boom Witzel S, et al. 2005. Loss of imprinting of Igf2 alters intestinal maturation and tumorigenesis in mice. *Science* 307:1976–78
99. Sakatani T, Wei M, Katoh M, Okita C, Wada D, et al. 2001. Epigenetic heterogeneity at imprinted loci in normal populations. *Biochem. Biophys. Res. Commun.* 283:1124–30
100. Sandovici I, Kassovska-Bratinova S, Loredo-Osti JC, Leppert M, Suarez A, et al. 2005. Interindividual variability and parent of origin DNA methylation differences at specific human Alu elements. *Hum. Mol. Genet.* 14:2135–43
101. Sandovici I, Leppert M, Hawk PR, Suarez A, Linares Y, Sapienza C. 2003. Familial aggregation of abnormal methylation of parental alleles at the IGF2/H19 and IGF2R differentially methylated regions. *Hum. Mol. Genet.* 12:1569–78
102. Schieve LA, Meikle SF, Ferre C, Peterson HB, Jeng G, Wilcox LS. 2002. Low and very low birth weight in infants conceived with use of assisted reproductive technology. *N. Engl. J. Med.* 346:731–37
103. Snoeck A, Remacle C, Reusens B, Hoet JJ. 1990. Effect of a low protein diet during pregnancy on the fetal rat endocrine pancreas. *Biol. Neonate* 57:107–18
104. Song F, Smith JF, Kimura MT, Morrow AD, Matsuyama T, et al. 2005. Association of tissue-specific differentially methylated regions (TDMs) with differential gene expression. *Proc. Natl. Acad. Sci. USA* 102:3336–41
105. Stover PJ, Garza C. 2006. Nutrition and developmental biology—implications for public health. *Nutr. Rev.* 64:S60–71; discussion S72–91
106. Susser M. 1991. Maternal weight gain, infant birth weight, and diet: causal sequences. *Am. J. Clin. Nutr.* 53:1384–96
107. Suter CM, Martin DI, Ward RL. 2004. Germline epimutation of MLH1 in individuals with multiple cancers. *Nat. Genet.* 36:497–501
108. Sutter NB, Scalzo D, Fiering S, Groudine M, Martin DI. 2003. Chromatin insulation by a transcriptional activator. *Proc. Natl. Acad. Sci. USA* 100:1105–10
109. Tamashiro KL, Wakayama T, Akutsu H, Yamazaki Y, Lachey JL, et al. 2002. Cloned mice have an obese phenotype not transmitted to their offspring. *Nat. Med.* 8:262–67
110. Trichopoulos D. 1990. Hypothesis: Does breast cancer originate in utero? *Lancet* 335:939–40
111. Ulrey CL, Liu L, Andrews LG, Tollefsbol TO. 2005. The impact of metabolism on DNA methylation. *Hum. Mol. Genet.* 14(Spec. No. 1):R139–47
112. Vadlamudi S, Kalhan SC, Patel MS. 1995. Persistence of metabolic consequences in the progeny of rats fed a HC formula in their early postnatal life. *Am. J. Physiol.* 269:E731–38
113. Van den Veyver I. 2002. Genetic effects of methylation diets. *Annu. Rev. Nutr.* 22:255–82
114. Waddington CH. 1968. The basic ideas of biology. In *Towards a Theoretical Biology*, ed. CH Waddington, pp. 1–31. Edinburgh: Edinburgh Univ. Press

115. Walsh CP, Bestor TH. 1999. Cytosine methylation and mammalian development. *Genes Dev.* 13:26–34
116. Waterland R, Garza CG. 2002. Potential for metabolic imprinting by nutritional perturbation of epigenetic gene regulation. In *Public Health Issues in Infant and Child Nutrition*, ed. R Black, KF Michaelson, pp. 317–33. New York: Lippincott Williams & Wilkins
117. Waterland RA. 2005. Does nutrition during infancy and early childhood contribute to later obesity via metabolic imprinting of epigenetic gene regulatory mechanisms? In *Feeding During Late Infancy and Early Childhood: Impact on Health*, ed. OS Hernell, J Schmitz, pp. 157–74. Vevey, Switzerland: Nestle Nutr.
118. Waterland RA. 2006. Assessing the effects of high methionine intake on DNA methylation. *J. Nutr.* 136:1706–10S
119. Waterland RA, Dolinoy DC, Lin JR, Smith CA, Shi X, Tahiliani KG. 2006. Maternal methyl supplements increase offspring DNA methylation at Axin fused. *Genesis* 44:401–6
120. Waterland RA, Garza C. 1999. Potential mechanisms of metabolic imprinting that lead to chronic disease. *Am. J. Clin. Nutr.* 69:179–97
121. Waterland RA, Garza C. 2002. Early postnatal nutrition determines adult pancreatic glucose-responsive insulin secretion and islet gene expression in rats. *J. Nutr.* 132:357–64
122. Waterland RA, Jirtle RL. 2003. Transposable elements: targets for early nutritional effects on epigenetic gene regulation. *Mol. Cell. Biol.* 23:5293–300
123. Waterland RA, Jirtle RL. 2004. Early nutrition, epigenetic changes at transposons and imprinted genes, and enhanced susceptibility to adult chronic diseases. *Nutrition* 20:63–68
124. Waterland RA, Lin JR, Smith CA, Jirtle RL. 2006. Post-weaning diet affects genomic imprinting at the insulin-like growth factor 2 (Igf2) locus. *Hum. Mol. Genet.* 15:705–16
125. Weaver IC, Cervoni N, Champagne FA, D'Alessio AC, Sharma S, et al. 2004. Epigenetic programming by maternal behavior. *Nat. Neurosci.* 7:847–54
126. Weksberg R, Smith AC, Squire J, Sadowski P. 2003. Beckwith-Wiedemann syndrome demonstrates a role for epigenetic control of normal development. *Hum. Mol. Genet.* 12(Spec. No. 1):R61–68
127. Whitelaw E, Martin DI. 2001. Retrotransposons as epigenetic mediators of phenotypic variation in mammals. *Nat. Genet.* 27:361–65
128. Whitelaw NC, Whitelaw E. 2006. How lifetimes shape epigenotype within and across generations. *Hum. Mol. Genet.* 15(Spec. No. 2):R131–37
129. Willett WC. 2002. Balancing life-style and genomics research for disease prevention. *Science* 296:695–98
130. Wolff GL, Kodell RL, Moore SR, Cooney CA. 1998. Maternal epigenetics and methyl supplements affect agouti gene expression in *Avy/a* mice. *FASEB J.* 12:949–57
131. Wolff GL, Roberts DW, Mountjoy KG. 1999. Physiological consequences of ectopic agouti gene expression: the yellow obese mouse syndrome. *Physiol. Genomics* 1:151–63
132. Wong AH, Gottesman II, Petronis A. 2005. Phenotypic differences in genetically identical organisms: the epigenetic perspective. *Hum. Mol. Genet.* 14(Spec. No. 1):R11–18
133. Wren JD, Garner HR. 2005. Data-mining analysis suggests an epigenetic pathogenesis for type 2 diabetes. *J. Biomed. Biotechnol.* 2005:104–12
134. Ying AK, Hassanain HH, Roos CM, Smiraglia DJ, Issa JJ, et al. 2000. Methylation of the estrogen receptor-alpha gene promoter is selectively increased in proliferating human aortic smooth muscle cells. *Cardiovasc. Res.* 46:172–79
135. Young LE, Fernandes K, McEvoy TG, Butterwith SC, Gutierrez CG, et al. 2001. Epigenetic change in IGF2R is associated with fetal overgrowth after sheep embryo culture. *Nat. Genet.* 27:153–54

Taste Receptor Genes

Alexander A. Bachmanov and Gary K. Beauchamp

Monell Chemical Senses Center, Philadelphia, Pennsylvania 19104;
email: bachmanov@monell.org, beauchamp@monell.org

Annu. Rev. Nutr. 2007. 27:389–414

First published online as a Review in Advance on April 19, 2007

The *Annual Review of Nutrition* is online at http://nutr.annualreviews.org

This article's doi:
10.1146/annurev.nutr.26.061505.111329

0199-9885/07/0821-0389$20.00

Key Words

gustatory, sweet, bitter, umami, salty, sour

Abstract

In the past several years, tremendous progress has been achieved with the discovery and characterization of vertebrate taste receptors from the T1R and T2R families, which are involved in recognition of bitter, sweet, and umami taste stimuli. Individual differences in taste, at least in some cases, can be attributed to allelic variants of the T1R and T2R genes. Progress with understanding how T1R and T2R receptors interact with taste stimuli and with identifying their patterns of expression in taste cells sheds light on coding of taste information by the nervous system. Candidate mechanisms for detection of salts, acids, fat, complex carbohydrates, and water have also been proposed, but further studies are needed to prove their identity.

Contents

INTRODUCTION

The major focus of this review is on the mammalian taste receptors from the T1R and T2R families. We also briefly discuss other candidate taste receptors in mammals.

Taste System

In the common language, the word "taste" is often used to describe sensations arising from the oral cavity. However, the biological definition of taste, or gustation, is narrower and includes only sensations mediated by a specialized anatomically and physiologically defined chemosensory gustatory system. Along with taste sensations, food usually simultaneously evokes other sensations, e.g., odor, touch, temperature, and irritation. Although it is not always easy to separate all these sensations perceptually, the nongustatory components are sensed by different systems, olfaction and somatosensation.

The gustatory system in mammals includes taste receptor cells (TRCs) organized in taste buds located within gustatory papillae. Most of the taste papillae belong to three types—fungiform, foliate, and vallate—and are located in the tongue. There is also a substantial number of nonlingual taste papillae in the palate, oropharynx, larynx, epiglottis, and the upper esophagus. Apical ends of the TRCs are exposed to the oral cavity and interact with taste stimuli, usually water-soluble chemicals. This interaction generates signals that are transmitted to the brain via branches of three cranial nerves, VII (facial), IX (glossopharyngeal), and X (vagus). One branch of the VII nerve, the chorda tympani nerve, sends fibers to the anterior part of the tongue including fungiform papillae and possibly to the anterior portion of the foliate papillae. The other branch of the VII nerve, the greater petrosal nerve, sends fibers to the taste buds on the soft palate. Axons of the glossopharyngeal nerve innervate vallate and foliate papillae, and possibly taste buds in the pharynx. Axons of the vagus nerve innervate taste buds in the epiglottis, larynx, and the upper esophagus

(170). These first-order ganglionic neurons terminate in the rostral part of nucleus of the solitary tract in the medulla. The upper-order projections from the nucleus of the solitary tract include parabrachial nucleus, thalamic taste area, insular-opecular (primary) taste cortex, caudolateral orbitofrontal (secondary) cortical taste area, amygdala, hypothalamus, and basal ganglia (144). This wide representation of taste information in the brain probably serves necessary to integrate it with interoceptive (hunger, satiety, specialized appetites) and exteroceptive (vision, olfaction, somatosensation) signals and to generate behavioral responses to taste stimuli. Central taste processing results in perception of several different aspects of taste: quality, intensity, hedonics (pleasantness or unpleasantness), location, and persistence.

Nutrition, Taste Reception, and Taste Receptors

The survival of all animals depends on consumption of nutrients. However, sources of nutrients often also contain toxic substances. Taste helps animals to decide whether a food is beneficial for them and should be consumed or whether it is dangerous for them and should be rejected. Probably, taste evolved to insure animals choose food appropriate for body needs.

The current consensus is that human taste sensations can be divided into five qualities: bitter, sour, salty, sweet, and umami (savory; the prototypical stimulus being the amino acid glutamate). Aversive bitter taste often indicates presence of toxins in food. Bitter and sour tastes may also signal spoiled food. The main salty taste stimuli are sodium salts, but some nonsodium salts also have a salty taste component. This suggests that salty taste signals the presence of either sodium or minerals in general. For some species, consummatory responses to salty taste stimuli differ widely between sodium-replete and -deplete animals. Concentrated salt solutions, which are aversive to sodium- or mineral-replete animals, can be palatable to animals with depletion. The most common natural sweet taste stimuli are sugars, which indicate the presence of carbohydrates in food. The most common umami taste stimulus is L-glutamate, which may indicate the presence of protein. Other important nutrients include lipids, calcium, and water, but the existence of taste qualities corresponding to them is debatable.

TRC: taste receptor cell

GPCR: G protein–coupled receptor

The existence of several different taste qualities implies that each taste quality has a specific coding mechanism mediated by specialized taste receptors. Current data support this hypothesis. Reception of taste qualities that humans describe as sweet, umami, and bitter involves proteins from the T1R and T2R families. Candidate receptors have been proposed for salty and sour tastes.

Traditionally, human sensations are used to describe the main five taste qualities. Although there are many studies showing that the mechanisms underlying perception of particular taste qualities are similar in human and nonhuman animals, applying terms for human sensations to nonhuman animals should be used with caution. It is more accurate to describe taste quality perception by nonhuman animals using chemical names of taste stimuli (e.g., sodium taste, or sucroselike taste), but for brevity we use in this review human descriptors for taste qualities.

What Are Taste Receptors?

Taste receptors function as chemoreceptors that interact with taste stimuli, or ligands, to initiate an afferent signal transmitted to the brain, which results in taste perception. Because many taste ligands do not easily permeate cell membranes, taste receptors are believed to be a part of the TRC membranes. Consistent with this belief, T1R and T2R receptors belong to a superfamily of G protein–coupled receptors (GPCRs) with characteristic seven domains spanning the plasma membrane. However, some other taste stimuli can penetrate cell membranes; these include sodium, protons, and some bitter and sweet compounds. These compounds may interact with intracellular targets to activate TRC, and therefore the definition of what would be a taste receptor for such ligands is less clear.

Although a number of proteins have been suggested to function as taste receptors, not all of them have been unanimously accepted as such. We believe that to prove that a molecule functions as a taste receptor, several criteria must be met: (*a*) the molecular identity of the candidate receptor should be established, (*b*) its expression in TRCs should be confirmed, (*c*) appropriate ligands should be identified, and (*d*) changes in taste function resulting from changes in the taste receptor should be demonstrated.

Nomenclature and Classification of Taste Receptor Genes and Proteins

Publications on taste receptors have a number of discrepancies in naming genes and proteins [e.g., see **Supplemental Tables 1** and **2** (for all Supplemental Material, follow the Supplemental Material link from the Annual Reviews home page at **http://www.annualreviews.org**)]. This creates difficulties in comparing descriptions of the same gene that has different names in different publications. This situation is also common with other types of genes and may become especially confusing with large gene families present in multiple species, such as taste receptor genes. This problem resulted in attempts to unify gene and protein nomenclature (157).

The confusion with identification of taste receptor genes and proteins underscores the importance of following nomenclature rules. Guidelines for human, mouse, and rat gene nomenclature are accessible on the Internet (3, 5). For the two best-characterized families of taste receptors, T1R and T2R, standard gene names follow the following description: "taste receptor, type 1, member 1" (with corresponding type and member numbers). A corresponding gene symbol abbreviates this name to *Tas1r1* (in mouse or rat) or *TAS1R1* (in human); a corresponding protein symbol is T1R1 (uppercase letters and not italicized). For brevity, and especially when we refer to both human (*TAS . . . R*) and rodent (*Tas . . . r*) genes, we describe them as T . . . R genes. Besides differences in symbol letters (upper- or lowercase), human and mouse T2R genes can also be distinguished by member number: The human genes have member numbers smaller than 100 (*TAS2R1–TAS2R65*), whereas the mouse genes have member numbers higher than 100 (*Tas2r102–Tas2r146*). Genes and proteins of other species can be distinguished by adding a lowercase letter indicating species, e.g., *rTas2r123* for rat. Lists of human and mouse taste receptor genes, including their names, symbols, and synonyms, can be found in **Supplemental Tables 1** and **2**, and can also be found in the human (2) and mouse (4) genome databases. A compilation of human and mouse T2R gene symbols, alternative symbols, and GenBank accession numbers is published in (7). An ultimate identifier of a gene is its nucleotide sequence, which should be used if gene identity is not certain.

Several classification systems have been proposed for the GPCR superfamily. One of the most frequently used includes GPCRs of different vertebrate and invertebrate species and groups them into six classes (clans): A, B, C, D, E, and F (1). According to this classification, T1Rs belong to class C (metabotropic glutamate/pheromone) GPCRs. T2Rs are described either as a separate putative family (1) or as distantly related to class A (rhodopsinlike) GPCRs (6). More recently, the GRAFTS (glutamate-rhodopsin-adhesion-frizzled/taste2-secretin) classification system was developed based on phylogenetic analyses of transmembrane parts of human GPCRs (58). According to this classification, T1Rs belong to the glutamate family. T2Rs form a distinct cluster within the frizzled/taste2 family; the second cluster of this family includes the frizzled receptors involved in cell proliferation and development.

T1R RECEPTORS

Discovery

The discovery of three mammalian T1R receptors resulted from two converging lines of studies. The first line was related to identification of a genetic locus that affects saccharin preference in mice (the *Sac* locus). In 1974, using long-term two-bottle tests, Fuller (60) showed that differences in saccharin preferences between the C57BL/6 and DBA/2 inbred strains largely depend on a single locus, *Sac*, with a dominant Sac^b allele present in the C57BL/6 strain that was associated with higher saccharin preference and a recessive Sac^d allele present in the DBA/2 strain that was associated with lower saccharin preference. Subsequent studies confirmed this finding in the BXD recombinant inbred strains, and in crosses between the C57BL/6 and DBA/2 and between the C57BL/6 and 129 strains (16, 23, 26, 113, 115, 133). In addition to sweetener preferences, the *Sac* genotype influenced the afferent responses of gustatory nerves to sweeteners (16, 98), which indicated that the *Sac* gene is involved in peripheral taste transduction and may encode a sweet taste receptor. The *Sac* locus has been mapped to the subtelomeric region of mouse chromosome 4 (16, 26, 115, 133).

The second line of studies stemmed from analyses of a taste-bud-enriched cDNA library (72), which resulted in a discovery of two putative G protein–coupled taste receptors, T1R1 and T1R2 (71). Localization of the *Tas1r1* gene in the distal part of mouse chromosome 4, near the *Sac* locus, suggested that *Tas1r1* and *Sac* were identical. However, a high-resolution genetic mapping study rejected this possibility by showing distinct locations for *Tas1r1* and *Sac* (98). A positional cloning study at the Monell Chemical Senses Center has shown that the *Sac* locus corresponds to a novel gene, *Tas1r3*, which is the third member of the *Tas1r* family (14, 97, 137). These studies restricted the genomic position of the *Sac* locus to a critical interval not exceeding 194 kb and identified genes within this region. One of these genes, *Tas1r3*, was the most likely candidate for the *Sac* locus based on the effects of the *Sac* genotype on peripheral sweet taste responsiveness (16, 98) and the involvement of a G protein–coupled mechanism in sweet taste transduction (171). *Tas1r3* sequence variants were associated with sweetener preference phenotypes in genealogically diverse mouse strains (14, 137). Substitution of *Tas1r3* alleles in congenic mice resulted in phenotypical changes attributed to the *Sac* locus (14). These data provided evidence for the identity of *Sac* and *Tas1r3* and for the role of the T1R3 receptor in sweet taste.

Several other studies provided additional evidence that *Sac* and *Tas1r3* are identical:

1. A phenotype rescue transgenic experiment, in which a genomic clone containing the *Tas1r3* gene from the C57BL/6 mouse strain with a dominant *Sac* allele determining higher sweetener preference was incorporated in the genome of mice carrying a recessive *Sac* allele (from the 129X1/Sv strain) determining lower sweetener preference. The transgenic mice had higher taste preferences for sucrose and saccharin (but not for nonsweet taste solutions) compared with the 129X1/Sv mice (127).
2. Genetically engineered mice lacking the *Tas1r3* gene had diminished or abolished taste responses to sweeteners (46, 179).
3. Cells with heterologously expressed T1R2 + T1R3 proteins responded to sucrose and saccharin more strongly when the C57BL/6 *Tas1r3* allele was used compared with cell responses when 129X1/Sv *Tas1r3* allele was used (126).
4. An in vitro study (130) has shown that binding of several sweeteners to the extracellular N-terminal domain of the T1R3 protein was reduced when isoleucine at position 60 [a predicted sweetener-sensitive allele of the *Sac/Tas1r3* gene (137)] was substituted

to threonine (a predicted hyposensitive allele of the *Sac/Tas1r3* gene).

Additional evidence that the three T1R proteins function as taste receptors included the demonstration that: (*a*) T1Rs are expressed in taste receptor cells (46, 71, 86, 91, 92, 99, 101, 107, 120, 123, 127, 137, 147); (*b*) cell cultures with heterologously expressed T1Rs respond to taste stimuli (100, 126, 127, 179); and (*c*) targeted mutations of the *Tas1r* genes affect taste responses of the genetically engineered mice (46, 179).

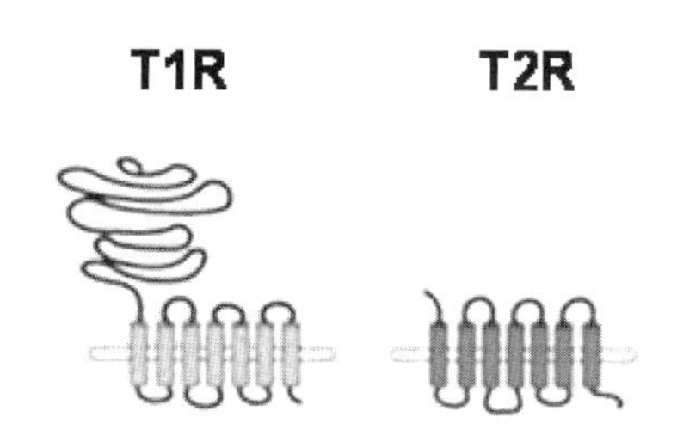

Figure 1

Conformation of T1R and T2R proteins. Both T1R and T2R proteins are predicted to have seven transmembrane domains. The T1R proteins consist of ~850 amino acids and have a large extracellular N-terminus. The T2R proteins consist of ~300–330 amino acids and have a short extracellular N-terminus.

Genomic Organization

The three mouse *Tas1r* genes are located in the distal chromosome 4 in the order *Tas1r2* (70.0 cM or 139 Mb, NCBI Build 36)—*Tas1r1* (81.5 cM or 151 Mb)—*Tas1r3* (83.0 cM or 155 Mb). Their human orthologs reside in a region of conserved synteny in the short arm of human chromosome 1 in the same order: *TAS1R2* (1p36.13)—*TAS1R1* (1p36.23)—*TAS1R3* (1p36.33) (see **Supplemental Figure 1**).

The mouse *Tas1r* genes contain six coding exons (**Supplemental Figure 2**) and are translated into 842–858-amino acid proteins. The T1R proteins (**Figure 1**) have a predicted secondary structure that includes seven transmembrane helices forming a heptahelical domain and a large extracellular N-terminus composed of a Venus flytrap module and a cysteine-rich domain connected to the heptahelical domain (134). There is evidence for alternative splicing of the T1R1 (**Supplemental Figure 3**), T1R2 (123), and T1R3 (92, X. Li and D. Reed, unpublished data) genes.

Tissue Expression

The main sites of expression of the T1R genes are TRC of the taste buds. In mice, rats, humans, pigs, and cats, the T1R3 gene is expressed in all types of taste buds (46, 91, 92, 99, 107, 120, 123, 127, 137, 147). Initial studies have shown that in mice and rats, the T1R1 gene is predominantly expressed in the fungiform and palate taste buds, is expressed in a smaller percentage of the foliate taste buds, and is rarely expressed in the circumvallate taste buds. The T1R2 gene is predominantly expressed in the circumvallate and foliate taste buds, is expressed in a smaller percentage of the palate taste buds, and is rarely expressed in the fungiform taste buds (71, 91, 123, 127). T1R1 and T1R2 are rarely coexpressed in the same TRC (71, 127). The T1R genes are not coexpressed with the T2R genes (127). In mice and rats, there are three main patterns of coexpression of the T1R genes in TRC: The first pattern is coexpression of T1R1 and T1R3 (in fungiform and palate taste buds), the second pattern is coexpression of T1R2 and T1R3 (in circumvallate, foliate and palate taste buds), and the third pattern is expression of only T1R3 (in fungiform and palate taste buds) (120, 123, 127).

Coexpression of T1R3 with either T1R1 or T1R2 in the same TRC suggested that they may function as heterodimers, which is believed to commonly occur with GPCRs (134). This pattern of coexpression also suggested that taste responses to sweeteners mediated by the T1R2 + T1R3 receptor combination should predominantly occur in the glossopharyngeal nerve that innervates the circumvallate taste buds, and that umami/L–amino acid taste responses mediated by the T1R1 + T1R3 receptor combination should predominantly occur in the chorda tympani nerve that innervates fungiform taste buds. However, this does not correspond to results of electrophysiological studies that show that both chorda tympani and glossopharyngeal nerves respond to sweet and umami taste stimuli (47, 74, 131, 132).

A subsequent study in mice has shown that TRCs in both fungiform and circumvallate papillae express each T1R receptor alone and in all possible combinations (T1R1 + T1R2, T1R1 + T1R3, T1R2 + T1R3, and T1R1 + T1R2 + T1R3) (86). Similarly, it was found that human fungiform taste buds express all three T1R genes, with some fungiform TRC coexpressing T1R2 and T1R3 (101). These results are in a better agreement with electrophysiological responsiveness of the chorda tympani and glossopharyngeal nerves. They also suggest the existence of T1R1 + T1R2 heterodimers and homodimers for each T1R receptor. Coexpression of the T1R1 and T2R genes in mice has also been reported (86).

Ligands

T1R receptor-ligand interactions were characterized in two types of studies. In vitro heterologous expression experiments analyzed responses to taste stimuli in cells transfected with T1Rs. In vivo experiments examined effects of *Tas1r* genotypes on taste responses in mice. Two types of gene variation were studied in vivo: targeted mutations disrupting a gene (46, 179) and natural allelic variation (78) (these results are summarized in **Supplemental Table 3**).

Heterologously expressed T1R2 + T1R3 responds to a large number of sweeteners. The in vitro system reproduces in vivo species differences in sweet taste sensitivity. Several sweeteners (aspartame, cyclamate, neohesperidin dihydrochalcone, neotame, and sweet proteins) are perceived as sweet by humans but not rodents (e.g., 17, 48, 77). Correspondingly, human—but not rodent—T1R2 + T1R3 responds to these sweeteners. Heterologously expressed T1R1 + T1R3 functions as a broadly tuned L-amino acid receptor in mice and as a more narrowly tuned umami receptor in humans.

Experiments involving heterologous expression of combinations of T1Rs from different species (including interspecies receptor chimeras and receptors with mutations created at the interspecies variant sites) characterized the functional importance of different domains of T1R proteins. These studies have shown that human T1R1 determines higher T1R1 + T1R3 receptor selectivity for glutamate relative to the mouse receptor (126). Human T1R2 confers responsiveness of the T1R2 + T1R3 receptor to aspartame, glycyrrhizic acid, neotame, thaumatin, brazzein, and monellin (83, 126, 169, 179). The extracellular N-terminal domain of T1R2 is involved in recognition of aspartame (80, 176), neotame (176), D-tryptophan, and sucrose (80). The transmembrane domain of T1R2 is required for G-protein coupling of the T1R2 + T1R3 receptor (176). Responsiveness of the T1R2 + T1R3 receptor to cyclamate and neohesperidin dihydrochalcone, and its sensitivity to a sweet taste inhibitor lactisole, depend on the presence of human T1R3 (83, 178), specifically its transmembrane domain (81, 82, 169, 176). The cysteine-rich region of T1R3 is involved in recognition of brazzein and monellin (83).

For some ligands, interaction with both T1R2 and T1R3 receptor subunits has been demonstrated. Responsiveness to brazzein and monellin depends on interaction with both human T1R2 and human T1R3 (83). Binding assays have shown that N-terminal domains of mouse T1R2 and T1R3 bind sweeteners (glucose, sucrose, and sucralose), though with distinct affinities and conformational changes: Relative to T1R2, T1R3 binds sucrose with higher affinity and glucose with lower affinity (130).

Consistent with the in vitro results, *Tas1r1* knockout mice are deficient in taste responses to L-amino acids and umami stimuli, *Tas1r2* knockout mice are deficient in taste responses to sweeteners, and *Tas1r3* knockout mice are deficient in taste responses to all these stimuli (46, 179). Variation of naturally occurring *Tas1r3* alleles in inbred mouse strains (78) has a pattern of effects not completely identical to effects of *Tas1r3* disruption in knockout mice. *Tas1r3* allelic variation affects taste responses to sweeteners (including D-amino acids) but not to L-amino acids, nonchiral glycine, or umami taste stimuli. This pattern is more similar to changes found in *Tas1r2* knockout mice. The likely reason for this is that the null allele of *Tas1r3* prevents the formation of heteromeric receptors with both T1R1 and T1R2, thus affecting responses to all ligands of these receptors. Natural allelic variation of *Tas1r3* affects binding affinity of the T1R3 protein for sweeteners (130), but it does not affect responses of heterologously expressed T1R1 + T1R3 to amino acids (126), which corresponds to effects of *Tas1r3* polymorphisms in vivo. The lack of effect of the natural allelic variation of *Tas1r3* on taste responses to ligands of the T1R1 + T1R3 receptor can be explained by several possible mechanisms: (*a*) ligand binding to the T1R3 receptor at a site that is not affected by the polymorphic variants, (*b*) ligand binding to the T1R1 receptor, or (*c*) the existence of another taste receptor binding these ligands.

In *Tas1r2* and *Tas1r3* knockout mice, concentrated solutions of sugars elicited reduced, but not completely eliminated, taste responses (46, 179). These residual responses were completely eliminated in *Tas1r2*/*Tas1r3* double-knockout mice (179). This suggests that T1R2 and T1R3 may function on their own as low-affinity sugar receptors, probably as homodimers. Consistent with this hypothesis, heterologously expressed T1R3 alone responded to 0.5 M sucrose, but not to lower sucrose concentrations (<0.3 M) or to artificial sweeteners (179). Heterologously expressed T1R3 alone was also reported to respond to a sugar trehalose (8); however, another study reported that trehalose induced significant receptor-independent rises in Ca^{2+}, and thus its use in a heterologous system was impractical (179). No responses to sweeteners were reported in cells with heterologously expressed T1R2 alone.

The data on ligand specificity of the T1R receptors suggest that perception of most of sweet and umami taste stimuli occurs via activation of these receptors. This is consistent with results of some human perception studies (31, 32). However, the existence of additional sweet or umami taste receptors is not precluded, and several candidates are described in a following section.

Allelic Variation of T1R Genes and Its Role in Individual Variation in Taste Responses

Within-species variation of the T1R genes has been examined in individual humans of different ethnicities and in strains of rats and mice. In rats and mice, the association of variants of the *Tas1r3* gene with sweetener taste responses has been analyzed.

Humans. Humans differ in perception of sweet taste, but genetic determination of this variation has not been unequivocally established (138, 140). In humans of African, Asian, European, and Native American origin, all three *TAS1R* genes have multiple polymorphisms, which include those resulting in amino acid changes of T1R proteins and even in a premature stop codon in *TAS1R1*. The majority of amino acid sequence variation occurs in the N-terminus extracellular domain, where taste ligands are likely to bind the taste receptors. *TAS1R2* was particularly diverse compared with other human genes: Its rate of polymorphisms was higher than average, in the top 5% to 10% of all human genes surveyed. Thus, *TAS1R* variation in human populations was predicted to contribute more to variation in sweet taste (which depends on *TAS1R2* and *TAS1R3*) than to variation in umami taste (which depends on *TAS1R1* and *TAS1R3*) (89).

Rats. Several rat strains with different saccharin preferences did not differ in protein sequence of T1R3. Some nonprotein-coding *Tas1r3* variants found among these strains were not associated with marked differences in *Tas1r3* expression and thus are unlikely to affect T1R3 function. Therefore, the prominent rat strain differences in saccharin preferences depend on genes other than *Tas1r3* (107).

Mice. In initial studies that identified the mouse *Tas1r3* gene, several polymorphisms associated with sweetener preferences were detected (91, 120, 123, 127, 147). However, these studies lacked proper quantitative analyses of gene-phenotype associations. Reed et al. (137) conducted a comprehensive quantitative analysis of the *Tas1r3* sequence variants associated with saccharin preference using 30 genealogically diverse inbred mouse strains. Of the 89 polymorphisms detected within the ~6.7 kb genomic region including the *Tas1r3* gene, eight were significantly associated with saccharin preferences. An absence of differences in the *Tas1r3* gene expression in the taste tissues of mice with different *Tas1r3* alleles suggested that the receptor function is likely to be affected by polymorphisms that change amino acid sequence of the T1R3 protein. A coding polymorphism with the strongest association with saccharin preferences resulted in the amino acid substitution of isoleucine to threonine at position 60 (I60T) in the extracellular N-terminus of the predicted T1R3 protein. Modeling of the T1R3 protein using the structure of the related mGluR1 receptor as a prototype has suggested that the I60T substitution introduces an extra N-terminal glycosylation site, which could affect dimerization of the receptor (120). However, this was not confirmed in a coimmunoprecipitation experiment (126). It was also suggested that this type of polymorphism could affect ligand binding (137). This prediction was subsequently confirmed in an in vitro study showing that a corresponding site-directed mutation changes binding affinity of the T1R3 protein to several sweeteners (130).

Other Candidate Receptors for Sweet and Umami Tastes

Several molecules have been proposed as candidate mammalian taste receptors for umami or glutamate taste, including splice variants of metabotropic glutamate receptors, mGluR4 and mGluR1, and the N-methyl-D-aspartate-type glutamate ion channel receptor (30, 39a, 148, 160). Some sweet-tasting compounds can penetrate TRC membrane and act on intracellular targets (125). Thus, these biological molecules may function as intracellular receptors of such compounds.

PROP: 6-n-propyl-2-thiouracil

T2R RECEPTORS

Discovery

The existence of a family of bitter taste receptors was predicted more than ten years ago by I. Lush, a geneticist who studied mouse strain differences in bitter taste avoidance, and who suggested that a cluster of bitterness-tasting genes "have evolved from one original bitterness gene by a process of local duplication and differentiation" (115). The T2R genes were discovered in 2000 by two groups. These discoveries were based on analyses of the recently released human genome sequences in the genome regions linked to bitter taste responsiveness in humans and mice. Adler et al. (6) examined a region of human chromosome 5 linked to perception of a bitter compound 6-n-propyl-2-thiouracil (PROP) (139) and discovered a novel GPCR, *TAS2R1*. Similarity searches of genomic DNA revealed additional related genes in human chromosomes 7 and 12. Although the *TAS2R1* gene is a candidate for the PROP sensitivity locus, which suggests that this is a bitter taste receptor for PROP, this relationship has not been experimentally proven yet, and T2R1 ligands are still not known. Matsunami et al. (118) examined a region of human chromosome 12 with

PLCβ2: phospholipase Cβ2

conserved synteny to a region of mouse chromosome 6 containing the sucrose octaacetate aversion (*Soa*) locus (13, 36, 115) and discovered *TAS2R* genes based on their weak similarity to a vomeronasal receptor gene. Several subsequent publications have identified additional human, rat, and mouse *TAS2R* genes (42, 43, 174).

Genomic Organization

Current genomic databases (2, 4) list 43 human *TAS2R* genes (38 intact genes and 5 pseudogenes; **Supplemental Table 1**) on chromosomes 5, 7, and 12 (**Supplemental Figure 1**) and 40 mouse *Tas2r* genes (35 intact genes and 5 pseudogenes; **Supplemental Table 2**) on chromosomes 2, 6, and 15. The T2R genes are intronless (**Supplemental Figure 2**) and encode ~300–330 amino acid GPCR proteins with a short N-terminal extracellular domain (**Figure 1**).

Tissue Expression

The main sites of expression of the T2R genes in mammals are TRCs of the circumvallate, foliate, palate, and epiglottis taste buds, and to a lesser degree fungiform taste buds (6, 9, 21, 33, 34, 93, 118). In mammals, T2R and T1R genes are expressed in different subsets of TRC (127) (but see 86).

It appears that multiple T2Rs are coexpressed in the same TRC, and possibly nearly all T2Rs are expressed in each T2R-positive TRC (6). The largely overlapping expression of the T2R genes within individual TRCs has been confirmed in a transgenic "rescue" experiment. In bitter taste–deficient phospholipase Cβ2 (PLCβ2) knockout mice, PLCβ2 was reintroduced under the control of three different *Tas2r* gene promoters. Responsiveness to all bitter taste stimuli examined (presumably acting on different T2R receptors) was restored in each of the transgenic lines produced with different constructs (124). However, results of another study (118) suggested that different TRCs may express different T2Rs.

The pattern of T2R expression has implications for bitter taste coding. Coexpression of multiple T2Rs in the same TRCs (6, 124) is consistent with behavioral discrimination and generalization data in primates and rats suggesting an identical taste quality perception of different bitter compounds (10, 154) and with neurophysiological data showing that responses to different bitter taste stimuli activate similar groups of neurons in the rat nucleus of the solitary tract (37) and in the primate cortex (152). On the other hand, expression of different T2Rs in different TRCs (118) is consistent with neurophysiological data showing that different bitter taste stimuli activate different TRCs (35) and afferent peripheral gustatory neurons (45) in rats and with the lack of conditioned taste aversion generalization between some bitter taste stimuli in hamsters (56). These latter data suggest that the taste system can discriminate among different bitter taste stimuli. It was proposed that a discrepancy between expression of multiple T2Rs in the same TRC and selective responses of TRCs to bitter tastants might be due to differences in levels of expression of the same T2R in different TRCs. This would result in variation among individual T2R-expressing cells in their sensitivity to bitter tastants, although each of these TRCs still would respond to multiple bitter ligands (38).

Ligands

The number of compounds perceived by humans as bitter (65) is much larger than the number of human *TAS2R* genes, implying that each human T2R responds to more than one bitter ligand (22). The same is likely to be true for other species. Some T2Rs interact with a wide range of bitter-tasting ligands (e.g., *TAS2R14* and *TAS2R16*; see **Supplemental Table 4**), which supports this expectation. However, some other T2Rs appear to have narrow ligand specificities. It has been suggested that different T2R alleles may have different profiles of ligand specificity (87, 122). Thus, the repertoire of bitter taste receptors may be not limited by a number of the T2R genes, but may involve as many receptors as there are T2R alleles (122).

Ligands have been determined for only a relatively small number of T2Rs in four vertebrate species: humans, chimpanzees, rats, and mice (**Supplemental Table 4**). All of the compounds that interact with T2Rs evoke bitter taste sensation in humans. The T2R ligand specificities have been determined predominantly using in vitro studies. For the following six T2Rs, ligand specificity was examined both in vitro and in vivo with matching results, which provides compelling evidence that these T2Rs function as bitter taste receptors.

Mouse *Tas2r105* gene is located in the genomic region of the *Cyx* (cycloheximide tasting) locus (11, 114) on distal chromosome 6. *Tas2r105* coding sequence variants are associated with behavioral sensitivity to cycloheximide in several inbred mouse strains (39, 128). Cells heterologously expressing *Tas2r105* respond to cycloheximide. Expression of a *Tas2r105* allele from a cycloheximide taster strain results in higher cell responsiveness than does expression of an allele from a nontaster strain (39). *Tas2r105* knockout mice show selective impairment in neural and behavioral responses to cycloheximide but not to other bitter or nonbitter taste stimuli (124).

Although these data provide strong evidence that the *Tas2r105* gene is identical to the *Cyx* locus and encodes a receptor binding cycloheximide, some other data do not agree with this hypothesis. Chandrashekar et al. (39) examined strain distribution patterns of *Tas2r105* genotypes and *Cyx* phenotypes in BXD recombinant inbred strains and found a tight linkage but not perfect concordance between these loci; they have explained this discordance by ambiguity in designation of the *Cyx* phenotype of the BXD strains by Lush & Holland (114). However, the study of Lush & Holland (114) has shown a clearly dichotomous strain distribution pattern of the BXD strains. But, strangely, the progenitors of the BXD strains had similar responsiveness to cycloheximide: The average preference scores for 1 μM cycloheximide were 22% in the C57BL/6 inbred strain and 29% for the DBA/2 strain. Both progenitor strains were similar to a group of BXD strains that formed a cluster of sensitive strains with an average preference score for 1 μM cycloheximide of 18%, as opposed to a group of relatively insensitive BXD strains with an average preference score 41% (114). Consistent with these data, no differences were found between C57BL/6 and DBA/2 strains in brief-access responses to cycloheximide in a recent study (29). In addition, preference scores for cycloheximide were continuously distributed among 27 inbred strains (114), which does not allow them to be categorized as tasters and nontasters. Thus, analysis of *Tas2r105* sequence variants between strains assumed to be tasters (CBA/Ca, BALB/c, C3H/He, and DBA/2) and nontasters (C57BL/6 and 129/Sv) (39) is questionable. An additional limitation of this analysis is that the four taster strains have shared genealogy (20) and thus are likely to share many parts of the genome due to identity-by-descent, and not necessarily because of a true genotype-phenotype association. These inconsistencies require additional studies to resolve. A quantitative analysis of genotype-phenotype associations in genealogically diverse strains (e.g., 137) would provide more conclusive data.

Orthologous human *TAS2R4* and mouse *Tas2r108* respond to denatonium and PROP in a heterologous system (39). Transgenic expression of each gene in the chemosensory neurons of *Caenorhabditis elegans* affected behavioral responses of worms to denatonium and PROP (44).

Human *TAS2R16* responds to β-glucopyranosides in the heterologous expression system (34). Naturally occurring human *TAS2R16* alleles have different responsiveness to several β-glucopyranosides in vitro (69, 153). It is unknown whether these alleles are also associated with human perception

PTC: phenylthiocarbamide

of β-glucopyranoside bitterness. Although wild-type mice are indifferent to phenyl-β-D-glucopyranoside, mice with a human *TAS2R16* transgene expressed in bitter-sensing cells under control of the mouse *Tas2r119* promoter avoid phenyl-β-D-glucopyranoside in behavioral tests. Mice with human *TAS2R16* transgene expressed in sweet-sensing cells under control of the mouse *Tas1r2* promoter show preference for phenyl-β-D-glucopyranoside (124). Transgenic expression of human *TAS2R16* in the chemosensory neurons of *C. elegans* affected behavioral responses of worms to phenyl-β-D-glucopyranoside (44).

Human *TAS2R38* was demonstrated in a positional cloning study (88) as a gene identical to a human phenylthiocarbamide (PTC) bitter taste sensitivity locus on chromosome 7q (50). *TAS2R38* has three common missense single nucleotide polymorphisms resulting in substitutions of proline to alanine at amino acid position 49 (P49A), alanine to valine at position 262 (A262V), and valine to isoleucine at position 296 (V296I). These polymorphisms give rise to several haplotypes, the most common of which are PAV (PTC-sensitive allele) and AVI (PTC-insensitive allele) (88, 173). *TAS2R38* genotypes are associated with human perception of PTC and PROP bitterness (33, 52, 121, 135). Cells heterologously expressing the sensitive PAV alleles of *TAS2R38* respond to thioamides (including PTC and PROP). PTC and PROP responses of cells heterologously expressing different alleles of *TAS2R38* correlate with psychophysical responses of individuals carrying these alleles (33). Although wild-type mice do not show strong lick suppression in response to PTC solutions in brief-access tests (128), mice with a taster (PAV) allele of human *TAS2R38* transgenically expressed in bitter-sensing cells under the control of a mouse *Tas2r* promoter show strong aversion to PTC (124).

Although a PTC nontaster allele of human *TAS2R38* (AVI) is expressed in taste buds, it does not respond to taste stimuli in vitro (33). Because taster and nontaster alleles of *TAS2R38* are maintained by balanced selection (173), it was suggested that the nontaster allele may serve as a receptor for as yet unidentified toxic bitter substances other than PTC (87, 173).

Allelic variants of chimpanzee *TAS2R38*, an ortholog of human *TAS2R38*, are also associated with taste sensitivity to PTC in individual animals. A taster allele of chimpanzee *TAS2R38* responds to PTC in vitro (172).

Allelic Variation of T2R Genes and Its Role in Individual Variation in Taste Responses

Humans. Individual humans differ in bitter taste perception, and some of this variation has a genetic component (140). Human *TAS2R* genes have substantial diversity of coding sequence (87, 122, 161, 167), which suggests that *TAS2R* polymorphisms may be responsible for the genetic component of individual differences in bitter taste.

However, this relationship has been demonstrated only for one gene, *TAS2R38*. It is located on chromosome 7, where linkages for PTC and PROP taste sensitivity have been detected (40, 41, 50, 135, 139). Allelic variants of *TAS2R38* explain more than 50% of phenotypical variation in PTC sensitivity (88) and are also associated with human perception of PROP bitterness (33, 52, 121, 135).

Significant or suggestive linkages have been also detected on chromosomes 1, 3, 10, and 16 for PTC taste sensitivity (50) and on chromosome 5 for PROP taste sensitivity (139). The PROP sensitivity locus on human chromosome 5 (139) includes the *TAS2R1* gene but no other *TAS2R* genes. However, the identity of the PROP sensitivity locus and the *TAS2R1* gene has not yet been proven. The PTC sensitivity loci in chromosomes 1, 3, 10, and 16 (50) contain no *TAS2R* genes. Identification of genes corresponding to the genetic loci for bitter taste sensitivity, and matching variation in *TAS2R* sequences with individual variation in bitter taste perception, are important areas for future studies.

Hamsters, rats, and mice. Strain differences in behavioral responses to bitter taste stimuli were found in rats (159) and hamsters (57), but most research on genetics of taste has been conducted in mice. Mouse strains differ in behavioral and neural responses to bitter taste stimuli (e.g., 27, 29, 76, 108–112, 114). Several linked genetic loci on mouse chromosome 6, in a *Tas2r* gene–cluster region, are responsible for variation in aversion to bitter-tasting quinine (*Qui*), cycloheximide (*Cyx*), copper glycinate (*Glb*), and acetylated sugars, sucrose octaacetate and raffinose undecaacetate (*Soa/Rua*) (11, 13, 26, 36, 66, 67, 76, 108, 110, 112, 114, 115, 129, 168).

A few studies conducted so far have detected considerable variation in sequences of the mouse *Tas2r* genes (39, 128, 129). All this strongly suggests that the genetic variation in taste responses to the bitter compounds is due to polymorphisms of the *Tas2r* genes, as was predicted by Lush et al. (115). However, this relationship has been demonstrated only for the *Tas2r105* gene corresponding to the *Cyx* locus (39, 124, 128), although with some inconsistencies (see Ligands section, above). There is also evidence for additional linkages of mouse bitter taste responses outside the *Tas2r* regions (68, 95, 129).

Other Candidate Receptors for Bitter Taste

In addition to activation of T2R receptor proteins, some bitter compounds can interact with ion channels in the cell membrane or with intracellular targets (125, 145, 150). Thus, these proteins may also function as receptors for these compounds.

OTHER TASTE RECEPTORS

Candidate Sour Taste Receptors

A commonly accepted view is that the taste receptors for sour (H^+) and salty (Na^+) tastes are ion channels (25, 49). Several candidate sour (acid) taste receptors have been proposed in recent years. One of these genes is a neuronal (degenerin) amiloride-sensitive cation channel 1 (see ACCN1 sidebar). It has been proposed as a sour taste receptor in rat (102, 105, 162–164). However, this channel is not expressed in mouse taste buds (143), and behavioral (90) and physiological (143) responses to sour taste stimuli are unaltered in mice lacking the *Accn1* gene. HCN1 and HCN4, members of a family of hyperpolarization-activated cyclic nucleotide-gated (HCN) channels (see HCN sidebar), were also proposed as putative sour receptors (156). However, Ca^{2+} responses of taste cells to acids were not inhibited by Cs^+, an inhibitor of HCN channels (141). Acid taste transduction involves intracellular acidification of TRC (116, 141), which is expected to affect acid-sensitive ion channel(s). Several two-pore domain potassium leak conductance channels from the K_2P family are sensitive to intracellular acidification and thus were examined as candidate acid taste transducers. Based on the gene expression pattern and pharmacological analysis, TASK-1 appears to be the most likely candidate (see TASK-1 sidebar), although other K_2P channels cannot be excluded (142). The Na^+-H^+-exchanger isoform 1 (NHE-1) (see NHE-1 sidebar) was also suggested to be involved in sour taste transduction based on its gene expression and pharmacological analyses (165).

Finally, the most recent studies suggest that the *Pkd1l3* and *Pkd2l1* genes (see PKD1L3 and PKD2L1 sidebar) participate in reception of sourness (73, 79, 106). However, their role in behavioral taste responses to sourness has not yet been demonstrated. In addition, some questions arising from the most recent studies have not been resolved. For example, acids activate the *Pdk2l1* protein in vitro only when it is coexpressed with *Pkd1l3* (79). Yet, disruption of *Pdk2l1*-expressing cells in the fungiform papillae abolishes CT responses to acids (73) despite lack of *Pkd1l3* expression in these cells (73,

ACCN1

In humans, the neuronal (degenerin) amiloride-sensitive cation channel 1 is encoded by the *ACCN1* gene on chromosome 17q11 [gene name: amiloride-sensitive cation channel 1, neuronal (degenerin); other symbols: *ACCN, ASIC2a, ASIC2, BNC1, BNaC1, hBNaC1* and *MDEG*]. In the mouse, it is encoded by the *Accn1* gene on chromosome 11 [gene name: amiloride-sensitive cation channel 1, neuronal (degenerin); other symbols: *ASIC2, BNaC1a, BNC1, Mdeg*]. *Accn1* is a member of a family of voltage-insensitive cation channels involved in mechanosensitivity and acid sensitivity. Its mRNA exists as two splice variants, described as ASIC2a and ASIC2b (166).

HCN

The human *HCN1* gene is on chromosome 5p12 (gene name: hyperpolarization activated cyclic nucleotide-gated potassium channel 1; other names: *BCNG1, BCNG-1, HAC-2*). The mouse *Hcn1* gene is on chromosome 13 (gene name: hyperpolarization-activated, cyclic nucleotide-gated K^+ 1; other names: *Bcng1, HAC2*). The human *HCN4* gene is on chromosome 15q24 (gene name: hyperpolarization activated cyclic nucleotide-gated potassium channel 4). The mouse *Hcn4* gene is on chromosome 9 (gene name: hyperpolarization-activated, cyclic nucleotide-gated K^+ 4).

TASK-1

In humans, the TASK-1 channel protein is encoded by the *KCNK3* gene on chromosome 2p23 (gene name: potassium channel, subfamily K, member 3; other names: *TASK, TASK-1*). Its mouse ortholog is *Kcnk3* on chromosome 5 (gene name: potassium channel, subfamily K, member 3; other names: *cTBAK-1*).

79). This suggests the existence of another, yet unknown partner for heteromerization with *Pdk2l1*.

Candidate Salty Taste Receptors

A large number of studies suggested that at least in rodents, Na^+ taste reception involves the selective epithelial amiloride-sensitive sodium channel, ENaC, which is a member of the degenerin/ENaC superfamily of ion channels (for reviews, see 28, 103). In humans, there are four ENaC channel subunits, α, β, γ, and δ. Mice and rats lack the ENaC δ subunit (85) (see ENaC sidebar). A variant of a vanilloid (capsaicin) receptor-1 has been proposed as an amiloride-insensitive salt taste receptor in rodents (117) (see TRPV1 sidebar). However, the evidence for ENaC or other candidate salt taste receptors in vertebrate is not as convincing as it is for the T1R and T2R receptors. The strongest evidence for involvement of degenerin/ENaC channel genes in Na^+ taste responses was found for the *ppk11* and *ppk19* genes in *Drosophila* (104).

Taste Detection of Lipids

The predominant orosensory cue for fat itself is its texture (119). Fat may also be detected by the presence of its decomposition products or impurities (136), which can activate olfactory or gustatory systems. Recent data suggest that taste may play a more important role in detection of dietary lipids than was previously believed. Dietary lipids consist mainly of triglycerides, but the lingual lipase hydrolyzes triglycerides and releases free fatty acids in the oral cavity where they can access TRCs and affect their function. Free fatty acids were shown to inhibit the delayed rectifying potassium channels in rat TRCs (63). In addition, the fatty acid transporter CD36 is expressed in TRCs and may be involved in oral detection of fatty acids (59, 94, 177) (see CD36 sidebar).

Taste Detection of Complex Carbohydrates

Rats and some other species may also perceive a taste of polysaccharides and starch, which is qualitatively distinct from the taste of sugars (151). A molecular mechanism of gustatory reception of these complex carbohydrates is unknown, but there is evidence that it does not involve the T1R3 receptor (75).

Taste Detection of Water

Water consumption is crucial for animals' survival and is regulated by thirst, a specialized water appetite. This suggests that animals have mechanisms for chemosensory detection of water or hypo-osmotic fluids. Consistent with this, water can evoke taste responses (62). It was suggested that TRCs act as osmotic sensors and that transduction of hypo-osmotic stimuli involves water influx through aquaporins followed by activation of volume-regulated anion channels (62). Several aquaporin molecules are expressed in TRC, with the apically expressed AQP5 being the most likely candidate for water taste transduction (62, 64) (see AQP5 sidebar).

Taste perception of water by humans largely depends on the adaptation state of the oral cavity. Adaptation to different taste solutions (and probably to saliva) affects how water is perceived (18). Water elicits a strong sweet taste when it is applied to the oral cavity after exposure to sweet taste blockers. This phenomenon has been labeled "sweet water aftertaste" (51). This adaptation-dependent perception of water taste could involve central mechanisms, intracellular adaptation within TRC, or interactions at the receptor level. A recent in vitro study with a heterologously expressed T1R2 + T1R3 receptor demonstrated that sweet water aftertaste is explained by interactions at the receptor level. This study suggested that the sweet taste receptor shifts from an inactive state (when it is exposed to a sweet taste inhibitor) to an active state (upon rinsing with water), which initiates transduction events and results in perception of sweetness (61).

NHE-1

In humans, the NHE-1 protein is encoded by the *SLC9A1* gene on chromosome 1p36 [gene name: solute carrier family 9 (sodium/hydrogen exchanger), member 1 (antiporter, Na^+/H^+, amiloride sensitive); other symbols: *APNH, NHE1*]. Its mouse ortholog is *Slc9a1* on chromosome 4 [gene name: solute carrier family 9 (sodium/hydrogen exchanger), member 1; other symbols: antiporter, *Apnh*, Na^+/H^+, amiloride sensitive, *Nhe1*].

PKD1L3 AND PKD2L1

The human *PKD1L3* gene is on chromosome 16q22 (gene name: polycystic kidney disease 1-like 3); its mouse ortholog is *Pkd1l3* on chromosome 8 (gene name: polycystic kidney disease 1 like 3). The human *PKD2L1* gene is on chromosome 10q24 (gene name: polycystic kidney disease 2-like 1; other symbols: *PKD2L, PKDL*). Its mouse ortholog is *Pkd2l1* on chromosome 19 (gene name: polycystic kidney disease 2-like 1; other symbols: *PCL, PKD2L, Pkdl*, polycystin-L, *TRPP3*).

ENaC

The four human ENaC channel subunits, α, β, γ, and δ, are encoded respectively by four genes: *SCNN1A* (alias: *ENaCa*) on chromosome 12p13, closely linked *SCNN1B* (alias: *ENaCb*) and *SCNN1G* (alias: *ENaCg*) on chromosome 16p12, and *SCNN1D* (aliases: *dNaCh, ENaCd*) on chromosome 1p36 (gene names: sodium channel, nonvoltage-gated 1 alpha, beta, gamma, or delta; *SCNN1B* is also known as a gene responsible for Liddle syndrome). The three mouse ENaC channel subunits, α, β, and γ, are encoded respectively by three genes: *Scnn1a* on chromosome 6, and closely linked *Scnn1b* and *Scnn1g* on chromosome 7 (gene names: sodium channel, nonvoltage-gated, type I, alpha, beta, or gamma).

TASTE RECEPTORS IN NONTASTE TISSUES AND INTERNAL CHEMOSENSATION

Some substances detected by the gustatory system as taste stimuli also need to be detected inside the body for homeostatic regulation. There are interoceptive mechanisms for detecting sodium, pH, glucose, and amino acids in different internal organs, such as the kidney, pancreas, gut, and brain. This raises the possibility that the same receptors can serve as

TRPV1

Human vanilloid receptor-1 is encoded by the *TRPV1* gene on chromosome 17p13 (gene name: transient receptor potential cation channel, subfamily V, member 1; previous name: vanilloid receptor subtype 1; previous symbol: *VR1*). Its mouse ortholog is *Trpv1* on chromosome 11 (gene name: transient receptor potential cation channel, subfamily V, member 1; other names: capsaicin receptor, *OTRPC1*, *VR-1*).

CD36

Human *CD36* gene is on chromosome 7q11 (gene name: CD36 molecule; previous names: CD36 antigen, collagen type I receptor, thrombospondin receptor; other symbols: *SCARB3*, *GPIV*, *FAT*, *GP4*, *GP3B*). Its mouse ortholog is *Cd36* on chromosome 5 (gene name: CD36 antigen; other symbols: *FAT*, fatty acid translocase, *Scarb3*).

AQP5

Human *AQP5* gene is on chromosome 12q13 (gene name: aquaporin 5); its mouse ortholog is *Aqp5* on chromosome 15 (gene name: aquaporin 5).

taste receptors and interoceptors. Although in some cases taste and interoception use different receptor mechanisms [e.g., for detection of glucose and sodium by brain (70, 96)], there are examples of sharing the same receptor protein by the two systems. The *Pkd2l1* channel is involved in pH sensing by the TRC and by neurons in the spinal cord (73). ENaC may also be a shared mechanism for sodium detection by TRC and other body tissues.

A number of studies have detected expression of the T1R and T2R genes in nontaste tissues. The T1R genes were found in testis (91, 92, 120), brain, thymus (120), gastrointestinal tract, enteroendocrine cells (24, 53, 120, 146), kidney, lymphocytes (92), liver, and pancreas (158). The T2R genes were found in testis (118), gastrointestinal tract, enteroendocrine cells (146, 174, 175), and nasal respiratory epithelium (55). This suggests that the taste receptors may be involved in the chemosensory function of these organs (155).

Ectopic expression of olfactory receptor genes similarly has raised questions about the role they play in nonolfactory tissues. A recent systematic analysis of olfactory receptor expression in different tissues suggested that only small olfactory receptor subsets might play functional roles in different tissues, while most of them are likely to be under a neutral transcription control (54). Similarly, caution should be exerted when offering a functional interpretation for ectopic expression of taste receptors until more comprehensive studies are conducted.

PRACTICAL APPLICATIONS OF TASTE RECEPTOR STUDIES

There is substantial interest in developing novel taste stimuli and taste modifiers for humans and other animals. For humans, areas of interest include making food and drinks healthier without sacrificing their palatability and making oral medications more acceptable to patients. A substantial demand exists for artificial sweet and umami compounds, enhancers of salty, sweet, and umami taste, blockers of bitter taste, and pharmaceutical compounds with improved sensory properties. There is also a demand for improvement in the taste quality of food for companion and farm animals and for developing nonlethal repellents of wild animals, e.g., nontoxic chemicals with aversive taste. Development of such products has been hampered by lack of knowledge of the molecular identity of the taste receptors. Discovery of taste receptors, characterization of their active sites involved in interactions with agonists and antagonists, and development of high-throughput techniques for in vitro screening of taste stimuli will facilitate the design of novel taste-active compounds.

Allelic variation of human taste receptors can affect food perception, choice, and consumption. As a result, it can influence nutrition and potentially predispose individuals to certain diseases (e.g., 19). Thus, some taste receptor alleles can be disease risk factors. Genotypes of these receptors may be useful as biological markers to identify predispositions to some diseases and to suggest interventions for disease prevention. Available data provide some examples for the role of taste receptor variation in human nutrition and health.

Sensitive alleles of human *TAS2R38* receptor respond to PTC, PROP, and related compounds that contain a thiourea (N – C = S) moiety. Some plants consumed by humans contain glucosinolates, compounds that also contain the thiourea moiety. A recent study has shown that *TAS2R38* genotype affects perception of bitterness of glucosinolate-containing plants, such as broccoli, turnip, and horseradish (149). Allelic variation of *TAS2R38* may have even more widespread effects on food choice, as it was shown to be associated with preferences for sucrose and sweet-tasting beverages and foods in children (but not adults) (121).

Taste receptor variation may be a biomarker of predisposition to alcoholism. Ethanol flavor has bitter and sweet taste components. Variation in bitter and sweet taste responsiveness is associated with perception of ethanol flavor and consumption of alcoholic beverages (12). In mice, allelic variation of the *Tas1r3* sweet taste receptor gene is associated with voluntary ethanol consumption (15). Although hedonic responses to sweet taste are considered as one of the biomarkers of predisposition to alcoholism in humans (84), genes responsible for this association are still unknown. Higher sensitivity to ethanol bitterness may protect against excess alcohol consumption. Consistent with this hypothesis, individuals carrying one or two sensitive (PAV) alleles of the PTC receptor gene, *TAS2R38*, had lower yearly consumption of alcoholic beverages than did individuals homozygous for the insensitive allele, AVI (52). Similarly, there is an association between risk of alcohol dependence and *TAS2R16* (β-glucopyranosides receptor) polymorphisms: An ancestral K172 allele, which is less sensitive to β-glucopyranosides in vitro, is associated with increased risk of alcohol dependence (69).

CONCLUDING REMARKS

Taste receptors function as one of the interfaces between internal and external milieus. Tremendous progress has been achieved in the past few years with the discovery of the T1R and T2R receptors and the understanding of their function. Individual differences in taste, at least in some cases, can be attributed to allelic variants of the taste receptor genes. Understanding how taste receptors interact with taste stimuli and identifying their patterns of expression in taste cells shed light on coding of taste information by the nervous system.

However, many challenging tasks remain before we fully understand how taste works. Much of this important future research must be done with taste receptor genes. The important questions to be addressed include finding genes that encode a complete repertoire of taste receptors for different taste qualities, as well as genes that encode proteins involved in taste transduction and transmission, taste bud cell turnover, and connectivity between taste cells and afferent nerves. Studies of allelic variation of taste receptors will help to elucidate individual differences in taste perception, food choice, nutrition, and health, and to understand functional organization of receptor domains and their ligand specificities.

ACKNOWLEDGMENTS

Research by the authors is supported by NIH grants R01DC00882 and R01AA11028 and an Ajinomoto Amino Acid Research Program Focused Research grant.

LITERATURE CITED

1. GPCRDB. *Information system for G protein-coupled receptors (GPCRs).* Accessed March 27, 2007. Nijmegen, Netherlands: GPCRDB Inform. Syst. **http://www.gpcr.org/7tm/**
2. Human Genome Database. Accessed March 27, 2007. Baltimore, MD: GDB. **http://www.gdb.org**
3. The Human Genome Organisation (HUGO) Gene Nomenclature Committee. Accessed March 27, 2007. London: HUGO. **http://www.gene.ucl.ac.uk/nomenclature/**
4. Mouse Genome Informatics. Accessed March 27, 2007. Bar Harbor, ME: Jackson Lab. **http://www.informatics.jax.org**
5. Rules for Nomenclature of Genes, Genetic Markers, Alleles, and Mutations in Mouse and Rat. Accessed March 27, 2007. Bar Harbor, ME: Jackson Lab. **http://www.informatics.jax.org/mgihome/nomen/gene.shtml**
6. Adler E, Hoon MA, Mueller KL, Chandrashekar J, Ryba NJP, Zuker CS. 2000. A novel family of mammalian taste receptors. *Cell* 100:693–702
7. Andres-Barquin PJ, Conte C. 2004. Molecular basis of bitter taste: the T2R family of G protein-coupled receptors. *Cell Biochem. Biophys.* 41:99–112
8. Ariyasu T, Matsumoto S, Kyono F, Hanaya T, Arai S, et al. 2003. Taste receptor T1R3 is an essential molecule for the cellular recognition of the disaccharide trehalose. *In Vitro Cell Dev. Biol. Anim.* 39:80–88
9. Asano-Miyoshi M, Abe K, Emori Y. 2001. IP(3) receptor type 3 and PLCbeta2 are coexpressed with taste receptors T1R and T2R in rat taste bud cells. *Chem. Senses* 26:259–65
10. Aspen J, Gatch MB, Woods JH. 1999. Training and characterization of a quinine taste discrimination in rhesus monkeys. *Psychopharmacology (Berl.)* 141:251–57
11. Azen EA, Lush IE, Taylor BA. 1986. Close linkage of mouse genes for salivary proline-rich proteins (PRPs) and taste. *Trends Genet.* 2:199–200
12. Bachmanov AA, Kiefer SW, Molina JC, Tordoff MG, Duffy VB, et al. 2003. Chemosensory factors influencing alcohol perception, preferences, and consumption. *Alcohol. Clin. Exp. Res.* 27:220–31
13. Bachmanov AA, Li X, Li S, Neira M, Beauchamp GK, Azen EA. 2001. High-resolution genetic mapping of the sucrose octaacetate taste aversion (*Soa*) locus on mouse chromosome 6. *Mamm. Genome* 12:695–99
14. Bachmanov AA, Li X, Reed DR, Ohmen JD, Li S, et al. 2001. Positional cloning of the mouse saccharin preference (*Sac*) locus. *Chem. Senses* 26:925–33
15. Bachmanov AA, Reed DR, Li X, Li S, Beauchamp GK, Tordoff MG. 2002. Voluntary ethanol consumption by mice: genome-wide analysis of quantitative trait loci and their interactions in a C57BL/6ByJ × 129P3/J F2 intercross. *Genome Res.* 12:1257–68
16. Bachmanov AA, Reed DR, Ninomiya Y, Inoue M, Tordoff MG, et al. 1997. Sucrose consumption in mice: major influence of two genetic loci affecting peripheral sensory responses. *Mamm. Genome* 8:545–48
17. Bachmanov AA, Tordoff MG, Beauchamp GK. 2001. Sweetener preference of C57BL/6ByJ and 129P3/J mice. *Chem. Senses* 26:905–13
18. Bartoshuk LM. 1977. Water taste in mammals. In *Drinking Behavior: Oral Stimulation, Reinforcement, and Preference*, ed. JAWM Weijnen, J Mendelson, pp. 317–39. New York: Plenum

19. Basson MD, Bartoshuk LM, Dichello SZ, Panzini L, Weiffenbach JM, Duffy VB. 2005. Association between 6-n-propylthiouracil (PROP) bitterness and colonic neoplasms. *Dig. Dis. Sci.* 50:483–89
20. Beck JA, Lloyd S, Hafezparast M, Lennon-Pierce M, Eppig JT, et al. 2000. Genealogies of mouse inbred strains. *Nat. Genet.* 24:23–25
21. Behrens M, Brockhoff A, Kuhn C, Bufe B, Winnig M, Meyerhof W. 2004. The human taste receptor hTAS2R14 responds to a variety of different bitter compounds. *Biochem. Biophys. Res. Commun.* 319:479–85
22. Behrens M, Meyerhof W. 2006. Bitter taste receptors and human bitter taste perception. *Cell Mol. Life Sci.* 63:1501–9
23. Belknap JK, Crabbe JC, Plomin R, McClearn GE, Sampson KE, et al. 1992. Single-locus control of saccharin intake in BXD/Ty recombinant inbred (RI) mice: some methodological implications for RI strain analysis. *Behav. Genet.* 22:81–100
24. Bezencon C, le Coutre J, Damak S. 2007. Taste-signaling proteins are coexpressed in solitary intestinal epithelial cells. *Chem. Senses.* 32:41–49
25. Bigiani A, Ghiaroni V, Fieni F. 2003. Channels as taste receptors in vertebrates. *Prog. Biophys. Mol. Biol.* 83:193–225
26. Blizard DA, Kotlus B, Frank ME. 1999. Quantitative trait loci associated with short-term intake of sucrose, saccharin and quinine solutions in laboratory mice. *Chem. Senses* 24:373–85
27. Boughter JD, Bachmanov AA. 2007. Behavioral genetics and taste. *BMC Neurosci.* In press
28. Boughter JD Jr, Gilbertson TA. 1999. From channels to behavior: an integrative model of NaCl taste. *Neuron* 22:213–15
29. Boughter JD Jr, Raghow S, Nelson TM, Munger SD. 2005. Inbred mouse strains C57BL/6J and DBA/2J vary in sensitivity to a subset of bitter stimuli. *BMC Genet.* 6:36
30. Brand JG. 2000. Receptor and transduction processes for umami taste. *J. Nutr.* 130:942–45S
31. Breslin PA, Beauchamp GK, Pugh EN Jr. 1996. Monogeusia for fructose, glucose, sucrose, and maltose. *Percept. Psychophys.* 58:327–41
32. Breslin PA, Kemp S, Beauchamp GK. 1994. Single sweetness signal. *Nature* 369:447–48
33. Bufe B, Breslin PA, Kuhn C, Reed DR, Tharp CD, et al. 2005. The molecular basis of individual differences in phenylthiocarbamide and propylthiouracil bitterness perception. *Curr. Biol.* 15:322–27
34. Bufe B, Hofmann T, Krautwurst D, Raguse JD, Meyerhof W. 2002. The human TAS2R16 receptor mediates bitter taste in response to beta-glucopyranosides. *Nat. Genet.* 32:397–401
35. Caicedo A, Roper SD. 2001. Taste receptor cells that discriminate between bitter stimuli. *Science* 291:1557–60
36. Capeless CG, Whitney G, Azen EA. 1992. Chromosome mapping of *Soa*, a gene influencing gustatory sensitivity to sucrose octaacetate in mice. *Behav. Genet.* 22:655–63
37. Chan CY, Yoo JE, Travers SP. 2004. Diverse bitter stimuli elicit highly similar patterns of Fos-like immunoreactivity in the nucleus of the solitary tract. *Chem. Senses* 29:573–81
38. Chandrashekar J, Hoon MA, Ryba NJ, Zuker CS. 2006. The receptors and cells for mammalian taste. *Nature* 444:288–94
39. Chandrashekar J, Mueller KL, Hoon MA, Adler E, Feng L, et al. 2000. T2Rs function as bitter taste receptors. *Cell* 100:703–11
39a. Chaudhari N, Landin AM, Roper SO. 2000. Ametabotropic glutamate receptor variant functions as a taste receptor. *Nat. Neurosci.* 3:113–19

40. Chautard-Freire-Maia EA. 1974. Linkage relationships between 22 autosomal markers. *Ann. Hum. Genet.* 38:191–98
41. Conneally PM, Dumont-Driscoll M, Huntzinger RS, Nance WE, Jackson CE. 1976. Linkage relations of the loci for Kell and phenylthiocarbamide taste sensitivity. *Hum. Hered.* 26:267–71
42. Conte C, Ebeling M, Marcuz A, Andres-Barquin PJ. 2003. Identification of the T2R repertoire of taste receptor genes in the rat genome sequence. *Genome Lett.* 2:155–61
43. Conte C, Ebeling M, Marcuz A, Nef P, Andres-Barquin PJ. 2002. Identification and characterization of human taste receptor genes belonging to the TAS2R family. *Cytogenet. Genome Res.* 98:45–53
44. Conte C, Guarin E, Marcuz A, Andres-Barquin PJ. 2006. Functional expression of mammalian bitter taste receptors in *Caenorhabditis elegans*. *Biochimie* 88:801–6
45. Dahl M, Erickson RP, Simon SA. 1997. Neural responses to bitter compounds in rats. *Brain Res.* 756:22–34
46. Damak S, Rong M, Yasumatsu K, Kokrashvili Z, Varadarajan V, et al. 2003. Detection of sweet and umami taste in the absence of taste receptor T1r3. *Science* 301:850–53
47. Danilova V, Hellekant G. 2003. Comparison of the responses of the chorda tympani and glossopharyngeal nerves to taste stimuli in C57BL/6J mice. *BMC Neurosci.* 4:5
48. Danilova V, Hellekant G, Tinti JM, Nofre C. 1998. Gustatory responses of the hamster *Mesocricetus auratus* to various compounds considered sweet by humans. *J. Neurophysiol.* 80:2102–12
49. Desimone JA, Lyall V. 2006. Taste receptors in the gastrointestinal tract III. Salty and sour taste: sensing of sodium and protons by the tongue. *Am. J. Physiol. Gastrointest. Liver Physiol.* 291:G1005–10
50. Drayna D, Coon H, Kim UK, Elsner T, Cromer K, et al. 2003. Genetic analysis of a complex trait in the Utah Genetic Reference Project: a major locus for PTC taste ability on chromosome 7q and a secondary locus on chromosome 16p. *Hum. Genet.* 112:567–72
51. DuBois GE. 2004. Unraveling the biochemistry of sweet and umami tastes. *Proc. Natl. Acad. Sci. USA* 101:13972–73
52. Duffy VB, Davidson AC, Kidd JR, Kidd KK, Speed WC, et al. 2004. Bitter receptor gene (TAS2R38), 6-n-propylthiouracil (PROP) bitterness and alcohol intake. *Alcohol. Clin. Exp. Res.* 28:1629–37
53. Dyer J, Salmon KS, Zibrik L, Shirazi-Beechey SP. 2005. Expression of sweet taste receptors of the T1R family in the intestinal tract and enteroendocrine cells. *Biochem. Soc. Trans.* 33:302–5
54. Feldmesser E, Olender T, Khen M, Yanai I, Ophir R, Lancet D. 2006. Widespread ectopic expression of olfactory receptor genes. *BMC Genomics* 7:121
55. Finger TE, Bottger B, Hansen A, Anderson KT, Alimohammadi H, Silver WL. 2003. Solitary chemoreceptor cells in the nasal cavity serve as sentinels of respiration. *Proc. Natl. Acad. Sci. USA* 100:8981–86
56. Frank ME, Bouverat BP, MacKinnon BI, Hettinger TP. 2004. The distinctiveness of ionic and nonionic bitter stimuli. *Physiol. Behav.* 80:421–31
57. Frank ME, Wada Y, Makino J, Mizutani M, Umezawa H, et al. 2004. Variation in intake of sweet and bitter solutions by inbred strains of golden hamsters. *Behav. Genet.* 34:465–76
58. Fredriksson R, Lagerstrom MC, Lundin LG, Schioth HB. 2003. The G-protein-coupled receptors in the human genome form five main families. Phylogenetic analysis, paralogon groups, and fingerprints. *Mol. Pharmacol.* 63:1256–72

59. Fukuwatari T, Kawada T, Tsuruta M, Hiraoka T, Iwanaga T, et al. 1997. Expression of the putative membrane fatty acid transporter (FAT) in taste buds of the circumvallate papillae in rats. *FEBS Lett.* 414:461–64
60. Fuller JL. 1974. Single-locus control of saccharin preference in mice. *J. Heredity* 65:33–36
61. Galindo-Cuspinera V, Winnig M, Bufe B, Meyerhof W, Breslin PA. 2006. A TAS1R receptor-based explanation of sweet "water-taste." *Nature* 441:354–57
62. Gilbertson TA, Baquero AF, Spray-Watson KJ. 2006. Water taste: the importance of osmotic sensing in the oral cavity. *J. Water Health* 4(Suppl. 1):35–40
63. Gilbertson TA, Fontenot DT, Liu L, Zhang H, Monroe WT. 1997. Fatty acid modulation of K+ channels in taste receptor cells: gustatory cues for dietary fat. *Am. J. Physiol.* 272:C1203–10
64. Gilbertson TA, Kim I, Siears NL, Zhang H, Liu L. 1999. The water response in taste cells: expression of aquaporin-1, -2 and -5 and the characterization of hypoosmic-induced currents in mammalian taste cells. *Chem. Senses* 24:596 (Abstr.)
65. Glendinning JI. 1994. Is the bitter rejection response always adaptive? *Physiol. Behav.* 56:1217–27
66. Harder DB, Capeless CG, Maggio JC, Boughter JD, Gannon KS, et al. 1992. Intermediate sucrose octa-acetate sensitivity suggests a third allele at mouse bitter taste locus *Soa* and *Soa-Rua* identity. *Chem. Senses* 17:391–401
67. Harder DB, Whitney G. 1985. Evidence for a third allele at the Soa locus controlling sucrose octaacetate tasting in mice. *Behav. Genet.* 15:594
68. Harder DB, Whitney G. 1998. A common polygenic basis for quinine and PROP avoidance in mice. *Chem. Senses* 23:327–32
69. Hinrichs AL, Wang JC, Bufe B, Kwon JM, Budde J, et al. 2006. Functional variant in a bitter-taste receptor (hTAS2R16) influences risk of alcohol dependence. *Am. J. Hum. Genet.* 78:103–11
70. Hiyama TY, Watanabe E, Ono K, Inenaga K, Tamkun MM, et al. 2002. Na(x) channel involved in CNS sodium-level sensing. *Nat. Neurosci.* 5:511–12
71. Hoon MA, Adler E, Lindemeier J, Battey JF, Ryba NJ, Zuker CS. 1999. Putative mammalian taste receptors: a class of taste-specific GPCRs with distinct topographic selectivity. *Cell* 96:541–51
72. Hoon MA, Ryba NJP. 1997. Analysis and comparison of partial sequences of clones from a taste-bud-enriched cDNA library. *J. Dental Res.* 76:831–38
73. Huang AL, Chen X, Hoon MA, Chandrashekar J, Guo W, et al. 2006. The cells and logic for mammalian sour taste detection. *Nature* 442:934–38
74. Inoue M, Beauchamp GK, Bachmanov AA. 2004. Gustatory neural responses to umami taste stimuli in C57BL/6ByJ and 129P3/J mice. *Chem. Senses* 29:789–95
75. Inoue M, Glendinning JI, Theodorides ML, Harkness S, Li X, et al. 2007. Allelic variation of the *Tas1r3* taste receptor gene selectively affects taste responses to sweeteners: evidence from 129.B6-*Tas1r3* congenic mice. Submitted
76. Inoue M, Li X, McCaughey SA, Beauchamp GK, Bachmanov AA. 2001. *Soa* genotype selectively affects mouse gustatory neural responses to sucrose octaacetate. *Physiol. Genom.* 5:181–86
77. Inoue M, McCaughey SA, Bachmanov AA, Beauchamp GK. 2001. Whole-nerve chorda tympani responses to sweeteners in C57BL/6ByJ and 129P3/J mice. *Chem. Senses* 26:915–23
78. Inoue M, Reed DR, Li X, Tordoff MG, Beauchamp GK, Bachmanov AA. 2004. Allelic variation of the *Tas1r3* taste receptor gene selectively affects behavioral and neural taste

responses to sweeteners in the F_2 hybrids between C57BL/6ByJ and 129P3/J mice. *J. Neurosci.* 24:2296–303

79. Ishimaru Y, Inada H, Kubota M, Zhuang H, Tominaga M, Matsunami H. 2006. Transient receptor potential family members PKD1L3 and PKD2L1 form a candidate sour taste receptor. *Proc. Natl. Acad. Sci. USA* 103:12569–74
80. Jiang P, Cui M, Ji Q, Snyder L, Liu Z, et al. 2005. Molecular mechanisms of sweet receptor function. *Chem. Senses* 30(Suppl. 1):i17–18
81. Jiang P, Cui M, Zhao B, Liu Z, Snyder LA, et al. 2005. Lactisole interacts with the transmembrane domains of human T1R3 to inhibit sweet taste. *J. Biol. Chem.* 280:15238–46
82. Jiang P, Cui M, Zhao B, Snyder LA, Benard LM, et al. 2005. Identification of the cyclamate interaction site within the transmembrane domain of the human sweet taste receptor subunit T1R3. *J. Biol. Chem.* 280:34296–305
83. Jiang P, Ji Q, Liu Z, Snyder LA, Benard LM, et al. 2004. The cysteine-rich region of T1R3 determines responses to intensely sweet proteins. *J. Biol. Chem.* 279:45068–75
84. Kampov-Polevoy AB, Eick C, Boland G, Khalitov E, Crews FT. 2004. Sweet liking, novelty seeking, and gender predict alcoholic status. *Alcohol. Clin. Exp. Res.* 28:1291–98
85. Kellenberger S, Schild L. 2002. Epithelial sodium channel/degenerin family of ion channels: a variety of functions for a shared structure. *Physiol. Rev.* 82:735–67
86. Kim MR, Kusakabe Y, Miura H, Shindo Y, Ninomiya Y, Hino A. 2003. Regional expression patterns of taste receptors and gustducin in the mouse tongue. *Biochem. Biophys. Res. Commun.* 312:500–6
87. Kim U, Wooding S, Ricci D, Jorde LB, Drayna D. 2005. Worldwide haplotype diversity and coding sequence variation at human bitter taste receptor loci. *Hum. Mutat.* 26:199–204
88. Kim UK, Jorgenson E, Coon H, Leppert M, Risch N, Drayna D. 2003. Positional cloning of the human quantitative trait locus underlying taste sensitivity to phenylthiocarbamide. *Science* 299:1221–25
89. Kim UK, Wooding S, Riaz N, Jorde LB, Drayna D. 2006. Variation in the human TAS1R taste receptor genes. *Chem. Senses* 31:599–611
90. Kinnamon SC, Price MP, Stone LM, Lin W, Welsh MJ. 2000. The acid sensing ion channel BNC1 is not required for sour taste transduction. *13th Internat. Symp. Olfact. Taste* XIII:80 (Abstr.)
91. Kitagawa M, Kusakabe Y, Miura H, Ninomiya Y, Hino A. 2001. Molecular genetic identification of a candidate receptor gene for sweet taste. *Biochem. Biophys. Res. Commun.* 283:236–42
92. Kiuchi S, Yamada T, Kiyokawa N, Saito T, Fujimoto J, Yasue H. 2006. Genomic structure of swine taste receptor family 1 member 3, TAS1R3, and its expression in tissues. *Cytogenet. Genome Res.* 115:51–61
93. Kuhn C, Bufe B, Winnig M, Hofmann T, Frank O, et al. 2004. Bitter taste receptors for saccharin and acesulfame K. *J. Neurosci.* 24:10260–65
94. Laugerette F, Passilly-Degrace P, Patris B, Niot I, Febbraio M, et al. 2005. CD36 involvement in orosensory detection of dietary lipids, spontaneous fat preference, and digestive secretions. *J. Clin. Invest.* 115:3177–84
95. Le Roy I, Pager J, Roubertoux PL. 1999. Genetic dissection of gustatory sensitivity to bitterness (sucrose octaacetate) in mice. *CR Acad. Sci. III* 322:831–36
96. Levin BE, Routh VH, Kang L, Sanders NM, Dunn-Meynell AA. 2004. Neuronal glucosensing: What do we know after 50 years? *Diabetes* 53:2521–28

97. Li X, Bachmanov AA, Li S, Chen Z, Tordoff MG, et al. 2002. Genetic, physical and comparative map of the subtelomeric region of mouse chromosome 4. *Mamm. Genome* 13:5–19
98. Li X, Inoue M, Reed DR, Huque T, Puchalski RB, et al. 2001. High-resolution genetic mapping of the saccharin preference locus (*Sac*) and the putative sweet taste receptor (T1R1) gene (*Gpr70*) to mouse distal chromosome 4. *Mamm. Genome* 12:13–16
99. Li X, Li W, Wang H, Cao J, Maehashi K, et al. 2005. Pseudogenization of a sweet-receptor gene accounts for cats' indifference toward sugar. *PLoS Genet.* 1:27–35
100. Li X, Staszewski L, Xu H, Durick K, Zoller M, Adler E. 2002. Human receptors for sweet and umami taste. *Proc. Natl. Acad. Sci. USA* 99:4692–96
101. Liao J, Schultz PG. 2003. Three sweet receptor genes are clustered in human chromosome 1. *Mamm. Genome* 14:291–301
102. Lin W, Ogura T, Kinnamon SC. 2002. Acid-activated cation currents in rat vallate taste receptor cells. *J. Neurophysiol.* 88:133–41
103. Lindemann B. 1997. Sodium taste. *Curr. Opin. Nephrol. Hypertens.* 6:425–29
104. Liu L, Leonard AS, Motto DG, Feller MA, Price MP, et al. 2003. Contribution of *Drosophila* DEG/ENaC genes to salt taste. *Neuron* 39:133–46
105. Liu L, Simon SA. 2001. Acidic stimuli activates two distinct pathways in taste receptor cells from rat fungiform papillae. *Brain Res.* 923:58–70
106. LopezJimenez ND, Cavenagh MM, Sainz E, Cruz-Ithier MA, Battey JF, Sullivan SL. 2006. Two members of the TRPP family of ion channels, Pkd1l3 and Pkd2l1, are co-expressed in a subset of taste receptor cells. *J. Neurochem.* 98:68–77
107. Lu K, McDaniel AH, Tordoff MG, Li X, Beauchamp GK, et al. 2005. No relationship between sequence variation in protein coding regions of the *Tas1r3* gene and saccharin preference in rats. *Chem. Senses* 30:231–40
108. Lush IE. 1981. The genetics of tasting in mice. I. Sucrose octaacetate. *Genet. Res.* 38:93–95
109. Lush IE. 1982. The genetics of tasting in mice. II. Strychnine. *Chem. Senses* 7:93–98
110. Lush IE. 1984. The genetics of tasting in mice. III. Quinine. *Genet. Res.* 44:151–60
111. Lush IE. 1986. Differences between mouse strains in their consumption of phenylthiourea (PTC). *Heredity* 57:319–23
112. Lush IE. 1986. The genetics of tasting in mice. IV. The acetates of raffinose, galactose and b-lactose. *Genet. Res.* 47:117–23
113. Lush IE. 1989. The genetics of tasting in mice. VI. Saccharin, acesulfame, dulcin and sucrose. *Genet. Res.* 53:95–99
114. Lush IE, Holland G. 1988. The genetics of tasting in mice. V. Glycine and cycloheximide. *Genet. Res.* 52:207–12
115. Lush IE, Hornigold N, King P, Stoye JP. 1995. The genetics of tasting in mice. VII. Glycine revisited, and the chromosomal location of *Sac* and *Soa*. *Genet. Res.* 66:167–74
116. Lyall V, Alam RI, Phan DQ, Ereso GL, Phan TH, et al. 2001. Decrease in rat taste receptor cell intracellular pH is the proximate stimulus in sour taste transduction. *Am. J. Physiol. Cell Physiol.* 281:C1005–13
117. Lyall V, Heck GL, Vinnikova AK, Ghosh S, Phan TH, et al. 2004. The mammalian amiloride-insensitive nonspecific salt taste receptor is a vanilloid receptor-1 variant. *J. Physiol.* 558:147–59
118. Matsunami H, Montmayeur JP, Buck LB. 2000. A family of candidate taste receptors in human and mouse. *Nature* 404:601–4
119. Mattes RD. 2005. Fat taste and lipid metabolism in humans. *Physiol. Behav.* 86:691–97

120. Max M, Shanker YG, Huang L, Rong M, Liu Z, et al. 2001. *Tas1r3*, encoding a new candidate taste receptor, is allelic to the sweet responsiveness locus *Sac*. *Nat. Genet.* 28:58–63
121. Mennella JA, Pepino MY, Reed DR. 2005. Genetic and environmental determinants of bitter perception and sweet preferences. *Pediatrics* 115:e216–22
122. Meyerhof W. 2005. Elucidation of mammalian bitter taste. *Rev. Physiol. Biochem. Pharmacol.* 154:37–72
123. Montmayeur JP, Liberles SD, Matsunami H, Buck LB. 2001. A candidate taste receptor gene near a sweet taste locus. *Nat. Neurosci.* 4:492–98
124. Mueller KL, Hoon MA, Erlenbach I, Chandrashekar J, Zuker CS, Ryba NJ. 2005. The receptors and coding logic for bitter taste. *Nature* 434:225–29
125. Naim M, Nir S, Spielman AI, Noble AC, Peri I, et al. 2002. Hypothesis of receptor-dependent and receptor-independent mechanisms for bitter and sweet taste transduction: implications for slow taste onset and lingering aftertaste. In *Chemistry of Taste: Mechanisms, Behaviors, and Mimics. ACS Symposium Series; 825*, ed. P Given, D Parades, pp. 2–17. Washington, DC: Am. Chem. Soc.
126. Nelson G, Chandrashekar J, Hoon MA, Feng L, Zhao G, et al. 2002. An amino-acid taste receptor. *Nature* 416:199–202
127. Nelson G, Hoon MA, Chandrashekar J, Zhang Y, Ryba NJ, Zuker CS. 2001. Mammalian sweet taste receptors. *Cell* 106:381–90
128. Nelson TM, Munger SD, Boughter JD Jr. 2003. Taste sensitivities to PROP and PTC vary independently in mice. *Chem. Senses* 28:695–704
129. Nelson TM, Munger SD, Boughter JD Jr. 2005. Haplotypes at the Tas2r locus on distal chromosome 6 vary with quinine taste sensitivity in inbred mice. *BMC Genet.* 6:32
130. Nie Y, Vigues S, Hobbs JR, Conn GL, Munger SD. 2005. Distinct contributions of T1R2 and T1R3 taste receptor subunits to the detection of sweet stimuli. *Curr. Biol.* 15:1948–52
131. Ninomiya Y, Kajiura H, Mochizuki K. 1993. Differential taste responses of mouse chorda tympani and glossopharyngeal nerves to sugars and amino acids. *Neurosci. Lett.* 163:197–200
132. Ninomiya Y, Nakashima K, Fukuda A, Nishino H, Sugimura T, et al. 2000. Responses to umami substances in taste bud cells innervated by the chorda tympani and glossopharyngeal nerves. *J. Nutr.* 130:950–53S
133. Phillips TJ, Crabbe JC, Metten P, Belknap JK. 1994. Localization of genes affecting alcohol drinking in mice. *Alcohol. Clin. Exp. Res.* 18:931–41
134. Pin JP, Galvez T, Prezeau L. 2003. Evolution, structure, and activation mechanism of family 3/C G-protein-coupled receptors. *Pharmacol. Ther.* 98:325–54
135. Prodi DA, Drayna D, Forabosco P, Palmas MA, Maestrale GB, et al. 2004. Bitter taste study in a sardinian genetic isolate supports the association of phenylthiocarbamide sensitivity to the TAS2R38 bitter receptor gene. *Chem. Senses* 29:697–702
136. Ramirez I. 1992. Chemoreception for fat: Do rats sense triglycerides directly? *Appetite* 18:193–206
137. Reed DR, Li S, Li X, Huang L, Tordoff MG, et al. 2004. Polymorphisms in the taste receptor gene (*Tas1r3*) region are associated with saccharin preference in 30 mouse strains. *J. Neurosci.* 24:938–46
138. Reed DR, McDaniel AH. 2006. The human sweet tooth. *BMC Oral Health* 6(Suppl. 1):S17

139. Reed DR, Nanthakumar E, North M, Bell C, Bartoshuk LM, Price RA. 1999. Localization of a gene for bitter-taste perception to human chromosome 5p15. *Am. J. Hum. Genet.* 64:1478–80
140. Reed DR, Tanaka T, McDaniel AH. 2006. Diverse tastes: genetics of sweet and bitter perception. *Physiol. Behav.* 88:215–26
141. Richter TA, Caicedo A, Roper SD. 2003. Sour taste stimuli evoke Ca2+ and pH responses in mouse taste cells. *J. Physiol.* 547:475–83
142. Richter TA, Dvoryanchikov GA, Chaudhari N, Roper SD. 2004. Acid-sensitive two-pore domain potassium (K2P) channels in mouse taste buds. *J. Neurophysiol.* 92:1928–36
143. Richter TA, Dvoryanchikov GA, Roper SD, Chaudhari N. 2004. Acid-sensing ion channel-2 is not necessary for sour taste in mice. *J. Neurosci.* 24:4088–91
144. Rolls ET, Scott TR. 2003. Central taste anatomy and neurophysiology. In *Handbook of Olfaction and Gustation*, ed. RL Doty, pp. 679–705. New York: Marcel Dekker
145. Rosenzweig S, Yan W, Dasso M, Spielman AI. 1999. Possible novel mechanism for bitter taste mediated through cGMP. *J. Neurophysiol.* 81:1661–65
146. Rozengurt N, Wu SV, Chen MC, Huang C, Sternini C, Rozengurt E. 2006. Colocalization of the alpha-subunit of gustducin with PYY and GLP-1 in L cells of human colon. *Am. J. Physiol. Gastrointest. Liver Physiol.* 291:G792–802
147. Sainz E, Korley JN, Battey JF, Sullivan SL. 2001. Identification of a novel member of the T1R family of putative taste receptors. *J. Neurochem.* 77:896–903
148. San Gabriel A, Uneyama H, Yoshie S, Torii K. 2005. Cloning and characterization of a novel mGluR1 variant from vallate papillae that functions as a receptor for L-glutamate stimuli. *Chem. Senses* 30(Suppl. 1):i25–26
149. Sandell MA, Breslin PA. 2006. Variability in a taste-receptor gene determines whether we taste toxins in food. *Curr. Biol.* 16:R792–94
150. Sawano S, Seto E, Mori T, Hayashi Y. 2005. G-protein-dependent and -independent pathways in denatonium signal transduction. *Biosci. Biotechnol. Biochem.* 69:1643–51
151. Sclafani A. 2004. The sixth taste? *Appetite* 43:1–3
152. Scott TR, Giza BK, Yan J. 1999. Gustatory neural coding in the cortex of the alert cynomolgus macaque: the quality of bitterness. *J. Neurophysiol.* 81:60–71
153. Soranzo N, Bufe B, Sabeti PC, Wilson JF, Weale ME, et al. 2005. Positive selection on a high-sensitivity allele of the human bitter-taste receptor TAS2R16. *Curr. Biol.* 15:1257–65
154. Spector AC, Kopka SL. 2002. Rats fail to discriminate quinine from denatonium: implications for the neural coding of bitter-tasting compounds. *J. Neurosci.* 22:1937–41
155. Sternini C. 2007. Taste receptors in the gastrointestinal tract. IV. Functional implications of bitter taste receptors in gastrointestinal chemosensing. *Am. J. Physiol. Gastrointest. Liver Physiol.* 292:G457–61
156. Stevens DR, Seifert R, Bufe B, Muller F, Kremmer E, et al. 2001. Hyperpolarization-activated channels HCN1 and HCN4 mediate responses to sour stimuli. *Nature* 413:631–35
157. Tamames J, Valencia A. 2006. The success (or not) of HUGO nomenclature. *Genome Biol.* 7:402
158. Taniguchi K. 2004. Expression of the sweet receptor protein, T1R3, in the human liver and pancreas. *J. Vet. Med. Sci.* 66:1311–14
159. Tobach E, Bellin JS, Das DK. 1974. Differences in bitter taste perception in three strains of rats. *Behav. Genet.* 4:405–10

160. Toyono T, Seta Y, Kataoka S, Kawano S, Shigemoto R, Toyoshima K. 2003. Expression of metabotropic glutamate receptor group I in rat gustatory papillae. *Cell Tissue Res.* 313:29–35
161. Ueda T, Ugawa S, Ishida Y, Shibata Y, Murakami S, Shimada S. 2001. Identification of coding single-nucleotide polymorphisms in human taste receptor genes involving bitter tasting. *Biochem. Biophys. Res. Commun.* 285:147–51
162. Ugawa S. 2003. Identification of sour-taste receptor genes. *Anat. Sci. Int.* 78:205–10
163. Ugawa S, Minami Y, Guo W, Saishin Y, Takatsuji K, et al. 1998. Receptor that leaves a sour taste in the mouth. *Nature* 395:555–56
164. Ugawa S, Yamamoto T, Ueda T, Ishida Y, Inagaki A, et al. 2003. Amiloride-insensitive currents of the acid-sensing ion channel-2a (ASIC2a)/ASIC2b heteromeric sour-taste receptor channel. *J. Neurosci.* 23:3616–22
165. Vinnikova AK, Alam RI, Malik SA, Ereso GL, Feldman GM, et al. 2004. Na+-H+ exchange activity in taste receptor cells. *J. Neurophysiol.* 91:1297–313
166. Waldmann R, Lazdunski M. 1998. H(+)-gated cation channels: neuronal acid sensors in the NaC/DEG family of ion channels. *Curr. Opin. Neurobiol.* 8:418–24
167. Wang X, Thomas SD, Zhang J. 2004. Relaxation of selective constraint and loss of function in the evolution of human bitter taste receptor genes. *Hum. Mol. Genet.* 13:2671–78
168. Whitney G, Harder DB. 1986. Single locus control of sucrose octaacetate tasting among mice. *Behav. Genet.* 16:559–74
169. Winnig M, Bufe B, Meyerhof W. 2005. Valine 738 and lysine 735 in the fifth transmembrane domain of rTas1r3 mediate insensitivity towards lactisole of the rat sweet taste receptor. *BMC Neurosci.* 6:22
170. Witt M, Reutter K, Miller IJ. 2003. Morphology of peripheral taste system. In *Handbook of Olfaction and Gustation*, ed. RL Doty, pp. 651–77. New York: Marcel Dekker
171. Wong GT, Gannon KS, Margolskee RF. 1996. Transduction of bitter and sweet taste by gustducin. *Nature* 381:796–800
172. Wooding S, Bufe B, Grassi C, Howard MT, Stone AC, et al. 2006. Independent evolution of bitter-taste sensitivity in humans and chimpanzees. *Nature* 440:930–34
173. Wooding S, Kim UK, Bamshad MJ, Larsen J, Jorde LB, Drayna D. 2004. Natural selection and molecular evolution in PTC, a bitter-taste receptor gene. *Am. J. Hum. Genet.* 74:637–46
174. Wu SV, Chen MC, Rozengurt E. 2005. Genomic organization, expression, and function of bitter taste receptors (T2R) in mouse and rat. *Physiol. Genomics* 22:139–49
175. Wu SV, Rozengurt N, Yang M, Young SH, Sinnett-Smith J, Rozengurt E. 2002. Expression of bitter taste receptors of the T2R family in the gastrointestinal tract and enteroendocrine STC-1 cells. *Proc. Natl. Acad. Sci. USA* 99:2392–97
176. Xu H, Staszewski L, Tang H, Adler E, Zoller M, Li X. 2004. Different functional roles of T1R subunits in the heteromeric taste receptors. *Proc. Natl. Acad. Sci. USA* 101:14258–63
177. Zhang X, Fitzsimmons RL, Cleland LG, Ey PL, Zannettino AC, et al. 2003. CD36/fatty acid translocase in rats: distribution, isolation from hepatocytes, and comparison with the scavenger receptor SR-B1. *Lab Invest.* 83:317–32
178. Zhang Y, Hoon MA, Chandrashekar J, Mueller KL, Cook B, et al. 2003. Coding of sweet, bitter, and umami tastes. Different receptor cells sharing similar signaling pathways. *Cell* 112:293–301
179. Zhao GQ, Zhang Y, Hoon MA, Chandrashekar J, Erlenbach I, et al. 2003. The receptors for mammalian sweet and umami taste. *Cell* 115:255–66

The Ketogenic Diet and Brain Metabolism of Amino Acids: Relationship to the Anticonvulsant Effect

Marc Yudkoff,[1] Yevgeny Daikhin,[1]
Torun Margareta Melø,[2] Ilana Nissim,[1]
Ursula Sonnewald,[2] and Itzhak Nissim[1]

[1]Children's Hospital of Philadelphia and Department of Pediatrics, University of Pennsylvania School of Medicine, Philadelphia, Pennsylvania, [2]Department of Neuroscience, Norwegian University of Science and Technology, NTNU, N-7489, Trondheim, Norway; email: yudkoff@email.chop.edu

Annu. Rev. Nutr. 2007. 27:415–30

First published online as a Review in Advance on April 19, 2007

The *Annual Review of Nutrition* is online at http://nutr.annualreviews.org

This article's doi:
10.1146/annurev.nutr.27.061406.093722

0199-9885/07/0821-0415$20.00

Key Words

ketosis, brain amino acid metabolism, epilepsy, anticonvulsant therapy

Abstract

In many epileptic patients, anticonvulsant drugs either fail adequately to control seizures or they cause serious side effects. An important adjunct to pharmacologic therapy is the ketogenic diet, which often improves seizure control, even in patients who respond poorly to medications. The mechanisms that explain the therapeutic effect are incompletely understood. Evidence points to an effect on brain handling of amino acids, especially glutamic acid, the major excitatory neurotransmitter of the central nervous system. The diet may limit the availability of oxaloacetate to the aspartate aminotransferase reaction, an important route of brain glutamate handling. As a result, more glutamate becomes accessible to the glutamate decarboxylase reaction to yield gamma-aminobutyric acid (GABA), the major inhibitory neurotransmitter and an important antiseizure agent. In addition, the ketogenic diet appears to favor the synthesis of glutamine, an essential precursor to GABA. This occurs both because ketone body carbon is metabolized to glutamine and because in ketosis there is increased consumption of acetate, which astrocytes in the brain quickly convert to glutamine. The ketogenic diet also may facilitate mechanisms by which the brain exports to blood compounds such as glutamine and alanine, in the process favoring the removal of glutamate carbon and nitrogen.

Contents

INTRODUCTION

The development of effective antiepileptic drugs has been a major achievement of neuroscience research. Unfortunately, these medications often fail completely to control convulsions or they cause obnoxious and even incapacitating side effects (13). This therapeutic limitation has prompted a continuing search for new drugs and alternate treatments.

One such intervention is the ketogenic diet, which clinicians commonly recommend when drug therapy proves suboptimal (35, 133, 134, 140). The diet can be remarkably effective—at least 50% of patients experience a reduction in seizure frequency of 50%, and many show complete and sustained remission (36, 55, 61, 78, 117, 123). The diet has been shown effective against different forms of epilepsy and in different patient cohorts, including adolescents and older individuals (56, 57, 65). Even a milder form of a low-carbohydrate diet (e.g., Atkins diet) may have a therapeutic effect (55).

An advantage of the diet is the relative absence of side effects, particularly the obtundation, memory loss, and other cognitive deficits that often accompany administration of antiepileptic drugs. There are no major effects on growth or weight (124). Hyperlipidemia may occur (58), but it is unclear if this perturbation is atherogenic. A recent review (9) of low-carbohydrate diets found no cogent evidence of major adverse effects on blood pressure, blood glucose, serum insulin, or blood lipids.

A ketogenic diet provides 80%–90% of calories as lipid, most frequently long-chain triglycerides, with the remainder deriving primarily from protein (61, 114). An alternate approach is to furnish lipid as medium-chain triglycerides, a more palatable strategy, but one that can cause diarrhea and cramping. Induction of ketosis traditionally is accomplished with a brief (24- to 48-hour) period of fasting, but a recent report suggests that gradual introduction of a high-fat diet results in brisk ketosis (>1.5 mM) and a robust therapeutic effect (4). A diet that provides a greater fraction of fat (>60%) as the polyunsaturated or monounsaturated species affords more intense ketosis (37).

An important and unresolved issue is whether the antiepileptic effect derives from a direct action of ketone bodies on brain physiology or results from a limitation of dietary carbohydrate and/or caloric restriction, both of which lower the blood glucose concentration. Caloric restriction confers seizure control in EL mice, a model of human multifactorial idiopathic epilepsy (43, 67). Dietary caloric restriction lowers neuronal activity in the dentate gyrus (8) and protects rats against the action of pentylenetetrazole, a convulsant (29). Extreme caloric restriction (50%) lowers seizures as effectively as the ketogenic diet and does so without greatly increasing blood ketones (8, 29).

The ketogenic diet is today an accepted therapeutic modality, but formidable scientific and ethical obstacles complicate performance of carefully controlled, long-term clinical studies of efficacy. An unresolved issue is the nature of the many physiologic and biochemical responses of brain function that the diet presumably evokes. Research suggests several hypothetical mechanisms: (*a*) A high-fat, low-carbohydrate diet favors production of 3-OH-butyric acid and acetoacetic acid, the "ketone bodies," perhaps acidifying the brain parenchyma and inhibiting neuronal H^+-sensitive ion channels. However, there is no cogent evidence that such acidification occurs (1). (*b*) Ketosis may hyperpolarize neuronal membranes through an effect of ketone bodies or long-chain fatty acids on adenosine triphosphate (ATP)-sensitive K^+ channels (120). (*c*) Fatty acids may directly inhibit neuronal function (21); (*d*) acetone, which quickly enters brain (40), diminishes seizure threshold and severity (62); (*e*) glucose, even in physiologic concentration, may increase neuronal excitability (11), and hyperglycemia lowers the seizure threshold (103). Conversely, a diminution of blood glucose, which ought to occur with a low-carbohydrate diet, might lower neuronal excitability and thereby attenuate an epileptic diathesis. However, it should be noted that a ketogenic diet enhances brain glucose transport (17), thereby maintaining central nervous system glucose concentrations even though blood levels are diminished. (*f*) Recent investigations in mice lacking dopamine-β-hydroxylase suggest that an intact noradenergic system is necessary to recruit the therapeutic effect (115), suggesting that the diet may alter metabolism and/or function of brain biogenic amines. (*g*) Increased concentrations of fatty acids enhance both the levels and the activity of mitochondrial uncoupling protein (71, 112, 113), a phenomenon that might explain the protective effect of the diet against disorders such as glutamate toxicity (77), traumatic brain injury (96), and Parkinsonism (119).

In addition to these effects, a ketogenic diet alters brain energy metabolism (23, 26, 31, 59, 86, 99, 138–142). Ketone bodies may be a more efficient fuel than glucose in terms of energy produced per mole of oxygen consumed (99). In isolated heart, the administration of 3-OH-butyrate significantly increased (2–10 times) the nicotinamide adenine dinucleotide, reduced form/nicotinamide adenine dinucleotide (NADH/NAD) ratio and diminished (2–4 times) the mitochondrial coenzyme Q couple (99). As a consequence, energy released from oxidation of mitochondrial NADH increased from –53 kJ/mol to –60 kJ/mol. The ability of ketone bodies to increase energy produced per mole of oxygen consumed may favor restoration of membrane potential following depolarization and may diminish free radical production (121, 122).

The partial substitution of ketone bodies for glucose as a fuel also may alter brain handling of amino acids like glutamate and gamma-aminobutyric acid (GABA), the major excitatory and inhibitory neurotransmitters, respectively (91). Thus, the anticonvulsant effect might enhance inhibitory versus excitatory tone in neurons. To understand how a high-fat and low-carbohydrate diet could affect brain amino acid metabolism, we must review interrelationships between cerebral handling of glucose, glutamate, and GABA.

BRAIN METABOLISM OF GLUCOSE

The human brain consumes more than 300 kcal/kg/day. Whole-body energy expenditure in adult humans is about one-tenth this value. The brain satisfies this voracious demand by extracting from blood about 10% of the glucose of the arterial blood, or 310 μmol/kg/min, and about 50% of oxygen in arterial blood, or 1560 μmol/kg/min (53). Since whole-body oxygen use is about 8000 μmol/kg/min, it follows that the brain, which comprises only 2% of body weight, utilizes nearly 20% of overall oxygen consumption. If glucose oxidation is complete, then the stoichiometry of glucose metabolism ($C_6H_{12}O_6 + 6O_2 \rightarrow 6\,CO_2 + 6\,H_2O$) requires that consumption of oxygen must exceed that of glucose by a factor of six rather than the observed ratio (1560/310) of about five. This discrepancy in part reflects the fact that brain glucose oxidation is incomplete, with some glucose being converted to lactate, not CO_2. In addition, a small component of overall oxygen consumption is applied not to glucose oxidation but to the synthesis of macromolecules (19, 66, 106).

Cerebral metabolism is intense for several reasons. Brain cells must maintain extraordinarily high cross-membrane gradients of ions and neurotransmitters. Depolarization of neurons partially dissipates such gradients, the restoration of which obliges vigorous consumption of ATP by astrocytes and neurons. Energy also goes to support the several anabolic functions of brain, including a very active rate of synthesis of proteins and lipids as well as the formation of a key intermediate, glutamine, the synthesis of which consumes ATP.

The oxidation of glucose provides essentially all energy needed to maintain cerebral function. Glycolysis may be relatively more prominent in some cells or in specific subcellular compartments. Thus, the filopodia of astrocytes are too narrow to accommodate mitochondria, and these cells will activate glycolysis (and glycogenolysis) in order to provide the energy that maintains their vital function of removing from the synaptic cleft much of the glutamate and K^+ that presynaptic neuronal terminals release upon depolarization (24, 46). The fate of the pyruvate generated via glycolysis remains a topic of active inquiry and debate. It may be that astrocytes do not immediately oxidize all pyruvate produced via glycolysis. Instead, they may convert some pyruvate to lactate and release the latter to the extracellular fluid, from which neurons extract it and oxidize it as a fuel. Neurons can respire on lactate (102), but they may require glucose as a substrate if they are to maintain large internal pools of glutamate and aspartate (125). Astrocytic release of lactate and subsequent neuronal oxidation may constitute a mechanism by which neuronal and metabolic activity are effectively coupled (33, 66).

Brain glucose metabolism is complex for yet another reason. Extremely rapid transamination of oxaloacetate and 2-oxo-glutarate—key intermediates of the tricarboxylic acid cycle—means that as glucose carbon traverses the cycle, it is in near immediate equilibrium with very large intracellular pools of aspartate and glutamate (72, 143). Extensive compartmentation of these pools has been shown (108, 128). The amino group of glutamate is transferred to glutamine, alanine, and GABA, all of which are present in high concentration in the nervous system. Thus, the flow of glucose carbon seldom, if ever, conforms to the "simple" sequence: glucose → pyruvate → tricarboxylic acid cycle → CO_2. Instead, glucose carbon passes through several amino acid pools, each of which pursues its own idiosyncratic fate, depending upon cell type and metabolic exigencies.

This interaction between metabolism of glucose and that of amino acids suggested to us (23, 31, 75, 138–142) that administration of a ketogenic diet might alter brain handling of neuroactive compounds such as glutamate and GABA. Our rationale was that a dietary regimen that sharply limits carbohydrate intake and obliges a shift in cerebral respiration to fuels other than glucose would have far-reaching implications for the handling of amino acids. Furthermore, we considered that the antiepileptic effect of the ketogenic diet could derive in part from a change in brain metabolism of glutamate. In order better to delineate this hypothetical effect, a short summary of brain glutamate handling is necessary.

BRAIN HANDLING OF GLUTAMATE

Glutamic acid is the major excitatory neurotransmitter (74, 91). In order to maximize the signal-to-noise ratio upon release of glutamate from presynaptic terminals, the glutamate concentration in the synaptic cleft must be maintained at a very low level. Another reason why brain cells keep synaptic glutamate low is that untoward accumulations of this amino acid excessively stimulate postsynaptic neurons, thereby causing the excitotoxicity that plays a role in diverse forms of brain injury, including hypoxia, traumatic brain injury, and epilepsy (82, 101, 131). The role of removing glutamate from the synapse falls primarily to astrocytes (24, 39, 47, 116), which have extremely effective

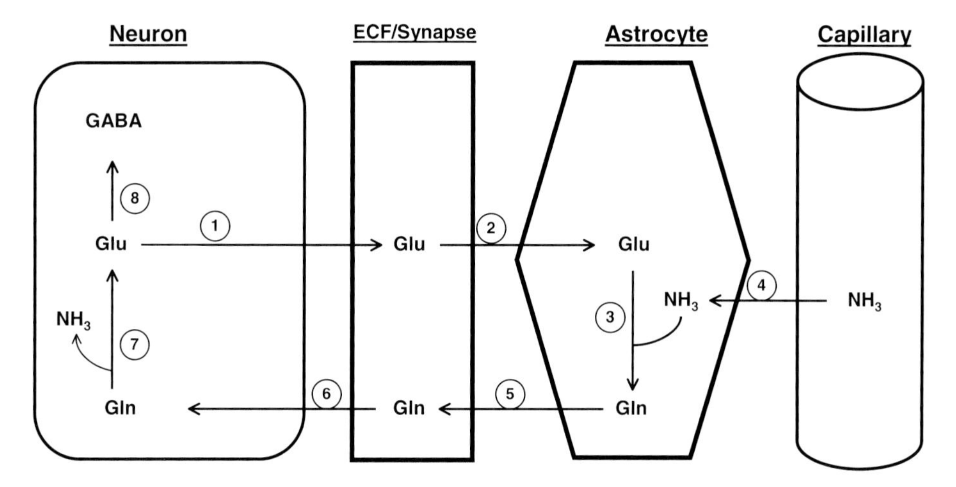

Figure 1

The glutamate-glutamine cycle. Glutamate is released (*1*) from presynaptic terminals into the ECF/synapse, where it stimulates postsynaptic glutamatergic receptors. High-affinity astrocytic transport systems (*2*) quickly remove glutamate from the synapse and convert it to glutamine in the astrocytic glutamine synthetase pathway (*3*). Ammonia diffuses from blood and neurons (*4*) to provide a coreactant for glutamine synthetase. Astrocytes release glutamine (*5*) via specific transport systems. Neurons subsequently take up the glutamine (*6*) via neutral amino acid transporters. Neuronal mitochondria then hydrolyze glutamine to glutamate (7), in the process completing the cycle. ECF, extracellular fluid; GABA, gamma-aminobutyric acid; Gln, glutamine; Glu, glutamate; NH_3, ammonia.

glutamate transporters on the cell surface (2). A relatively high astrocytic membrane potential facilitates uptake of glutamate via Na^+-dependent transport systems (32). In cerebellum, neuronal uptake may be important (84).

A mechanism must exist for the restoration of glutamate to neurons following glial uptake of this amino acid. Astrocytic transfer of glutamate to neurons would invite the risk of depolarization as this neurotransmitter traverses the extracellular fluid. Thus, a strategy evolved that involves astrocytic conversion of glutamate to glutamine via the glutamine synthetase reaction (glutamate + NH_3 + ATP $\rightarrow$ glutamine + ADP +P_i), an almost exclusively glial enzyme (69, 79). The coreactant ammonia derives from blood (20), although during periods of heightened activity, the oxidation of glutamate can yield ammonia (94). Specific transport systems enable the release of glutamine from astrocytes and subsequent uptake into neurons (16, 51), which hydrolyze this amino acid to glutamate and ammonia via phosphate-activated glutaminase (109).

The cycle starting with neuronal glutamate release, proceeding through glutamine formation in astrocytes and terminating in glutamine hydrolysis in neuronal mitochondria is termed the "glutamate-glutamine cycle" (GGC) (**Figure 1**). This anatomical and biochemical network has long been the central figuration in all formulations of brain amino acid metabolism (104).

A great deal of experimental evidence now supports the main elements of the GGC, but this model oversimplifies important aspects of brain amino acid handling. Thus, the model fails to account for the external sources of nitrogen that must be imported in order to maintain homeostasis. Losses of nitrogen from the system are inevitable, although the mechanisms by which brain exports nitrogen are not well understood. The uptake from blood to brain of either glutamine or glutamate is quite limited (44, 107).

Attention has centered on leucine as a probable external source of nitrogen to replace that lost from oxidative processes.

Leucine readily passes into brain, where it is quickly transaminated to yield glutamate and 2-oxo-isocaproic acid (ketoleucine) (6, 50, 137). Magnetic resonance spectroscopy studies utilizing [^{15}N]leucine as a metabolic probe suggest that leucine is the source of as much as one-third of all brain nitrogen (52). Valine and isoleucine, the other branched-chain amino acids, may increase this contribution to as high as 50%.

The GCC oversimplifies the fact that amino acids like glutamate, aspartate, and GABA not only are neurotransmitters, but also are pivotal metabolic intermediates through which glucose carbon must pass during its journey through the tricarboxylic acid cycle. This comes about because the transamination of 2-oxo-glutarate in the aspartate aminotransferase reaction affords a near-immediate articulation between the cycle and the very substantial pools of brain amino acids:

$$\alpha\text{-keto-glutarate} + \text{aspartate} \leftrightarrow \text{glutamate} + \text{oxaloacetate}$$

$$\text{glutamate} \rightarrow \text{GABA} + CO_2$$

We might anticipate that a shift in brain metabolism away from glucose to ketone bodies as metabolic substrate should invite changes in the handling of glutamate and related compounds. As we discuss in the section below, some experimental evidence suggests that precisely such an adaptation may occur.

INTERACTIONS OF METABOLISM OF KETONE BODIES AND OF GLUTAMIC ACID

Ingestion of a diet low in carbohydrate and high (80%–90% of calories) in lipid increases hepatic production of 3-OH-butyrate and acetoacetate from fatty acids. The liver does not consume ketone bodies. Instead, it exports them to peripheral tissues, among them the brain, which utilize ketone bodies as a metabolic substrate. Once the blood concentration of 3-OH-butyrate rises to 2–4 mM, the ketone bodies furnish as much as 70% of cerebral metabolic requirements, thereby replacing glucose as the major fuel (12, 85).

If ketosis is sufficiently intense and longstanding, the brain recruits monocarboxylate transporters that facilitate uptake of ketone bodies from blood (18, 93). Both neurons and glia accumulate and oxidize ketone bodies, with uptake being directly related to the blood concentration. It should be emphasized that at certain stages of development, ketone bodies are utilized not only as a metabolic substrate but also as a source of acetyl-CoA that is a precursor to myelin, especially during early development, when brain myelin synthesis is extremely high (41, 54, 63). It is noteworthy in this regard that the relatively high fat content of maternal milk favors ketosis (28, 76).

The initial step in ketone body oxidation is convertion of 3-OH-butyrate to acetoacetate via β-hydroxybutyrate dehydrogenase, a NAD-dependent enzyme. In the succinyl-coenzyme A (CoA) transferase reaction, a very active pathway in brain (38), acetoacetate becomes converted to acetoacetyl-CoA and succinate, the latter then being oxidized via succinate dehydrogenase of the tricarboxylic acid cycle. A thiolase then hydrolyzes acetoacetyl-CoA to acetyl-CoA, which condenses with oxaloacetate to yield citrate in the citrate synthase pathway.

It might be thought that whether brain consumes glucose or 3-OH-butyrate should make no difference to brain biochemistry and physiology. Oxidation of either fuel leads ultimately to the production of ATP via the electron transport chain. However, there are important differences in the biochemical mechanisms that mediate the oxidation of the two fuels. **Figure 2** (see color insert) illustrates salient features of the impact of ketone body oxidation on brain glutamate handling. Glucose metabolism presupposes flow through glycolysis to yield pyruvate, which mitochondria decarboxylate to acetyl-CoA in the pyruvate dehydrogenase reaction. In addition, glycolysis results in synthesis of NADH, which

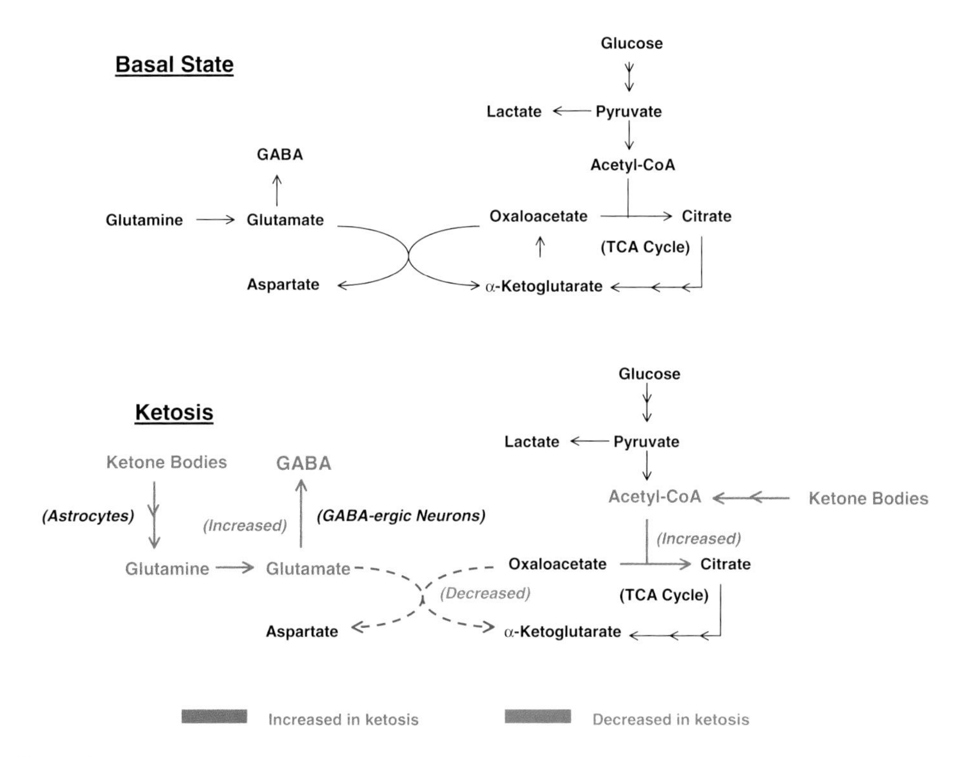

Figure 2

The impact of ketone body metabolism on brain handling of glutamate. Under basal conditions, glucose is the sole fuel of brain metabolism (*upper half of figure*). Glucose is converted to pyruvate via glycolysis, and pyruvate is converted to acetyl-CoA, which enters the tricarboxylic acid cycle. Glutamic acid is formed via transamination of α-ketoglutarate with aspartate. When an individual consumes a ketogenic diet and blood levels of 3-OH-butyrate and acetoacetate increase, the brain will consume these compounds as well as glucose (*lower half of figure*). Unlike glucose, the metabolism of which yields energy during conversion to pyruvate and lactate via glycolysis, the ketone bodies must be converted to acetyl-CoA, which is metabolized via citrate synthetase (acetyl-CoA + oxaloacetate → citrate + CoA), thereby diminishing the availability of oxaloacetate for transamination of glutamate to aspartate. More glutamate is then available to the glutamate decarboxylase pathway for the synthesis of GABA in GABA-ergic neurons. In addition, in ketosis there is increased blood acetate (or acetylcarnitine). Astrocytes, the major site of acetate consumption, convert this substrate to glutamine, which can be exported to GABA-ergic neurons, which convert this precursor to GABA, the major inhibitory neurotransmitter. The red lettering indicates pathways that are relatively more intense in ketosis, and the blue lettering indicates pathways that become relatively more attenuated.

the malate-aspartate shuttle transports to mitochondria.

In contrast to the oxidation of glucose, which involves glycolysis in the cytosol, the oxidation of ketone bodies occurs only in mitochondria and directly to acetyl-CoA, the concentration of which is increased in brain of ketotic mice (139). Ketone body metabolism does not involve formation of an intermediate such as pyruvate. As indicated above, when glucose is virtually the sole metabolic substrate of brain, glycolysis is not only a major route of astrocyte glucose metabolism, but the glia may convert some pyruvate to lactate and release the latter to the extracellular fluid (66). Thus, a salient metabolic difference between brain respiring solely on glucose and brain respiring on glucose/ketone bodies is that, in the latter instance, there is (*a*) enhanced formation of acetyl-CoA, (*b*) increased flux through the citrate synthetase reaction (acetyl-CoA + oxaloacetate → citrate), and (*c*) increased flux through the tricarboxylic acid cycle. This phenomenon was reflected in the recent study of Melo et al. (75), who administered [1-^{13}C]glucose and [1, 2-^{13}C]acetate in order to trace neuronal and glial metabolism, respectively, in rats that received a ketogenic diet for 21 days. Flux through glycolysis was diminished in neurons, and consumption of acetate was increased in astrocytes, the major site of brain acetate metabolism (5, 15, 130).

Both acetate consumption and glutamine synthesis are primarily glial functions (5, 15, 69, 79, 130), and blood acetate and acetylcarnitine probably increase in the ketotic individual (100). Thus, ketosis is associated with augmented astrocytic production of glutamine from acetate, as our groups independently demonstrated in studies with [1-^{13}C]acetate and [1, 2-^{13}C]acetate (75, 139).

As indicated above, acetyl-CoA must "enter" the tricarboxylic acid cycle via citrate synthetase, an extremely active reaction in brain with a maximal velocity that exceeds flow through pyruvate dehydrogenase by a factor of 10 (98). In synaptosomes, flux through pyruvate dehydrogenase scarcely equals overall metabolic rate (30). Intensified flow of acetyl-CoA through citrate synthetase (acetyl-CoA + oxaloacetate → citrate) tends to diminish the concentration of oxaloacetate, thereby limiting transamination of glutamate to aspartate, a major route of brain glutamate metabolism (31, 70, 72, 143, 138) (**Figure 2**). Transamination of glutamate to aspartate via aspartate aminotransferase, an equilibrium enzyme, depends in large measure upon the size of the oxaloacetate pool. If the latter if reduced in ketotic brain, then formation of aspartate will be diminished (26, 138).

We probed this hypothesis (138) by incubating cultured astrocytes with [^{15}N]glutamate and following appearance of label in [^{15}N]aspartate. In the presence of acetoacetate (5 mM), we noted a significant reduction in the glutamate → aspartate exchange. No change was observed with regard to the intra-astrocytic glutamate concentration, suggesting that glial uptake of glutamate was unaffected. Reductions in brain aspartate concentration have been seen in suckling mice that were injected with ketone bodies (118) and in rats on a high-fat diet (26). Our recent study of animals ketotic for 21 days did not show a diminution of total brain aspartate, but reduced production of [2-^{13}C]aspartate from [1-^{13}C]glucose (75).

Attenuated transamination of glutamate to aspartate in ketosis might contribute to an antiepileptic effect. Glutamate transamination to aspartate increases after depolarization (72, 90, 126), and extracellular aspartate increases postseizure (14, 27). Aspartate is an excitatory neurotransmitter that may have a role in the pathogenesis of hippocampal epilepsy (34, 68, 73, 97).

Reduced conversion of glutamate to aspartate might favor decarboxylation of glutamate to GABA (glutamate → GABA + CO_2). GABA is the major inhibitory neurotransmitter and a likely antiepileptic factor (25, 42, 48, 60, 64, 73, 83, 92, 132). It might be thought that the brain glutamate concentration (8–10 mM) saturates glutamate decarboxylase

(K_m 0.1–1.2 mM), but the glutamate level may be much lower in GABA-ergic neurons (110, 111), and less than 5% of total brain glutamate is precursor to GABA (87, 88) in GABA-ergic neurons, which constitute less than 20% of neurons. Furthermore, flux through glutamate decarboxylase (~0.5 nmol/min/mg protein) is rigorously controlled and much lower than maximal enzyme activity (3). Thus, small fluctuations of ambient internal glutamate affect GABA synthesis (89). Finally, several factors influence binding of glutamate to the decarboxylase, including Cl^- and aspartate (95, 135).

Studies in synaptosomes (31) showed an increase in GABA concentration as well as GABA synthesis upon exposure to a high (5 mM) concentration of acetoacetate. Thus, incubations with either L-[^{15}N]glutamine or L-[2, 3, 3, 4, 4-d_5]glutamine (0.5 mM each) were associated with sharply higher levels of [^{15}N]GABA or [$^2H_4$]GABA. The intrasynaptosomal level of aspartic acid was diminished in the presence of acetoacetate, suggesting a relative diversion of glutamate carbon from transamination and toward decarboxylation (31).

The source of GABA in these studies was glutamine, which neurons cleave to glutamate via phosphate-dependent glutaminase (109). Glutamine is an efficient GABA precursor that GABA-ergic terminals readily transport. Yudkoff et al. (139) found that ketosis increases brain [^{13}C]glutamine synthesis from injected [1-^{13}C]acetate. Melo et al. (75) reported increased formation of both [4, 5-^{13}C]glutamate and [4, 5-^{13}C]glutamine in epilepsy-prone animals (GAER rats) following intraperitoneal injections of [1, 2-^{13}C]acetate. The augmented ^{13}C-glutamine synthesis in part reflects heightened activity of pyruvate carboxylase, which in brain is a glial enzyme (105) that serves the anaplerotic function of restoring to the tricarboxylic acid cycle the carbon that is "lost" consequent to transamination of α-ketoglutarate to glutamate. Thus, in ketosis, overall astrocyte metabolism appeared to be increased, resulting in increased availability of glutamine, a good precursor to GABA, particularly at moments of heightened neuronal activity.

The latter point deserves some emphasis. The putative relationship between the ketogenic diet, the antiepileptic effect, and brain GABA synthesis may not necessarily imply an increased steady-state GABA concentration but an increased capacity for GABA synthesis. Indeed, Melo et al. (75) observed only a modest (~13%) and statistically insignificant increase of the GABA level in the cerebral cortex of ketotic rats. However, they found that ketosis caused a greater fraction of glutamate carbon to flow into GABA, a finding similar to that noted in synaptosomes (31). It may be that the antiepileptic effect derives from the capacity of the system to generate GABA in response to relatively intense neuronal depolarization.

Recent reports in humans suggest that the ketogenic diet might affect brain GABA metabolism. Wang et al. (129) utilized magnetic resonance spectroscopy to study brain GABA concentrations in three patients before and a few months after administration of a ketogenic diet. In one individual, the level of GABA did not increase and may even have declined by ~12% after three months of therapy. However, in the two other subjects, the brain GABA concentration increased by 52% and 34%, respectively. Dahlin et al. (22) measured amino acid levels in the cerebrospinal fluid of children at approximately four months after initiation of a ketogenic diet. They found a significant (~11%) increase of the GABA concentration. No significant change was observed in the spinal fluid level of either glutamate or aspartate, but the concentration of alanine was diminished significantly (by nearly 25%). Of note is the observation that the increase of GABA level was greatest in subjects who were rated "very good" responders to the diet. In these individuals, the pre- and postdiet levels were 4.47 and 4.8 μM, respectively. Similarly, in "good" responders, the cognate values were 3.24 and 3.77 μM. In contrast, in patients who failed to respond, the pre- and postspinal fluid GABA concentrations were 2.55 and 2.79 μM, respectively.

KETOGENIC DIET AND BRAIN AMINO ACID TRANSPORT

Ketosis increases the entry of leucine to brain as well as the concentration of branched-chain amino acids (140). These compounds enter brain via the L transporter, which exchanges large neutral amino acids for brain glutamine (7, 10, 49). A high brain glutamine concentration favors this process, although affinity of the transporter for glutamine is not high (136). Importation of leucine and other branched-chain amino acids might be favored in ketosis, when the blood:brain ratio for leucine is increased and that for glutamine may be decreased (139). The exit of glutamine from brain would favor removal of glutamate, especially during heightened neuronal activity, when glial uptake of glutamate and formation of glutamine are intense (45). This "loss" of nitrogen eventually would be compensated by transamination of newly imported leucine (50, 137), but the system would have at its disposal an accessory mechanism for the momentary removal of glutamate when synaptic concentrations of this neurotransmitter are high.

Trafficking of amino acids among brain cells and between brain and capillaries involves a dense and tightly controlled network of transporters (10, 45). Rates of amino acid exchange among these compartments depend on both intrinsic properties of the transporters and relative concentrations in brain and blood. These mechanisms have not been scrutinized in the context of the ketogenic diet, but such nutritional intervention likely alters these relationships. For example, we recently observed a sharp decrease in the brain:blood ratio in the concentration of alanine in animals after a short fast (142). Alanine may be an important shuttle of $-NH_2$ groups among brain cells (127), and sodium-dependent amino acid transporters are present on the abluminal surface of brain capillaries (81). Release of alanine and other neutral amino acids down a "favorable" concentration gradient in ketosis might abet removal from brain of glutamate N. Systems for the direct export of glutamate exist (45, 80) and could assume heightened importance in ketosis if blood levels of glutamate and aspartate are diminished.

ACKNOWLEDGMENT

Supported by grants HD269711, RR00240, U54RR019453, U54RR023567, and DK047870 from NIH.

LITERATURE CITED

1. Al-Mudallal AS, LaManna JC, Lust WD, Harik SI. 1996. Diet-induced ketosis does not cause cerebral acidosis. *Epilepsia* 37:258–61
2. Amara SG, Fontana AC. 2002. Excitatory amino acid transporters: keeping up with glutamate. *Neurochem. Int.* 41:313–18
3. Battaglioli G, Martin DL. 1990. Stimulation of synaptosomal γ-aminobutyric acid synthesis by glutamate and glutamine. *J. Neurochem.* 54:1179–87
4. Bergqvist AG, Schall JI, Gallagher PR, Cnaan A, Stallings VA. 2005. Fasting versus gradual initiation of the ketogenic diet: a prospective, randomized clinical trial of efficacy. *Epilepsia* 46:1810–19
5. Berl S, Takagaki G, Clarke DD, Waelsch H. 1962. Metabolic compartments in vivo. Ammonia and glutamic acid metabolism in brain and liver. *J. Biol. Chem.* 237:2562–69

6. Bixel MG, Hutson SM, Hamprecht B. 1997. Cellular distribution of branched-chain amino acid aminotransferase isoenzymes among rat brain glial cells in culture. *J. Histochem. Cytochem.* 45:685–94
7. Boado RJ, Li JY, Nagaya M, Zhang C, Pardridge WM. 1999. Selective expression of the large neutral amino acid transporter at the blood-brain barrier. *Proc. Natl. Acad. Sci. USA* 96:12079–84
8. Bough KJ, Schwartzkroin PA, Rho JM. 2003. Calorie restriction and ketogenic diet diminish neuronal excitability in rat dentate gyrus in vivo. *Epilepsia* 44:752–60
9. Bravata DM, Sanders L, Huang J, Krumholz HM, Olkin I, et al. 2003. Efficacy and safety of low-carbohydrate diets: a systematic review. *JAMA* 289:1837–50
10. Broer S, Brookes N. 2001. Transfer of glutamine between astrocytes and neurons. *J. Neurochem.* 77:705–19
11. Burdakov D, Gerasimenko O, Verkhratsky A. 2005. Physiological changes in glucose differentially modulate the excitability of hypothalamic melanin-concentrating hormone and orexin neurons in situ. *J. Neurosci.* 25:2429–33
12. Cahill GF Jr. 1998. Survival in starvation. *Am. J. Clin. Nutr.* 68:1–2
13. Camfield CR, Camfield CS. 1996. Antiepileptic drug therapy: When is epilepsy truly intractable? *Epilepsia* 37:S60–65
14. Carlson H, Ronne-Engstrum E, Ungerstedt U, Hillered L. 1992. Seizure-related elevations of extracellular amino acids in human focal epilepsy. *Neurosci. Lett.* 140:30–32
15. Cerdan S, Kunnecke B, Seelig J. 1990. Cerebral metabolism of [1, 2-^{13}C2]acetate as detected by in vivo and in vitro ^{13}C NMR. *J. Biol. Chem.* 265:12916–26
16. Chaudhry FA, Reimber RJ, Edward RH. 2002. The glutamine commute: Take the N line and transfer to the A. *J. Cell Biol.* 157:349–55
17. Cheng CM, Kelley B, Wang J, Strauss D, Eagles DA, Bondy CA. 2003. A ketogenic diet increases brain insulin-like growth factor receptor and glucose transporter gene expression. *Endocrinology* 144:2676–82
18. Chiry O, Pellerin L, Monnet-Tschudi F, Fishbein WN, Merezhinskaya N, et al. 2006. Expression of the monocarboxylate transporter MCT1 in the adult human brain cortex. *Brain Res.* 1070:65–70
19. Clarke DD, Sokoloff L. 1999. Circulation and energy metabolism of the brain. In *Basic Neurochemistry: Molecular, Cellular and Medical Aspects*, ed. GJ Siegel, BW Agranoff, RW Albers, SK Fisher, MD Uhler, pp. 637–69. Philadelphia: Lippincott-Raven. 6th ed.
20. Cooper AJL, McDonald JM, Gelbard AS, Gledhill RF, Duffy TE. 1979. The metabolic fate of ^{13}N-labeled ammonia in rat brain. *J. Biol. Chem.* 254:4982–92
21. Cunnane SC, Musa K, Ryan MA, Whiting S, Fraser DD. 2002. Potential role of polyunsaturates in seizure protection achieved with the ketogenic diet. *Prostaglandins Leukot. Essent. Fatty Acids* 67:131–35
22. Dahlin M, Elfving A, Ungerstedt U, Amark P. 2005. The ketogenic diet influences the levels of excitatory and inhibitory amino acids in the CSF in children with refractory epilepsy. *Epilepsy Res.* 64:115–25
23. Daikhin Y, Yudkoff M. 1998. Ketone bodies and brain glutamate and GABA metabolism. *Dev. Neurosci.* 20:358–64
24. Danbolt NC. 2001. Glutamate uptake. *Prog. Neurobiol.* 65:1–105
25. DeDeyn PP, Marescau B, MacDonald RL. 1990. Epilepsy and the GABA-hypothesis: a brief review and some samples. *Acta Neurol. Belg.* 90:65–81
26. DeVivo DC, Leckie MP, Ferrendelli JS, McDougal DB Jr. 1978. Chronic ketosis and cerebral metabolism. *Ann. Neurol.* 3:331–37

27. Do KQ, Klancnik J, Gahwiler BH. 1991. Release of EAA: animal studies and epileptic foci studies in humans. In *Excitatory Amino Acids*, ed. BS Meldrum, F Moroni, RP Simon, pp. 677–85. New York: Raven
28. Dombrowski GJ Jr, Swiatek KR, Chao KL. 1989. Lactate, 3-hydroxybutyrate and glucose as substrates for early postnatal rat brain. *Neurochem. Res.* 14:667–75
29. Eagles DA, Boyd SJ, Kotak A, Allan F. 2003. Calorie restriction of a high-carbohydrate diet elevates the threshold of PTZ-induced seizures to values equal to those seen with a ketogenic diet. *Epilepsy Res.* 54:41–52
30. Erecinska M, Dagani F. 1990. Relationships between the neuronal sodium/potassium pump and energy metabolism. Effects of K^+, Na^+ and adenosine triphosphate in isolated brain synaptosomes. *J. Gen. Physiol.* 95:591–616
31. Erecinska M, Nelson D, Daikhin Y, Yudkoff M. 1996. Regulation of GABA level in rat brain synaptosomes: fluxes through enzymes of the GABA shunt and effects of glutamate, calcium and ketone bodies. *J. Neurochem.* 67:2325–34
32. Erecinska M, Silver IA. 1990. Metabolism and role of glutamate in mammalian brain. *Prog. Neurobiol.* 35:245–96
33. Escartin C, Valette J, Lebon V, Bonvento G. 2006. Neuron-astrocyte interactions in the regulation of brain energy metabolism: a focus on NMR spectroscopy. *J. Neurochem.* 99:393–401
34. Fleck MW, Henze DA, Barrionuevo G, Palmer AM. 1993. Aspartate and glutamate mediate excitatory synaptic transmission in area CA1 of the hippocampus. *J. Neurosci.* 13:3944–55
35. Freeman J, Veggiotti P, Lanzi G, Tagliabue A, Perucca E. 2006. The ketogenic diet: from molecular mechanisms to clinical effects. *Epilepsy Res.* 68:145–80
36. Freeman JM, Vining EP, Pillas DJ, Pyzik PL, Casey JC, Kelly LM. 1998. The efficacy of the ketogenic diet—1998: a prospective evaluation of intervention in 150 children. *Pediatrics* 102:1358–63
37. Fuehrlein BS, Rutenberg MS, Silver JN, Warren MW, Theriaque DW, et al. 2004. Differential metabolic effects of saturated versus polyunsaturated fats in ketogenic diets. *J. Clin. Endocrinol. Metab.* 89:1641–45
38. Fukao T, Song XQ, Mitchell GA, Yamaguchi S, Sukegawa K, et al. 1997. Enzymes of ketone body utilization in human tissues: protein and messenger RNA levels of succinyl-coenzyme A (CoA):3-ketoacid CoA transferase and mitochondrial and cytosolic acetoacetyl-CoA thiolases. *Pediatr. Res.* 42:498–502
39. Gegelashvili G, Schousboe A. 1998. Cellular distribution and kinetic properties of high-affinity glutamate transporters. *Brain Res. Bull.* 45:233–38
40. Gerasimov MR, Ferrieri RA, Pareto D, Logan J, Alexoff D, Ding YS. 2005. Synthesis and evaluation of inhaled [^{11}C]butane and intravenously injected [^{11}C]acetone as potential radiotracers for studying inhalant abuse. *Nucl. Med. Biol.* 32:201–8
41. Gerhart DZ, Enerson BE, Zhdankina OY, Leino RL, Drewes LR. 1997. Expression of monocarboxylate transporter MCT1 by brain endothelium and glia in adult and suckling rats. *Am. J. Physiol.* 273:E207–13
42. Gould EM, Curto KA, Craig CR, Fleming WW, Taylor DA. 1995. The role of GABA-A receptors in the subsensitivity of Purkinje neurons to GABA in genetic epilepsy-prone rats. *Brain Res.* 698:62–68
43. Greene AE, Todorova MT, McGowan R, Seyfried TN. 2001. Caloric restriction inhibits seizure susceptibility in epileptic EL mice by reducing blood glucose. *Epilepsia* 42:1371–78

44. Grill V, Björkhem M, Gutniak M, Lindqvist M. 1992. Brain uptake and release of amino acids in nondiabetic and insulin-dependent diabetic subjects: important role of glutamine release for nitrogen balance. *Metabolism* 41:28–32
45. Hawkins RA, O'Kane RL, Simpson IA, Vina JR. 2006. Structure of the blood-brain barrier and its role in the transport of amino acids. *J. Nutr.* 136:218–26S
46. Hertz L, Peng L, Dienel GA. 2007. Energy metabolism in astrocytes: high rate of oxidative metabolism and spatiotemporal dependence on glycolysis/glycogenolysis. *J. Cereb. Blood Flow Metab.* 27(2):219–49
47. Hertz L, Peng L, Westergaard N, Yudkoff M, Schousboe A. 1992. Neuronal-astrocytic interactions in metabolism of transmitter amino acids of the glutamate family. In *Drug Research Related to Neuroactive Amino Acids, Alfred Benzon Symposium 32*, ed. A Schousboe, NH Diemer, H Kofod, pp 30–48. Copenhagen: Munksgaard
48. Hovanics GE, DeLorey TM, Firestone LL, Quinlan JJ, Handforth A, et al. 1997. Mice devoid of gamma-aminobutyrate type A receptor beta3 subunit have epilepsy, cleft palate, and hypersensitive behavior. *Proc. Natl. Acad. Sci. USA* 94:4143–48
49. Huang Y, Zielke HR, Tildon JT, Zielke CL, Baab PJ. 1996. Elevation of amino acids in the interstitial space of the rat brain following infusion of large neutral amino and keto acids by microdialysis: leucine infusion. *Dev. Neurosci.* 18:415–19
50. Hutson SM, Wallin R, Hall TR. 1992. Identification of mitochondrial branched chain aminotransferase and its isoforms in rat tissues. *J. Biol. Chem.* 267:15681–86
51. Kanamori K, Ross BD. 2004. Quantitative determination of extracellular glutamine concentration in rat brain, and its elevation in vivo by system A transport inhibitor, alpha-(methylamino)isobutyrate. *J. Neurochem.* 90:203–10
52. Kanamori K, Ross BD, Kondrat RW. 1998. Rate of glutamate synthesis from leucine in rat brain measured in vivo by ^{15}N NMR. *J. Neurochem.* 70:1304–15
53. Kety SS, Schmidt CF. 1948. The nitrous oxide method for the quantitative determination of cerebral blood flow in man: theory, procedure, and normal values. *J. Clin. Invest.* 27:476–83
54. Koper JW, Lopes-Cardozo M, Van Golde LM. 1981. Preferential utilization of ketone bodies for the synthesis of myelin cholesterol in vivo. *Biochem. Biophys. Acta* 666:411–17
55. Kossoff EH, Krauss GL, McGrogan JR, Freeman JM. 2003. Efficacy of the Atkins diet as therapy for intractable epilepsy. *Neurology* 61:1789–91
56. Kossoff EH, Pyzik PL, McGrogan JR, Vining EP, Freeman JM. 2002. Efficacy of the ketogenic diet for infantile spasms. *Pediatrics* 109:780–83
57. Kossoff EH, Thiele EA, Pfeifer HH, McGrogan JR, Freeman JM. 2005. Tuberous sclerosis complex and the ketogenic diet. *Epilepsia* 46:1684–86
58. Kwiterovich PO Jr, Vining EP, Pyzik P, Skolasky R Jr, Freeman JM. 2003. Effect of a high-fat ketogenic diet on plasma levels of lipids, lipoproteins, and apolipoproteins in children. *JAMA* 290:912–20
59. Lapidot A, Haber S. 2002. Effect of endogenous β-hydroxybutyrate on brain glucose metabolism in fetuses of diabetic rabbits, studied by 13C magnetic resonance spectroscopy. *Dev. Brain Res.* 135:87–99
60. Lasley SM, Yan QS. 1994. Diminished potassium-stimulated GABA release in vivo in genetically epilepsy-prone rats. *Neurosci. Lett.* 175:145–48
61. Lefevre F, Aronson A. 2000. Ketogenic diet for the treatment of refractory epilepsy in children: a systematic review of efficacy. *Pediatrics* 105:E46
62. Likhodii SS, Serbanescu I, Cortez MA, Murphy P, Snead OC 3rd, Burnham WM. 2003. Anticonvulsant properties of acetone, a brain ketone elevated by the ketogenic diet. *Ann. Neurol.* 54:219–26

63. Lopes-Cardozo M, Koper JW, Klein W, Van Golde LM. 1984. Acetoacetate is a cholesterogenic precursor for myelinating rat brain and spinal cord. Incorporation of label from [3-14C]acetoacetate, [14C]glucose and 3H2O. *Biochem. Biophys. Acta* 794:350–52
64. Loscher W, Swark WS. 1985. Evidence for impaired GABAergic activity in the substantia nigra of amygdaloid kindled rats. *Brain Res.* 339:146–50
65. Mady MA, Kossoff EH, McGregor AL, Wheless JW, Pyzik PL, Freeman JM. 2003. The ketogenic diet: Adolescents can do it, too. *Epilepsia* 44:847–51
66. Magistretti PJ, Pellerin L, Rothman DL, Shulman RG. 1999. Energy on demand. *Science* 283:496–97
67. Mantis JG, Centeno NA, Todorova MT, McGowan R, Seyfried TN. 2004. Management of multifactorial idiopathic epilepsy in EL mice with caloric restriction and the ketogenic diet: role of glucose and ketone bodies. *Nutr. Metab.* 1:1–11
68. Martin D, Bustos GA, Bowe MA, Bray SD, Nadler JV. 1991. Autoreceptor regulation of glutamate and aspartate release from slices of the hippocampal CA1 area. *J. Neurochem.* 56:1647–55
69. Martinez-Hernandez A, Bell KP, Norenberg MD. 1977. Glutamine synthetase: glial localization in brain. *Science* 195:1356–58
70. Mason GF, Gruetter R, Rothman DL, Behar KL, Shulman RG, Novotny EJ. 1995. Simultaneous determination of the rates of the TCA cycle, glucose utilization, alpha-ketoglutarate/glutamate exchange, and glutamine synthesis in human brain by NMR. *J. Cereb. Blood Flow Metab.* 15:12–25
71. Mattson MP, Liu D. 2003. Mitochondrial potassium channels and uncoupling proteins in synaptic plasticity and neuronal cell death. *Biochem. Biophys. Res. Comm.* 304:539–49
72. McKenna MC, Tildon JT, Stevenson JH, Boatright R, Huang S. 1993. Regulation of energy metabolism in synaptic terminals and cultured rat brain astrocytes: Differences revealed using aminooxyacetate. *Dev. Neurosci.* 15:320–29
73. Meldrum BS. 1994. The role of glutamate in epilepsy and other CNS disorders. *Neurology* 44:S14–23
74. Meldrum BS. 2000. Glutamate as a neurotransmitter in the brain: review of physiology and pathology. *J. Nutr.* 130:1007–15S
75. Melo TM, Nehlig A, Sonnewald U. 2006. Neuronal-glial interactions in rats fed a ketogenic diet. *Neurochem. Int.* 48:498–507
76. Nehlig A, Pereira de Vasconcelos A. 1993. Glucose and ketone body utilization by the brain of neonatal rats. *Progr. Neurobiol.* 40:163–221
77. Noh HS, Kim DW, Cho GJ, Choi WS, Kang SS. 2006. Increased nitric oxide caused by the ketogenic diet reduces the onset time of kainic acid-induced seizures in ICR mice. *Brain Res.* 1075:193–200
78. Nordli DR Jr, Kuroda MM, Carroll J, Koenigsberger DY, Hirsch LJ, et al. 2001. Experience with the ketogenic diet in infants. *Pediatrics* 108:129–33
79. Norenberg MD, Martinez-Hernandez A. 1979. Fine structural localization of glutamine synthetase in astrocytes of rat brain. *Brain Res.* 161:303–10
80. O'Kane RL, Martinez-Lopez I, DeJoseph MR, Vina JR, Hawkins RA. 1999. Na(+)-dependent glutamate transporters (EAAT1, EAAT2, and EAAT3) of the blood-brain barrier. A mechanism for glutamate removal. *J. Biol. Chem.* 274:31891–95
81. O'Kane RL, Vina JR, Simpson I, Hawkins RA. 2004. Na+-dependent neutral amino acid transporters A, ASC, and N of the blood-brain barrier: mechanisms for neutral amino acid removal. *Am. J. Physiol. Endocrinol. Metab.* 287:E622–29
82. Olney JW. 2003. Excitotoxicity, apoptosis and neuropsychiatric disorders. *Curr. Opin. Pharmacol.* 3:101–9

83. Olsen RW, Avoli M. 1997. GABA and epileptogenesis. *Epilepsia* 38:399–407
84. Olstad E, Qu H, Sonnewald U. 2007. Glutamate is preferred over glutamine for intermediary metabolism in cultured cerebellar neurons. *J. Cereb. Blood Flow Metab.* 27:811–20
85. Owen OE, Morgan AP, Kemp HG, Sullivan JM, Herrera MG, Cahill GF. 1967. Brain metabolism during fasting. *J. Clin. Invest.* 46:1589–95
86. Pan JW, Bebin EM, Chu WJ, Hetherington HP. 1999. Ketosis and epilepsy: ^{31}P spectroscopic imaging at 4.1T. *Epilepsia* 40:703–7
87. Patel AJ, Balazs R, Richter D. 1970. Contribution of the GABA bypath to glucose oxidation, and the development of compartmentation in the brain. *Nature* 226:1160–61
88. Patel AJ, Johnson AL, Balazs R. 1974. Metabolic compartmentation of glutamate associated with the formation of γ-aminobutyrate. *J. Neurochem.* 23:1271–79
89. Paulsen RE, Fonnum F. 1989. Role of glial cells for the basal and Ca^{2+}-dependent K^{+}-evoked release of transmitter amino acids investigated by microdialysis. *J. Neurochem.* 52:1823–29
90. Peng L, Hertz L. 1993. Potassium-induced stimulation of oxidative metabolism of glucose in cultures of intact cerebellar granule cells but not in corresponding cells with dendritic degeneration. *Brain Res.* 629:331–34
91. Petroff OA. 2002. GABA and glutamate in the human brain. *Neuroscientist* 8:562–73
92. Petroff OA, Rothman D, Behar KL, Mattson RH. 1996. Low brain GABA level is associated with poor seizure control. *Ann. Neurol.* 40:908–11
93. Pierre K, Pellerin L. 2005. Monocarboxylate transporters in the central nervous system: distribution, regulation and function. *J. Neurochem.* 94:1–14
94. Plaitakis A, Zaganas I. 2001. Regulation of human glutamate dehydrogenases: implications for glutamate, ammonia and energy metabolism in brain. *J. Neurosci. Res.* 66:899–908
95. Porter TG, Martin DL. 1988. Stability and activation of glutamate apodecarboxylase from pig brain. *J. Neurochem.* 51:1886–91
96. Prins ML, Lee SM, Fujima LS, Hovda DA. 2004. Increased cerebral uptake and oxidation of exogenous bHB improves ATP following traumatic brain injury in adult rats. *J. Neurochem.* 90:666–72
97. Raiteri M, Marchi M, Costi A, Volpe G. 1990. Endogenous aspartate release in the rat hippocampus inhibited by M2 "cardiac" muscarinic receptors. *Eur. J. Pharmacol.* 177:181–87
98. Ratnakumari L, Murthy CRK. 1989. Activities of pyruvate dehydrogenase, enzymes of citric acid cycle, and aminotransferases in the subcellular fractions of cerebral cortex in normal and hyperammonemic rats. *Neurochem. Res.* 14:221–28
99. Sato K, Kashiwaya Y, Keon CA, Tsuchiya N, King MT, et al. 1995. Insulin, ketone bodies, and mitochondrial energy transduction. *FASEB J.* 9:651–58
100. Scheppach W, Pomare EW, Elia M, Cummings JH. 1991. The contribution of the large intestine to blood acetate in man. *Clin. Sci.* 80:177–82
101. Schousboe A, Waagepetersen HS. 2005. Role of astrocytes in glutamate homeostasis: implications for excitotoxicity. *Neurotox. Res.* 8:221–25
102. Schurr A, Miller JJ, Payne RS, Rigor BM. 1999. An increase in lactate output by brain tissue serves to meet the energy needs of glutamate-activated neurons. *J. Neurosci.* 19:34–39
103. Schwechter EM, Veliskova J, Velisek L. 2003. Correlation between extracellular glucose and seizure susceptibility in adult rats. *Ann. Neurol.* 53:91–101
104. Shank RP, Aprison MH. 1977. Present status and significance of the glutamine cycle in neural tissues. *Life Sci.* 28:837–42

105. Shank RP, Bennett GS, Freytag SO, Campbell GL. 1985. Pyruvate carboxylase: an astrocyte-specific enzyme implicated in the replenishment of amino acid neurotransmitter pools. *Brain Res.* 329:364–67
106. Siesjo BK. 1997. *Brain Energy Metabolism*. New York: Wiley
107. Smith QR, Momma S, Aoyagi M, Rapoport SI. 1987. Kinetics of neutral amino acid transport across the blood-brain barrier. *J. Neurochem.* 49:1651–58
108. Sonnewald U, Schousboe A, Qu H, Waagepetersen HS. 2004. Intracellular metabolic compartmentation assessed by 13C magnetic resonance spectroscopy. *Neurochem. Int.* 45:305–10
109. Sonnewald U, Westergaard N, Schousboe A, Svendsen JS, Unsgard G, Petersen SB. 1993. Direct demonstration by [^{13}C]NMR spectroscopy that glutamine from astrocytes is a precursor for GABA synthesis in neurons. *Neurochem. Int.* 22:19–29
110. Storm-Mathisen J, Leknes AK, Bore AT, Vaaland JL, Edminson P, et al. 1983. First visualization of glutamate and GABA in neurones by immunocytochemistry. *Nature* 301:517–20
111. Storm-Mathisen J, Ottersen OP. 1986. Antibodies against amino acid neurotransmitters. In *Neurohistochemistry: Modern Methods and Applications*, ed. P Paunula, H Paivarinta, S Soinila, pp. 107–36. New York: Liss
112. Sullivan PG, Dube C, Dorenbos K, Steward O, Baram TZ. 2003. Mitochondrial uncoupling protein-2 protects the immature brain from excitotoxic neuronal death. *Ann. Neurol.* 53:711–17
113. Sullivan PG, Rippy NA, Dorenbos K, Concepcion RC, Agarwal AK, Rho JM. 2004. The ketogenic diet increases mitochondrial uncoupling protein levels and activity. *Ann. Neurol.* 55:576–80
114. Swink TD, Vining EP, Freeman JM. 1997. The ketogenic diet. *Adv. Pediatr.* 44:297–329
115. Szot P, Weinshenker D, Rho JM, Storey TW, Schwartzkroin PA. 2001. Norepinephrine is required for the anticonvulsant effect of the ketogenic diet. *Brain Res. Dev. Brain Res.* 129:211–14
116. Takahashi M, Billups B, Rossi D, Sarantis M, Hamann M, Attwell D. 1997. The role of glutamate transporters in glutamate homeostasis in the brain. *J. Exper. Biol.* 200:401–9
117. Thiele EA. 2003. Assessing the efficacy of antiepileptic treatments: the ketogenic diet. *Epilepsia* 44:26–29
118. Thurston JH, Hauhart RE, Schiro JA. 1986. Beta-hydroxybutyrate reverses insulin-induced hypoglycemic coma in suckling-weanling mice despite low blood and brain glucose levels. *Metab. Brain Dis.* 1:63–82
119. Tieu K, Perier C, Caspersen C, Teismann P, Wu DC, et al. 2003. D-beta-hydroxybutyrate rescues mitochondrial respiration and mitigates features of Parkinson disease. *J. Clin. Invest.* 112:892–901
120. Vamecq J, Vallee L, Lesage F, Gressens P, Stables JP. 2005. Antiepileptic popular ketogenic diet: emerging twists in an ancient story. *Prog. Neurobiol.* 75:1–28
121. Veech RL. 2004. The therapeutic implications of ketone bodies: the effects of ketone bodies in pathological conditions: ketosis, ketogenic diet, redox states, insulin resistance, and mitochondrial metabolism. *Prostaglandins Leukot. Essent. Fatty Acids* 70:309–19
122. Veech RL, Chance B, Kashiwaya Y, Lardy HA, Cahill GF Jr. 2001. Ketone bodies, potential therapeutic uses. *IUBMB Life* 51:241–47
123. Vining EP. 1999. Clinical efficacy of the ketogenic diet. *Epilepsy Res.* 37:181–90
124. Vining EPG, Pyzik P, McGrogan J, Hladky H, Anand A, et al. 2002. Growth of children on the ketogenic diet. *Dev. Med. Child Neurol.* 44:796–802

125. Waagepetersen HS, Bakken IJ, Larsson OM, Sonnewald U, Schousboe A. 1998. Comparison of lactate and glucose metabolism in cultured neocortical neurons and astrocytes using ^{13}C-NMR spectroscopy. *Dev. Neurosci.* 20:310–20
126. Waagepetersen HS, Sonnewald U, Larsson OM, Schousboe A. 2000. Compartmentation of TCA cycle metabolism in cultured neocortical neurons revealed by ^{13}C MR spectroscopy. *Neurochem. Int.* 36:349–58
127. Waagepetersen HS, Sonnewald U, Larsson OM, Schousboe A. 2000. A possible role of alanine for ammonia transfer between astrocytes and glutamatergic neurons. *J. Neurochem.* 75:471–79
128. Waagepetersen HS, Sonnewald U, Schousboe A. 2003. Compartmentation of glutamine, glutamate, and GABA metabolism in neurons and astrocytes: functional implications. *Neuroscientist* 9:398–403
129. Wang ZJ, Bergqvist C, Hunter JV, Jin D, Wang DJ, et al. 2003. In vivo measurement of brain metabolites using two-dimensional double-quantum MR spectroscopy-exploration of GABA levels in a ketogenic diet. *Magn. Reson. Med.* 49:615–19
130. Waniewski RA, Martin DL. 1998. Preferential utilization of acetate by astrocytes is attributable to transport. *J. Neurosci.* 18:5225–33
131. Waxman EA, Lynch DR. 2005. N-methyl-D-aspartate receptor subtypes: multiple roles in excitotoxicity and neurological disease. *Neuroscientist* 11:37–49
132. White HS. 1997. Clinical significance of animal seizure models and mechanism of action studies of potential antiepileptic drugs. *Epilepsia* 38(Suppl. 1):S9–17
133. Wilder RM. 1921. Effects of ketonuria on the course of epilepsy. *Mayo Clin. Bull.* 2:307–10
134. Wilkins L. 1937. Epilepsy in childhood. III. Results with the ketogenic diet. *J. Pediatr.* 10:341–57
135. Wu JY. 1976. Purification, characterization and kinetic studies of GAD and GABA-T from mouse brain. In *GABA in Nervous System Function*, ed. E Roberts, TN Chase, DB Tower, pp. 7–55. New York: Raven
136. Yanagida O, Kanai Y, Chairoungdua A, Kim DK, Segawa H, et al. 2001. Human L-type amino acid transporter 1. LAT1: characterization of function and expression in tumor cell lines. *Biochem. Biophys. Acta* 1514:291–302
137. Yudkoff M, Daikhin Y, Nelson D, Nissim I, Erecinska M. 1996. Neuronal metabolism of branched-chain amino acids: flux through the aminotransferase pathway in synaptosomes. *J. Neurochem.* 66:2136–45
138. Yudkoff M, Daikhin Y, Nissim I, Grunstein R, Nissim I. 1997. Effects of ketone bodies on astrocyte amino acid metabolism. *J. Neurochem.* 69:682–92
139. Yudkoff M, Daikhin Y, Nissim I, Horyn O, Lazarow A, et al. 2005. Response of brain amino acid metabolism to ketosis. *Neurochem. Int.* 47:119–28
140. Yudkoff M, Daikhin Y, Nissim I, Lazarow A, Nissim I. 2001. Ketogenic diet, amino acid metabolism and seizure control. *J. Neurosci. Res.* 66:931–40
141. Yudkoff M, Daikhin Y, Nissim I, Lazarow A, Nissim I. 2004. Ketogenic diet, brain glutamate metabolism and seizure control. *Prostaglandins Leukot. Essential Fatty Acids* 70:277–85
142. Yudkoff M, Daikhin Y, Nissim I, Horyn O, Luhovyy B, et al. 2006. Short-term fasting, seizure control and brain amino acid metabolism. *Neurochem. Int.* 48:650–56
143. Yudkoff M, Nelson D, Daikhin Y, Erecinska M. 1994. Tricarboxylic acid cycle in rat brain synaptosomes. Fluxes and interactions with aspartate aminotransferase and malate/aspartate shuttle. *J. Biol. Chem.* 269:27414–20

Cumulative Indexes

Contributing Authors, Volumes 23–27

Chapter Titles, Volumes 23–27

Lipids

Proteins, Peptides, and Amino Acids

Vitamins

Comparative Nutrition

Special Topics